Manual of
Canine and Feline
Cardiology

Fifth Edition

Manual of
Canine and Feline
Cardiology

Fifth Edition

FRANCIS W. K. **SMITH, JR., DVM**
Diplomate, American College of Veterinary Internal Medicine (Cardiology and
    Small Animal Internal Medicine)
Vice President, VetMed Consultants, Inc.
Lexington, Massachusetts

Clinical Assistant Professor, Department of Medicine
Cummings School of Veterinary Medicine, Tufts University
North Grafton, Massachusetts

LARRY P. **TILLEY, DVM**
Diplomate, American College of Veterinary Internal Medicine (Small Animal
    Internal Medicine)
President, VetMed Consultants, Inc.
Santa Fe, New Mexico

MARK A. **OYAMA, DVM**
Diplomate, American College of Veterinary Internal Medicine (Cardiology)
Professor and Chief of Cardiology Service
Department of Clinical Studies
School of Veterinary Medicine
University of Pennsylvania
Philadelphia, Pennsylvania

MEG M. **SLEEPER, VMD**
Diplomate, American College of Veterinary Internal Medicine (Cardiology)
Clinical Professor, Cardiology
Department of Small Animal Clinical Sciences
College of Veterinary Medicine
University of Florida
Gainesville, Florida

ELSEVIER

ELSEVIER

3251 Riverport Lane
St. Louis, Missouri 63043

Previous editions copyrighted 2008, 2001, 1995, and 1985.

Library of Congress Cataloging-in-Publication Data

Manual of canine and feline cardiology / [edited by] Francis W.K. Smith, Jr., Larry P. Tilley, Mark A. Oyama, Meg M. Sleeper.
    p. ; cm.
  Includes bibliographical references and index.
  ISBN 978-0-323-18802-9 (hardcover : alk. paper) 1. Dogs—Diseases. 2. Cats—Diseases. 3. Veterinary cardiology. I. Smith, Francis W. K., Jr., editor. II. Tilley, Lawrence P., editor. III. Oyama, Mark A., editor. IV. Sleeper, Meg M., editor.
  [DNLM: 1. Dog Diseases. 2. Heart Diseases—veterinary. 3. Cat Diseases. SF 992.C37]
  SF992.C37M36 2016
  636.7'089612—dc23

                                                                                2015009116

Content Strategy Director: Penny Rudolph
Professional Content Development Manager: Jolynn Gower
Senior Content Development Specialist: Courtney Sprehe
Publishing Services Manager: Patricia Tannian
Senior Project Manager: Claire Kramer
Design Direction: Ashley Miner

Printed in the United States of America

Last digit is the print number: 9 8 7 6 5 4

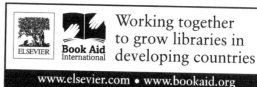

To May, Ben, and Jade. Thanks for being a
constant source of inspiration
and joy. Love always.

Francis W. K. Smith, Jr.

To my wife Jeri, my son Kyle,
my grandson Tucker.

To my late mother, Dorothy, who instilled
values in my brother, Steve, and in me
that have helped us throughout life.

To family and animals who represent
the purity of life.

Larry P. Tilley

To Lori, for her unwavering love and support.

Mark A. Oyama

For the many animals that have taught me
and made me the clinician and
the person I am today.

Meg M. Sleeper

Contributors

Jonathan A. Abbott, DVM, DACVIM (Cardiology)
Associate Professor, Small Animal Clinical Sciences, Virginia Maryland College of Veterinary Medicine, Virginia Tech, Blacksburg, Virginia; Associate Professor, Basic Sciences, Virginia Tech Carilion School of Medicine and Research Institute, Roanoke, Virginia
Acquired Valvular Disease

Janice McIntosh Bright, MS, DVM, DACVIM (Cardiology and SAIM)
Professor of Cardiology, Department of Clinical Sciences, College of Veterinary Medicine and Biomedical Sciences, Colorado State University, Fort Collins, Colorado
Pacemaker Therapy

Scott A. Brown, VMD, PhD
Josiah Meigs Distinguished Teaching Professor, Department of Physiology and Pharmacology, University of Georgia; Edward Gunst Professor of Small Animal Medicine, Small Animal Medicine and Surgery, University of Georgia College of Veterinary Medicine, Athens, Georgia
Systemic Hypertension

Clay A. Calvert, DVM, DACVIM (SAIM)
Professor, Small Animal Medicine and Surgery, College of Veterinary Medicine, University of Georgia, Athens, Georgia
Heartworm Disease

Kathleen E. Cavanagh, DVM, MET
Instructor, Distance Learning (OL), University of Guelph, Guelph, Ontario, Canada; Emergency Veterinarian, Niagara Veterinary Emergency Clinic, Thorold, Ontario, Canada; President, Matrix Multimedia, Ridgeville, Ontario, Canada; Veterinarian, Chippawa Animal Hospital, Niagara Falls, Ontario, Canada
Appendix 1: Canine and Feline Breed Predilections for Heart Disease

Amanda E. Coleman, DVM, DACVIM (Cardiology)
Assistant Professor of Cardiology, Small Animal Medicine and Surgery, University of Georgia, Athens, Georgia
Pericardial Disorders and Cardiac Tumors

Thomas K. Day, DVM, MS, DACVA, DACVECC, CVA
Criticalist, Anesthesiologist, Emergency Clinician, Veterinary Emergency Service/Veterinary Specialty Center, Middleton, Wisconsin
Anesthesia of the Cardiac Patient

Kenneth J. Drobatz, DVM, MSCE, DACVIM (SAIM)
Professor and Chief, Section of Critical Care, Department of Clinical Studies–Philadelphia, School of Veterinary Medicine; Director, Emergency Service, Mathew J. Ryan Veterinary Hospital of the University of Pennsylvania, School of Veterinary Medicine, University of Pennsylvania, Philadelphia, Pennsylvania
Cardiopulmonary Arrest and Resuscitation
Emergency Management and Critical Care

Lisa M. Freeman, DVM, PhD, DACVN
Professor, Department of Clinical Sciences, Cummings School of Veterinary Medicine, Tufts University, North Grafton, Massachusetts
Nutrition and Cardiovascular Disease

Virginia Luis Fuentes, MA, VetMB, PhD, DACVIM and ECVIM-CA (Cardiology)
Professor of Veterinary Cardiology, Veterinary Clinical Sciences, Royal Veterinary College, Hatfield, United Kingdom
Echocardiography and Doppler Ultrasound

Anna R. M. Gelzer, Dr.med.vet., PhD
Senior Lecturer in Cardiology, ECVIM-CA (Cardiology), Departments of Small Animal Medicine, The School of Veterinary Science, University of Liverpool, Neston, United Kingdom
Treatment of Cardiac Arrhythmias and Conduction Disturbances

Rebecca E. Gompf, DVM, MS, DACVIM (Cardiology)
Associate Professor of Cardiology, Small Animal Clinical Sciences, The University of Tennessee, Knoxville, Tennessee
History and Physical Examination

Rosemary A. Henik, DVM, MS, DACVIM (SAIM)
Specialist and Consultant, Veterinary Emergency Service and Veterinary Specialty Center, Madison, Wisconsin; Consultant/ Editor, Cardiopulmonary, VIN–Veterinary Information Network, Davis, California; Owner/Consultant, Cardiac Consultations for Companion Animals, Madison, Wisconsin
Systemic Hypertension

Lynelle R. Johnson, DVM, MS, PhD, DACVIM (SAIM)
Associate Professor, Department of Veterinary Medicine and Epidemiology, College of Veterinary Medicine, University of California, Davis, Davis, California
Cor Pulmonale and Pulmonary Thromboembolism

Marc S. Kraus, DVM, DACVIM (Cardiology, SAIM), DECVIM-CA (Cardiology)
Senior Lecturer in Cardiology, Departments of Small Animal Medicine, The School of Veterinary Science, University of Liverpool, Neston, United Kingdom
Treatment of Cardiac Arrhythmias and Conduction Disturbances

Kristin MacDonald, DVM, PhD, DACVIM (Cardiology)
Veterinary Cardiologist, VCA Animal Care Center of Sonoma County, Rohnert Park, California
Feline Cardiomyopathy

E. Christopher Orton, DVM, PhD, DACVS
Professor and Head, Department of Clinical Sciences, College of Veterinary Medicine and Biomedical Sciences, Colorado State University, Fort Collins, Colorado
Cardiac Surgery

Mark A. Oyama, DVM, DACVIM (Cardiology)
Professor and Chief of Cardiology Service, Department of Clinical Studies, School of Veterinary Medicine, University of Pennsylvania, Philadelphia, Pennsylvania
Genetic and Biomarker Testing of Cardiovascular Diseases
Canine Cardiomyopathy
Congenital Heart Disease
Appendix 2: Cardiopulmonary Drug Formulary

Brian A. Poteet, MS, DVM, DACVR
President, Radiology Consulting and Teleradiology, VitalRads, Cypress, Texas
Radiology of the Heart

Gregg S. Rapoport, DVM, DACVIM (Cardiology)
Assistant Professor of Cardiology, Small Animal Medicine and Surgery, College of Veterinary Medicine, University of Georgia, Athens, Georgia
Pericardial Disorders and Cardiac Tumors

John E. Rush, DVM, MS, DACVECC, DACVIM (Cardiology)
Professor, Department of Clinical Sciences, Cummings School of Veterinary Medicine, Tufts University, North Grafton, Massachusetts
Nutrition and Cardiovascular Disease

Carl D. Sammarco, BVSc, MRCVS, DACVIM (Cardiology)
Lecturer, Emergency and Critical Care, Department of Clinical Studies–Philadelphia, Matthew J. Ryan Veterinary Hospital, University of Pennsylvania, Philadelphia, Pennsylvania
Cardiovascular Effects of Systemic Diseases

Kari Santoro-Beer, DVM, DACVECC
Lecturer, Emergency and Critical Care, Department of Clinical Studies–Philadelphia, Matthew J. Ryan Veterinary Hospital, University of Pennsylvania, Philadelphia, Pennsylvania
Emergency Management and Critical Care

Donald P. Schrope, DVM, DACVIM (Cardiology)
Department Head, Department of Cardiology, Oradell Animal Hospital, Paramus, New Jersey
Cardiovascular Effects of Systemic Diseases

Meg M. Sleeper, VMD, DACVIM (Cardiology)
Clinical Professor, Cardiology, Department of
    Small Animal Clinical Sciences, College of
    Veterinary Medicine, University of Florida,
    Gainesville, Florida
    *Special Diagnostic Techniques for Evaluation of
    Cardiac Disease*
    Appendix 2: Cardiopulmonary Drug Formulary

**Francis W. K. Smith, Jr., DVM, DACVIM
(Cardiology, SAIM)**
Vice President, VetMed Consultants, Inc.,
    Lexington, Massachusetts; Clinical Assistant
    Professor, Department of Medicine,
    Cummings School of Veterinary Medicine,
    Tufts University, North Grafton, Massachusetts
    Electrocardiography
    Cardiovascular Effects of Systemic Diseases
    *Appendix 1: Canine and Feline Breed Predilections
    for Heart Disease*
    Appendix 2: Cardiopulmonary Drug Formulary

**Keith N. Strickland, DVM, DACVIM
(Cardiology)**
Department Head, Cardiology, Oradell Animal
    Hospital, Paramus, New Jersey
    Congenital Heart Disease
    Pathophysiology and Therapy of Heart Failure

Vincent J. Thawley, VMD, DACVECC
Staff Veterinarian–Emergency Services,
    Clinical Studies–Philadelphia, School
    of Veterinary Medicine, University of
    Pennsylvania, Philadelphia, Pennsylvania
    Cardiopulmonary Arrest and Resuscitation

**Justin D. Thomason, DVM, DACVIM
(Cardiology)**
Assistant Professor of Cardiology, Department
    of Clinical Sciences, Veterinary Health Center,
    Kansas State University, Manhattan, Kansas
    Heartworm Disease

Larry P. Tilley, DVM, DACVIM (SAIM)
President, VetMed Consultants, Inc., Santa Fe,
    New Mexico
    Electrocardiography
    Appendix 2: Cardiopulmonary Drug Formulary

Preface

In the last five years there have been a number of excellent textbook chapters and journal articles describing new findings in the field of canine and feline cardiology. However, for the practicing veterinarian and veterinary student, the amount of information is overwhelming. Many veterinarians and students have stated, in past surveys, the need to keep up with cardiovascular advances in the most time-effective way. The *Manual of Canine and Feline Cardiology*, now in its fifth edition, has been updated to continue to meet the need for a current textbook that can provide useful and practical information on cardiac disease in the dog and cat. We have worked hard to make this book a most reliable source for practicing cardiovascular medicine in the dog and cat. For the new edition, we have expanded the number of contributors, with each chapter written by an expert. We have also worked to conserve reading time by employing an easy-to-use format. The *Manual of Canine and Feline Cardiology* is unique as a quick reference with consistency of presentation.

This practical approach to the diagnosis and therapy of cardiac disease will be useful to a wide audience, from the veterinary student to the fully trained cardiologist. The approach is largely clinical and includes the practical as well as the most sophisticated methods for diagnosis and therapy.

Cardiovascular disorders in the dog and cat represent a substantial portion of diseases seen in the average veterinary practice. It is important for veterinary students and practitioners to understand the principles of diagnosis and treatment of the numerous cardiovascular disorders.

NEW TO THIS EDITION

Since the fourth edition of this textbook was published, there has been tremendous growth in the field of canine and feline cardiology. The fifth edition has been carefully revised, edited, and updated and also has a generous amount of new figures and charts, with the majority in color. New material includes the following:

- A new chapter on cardiac surgery
- A new chapter on pacemaker therapy
- A new chapter on genetic and biomarker testing of cardiovascular diseases

- A new chapter on nutrition and cardiovascular disease
- A table of canine and feline breed predilections for heart disease in Appendix 1

ORGANIZATION

Section 1 describes the methods of diagnosis of heart diseases in the dog and cat. The first six chapters follow the sequence that the veterinarian uses in approaching the patient: history and physical examination (Chapter 1), radiology of the heart (Chapter 2), electrocardiography (Chapter 3), echocardiography and Doppler ultrasound (Chapter 4), special diagnostic techniques for evaluation of cardiac diseases (Chapter 5), and genetics and biomarker testing of cardiac diseases (Chapter 6).

Section 2 presents, in a step-by-step fashion, a description of the various cardiac disorders that occur in the dog and cat, starting in each chapter with general considerations (e.g., definitions, incidence, pathophysiology, etiology), history, physical examination, electrocardiography, thoracic radiography, special diagnostic techniques, differential diagnosis, and finally, the therapeutic approach.

Section 3 includes chapters describing the treatment of cardiac failure and the treatment of arrhythmias and conduction disturbances and two separate chapters on cardiopulmonary arrest and resuscitation and on emergency management and critical care in cardiology. Chapters on anesthesia of the cardiac patient, cardiac surgery, and pacemaker therapy and a new chapter about nutrition and cardiovascular disease complete this section.

Appendix 1, Canine and Feline Breed Predilections for Heart Disease, represents the most current listing of breed-associated cardiac disorders.

Appendix 2, Cardiopulmonary Drug Formulary, contains extensive cardiopulmonary drug tables with indications, dosages, side effects, contraindications, and drug interactions. An extraordinary array of new cardiopulmonary drugs has become available, and both students and veterinarians have difficulty deciding which drugs from various drug classes should be prescribed.

Appendix 3, Echocardiographic Normal Values, by body weight and breed, represents an easy-to-refer-to list of normal values.

Appendix 4, Canine and Feline Genetic Tests for Breed Specific Cardiac Disease, is a new appendix.

The *Manual of Canine and Feline Cardiology*, fifth edition, will help to eliminate the aura of mystery that surrounds the diagnostic and therapeutic principles of veterinary cardiology. The teaching principles that are presented will allow even the novice to make an intelligent assessment of a cardiac case. This manual will be useful to a wide audience but comprehensive enough to serve as a reference for the advanced student and the veterinarian with expertise in cardiology.

Francis W. K. Smith, Jr., DVM
Larry P. Tilley, DVM
Mark A. Oyama, DVM
Meg M. Sleeper, VMD

Acknowledgments

The completion of this manual provides a welcome opportunity to recognize in writing the many individuals who have written this textbook. The authors have board certification and are uniquely qualified to give an update and review of their respective disciplines.

In addition to thanking veterinarians who have referred cases to us, we would like to express our gratitude to each of the veterinary students, interns, and residents whom we have had the pleasure of teaching. Their curiosity and intellectual stimulation have enabled us to grow and prompted us to undertake the task of writing this manual.

A special thank you goes to all of the staff in the production and editing department at Elsevier. For this edition, we would also like to thank Courtney Sprehe and Katie Stark, Content Development Specialists; Penny Rudolph, Content Strategy Director; and Claire Kramer, Senior Project Manager. All those at Elsevier were meticulous workers and kind people who made the final stages of preparing this book both inspiring and fun.

Francis W. K. Smith, Jr., DVM
Larry P. Tilley, DVM
Mark A. Oyama, DVM
Meg M. Sleeper, VMD

Contents

APPENDIXES

SECTION 1

DIAGNOSIS OF HEART DISEASE

History and Physical Examination

1

Rebecca E. Gompf

Despite the technical nature of many cardiovascular diagnostics, such as electrocardiography, radiography, and echocardiography, the history and physical examination remain the most crucial initial steps in the establishment of the correct diagnosis. Findings from a careful history and physical examination prompt the clinician to the probability or presence of heart disease. Results of the cardiovascular physical examination will usually allow the clinician to make a tentative diagnosis or formulate a specific differential diagnosis. The history and physical examination also provide important information regarding the stage of heart disease present, which may significantly affect therapy.

A good history and physical examination are invaluable in making a diagnosis of heart disease and helping to differentiate heart disease from pulmonary disease. Besides helping to make the diagnosis, a good history and physical examination help to tell the extent of the problem, the animal's response to previous therapy, the owner's ability to medicate the animal consistently, and the presence of other medical problems. Clinicians should obtain a thorough history and physical examination to properly diagnose and treat an animal with heart disease.

MEDICAL HISTORY

SIGNALMENT

AGE

Young animals usually have congenital diseases (e.g., patent ductus arteriosus [PDA]), whereas older animals usually have acquired diseases, such as degenerative diseases (e.g., mitral and tricuspid regurgitations) or neoplastic diseases (e.g., heart base tumor). There are exceptions because cardiomyopathies can occur in young dogs and cats (aged 6 months or younger) and older dogs can have congenital heart defects that were not diagnosed when they were young (e.g., PDA, atrial septal defect). Also, cardiac disease in older

animals can be modified or affected by other concurrent disease processes (e.g., collapsing trachea or other respiratory diseases and renal or liver disease).

BREED

Certain cardiac defects are more common in some breeds of animals; however, there can be regional differences in the rate of occurrence of cardiac problems. See the Appendix for a summary of some of the cardiac defects found in certain breeds of dogs and cats.

SEX

Males are more susceptible to certain cardiac diseases (e.g., male Cocker Spaniels to chronic valvular heart disease of the mitral valve and large-breed males to dilated cardiomyopathy). However, sick sinus syndrome occurs in the female Miniature Schnauzer, and PDA is more common in females of small breed dogs.

WEIGHT

The animal's weight influences several aspects of treatment, including the dose of cardiac medication, evaluation of the response to diuretic medication, and monitoring of cardiac cachexia. A Pickwickian syndrome (characterized by severe obesity, somnolence, and hypoventilation) can occur in an animal that is so obese that its ability to breathe is restricted.

UTILIZATION OF THE ANIMAL

Knowing how an animal is going to be used when giving a long-term prognosis for a cardiac disease is important. For example, hunting dogs with severe heartworm disease may not be able to hunt again after treatment. Also, some animals with congenital heart defects may have normal life spans and may make good pets; however, they should not be used for breeding purposes because the defect could be perpetuated.

The age, breed, and sex of the animal may help the clinician to make an accurate diagnosis; however, there are always exceptions to every rule. Clinicians should not ignore the fact that an animal could have an atypical problem for its age, breed, or sex.

HISTORY

- A good history will establish the presence of a cardiac problem, help to differentiate between cardiac and respiratory problems, and help to monitor the disease course and the response to therapy. It must be done carefully to prevent an owner from giving a misleading history. It includes several key questions, such as the reason the animal is being presented, the problems noted by the owner, the onset and duration of the problem(s), the progression of the disease, any known exposure to infectious diseases, the vaccination history, any current medications the animal is receiving, the animal's response to any medications that have been given, and the owner's ability to give the medication(s).
- The history will also define the animal's attitude and behavior because the owner will be asked whether the animal is listless and depressed or alert and playful. Does the animal tire easily with exercise?
- The patient's history should also cover the family history of the siblings and parents, especially if congenital disease is present in the patient. The owner will be asked about the health of other pets in the household, and the history will include the results of previous tests done on the patient.
- The history covers other relevant information that may help to identify the patient's problem(s), such as what and how much is being fed and the patient's appetite and water consumption. How frequently is the animal urinating, and does it have any diarrhea? Is there any vomiting or regurgitation? Has the patient had any seizures or syncopal episodes? What is the patient's reproductive status? Does the patient have any lameness or paresis? Is the patient coughing, sneezing, or having difficulty breathing? Does the animal rest comfortably, or is it restless? Has the patient had any previous trauma? Where is the animal housed (e.g., indoors, outdoors, fenced-in yard)? Does the animal have any diseases such as hyperthyroidism, chronic renal disease, respiratory disease or other diseases that can affect the heart or treatment of the animal's heart disease?

- Once a problem is identified by the history, more specific questions can be asked, including what is the character of the cough, when does it occur, and what stimuli evoke it. Common presenting complaints for cardiac disease include dyspnea or tachypnea, exercise intolerance, syncope, abdominal swelling, cyanosis, anorexia or decreased appetite, poor growth or performance, and a soft, moist cough if the animal has left-sided heart failure. Coughing by itself is *not* a primary complaint of heart disease.
- Other symptoms can be associated with cardiovascular disease. Polydipsia and polyuria are common in animals that are given diuretics or that have a concurrent disease (e.g., renal disease), whereas oliguria occurs with severe left-sided heart failure. Hemoglobinuria is found with the caval syndrome of heartworm disease.
- Cardiac drugs such as digitalis, diltiazem, and mexiletine can cause anorexia, vomiting, or diarrhea. Regurgitation occurs with congenital vascular ring anomalies. Right-sided heart failure can cause intestinal edema and a protein-losing enteropathy resulting in diarrhea. Cats with cardiomyopathy can have hemorrhagic enteritis resulting from thromboembolism of the gastric or mesenteric arteries.

KEY POINT

A good history will uncover all the animal's symptoms and problems whether they are due to a cardiac problem or to another concurrent problem. Also, by the end of a good history, an astute clinician will have a good idea as to the potential causes of the animal's problems.

SPECIFIC SYMPTOMS

COUGHING

- Previously, coughing has been ascribed as the most common complaint in dogs with significant heart disease. However, recent studies have shown that coughing in dogs with heart disease is due to concurrent respiratory disease and not to the heart disease itself. Cats rarely cough even when they have an enlarged left atrium.
- Coughing is a sudden, forced expiration and is a normal defense mechanism to clear debris from the tracheobronchial tree. It can originate from the larynx, pharynx, trachea, and bronchi but not from the smaller bronchi, bronchioles, and alveoli. A cardiac cough caused by left-sided heart failure occurs only when the pulmonary

Table 1.1   Characteristics of Coughs and Their Associated Causes in Dogs and Cats

Type of Cough	Causes
Acute	Tonsillitis, pharyngitis, tracheobronchitis, acute bronchitis, pleuritis, acute severe left-sided heart failure (dogs only)
Chronic	Heartworms, enlarged left atrium compressing trachea or main stem bronchus (dogs only), pulmonary neoplasia, asthma (cats only), chronic respiratory problems, chronic bronchitis (dogs only)
Acute onset, soft, moist that rapidly becomes worse in dogs with dyspnea	Pulmonary edema
Mild, intermittent cough, harsh, low pitched in dogs	Respiratory diseases
Loud, harsh, dry, sudden onset followed by gag in dogs	Tracheobronchitis
Honking, high pitched in dogs	Collapsing trachea or bronchi
Chronic, paroxysmal, loud, honking with excitement in dogs	Large airway disease
After drinking in dogs	Collapsing trachea, chronic tracheitis, tracheobronchitis, laryngeal paralysis, dysphagia
After eating in dogs	Pharyngeal dysfunction, megaesophagus, vascular ring anomalies, esophageal diverticula, esophageal foreign bodies, esophageal tumors
Without an inciting factor	Pulmonary or extrapulmonary disease

edema is peracute and severe enough that fluid accumulates in the airways. This cough is soft and moist sounding and produces blood-tinged sputum. An enlarged left atrium (in the absence of left-sided heart failure) may contribute to coughing by mechanical dorsal compression of the trachea or main stem bronchi, resulting in a cough of tracheal collapse. Table 1.1 lists some of the characteristic coughs in dogs and cats and their associated causes.

- Dogs and cats with pulmonary edema (cardiac or noncardiogenic) will have tachypnea or dyspnea and may have an acute onset of soft, moist coughing. Dogs with fulminant left-sided heart failure may have pink foam in the mouth and nose and be dyspneic, but they may or may not be coughing.
- Dogs with coughing as their primary problem should be radiographed and undergo other tests to find the cause of their coughing because it is uncommon to be due to heart disease or to left-sided heart failure. Dogs with a loud, harsh, dry cough of sudden onset followed by a nonproductive gag commonly have tracheobronchitis. Dogs with a honking, high-pitched cough often have a collapsing trachea or collapsed bronchi. Small breeds of dogs with large airway disease will have a chronic, paroxysmal cough that is hard, loud, and honking, and usually occurs with excitement. Dogs that cough after drinking may have cardiac disease, collapsing trachea, chronic tracheitis, tracheobronchitis, laryngeal paralysis, or other causes

of dysphagia. Dogs that cough without an inciting factor may have pulmonary or extrapulmonary disease. Dogs that cough after eating have pharyngeal dysphagia, megaesophagus, vascular ring anomalies, esophageal diverticula, esophageal foreign bodies, or esophageal tumors.

- Identifying the cause of the dog's coughing can be difficult. Radiographs, echocardiograms, fluoroscopy, transtracheal washes, and bronchoscopy should be done to try to find the cause. However, a cough that seems to respond to a therapeutic course of furosemide does not mean that the dog had heart failure because furosemide has both antiinflammatory and antitussive properties.
- It is unusual for cats with either left- or right-sided congestive heart failure to cough; however, they will cough with heartworm disease and with respiratory diseases such as asthma. If the clinician compresses the cat's trachea and the cat has a prolonged bout of coughing, then coughing is likely to be part of the cat's problem, and underlying respiratory problems should be pursued.

KEY POINT

The most common cause of coughing in dogs with murmurs is respiratory disease. Coughing is *not* caused by pulmonary edema unless the dog or cat is also tachypneic or dyspneic.

DYSPNEA

- Dyspnea is difficult, labored, or painful breathing. It is usually preceded by tachypnea (an increased rate of breathing), which owners may miss. It is a good idea to have the owner of a patient with cardiac disease learn to count his or her pet's respiratory rate at rest or sleeping. The respiratory rate should be less than 30 breaths per minute in a dog at rest, and if it goes over 50 breaths per minute, then the dog has tachypnea and should be examined by a veterinarian. Respiratory rate and effort have been shown to be the most reliable indication of left-sided heart failure and pulmonary edema.
- Dyspnea will occur whenever anything increases the amount of air that must be breathed by the animal. Box 1.1 lists the problems that can cause dyspnea. The usual cardiac cause of dyspnea in the dog is left-sided heart failure, which results in pulmonary edema. The usual cardiac causes of dyspnea in the cat are right-sided heart failure, which causes pleural effusion, and left-sided heart failure, which causes pulmonary edema. In patients with cardiac disease, dyspnea can be accompanied by stridor, which is a harsh, high-pitched respiratory sound. Other sounds include rhonchi, which sound like dry, coarse crackles. Also, dyspnea can be accompanied by wheezing, which is more typical of respiratory problems than cardiac problems. Table 1.2 lists the different types of dyspnea and the associated diseases or problems.
- Different types of dyspnea can be associated with certain problems or diseases. Acute dyspnea is usually caused by pulmonary edema (cardiac and noncardiac), severe pneumonia, airway obstruction, pneumothorax, or pulmonary embolism. Chronic, progressive dyspnea is caused by right-sided heart failure with ascites or pleural effusion, pericardial diseases, bronchial disease, lung diseases such as emphysema, pleural effusions, progressive anemia, and primary or secondary pulmonary neoplasia. Dyspnea at rest occurs with pneumothorax, pulmonary embolism, and severe left- or right-sided heart failure. Exertional dyspnea occurs after or during activity and can be associated with heart diseases, such as dilated cardiomyopathy, when the animal goes into heart failure. It can also be associated with chronic, obstructive lung disease. Expiratory dyspnea is prolonged, labored expiration and is caused by lower respiratory tract obstruction or disease. Inspiratory dyspnea is prolonged, and labored inspiration is due to upper airway obstruction. Mixed dyspnea is due to severe pulmonary edema caused by left-sided heart failure or severe pneumonia.

Box 1.1   Causes of Dyspnea

Acidosis
Anemia
Central nervous system disorders
Excitement
High altitude
Pain
Pericardial effusions
Pleural effusions
Primary cardiac diseases causing pulmonary edema
   or pleural effusion
Pulmonary edema (noncardiogenic)
Secondary cardiac diseases
Strenuous exercise
Thoracic wall problems (e.g., fractured ribs)

Table 1.2   Types of Dyspnea and Their Associated Diseases or Problems

Type of Dyspnea	Disease or Problem
Acute dyspnea	Pulmonary edema (cardiogenic and noncardiogenic), severe pneumonia, airway obstruction, pneumothorax, pulmonary embolism
Chronic, progressive dyspnea	Right-sided heart failure with ascites or pleural effusion, pericardial diseases, bronchial disease, lung diseases (e.g., emphysema), pleural effusions, progressive anemia, primary and secondary neoplasia
Dyspnea at rest	Pneumothorax, pulmonary embolism, severe left- or right-sided heart failure
Exertional dyspnea	Heart disease (e.g., dilated cardiomyopathy) or chronic obstructive lung disease
Expiratory dyspnea	Lower respiratory tract obstruction or disease
Inspiratory dyspnea	Upper airway obstruction
Mixed dyspnea	Pulmonary edema caused by left-sided heart failure or severe pneumonia
Orthopnea	Severe pulmonary edema, pericardial effusion, pleural effusion, diaphragmatic hernia, pneumothorax, severe pulmonary disease
Paroxysmal dyspnea	Arrhythmias (e.g., bradycardia or tachycardia)
Simple dyspnea or tachypnea	Fever, fear, pain, or excitement

- Orthopnea means that dyspnea occurs when the animal is lying down but not when standing. It is associated with severe pulmonary edema, pleural effusion, pericardial effusion, pneumothorax, diaphragmatic hernia, and severe respiratory problems. Paroxysmal dyspnea means that the dyspnea comes and goes. It can be associated with arrhythmias that cause either bradycardia or tachycardia. Simple dyspnea, or polypnea, is an increased rate of respiration caused by fever, fear, pain, or excitement. Cats with severe hyperthyroidism can also be dyspneic.
- Dyspnea that improves when treated with diuretics is suggestive of left-sided heart failure as the cause. Dyspnea that improves when treated with bronchodilators, antibiotics, or steroids is suggestive of respiratory disease as the cause.

KEY POINT

Dyspnea is a sign of significant cardiac, respiratory, or other systemic problems. It requires immediate diagnostic tests to identify the cause of the dyspnea so that specific therapy can be started. However, all tests should be done with minimal stress to the animal because these patients are fragile and stress could be fatal. Monitoring the animal's respiratory rate and effort at rest or during sleep is the most sensitive indicator of dyspnea and the onset of heart failure.

HEMOPTYSIS

- Hemoptysis is coughing up of blood. It is uncommon in animals because they usually swallow their sputum. Hemoptysis is a sign of severe pulmonary disease. The causes of hemoptysis are listed in Box 1.2. Cardiac causes of hemoptysis include severe pulmonary edema (e.g., ruptured chordae tendineae) and severe heartworm disease, usually with pulmonary embolism.

KEY POINT

Hemoptysis is a sign of a very serious underlying abnormality in the lungs, which may be caused by either a severe cardiac or respiratory problem.

SYNCOPE

- Syncope is a loss of consciousness caused by inadequate cerebral blood flow. It can recur and is usually brief. Syncope can be hard to differentiate from seizures. Animals usually fall over suddenly, get back up quickly, and are normal before and after the syncopal episode. Box 1.3 lists the causes of syncope in dogs and cats.
- In a dog with no other cardiac problems, syncope may be associated with severe bradycardias (e.g., third-degree heart block or sick sinus syndrome) or with marked sustained tachycardias (e.g., atrial or ventricular tachycardias), which are usually paroxysmal (i.e., they come and go).
- Small dogs with chronic, severe mitral regurgitation that cough when they get excited can have syncopal episodes. Dogs with severe subaortic stenosis, pulmonic stenosis, pulmonary hypertension, or tetralogy of Fallot can have arrhythmias associated with their ventricular hypertrophy and myocardial hypoxia. These arrhythmias will cause syncope. Syncope can

---

Box 1.2   Causes of Hemoptysis

Acute and chronic bronchitis
Chronic pulmonary granulomas
Clotting disorders
Disseminated intravascular coagulopathy
Lung abscesses
Lung lobe torsions
Oral or other neoplasia
Pulmonary embolism
Pulmonary fungal infections
Pulmonary neoplasia
Respiratory foreign bodies
Severe heartworm disease with pulmonary embolism
Severe pneumonia
Severe pulmonary edema (e.g., from ruptured chordae tendineae)
Trauma with severe pulmonary contusions

Box 1.3   Causes of Syncope in Dogs and Cats

Disease with poor cardiac output (e.g., dilated cardiomyopathy)
Severe bradycardia (e.g., complete heart block, sick sinus syndrome)
Severe sustained tachycardias (e.g., atrial or ventricular tachycardia)
Severe hypertrophic cardiomyopathy in cats
Systemic hypotension including arteriolar dilator therapy
Severe pulmonary hypertension
Severe subaortic stenosis
Severe pulmonic stenosis
Small dogs with severe mitral regurgitation that cough when excited
Tetralogy of Fallot

also occur in cats with severe hypertrophic cardiomyopathy. Animals with poor cardiac output caused by dilated cardiomyopathy can have syncope, especially if they also have arrhythmias such as atrial fibrillation or ventricular premature beats that further reduce their cardiac output. Cardiac medications such as vasodilators, especially arterial dilators, can result in systemic hypotension, which can also cause syncope.

KEY POINT

Syncope must be distinguished from seizures with a careful history and physical examination. Having the owner videotape an episode can also help the clinician distinguish between the two. Further tests such as Holter monitoring or event monitoring may be necessary to determine whether an arrhythmia is causing the syncope.

WEAKNESS AND EXERCISE INTOLERANCE

- Weakness and exercise intolerance are nonspecific signs of heart disease. Many diseases such as severe anemia, systemic diseases, metabolic diseases (e.g., hyperadrenocorticism), drug toxicities, and severe respiratory diseases can cause these signs. See Box 1.4 for causes of weakness and exercise intolerance.
- Because most animals do not exercise extensively, weakness and exercise intolerance are uncommon presenting complaints. Some owners think their animal is slowing down because of old age and not because of heart disease or other problems.
- Both complaints can be an early sign of decompensated heart failure because the heart cannot pump enough blood to the muscles on account of myocardial dysfunction (e.g., dilated cardiomyopathy or advanced mitral valve disease), obstruction to left ventricular outflow (e.g., subaortic stenosis or hypertrophic obstructive cardiomyopathy), inadequate ventricular filling (e.g., arrhythmias, pericardial diseases, hypertrophic cardiomyopathy), and decreased arterial oxygen (e.g., pulmonary edema or pleural effusion).

KEY POINT

Distinguishing between exercise intolerance caused by heart disease and other causes is important.

ASCITES

- Ascites is an accumulation of fluid in the abdomen. Ascites caused by cardiac problems is caused by either the inability of the right side

---

Box 1.4 Causes of Weakness and Exercise Intolerance

Cardiac disease with myocardial dysfunction (e.g., dilated cardiomyopathy)
Cardiac disease with obstruction to left ventricular outflow (e.g., subaortic stenosis, hypertrophic obstructive cardiomyopathy)
Decreased arterial oxygen (e.g., pulmonary edema, pleural effusion, or other pulmonary diseases)
Inadequate ventricular filling (e.g., arrhythmias, pericardial diseases)
Drug toxicities
Severe anemia
Severe metabolic disease
Severe respiratory diseases
Severe systemic diseases

---

of the heart to pump the blood presented to it or to pericardial disease, which prevents the blood from entering the right side of the heart. In either case the blood accumulates in the liver and spleen and causes congestion and increased venous pressure. Eventually fluid leaks out of the capsule of the liver, causing the ascites.
- Ascites is seen more frequently in dogs with right-sided heart failure because of acquired diseases (e.g., tricuspid regurgitation caused by chronic valvular heart disease, advanced heartworm disease, dilated cardiomyopathy, pericardial effusions, restrictive pericarditis) and congenital heart defects (e.g., tricuspid dysplasia, large ventricular septal defect, large atrial septal defect). See Figure 1.1 for an example of ascites and Box 1.5 for a list of causes of ascites in dogs. Ascites is less common in cats and is usually caused by tricuspid dysplasia but occasionally can be seen with other problems such as dilated cardiomyopathy.
- Large amounts of ascites will put pressure on the diaphragm, resulting in tachypnea or dyspnea. Ascites associated with right-sided heart failure is usually a protein-rich (modified) transudate and accumulates slowly.

KEY POINT

Decompensated heart diseases that result in ascites (e.g., pericardial effusion, some dilated cardiomyopathies, heartworm disease) may not have an associated murmur. Thus, any time ascites occurs, right-sided heart failure must be included in the differential diagnosis.

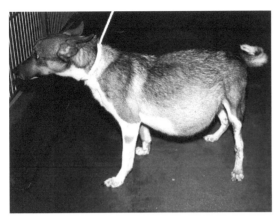

Figure 1.1 Notice the severe ascites in this dog with right-sided heart failure caused by severe pulmonic stenosis and severe tricuspid dysplasia.

Box 1.5   Causes of Ascites in Dogs

Advanced heartworm disease
Dilated cardiomyopathy
Large atrial septal defect
Large ventricular septal defect
Pericardial effusion
Restrictive pericarditis
Tricuspid dysplasia
Tricuspid regurgitation caused by chronic valvular
    heart disease

CYANOSIS

- Cyanosis is blue-tinged mucous membranes of the gums, tongue, eyes, ears, and other areas and is associated most commonly with right-to-left shunting congenital heart defects. Occasionally it is seen with severe left-sided heart failure or severe respiratory disease. It is rarely seen with abnormal hemoglobin production. Cyanosis is an insensitive way of detecting hypoxemia in dogs and cats because the oxygen saturation has to be very low to cause it and animals have darker mucous membranes, which makes cyanosis harder to detect until it is severe.
- Right-to-left shunting cardiac defects such as tetralogy of Fallot result in low oxygen saturation and high deoxygenated hemoglobin levels, which make affected animals cyanotic. These patients also have polycythemia, and the elevated number of red blood cells has increased amounts of reduced hemoglobin, which contributes to the cyanosis. Cyanosis becomes worse with exercise because the peripheral vascular resistance will decrease, although the pulmonary vascular pressure is unchanged so more deoxygenated venous blood will go systemically.

Cyanosis is a late finding in severe cardiac disease, except in right-to-left shunting congenital heart defects, so it is an insensitive indicator of membrane oxygenation and cardiac function.

WEIGHT LOSS

- Weight loss occurs in dogs with chronic, severe right-sided heart failure (e.g., severe tricuspid regurgitation, dilated cardiomyopathy, advanced heartworm disease). Weight loss in cats is usually associated with hyperthyroidism or infiltrative bowel disease, although cats with chronic right-sided heart failure can also lose weight. Cardiac cachexia is the loss of total body fat and lean body mass, especially skeletal muscle, despite a normal appetite and adequate therapy for the underlying heart disease. It can be a rapid loss of body condition in some dogs with dilated cardiomyopathy (Figure 1.2). See Box 1.6 for a list of the problems that contribute to cardiac cachexia in dogs.
- Weight loss is associated with ascites, malabsorption, congestion of the abdominal organs, lymphangiectasia, increased energy that is used for breathing, and medications that cause anorexia and vomiting. Dogs with ascites may have mild discomfort from the fluid, which makes them reluctant to eat. Also, the ascites and congested liver will compress the stomach so that the animal feels full after eating only a small amount of food. The fluid also restricts gastric emptying. Finally, if an unpalatable diet is fed, the animal is even more reluctant to eat and does not consume enough calories to keep from losing weight. Malabsorption caused by congestion of the intestines resulting from ascites also contributes to the weight loss.
- Right-sided heart failure causes congestion of the pancreas, which may decrease its function of secreting enzymes for digestion, resulting in maldigestion. Also, right-sided heart failure causes systemic venous and lymphatic hypertension, resulting in a secondary intestinal lymphangiectasia that produces a protein-losing enteropathy.
- Animals with right-sided heart failure and ascites have an increased effort of breathing and increased myocardial oxygen consumption that result from the decreased cardiac output. These two problems result in an increased use of energy and therefore calories by the heart and lungs. The activation of the sympathetic nervous system, which also results from the decreased cardiac output, causes increased energy use by the rest of the body.

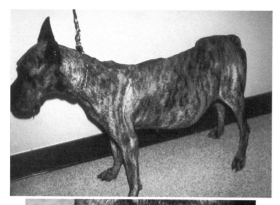

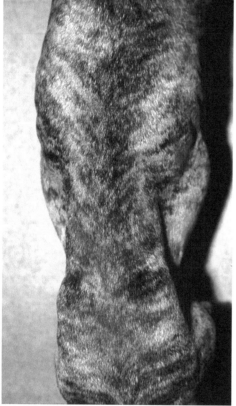

Figure 1.2 Great Dane with cardiac cachexia caused by dilated cardiomyopathy.

Box 1.6   Problems That Contribute to Cardiac Cachexia in Dogs

Ascites
Cardiac medications causing anorexia and vomiting
Electrolyte imbalance causing anorexia
Increased energy use by the body
Increased tumor necrosis factor
Malabsorption
Maldigestion
Protein-losing enteropathy

- Some cardiac medications such as digoxin, diltiazem, mexiletine, quinidine, and procainamide can cause anorexia or vomiting. Digoxin also has a direct effect on the small bowel, where it inhibits sugar and amino acid transport. The anorexia and vomiting also contribute to weight loss.
- Electrolytes, especially sodium and potassium, are adversely affected by diuretics, angiotensin-converting enzyme inhibitors, and digoxin. When potassium levels are abnormal, they contribute to anorexia and therefore weight loss.
- Dogs with chronic congestive heart failure have increased tumor necrosis factor, which inhibits the activity of lipoprotein lipase (hydrolyzes chylomicrons) and therefore interferes with the conversion of triglycerides to free fatty acids. This also will contribute to the animal's losing weight.

KEY POINT

Weight loss and cardiac cachexia are caused by multiple factors. It is important to make sure that an animal with ascites is being treated appropriately for heart failure and that the animal's digoxin levels, electrolytes, and renal function are being monitored. It is also important to calculate the animal's caloric requirement and make sure it is eating enough to meet its requirements (at least 60 kcal/kg daily). Special high-caloric diets and multiple small meals may be needed to ensure adequate caloric intake. The use of Puppy Chow, which is high in calories with a lower volume of food, has helped some patients maintain or gain weight. Appetite stimulants have been tried with varying success.

PARESIS

- Cats with acute posterior paresis (Figure 1.3) or paresis of one front leg (Figure 1.4) often have thromboembolism resulting from cardiomyopathy. The thrombi tend to form in the dilated left atrium or left ventricle, and pieces break off and lodge in the distal aorta or another artery. When the thrombus lodges in the aortic bifurcation, the cat will exhibit severe pain in the first few hours after the embolism, and the distal limbs will be cold and may be slightly swollen. The pads on the rear feet will be cyanotic (Figure 1.5). The cat's pulses cannot be detected, and the nails on the affected legs do not bleed when cut short.
- Acute posterior paresis is rare in dogs but it has been associated with emboli from severe, vegetative endocarditis of the aortic or mitral valve. Shifting leg lameness in dogs has also been associated with bacterial endocarditis.

Paresis in the rear limbs of the cat is usually caused by emboli that form in the left atrium resulting from left atrial enlargement that occurs with cardiomyopathies. Shifting leg lameness or posterior paresis in the dog can be caused by emboli from vegetations on either the mitral or aortic valve.

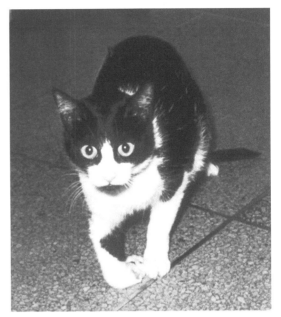

Figure 1.4 Cat with a front leg thrombus resulting from a left atrial thrombus caused by hypertrophic cardiomyopathy.

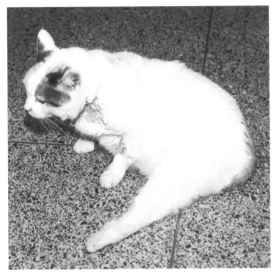

Figure 1.3 Cat with a saddle thrombus resulting from a left atrial thrombus caused by hypertrophic cardiomyopathy.

PHYSICAL EXAMINATION

OBSERVATION

- The animal's attitude and behavior can give clues to the severity and kind of problems that the animal is having. Note whether the animal is depressed or alert, listless or active. An animal that refuses to lie down may have severe pulmonary edema, pleural effusion, pericardial effusion, pneumothorax, diaphragmatic hernia, or respiratory disease (Box 1.7). An animal that stands with elbows abducted and head extended with open-mouth breathing and flared nostrils has severe respiratory distress and needs immediate therapy.
- The rate, rhythm, and effort of respirations can help determine the underlying problem. Tachypnea and panting are usually caused by excitement; however, expiratory dyspnea usually indicates lower airway disease, inspiratory dyspnea usually indicates upper airway disease, and mixed dyspnea can be caused by severe pulmonary edema or severe pneumonia. See Box 1.1 for the causes of dyspnea in animals.
- Noting the nature and type of coughing is helpful if it occurs during the course of the physical

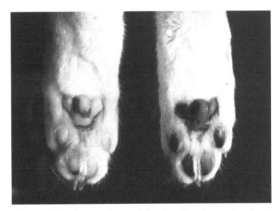

Figure 1.5 Comparison of the front and rear leg footpads in a cat with a saddle thrombus. Note the purple color of the rear leg caused by the complete occlusion of blood flow to the rear limbs secondary to the saddle thrombus and constriction of the collateral circulation.

examination. An animal that has a history of coughing and is not dyspneic is unlikely to have cardiac failure as the cause of coughing.
- The presence of dependent ventral edema can give the clinician an idea as to the source of the animal's problem. If edema is present in the neck, head, and forelimbs only, then it usually indicates an obstruction of the cranial vena cava or a mediastinal mass. If edema is present in the entire body, then pleural effusion with or without ascites is usually present. Other causes of edema (e.g., hypoproteinemia) should also be considered.

Box 1.7   Reasons That an Animal Will Not Lie Down

Diaphragmatic hernia
Pneumothorax
Severe pericardial effusion
Severe pleural effusion
Severe pulmonary edema
Severe respiratory disease

- An elevated temperature may occur with an infectious disease or subacute bacterial endocarditis. A subnormal temperature can occur with low cardiac output caused by severe heart failure in dogs or cats or with a saddle thrombus in cats.

KEY POINT

By observing an animal, a clinician can quickly determine the presence and severity of a respiratory or cardiac problem. Animals with severe dyspnea should be handled gently to avoid stress and should be treated immediately.

HEAD

- The eyes should be examined for changes that could indicate systemic diseases. Hypertension in cats will cause decreased pupillary responses due to retinal detachment or hemorrhage. A fundic examination may reveal papilledema (swelling of the optic disc) along with hemorrhage or retinal detachment. Retinal hemorrhages also can occur with polycythemia and bacterial endocarditis.
- Central retinal degeneration occurs in about one third of cats with dilated cardiomyopathy caused by taurine deficiency. The areas of degeneration are horizontal, linear, and hyper-reflective.
- The ears have no significant changes associated with the cardiovascular system. However, cyanosis can sometimes be recognized with evaluation of the color of the pinna.
- Examine the nose for signs of disease and for patency. Check each patient for any asymmetry and swellings, especially in the nasal and throat areas because these swellings could be obstructing airways and causing respiratory distress.
- The mucous membrane color and perfusion in the mouth should be noted. A perfusion time of greater than 2 seconds suggests decreased cardiac output; however, most animals with congestive heart failure have normal mucous membrane color until their heart failure is severe.

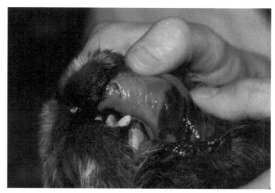

Figure 1.6 Hyperemic mucous membranes in a dog with polycythemia caused by tetralogy of Fallot.

Because of this, mucous membrane color and perfusion are insensitive ways to evaluate adequate circulation.
- Cyanosis of the mucous membranes is caused by hypoventilation or poor diffusion across the alveoli produced by multiple different factors (see the section on history discussed previously).
- Hyperemic mucous membranes (dark red to muddy) may indicate an increased packed cell volume (polycythemia), which can result from a chronic right-to-left vascular shunt (Figure 1.6).
- Pale mucous membranes indicate anemia or poor perfusion. The mucous membranes of the mouth should be compared with the posterior membranes (e.g., vagina, prepuce) because differential cyanosis can occur in a right-to-left shunting PDA. Also, check the oral cavity for severe dental tartar, gingivitis, or pyorrhea, which can serve as sources of sepsis leading to bacteremia and possibly endocarditis.

KEY POINT

Mucous membrane color and perfusion are insensitive signs of cardiac function, so when they are abnormal, the animal's cardiac or respiratory problem is severe.

NECK

- The jugular pulse should be evaluated while the animal is standing with its head in a normal position. Any pulse going over one third of the way up the neck is abnormal and can be due to any of several factors. See Box 1.8 for causes of abnormal jugular pulses. Arterial pulses can mimic a jugular pulse; however, when light pressure is applied to the area of the jugular pulse, the arterial pulse will continue, whereas the jugular pulse will stop.

> ### Box 1.8   Causes of Abnormal Jugular Pulses
>
> Arrhythmias
> Heartworm disease
> Pulmonary hypertension
> Pulmonic stenosis
> Right-sided heart failure (e.g., tricuspid regurgitation, dilated cardiomyopathy)

> ### Box 1.9   Causes of Distended Jugular Veins
>
> Right-sided heart failure (e.g., tricuspid regurgitation, dilated cardiomyopathy)
> Pericardial diseases
> Heart base tumor
> Mediastinal mass

- Abnormal jugular pulses occur in right-sided heart failure caused by tricuspid regurgitation or dilated cardiomyopathy, when the right ventricle contracts and the blood flows back into the right atrium and up the jugular veins because of the insufficient tricuspid valve. Abnormal jugular pulses also occur with pulmonic stenosis and pulmonary hypertension, when the right atrium contracts against a hypertrophied, noncompliant right ventricle so that only some of the blood enters the right ventricle and the rest goes back up the jugular veins.
- With heartworm disease, abnormal jugular pulses occur because there is both a stiff, hypertrophied right ventricle and tricuspid regurgitation, which both contribute to the jugular pulses.
- Arrhythmias such as second- or third-degree heart block or premature beats cause abnormal jugular pulses because the sequence of atrial and ventricular activation is disrupted. The right atrium contracts against a closed tricuspid valve, sending blood back up the jugular veins.
- The entire jugular vein can be distended, indicating increased systemic venous pressure caused by right-sided heart failure, pericardial disease, or obstruction of the cranial vena cava (e.g., heart base tumor). About 70% of dogs with right-sided heart failure have distended jugular veins, but they are rare in cats. Cats with left-sided heart failure may have distended jugular veins only when lying down, and the jugular veins return to normal when they sit or stand. See Box 1.9 for causes of jugular distension.
- Mediastinal masses such as lymphosarcoma can compress the cranial vena cava, causing a distended jugular vein; however, they also usually cause pleural effusion and head and neck edema.
- The hepatojugular reflex is a distension of the jugular veins that occurs when the abdomen is compressed for 10 to 30 seconds. It is caused by an increased return of blood to the right side of the abdomen. However, the right side of the heart is not normal and cannot handle the increased venous return, so the blood from the

cranial vena cava cannot enter the heart and the jugular veins become distended. This reflex is present with both right- and left-sided heart failure and indicates increased blood volume in the peripheral venous system caused by an inability of the heart to circulate the blood properly.
- A central venous pressure can be obtained in animals with distended jugular veins. It is most useful in the diagnosis of restrictive pericardial disease where less invasive tests have not confirmed the diagnosis.

KEY POINT

Jugular vein distention can be present with both right- and left-sided heart failure but may be present in only 70% of these cases. Abdominal ultrasound is a sensitive, noninvasive method of determining increased venous pressure by detecting distended hepatic veins; however, the ultrasound confirms only the presence of increased venous pressure and not the cause.

TRACHEAL PALPATION

- The trachea should be palpated for abnormalities such as collapsing, masses, or increased sensitivity. This part of the exam is best postponed until after auscultation of the thorax, because a cough may be elicited that makes auscultation difficult.
- Lymph nodes should be palpated to see if they are enlarged. The thyroids may be enlarged in cats with hyperthyroidism (thyroid slip). An old dog with a mass near the larynx and an associated thrill usually has thyroid carcinoma with an arteriovenous fistula causing the thrill (a murmur that can be felt as well as heard).

KEY POINT

Palpation of the neck can reveal primary or secondary problems that affect the heart and can mimic heart disease (collapsing trachea).

THORACIC PALPATION

- The apex beat (sometimes called the point of maximum intensity [PMI]) is where the cardiac impulse is felt strongest on the chest wall. It should be on the left side of the thorax between the fourth and sixth intercostal spaces. Shifting of the PMI is caused by cardiac enlargement, masses displacing the heart, collapsed lung lobes that allow the heart to shift, diaphragmatic hernias, pleural effusions associated with collapsed lung lobes or fibrin, or right lateral recumbency, which causes the heart to fall to the right. Pectus excavatum, a deformity of the sternum, can also shift the heart to the right (Box 1.10).
- A decreased intensity of heartbeat or heart sounds may be caused by obesity, pleural effusion, pericardial effusion, thoracic masses, severe pneumothorax, severe emphysema, diaphragmatic hernias, decreased left ventricular contractility with decreased cardiac output, or arrhythmias, which decrease cardiac filling and therefore cardiac output (Box 1.11).
- There can be an increased intensity of the PMI or heart sounds in young, thin animals or in animals with increased heart rates or with hyperdynamic states such as anemia, hyperthyroidism, or fever. Sometimes the heart appears to be beating on the chest wall. The heart is not actually hitting the chest wall; the appearance is caused by the increased wall tension of the thoracic wall for an indeterminate reason. It does not mean that the heart is contracting normally or better than normal.
- Loud cardiac murmurs can be palpated as thrills, which are caused by vibrations caused by blood flow. A thrill is always located where a murmur is loudest.

KEY POINT

It is important to locate both the PMI of the heartbeat and the presence of thrills caused by heart murmurs on the thoracic wall.

ABDOMINAL PALPATION

- Abdominal palpation is done to check for ascites, the presence of fluid in the abdomen. Ascites can be caused by right-sided heart failure as well as many other causes. The presence of ascites can be difficult to ascertain in obese animals. The clinician should put one hand on one side of the abdomen and the other hand on the other side, and then tap the abdomen. If a fluid wave is felt by the hand on the opposite side of the abdomen, then ascites is present. In

---

Box 1.10   Causes of Shifting of the Palpable Apex Beat or Point of Maximum Intensity

Cardiac enlargement
Collapsed lung lobes on the right
Diaphragmatic hernias
Pectus excavatum
Lying down in right lateral recumbency
Masses displacing the heart
Pleural effusions

Box 1.11   Causes of Changes in Heart Sounds

Decreased intensity caused by:
  Arrhythmias
  Decreased left ventricular cardiac output
  Diaphragmatic hernias
  Obesity
  Pleural or pericardial effusions
  Severe emphysema
  Severe pneumothorax
  Thoracic masses
Increased intensity caused by:
  Hyperdynamic states (e.g., anemia, hyperthyroidism, fever)
  Increased heart rates
  Young, thin animals

---

addition to ascites, check for signs of hepatomegaly and splenomegaly.
- The presence of ascites, splenomegaly, and hepatomegaly usually indicates right-sided heart failure caused by dilated cardiomyopathy, tricuspid regurgitation, heartworm disease, pericardial disease, or congenital heart disease. Ascites caused by right-sided heart failure is usually a protein-rich (modified) transudate that is seen on cytologic examination. Another possible cause of ascites is an obstruction of the posterior vena cava.
- Palpate the abdomen for any masses. Also palpate the kidneys because chronic renal failure can lead to systemic hypertension that can affect the heart.

KEY POINT

Ascites can be caused by right-sided heart failure or other heart problems, such as pericardial effusion; however, it can also be caused by other noncardiac problems. Further tests are indicated to determine the cause of ascites.

SKIN

- Palpate for evidence of edema caused by right-sided heart failure or venous obstruction.

FEMORAL PULSES

- Both femoral pulses should be felt with the dog or cat standing, and they should be compared with each other because one could be obstructed.
- It is difficult to palpate the femoral pulse in a normal cat; therefore the absence of palpable femoral pulses in a cat should not be interpreted as definite arterial obstruction.
- Partial or complete occlusion of the pulses so that they cannot be felt is usually caused by thromboembolism. In dogs this can occur with bacterial endocarditis of the mitral or aortic valves, hyperadrenocorticism, and protein-losing glomerulonephritis (especially amyloidosis). Cavalier King Charles Spaniels with chronic valvular heart disease of the mitral valve sometimes lack a pulse for unknown reasons. In cats, absent pulses are associated with cardiomyopathy but can also occasionally be caused by bacterial endocarditis or extracardiac disease.
- The femoral pulse rate should be taken. Normal rates in dogs are 70 to 180 beats/min. Puppies can have a normal rate of 220 beats/min. Normal rates in cats are 160 to 240 beats/min.
- The rhythm of the pulses should be noted. There should be a pulse for every heartbeat. Pulse deficits usually indicate incomplete ventricular filling, as seen with arrhythmias.
- Arterial pulse pressure (femoral pulse quality) is the difference between the arterial systolic pressure and the diastolic pressure. Pulse quality can normally vary depending on the animal's conformation, age, hydration, heart rate, cardiac function, and level of excitement or activity.
- The intensity of the pulse should be palpated. Normal pulses are strong and have a rapid rate of rise and fall. Table 1.3 lists the pulse quality and the cause for each type of pulse.
- Hypokinetic (weak) pulses are caused by decreased cardiac output (e.g., congestive heart failure, hypovolemia), decreased peripheral vascular resistance, increased arterial compliance, or slower rate of rise caused by delayed emptying of the left ventricle (e.g., subaortic stenosis). Dogs will have normal pulses until the stroke volume is markedly decreased with severe congestive heart failure, so pulses are an insensitive indicator of cardiac output.
- Hyperkinetic (strong) pulses rise and fall quickly and are caused by large left ventricular stroke volumes with rapid diastolic runoffs (e.g., PDA, aortic regurgitation). They are called "B-B shot" or "water-hammer" pulses.

Table 1.3 Types of Pulses and Their Associated Causes

Pulse	Cause
Absent pulses	Thromboembolism
Abrupt pulses	Mitral regurgitation
	Ventricular septal defects
Erratic pulses	Atrial fibrillation
Hypokinetic pulses	Heart failure
	Hypotension
	Hypovolemia
	Subaortic stenosis
Hyperkinetic pulses	Aortic regurgitation
	Fear
	Fever
	Patent ductus arteriosus
	Severe anemia
	Severe bradycardia
	Thyrotoxicosis
Pulse deficits	Arrhythmias
Pulsus alternans	Severe dilated cardiomyopathy
Pulsus bigeminus	Arrhythmias
Pulsus paradoxus	Cardiac tamponade

Fear, fever, severe bradycardia, thyrotoxicosis, and anemia can also produce this type of pulse.
- The pulses can be abrupt or jerky with chronic mitral valve disease and ventricular septal defects as a greater volume of blood is ejected in early systole.
- Pulsus alternans occurs when the pulse is alternately weak and then strong in patients with normal sinus rhythm. It is frequently associated with severe myocardial failure (e.g., dilated cardiomyopathy).
- Pulsus bigeminus occurs when weak pulses alternate with strong pulses. This is associated with arrhythmias such as ventricular bigeminy in which a normal heart beat alternates with a ventricular premature beat. The weak pulses occur because the premature beat causes the ventricles to contract before they are adequately filled so that a smaller than normal volume of blood is ejected by the left ventricle. The difference between the normal and abnormal pulses may be accentuated because the ventricles have more time to fill on the normal beats and so the normal pulses feel even stronger.
- Pulsus paradoxus is an alteration of the pulse strength during respiration caused by changes in ventricular filling. There is an increase in pulse strength on expiration and a decrease in strength on inspiration in normal animals; however, this change is exaggerated and easier to feel when cardiac tamponade is present.
- Pulses feel erratic when an animal has atrial fibrillation.

The quality of an animal's pulse is not a good indication of the severity of its cardiac problem because only very advanced heart disease will cause weak pulses; however, pulse deficits are good indicators of the presence of an arrhythmia.

PERCUSSION

- Percussion can be used to determine the presence of masses or fluid lines, especially in the thorax. It will clicit a hollow sound (hyperresonance) over the lungs and a dull sound (hyporesonant) over solid structures.
- If an area, especially a dorsal area, in the thorax sounds hyperresonant, then pneumothorax may be present.
- If an area, especially a ventral area, sounds hyporesonant, then pleural effusion may be present.

Percussion can be a rapid way of determining the presence or absence of pleural effusion.

STETHOSCOPE

- The main components of the stethoscope are the bell, diaphragm, tubing, and ear pieces. The bell transmits low-frequency (20-300 cycles per second [cps]) sounds when light pressure is used and high-frequency (300-1000 cps) sounds when firm pressure is used to apply it to the thorax. It is best for hearing third and fourth heart sounds. The diaphragm attenuates low frequencies and selectively transmits the high frequencies. It is best for hearing the first and second heart sounds.
- Most stethoscopes combine the bell and diaphragm into a dual-sided, combination-style chest piece. Some stethoscopes have the bell and diaphragm as one piece. With these stethoscopes, simple fingertip pressure allows one to switch from low- to high-frequency sounds. Unlike a traditional two-sided stethoscope, there is no interruption in sound, resulting in added convenience and efficiency in auscultation. For dogs and cats that weigh less than 15 lb, a pediatric stethoscope that has a smaller headpiece should be used.
- A practical tubing length on a stethoscope is approximately 14 to 18 inches. If the tubing is too long, it will attenuate all the heart and lung sounds.
- Ear pieces should angle forward to conform to the anatomy of the ear canals. A stethoscope with variable sizes of ear pieces is ideal because

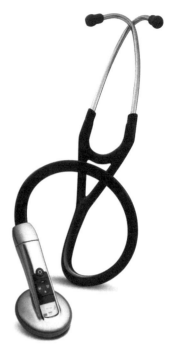

Figure 1.7 3M Littmann Electronic Stethoscope Model 3200. (Courtesy 3M, St. Paul, Minn.)

each person can find the correct-size earpiece that fits comfortably in the ear canal and shuts out extraneous sounds.
- In addition to electronic amplification of heart sounds and murmurs, electronic stethoscopes allow the user to record and play back sounds at either normal or half speed. This feature is useful for judging and timing the shape or quality of murmurs in patients with tachycardia and for judging the timing of transient heart sounds such as clicks or gallops. Some models also provide the ability to record graphic representations of sounds in a digital file format (i.e., a phonocardiogram) that can be stored on a computer, possibly even becoming part of the patient's medical record. One model of electronic stethoscope is the 3M Littman Model 3000 (Figure 1.7). It features useful ambient noise reduction circuitry that appears to overcome most, if not all, of the problems of background noise amplification that plagued previous models.

No one stethoscope works well for everyone. Ideally, a clinician should try various stethoscopes to find the one that works best for him or her and also find the ear piece size that best fits his or her ear canals.

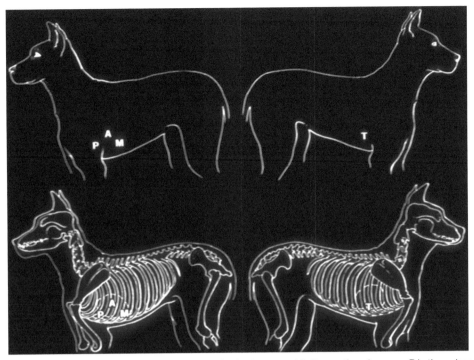

Figure 1.8 Areas of auscultation in the dog. *M* is the mitral valve area, *A* is the aortic valve area, *P* is the pulmonic valve area, and *T* is the tricuspid valve area. (From Gompf RE: The clinical approach to heart disease: history and physical examination. In Fox PR, ed: Canine and feline cardiology, New York, 1988, Churchill Livingstone.)

AUSCULTATION

- Auscultation of the heart is the most helpful part of the cardiac examination; it should be done carefully and systematically. The animal should be standing so that the heart is in its normal position. This avoids the problem of positional murmurs caused by the heart rubbing against the chest wall when an animal is lying down.
- Common artifacts that can be heard include respiratory clicks and murmurs, rumbles caused by shivering and twitching, and movement sounds such as crackling caused by rubbing of hair. Extraneous sounds will occur if auscultation is not performed in a quiet area.
- Be sure to auscultate the heart and lungs separately. Also, auscultate the entire thorax on both sides. Heart rate and rhythm should be identified. The effects of inspiration and expiration on heart rate, rhythm, and heart sounds should be noted. Also note the presence or absence of heart sounds.
- The areas of auscultation of the heart are shown in Figure 1.8. Table 1.4 lists the areas of auscultation.
- The pulmonic valve area is on the left side at the base of the heart. In the dog, it is between

Table 1.4 Areas of Auscultation in the Dog and Cat

Structure	Location
Mitral valve (left apex)	Dog—left side, fifth intercostal space at costochondral junction
	Cat—left side, fifth to sixth intercostal space near sternum
Aortic valve (left base)	Dog—left side, fourth intercostal space just above costochondral junction
	Cat—left side, second to third intercostal space just dorsal to pulmonic area
Pulmonic valve (left base)	Dog—left side, between second and fourth intercostal space just above sternum
	Cat—left side, second to third intercostal space one third of the way up from sternum
Tricuspid valve (right apex)	Dog—right side, third to fifth intercostal space near costochondral junction
	Cat—right side, fourth to fifth intercostal space near sternum

the second and the fourth intercostal spaces just above the sternum. In the cat, it is located at the second to the third intercostal space, one third to one half of the way up the thorax from the sternum.

- The aortic valve area is on the left side at the base of the heart. In the dog, it is at the fourth intercostal space, just above the costochondral junction. In the cat, it is at the second to third intercostal space, just dorsal to the pulmonic area.
- In cats and small dogs, it may be impossible to distinguish the pulmonic and aortic areas, so these two areas are referred to as the left heart base.
- The mitral valve area is on the left side. In the dog, it is at the fifth intercostal space at the costochondral junction. In the cat, it is at the fifth to the sixth intercostal space, one fourth of the way up the thorax from the sternum. In cats and small dogs, this area may also be referred to as the left heart apex.
- The tricuspid valve area is on the right side. In the dog, it is at the third to the fifth intercostal space near the costochondral junction. In the cat, it is at the fourth or fifth intercostal space, at a level opposite the mitral area. It may also be referred to as the right heart apex.

- Note the areas in which murmurs are loudest (PMI) and where they radiate.
- Alternative areas of auscultation include the thoracic inlets for radiation of the murmur of subaortic stenosis and the left axillary area for murmurs of PDA. Also, congenital defects have an area where they are heard the loudest and other areas where they are softer (referred to as areas of radiation).

KEY POINT

Auscultate the lungs and heart separately to avoid missing or confusing any abnormal sounds. Auscultate all valve areas in all animals. Congenital heart defects have been missed when clinicians listen only to the mitral valve area in a young animal.

NORMAL HEART SOUNDS

- Heart sounds are caused by the abrupt acceleration or deceleration of blood and the vibrations of the heart and vessels.
- The first heart sound (S_1) (Figure 1.9) is caused by passive closure of the mitral (left

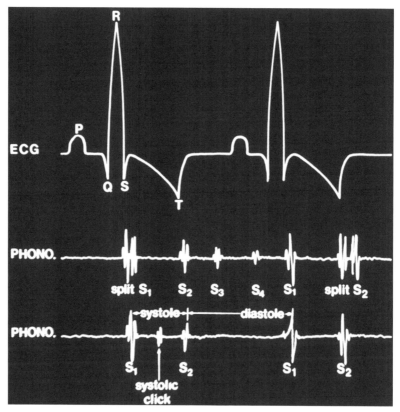

Figure 1.9   Heart sounds and their relationship to the ECG. The first heart sound is S_1. The second heart sound is S_2. The third heart sound is S_3, and the fourth is S_4. (From Gompf RE: The clinical approach to heart disease: history and physical examination. In Fox PR, ed: Canine and feline cardiology, New York, 1988, Churchill Livingstone.)

atrioventricular) and tricuspid (right atrioventricular) valves, resulting in the sudden acceleration and deceleration of blood. It has four parts that can be seen on a phonocardiogram.

- S_1 is longer, louder, duller, and lower pitched than the second heart sound (S_2). It is loudest over the mitral and tricuspid areas and in young, thin animals and those with high sympathetic tone (e.g., fear), tachycardia, systemic hypertension, anemia, or mitral regurgitation. The intensity of S_1 decreases because of obesity, pleural or pericardial effusion, thoracic masses, diaphragmatic hernias, bradycardia, emphysema, shock, and insufficient filling of the ventricles.
- S_1 varies in intensity with arrhythmias.
- Splitting of S_1 (see Figure 1.9) is caused by asynchronous closure of the mitral and tricuspid valves. It can be split normally in large breeds of dogs or abnormally with right bundle branch block, atrial or ventricular premature beats, cardiac pacing, or stenosis of the mitral or tricuspid valve. The arterial pulse occurs just after S_1, and the precordial impact occurs simultaneously with S_1.
- Box 1.12 lists the causes of changes in S_1.
- S_2 (see Figure 1.9) is produced by passive closure of the aortic and pulmonic valves. It is short, high pitched, and sharp. It is loudest over the aortic and pulmonic areas.
- A split S_2 (see Figure 1.9) is caused by closure of the pulmonic valve after the aortic valve. This occurs in pulmonary hypertension (e.g., severe heartworm disease or right-to-left PDA), right bundle branch block, ventricular premature beats originating in the left ventricle, atrial septal defect, pulmonic stenosis, and mitral stenosis.
- Paradoxical splitting of S_2 is caused by delayed closure of the aortic valve. This results from left bundle branch block, premature beats originating from the right ventricle, subaortic stenosis, severe systemic hypertension, and left ventricular failure.
- S_2 may be absent in arrhythmias where there is incomplete filling of the ventricles and insufficient pressure to open the semilunar valves.
- Box 1.13 lists the causes of changes in S_2.

KEY POINT

It is critical to identify the first and second heart sounds in all patients and use auscultation as an effective tool in the diagnosis of heart disease. If extraneous sounds are present, then the clinician may need to move to another area of the thorax to identify these sounds properly.

Box 1.12   Causes of Changes in the First Heart Sound (S_1)

Loud S_1
　Anemia
　Excitement
　Exercise
　Fear
　Fever
　Hyperthyroidism
　Mitral regurgitation
　Positive inotropic agents
　Pregnancy
　Systemic hypertension
　Tachycardia
　Thin animals
Soft S_1
　Bradycardias
　Decreased cardiac output
　Diaphragmatic hernias
　Emphysema
　Hypothyroidism
　Left bundle branch block
　Negative inotropic agents
　Obesity
　Pericardial effusion
　Pleural effusion
　Severe aortic or mitral regurgitation
　Severe heart failure
　Shock
　Thoracic masses
Variable S_1
　Arrhythmias
Split S_1
　Atrial or ventricular premature beats
　Cardiac pacing
　Right bundle branch block
　Stenosis of mitral or tricuspid valve

ABNORMAL HEART SOUNDS

- The third heart sound (S_3) (see Figure 1.9) is caused by rapid ventricular filling and is not heard in normal dogs or cats. It is lower pitched than the S_2 and is heard best in the mitral valve area. It occurs during diastole after S_2.
- S_3 in dogs indicates dilated ventricles, which most commonly occur with dilated cardiomyopathy, decompensated mitral or tricuspid regurgitation, large ventricular or atrial septal defects, and large PDA. In cats it is associated with dilated cardiomyopathy, severe anemia, and severe hyperthyroidism.
- Table 1.5 lists the causes of abnormal heart sounds.
- The fourth heart sound (S_4) (see Figure 1.9) is caused by atrial contraction into an already overdistended ventricle or into a stiff ventricle

Box 1.13 Causes of Changes in the Second Heart Sound (S_2)

Loud S_2
  Atrial septal defect
  Mild valvular pulmonic stenosis
  Patent ductus arteriosus
  Pulmonary embolism
  Pulmonary hypertension
  Systemic hypertension
  Valvular aortic stenosis
  Ventricular septal defect
Soft S_2
  Dilated cardiomyopathy
  Hypothyroidism
  Marked aortic regurgitation
  Shock
  Significant pulmonic stenosis
  Valvular aortic stenosis
Split S_2
  Atrial septal defect
  Heartworms
  Mitral stenosis
  Pulmonary hypertension—moderate to severe
  Pulmonic stenosis
  Right bundle branch block
  Right to left patent ductus arteriosus
  Ventricular premature beat from left ventricle
Paradoxical split S_2
  Left bundle branch block
  Left ventricular failure
  Severe systemic hypertension
  Significant aortic regurgitation
  Subaortic stenosis
  Ventricular premature beat from right ventricle
Absent S_2
  Arrhythmias

Table 1.5 Causes of Abnormal Heart Sounds

Sound	Cause
Gallop sounds	
S_3	Decompensated mitral or tricuspid regurgitation
	Dilated cardiomyopathy
	Large atrial septal defect
	Large patent ductus arteriosus
	Large ventricular septal defect
	Severe anemia in cats
	Severe hyperthyroidism in cats
	Significant aortic regurgitation
S_4	Anemia
	Hypertrophic cardiomyopathy
	Dogs with ruptured chordae tendineae
	Pulmonary hypertension
	Systemic hypertension
	Third-degree heart block
	Thyrotoxicosis
Systolic click	Mitral valve prolapse
Ejection sounds	Anemia
	Atrial septal defect
	Dilation of great vessels
	Exercise
	Heartworms
	Hyperthyroidism
	Pulmonary embolism
	Pulmonary hypertension
	Systemic hypertension
	Valvular aortic stenosis
	Valvular pulmonic stenosis

in dogs and cats. It is heard best over the aortic or pulmonic areas, but sometimes it can be heard over the mitral valve area. It occurs in diastole just before S_1.

- S_4 is present in dogs or cats when the atrium is dilated in response to ventricular diastolic dysfunction, such as hypertrophic cardiomyopathy or third-degree heart block. It may also be heard in dogs with ruptured chordae tendineae.
- A gallop rhythm is an S_3, an S_4, or a combination (summation) of the two. Gallops have a low frequency and can be difficult to hear. A gallop can be an early sign of heart failure, preceding clinical signs.
- Systolic clicks are short, mid- to high-frequency clicking noises that occur in systole between S_1 and S_2 (see Figure 1.9). They are usually loudest over the mitral and tricuspid areas. A systolic

click may come and go and may change its position in systole (gets closer to or further away from S_2) and may change its intensity.
- A systolic click can be hard to differentiate from a gallop, especially if the animal's heart rate is fast.
- The precise cause of the click is unknown, but it may be caused by the mitral valve buckling into the left atrium (mitral valve prolapse) in dogs with early mitral regurgitation because many of these animals have a mitral regurgitation murmur later in life. This is a benign finding and not usually associated with heart failure.
- Ejection sounds are high-frequency sounds generated in early systole caused by hypertension, dilation of the great vessels, or opening of abnormal semilunar valves such as in valvular pulmonic stenosis. These sounds are easily missed and misinterpreted as early systolic murmurs.

KEY POINT

The presence of a gallop is an indication of cardiac disease in small animals.

ARRHYTHMIAS HEARD ON AUSCULTATION

- Sinus arrhythmia has a cyclical pattern. The heart rate will increase during inspiration and decrease during expiration owing to changes in vagal tone. The intensity of the pulse and heart sounds may vary. It is normal in dogs, but in cats it is usually associated with heart disease. Sinus arrhythmia occurs at normal heart rates in dogs and cats and tends to disappear as the heart rate increases.
- Arrhythmias that increase the heart rate (tachycardias) include both atrial and ventricular arrhythmias. Sinus and atrial tachycardias are rapid and regular. All the heart sounds are of a uniform intensity, but an atrial tachycardia tends to be intermittent.
- Animals with atrial fibrillation have a rapid, irregular rhythm with heart sounds that vary in intensity. Pulse deficits are present. Atrial fibrillation has been described as being irregularly irregular and is rarely mistaken for other tachycardias.
- Ventricular tachycardias are usually intermittent and tend to be more regular than atrial fibrillation. However, an animal with multifocal ventricular tachycardia can sound like a dog with atrial fibrillation. Pulse deficits are frequently present with ventricular tachycardias. An electrocardiogram is necessary to distinguish among sinus, atrial, and ventricular tachycardia.
- Atrial and ventricular premature beats generate extra sounds that mimic S_3 and S_4. It is difficult to differentiate between the two types of premature beats, as well as between S_3 and S_4 during physical examination. An electrocardiogram and phonocardiogram may be necessary. Both atrial and ventricular premature beats interrupt the normal rhythm and are usually followed by a pause. Usually only S_1 is heard with a premature beat, and S_2 is absent. However, sometimes S_1 and S_2 can be heard close together. Premature beats can also cause a split S_1 or S_2.
- Arrhythmias that decrease the heart rate are called bradycardias; examples include sinus bradycardia and heart blocks. Sinus bradycardia has a very slow rhythm. The heart sounds may vary. The heart rate in dogs is between 50 and 70 beats/min, depending on the size of the dog. The heart rate in cats is less than 120 beats/min.
- Second- and third-degree heart blocks result in slow heart rates. The heart sounds will vary in intensity. S_4 may be present in third-degree block. The pulses will be slow and hyperkinetic, but there are no pulse deficits. A jugular pulse is usually present. Extra sounds may be generated by escape beats. An electrocardiogram is necessary to diagnose the type of bradycardia present.
- Unexpected pauses can occur with sinoatrial (or sinus) arrest. Sinus arrest occurs when an

impulse does not leave the sinoatrial node. The pause continues until the next normal beat or an escape beat occurs. The heart sound following a pause may be louder than usual because the ventricles have had longer to fill and eject a larger amount of blood. An electrocardiogram is necessary to diagnose sinus arrest.
- Sick sinus syndrome will have long pauses where the heart is not beating at all. If the pause lasts long enough, the dog will faint. Sometimes there are also periods of tachycardia, which gives it the name "bradycardia/tachycardia syndrome." Sick sinus syndrome was first described in older female Miniature Schnauzers but has been found in multiple breeds of dogs.

MURMURS

- Murmurs are caused by turbulent blood flow through the heart and vessels. The turbulence can be caused by disruptions of blood flow through holes in the heart (e.g., ventricular or atrial septal defect), a stenotic valve (e.g., aortic, pulmonic, mitral, or tricuspid stenosis), an insufficient valve (e.g., mitral, tricuspid, aortic, or pulmonic regurgitation), or an abnormal arterial venous connection near the heart (e.g., PDA), or it can be caused by altered blood viscosity or changes in blood vessel diameter. Table 1.6 lists the types of murmurs and their causes.

Table 1.6 Types of Heart Murmurs and Their Causes

Murmur	Cause
Physiologic	Anemia
	Athletic heart
	Fever
	Hypoproteinemia
	Hypertension
	Hyperthyroidism
	Pregnancy
Innocent	No known cause
Pathologic	Aortic regurgitation
	Aorticopulmonary septal defect
	Arteriovenous fistula
	Atrial septal defect
	Mitral dysplasia
	Mitral regurgitation
	Mitral stenosis
	Patent ductus arteriosus
	Pulmonic regurgitation
	Pulmonic stenosis
	Subaortic stenosis
	Tetralogy of Fallot
	Tricuspid dysplasia
	Tricuspid regurgitation
	Tricuspid stenosis
	Ventricular septal defect

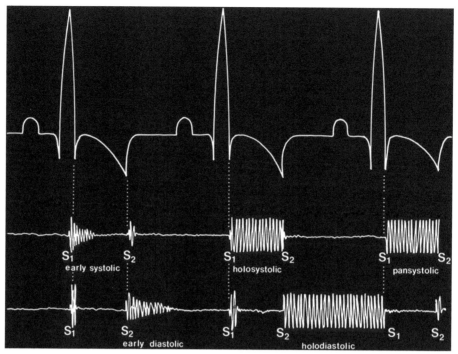

Figure 1.10   Timing and duration of murmurs. (From Gompf RE: The clinical approach to heart disease: history and physical examination. In Fox PR, ed: Canine and feline cardiology, New York, 1988, Churchill Livingstone.)

- Functional murmurs are divided into physiologic and innocent murmurs. Physiologic murmurs have a known cause, such as increased cardiac output or decreased blood viscosity and occur with anemia, hypoproteinemia, fever, increased blood pressure, pregnancy, hyperthyroidism, or an athletic heart. These are high-frequency murmurs that occur in the early to midsystolic phase, are loudest over the aortic and pulmonic areas, and rarely radiate to other areas.
- Innocent murmurs have no known cause and are not associated with any cardiac problem. These murmurs are soft systolic murmurs (no louder than grade 3) and usually occur in young animals. They can be located over any valve area but are most frequent over the mitral and aortic areas. Also, these murmurs should disappear by the time of the animal's last vaccinations (5 months of age).
- Pathologic murmurs are caused by underlying heart or vessel disease, such as stenosis of valves, outflow tract, or great vessels; valvular regurgitation; or abnormal intracardiac or extracardiac shunts. Refer to individual defects in the following chapters for a description of the murmurs associated with each defect.
- A murmur should be described with the following classification. First, the murmur should be identified as to its timing in the cardiac cycle (e.g., systolic, diastolic, continuous). Also, the duration of the murmur (e.g., early systolic, holosystolic, pansystolic) should be noted (Figures 1.10 and 1.11). Second, the site at which the murmur is loudest (PMI) (e.g., valve area) and where it radiates because of blood flow through the defect (e.g., other valve areas where it can be heard) should be noted. Third, the intensity or loudness of the murmur can be evaluated on the basis of the following scale: grade 1/6 can only be heard after listening for several minutes and sounds like a prolonged S_1; grade 2/6 is very soft but can be heard immediately; grade 3/6 is low to moderate in intensity; grade 4/6 is very loud, but a thrill cannot be palpated on the thorax; grade 5/6 is very loud, and a thrill can be palpated on the thorax; grade 6/6 can be heard without a stethoscope or with the stethoscope slightly off the thoracic wall. In general, the loudness of a murmur may not indicate the severity of the underlying problem. Fourth, the other areas where the murmur is heard should also be identified. These are the areas of radiation of the murmur and can help to identify the cause of the murmur. These four classifications should be used in the description of all murmurs.
- These additional descriptions can also aid in the diagnosis of the underlying problem. The quality or shape of the murmur is subjective but can be evaluated according to graphic appearance on phonocardiogram (see Figures 1.10 and 1.11).

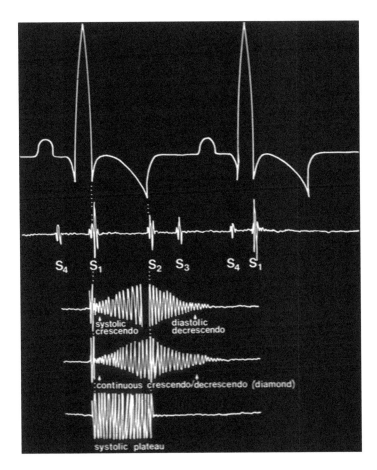

Figure 1.11 Timing and quality of murmurs. (From Gompf RE: The clinical approach to heart disease: history and physical examination. In Fox PR, ed: Canine and feline cardiology, New York, 1988, Churchill Livingstone.)

Regurgitant murmurs are plateau shaped (e.g., equal loudness throughout). Ejection murmurs are usually decrescendo, crescendo, or diamond shaped. Machinery or continuous murmurs are diamond shaped and peak at S2, continuing through all of systole and most of diastole. Blowing murmurs are decrescendo murmurs (e.g., decrease in intensity). The pitch or frequency of the murmur can also be described. Some murmurs are high, medium, or low pitched, or a mix. Also, they can be harsh, blowing, or musical.

OTHER SOUNDS AUSCULTATED IN THE THORAX

- Normal respiratory sounds include referred sounds from the trachea that are commonly heard over the lungs. Vesicular sounds are caused by air moving through the small bronchi and are louder on inspiration. Bronchial sounds are caused by air moving through the large bronchi and trachea and are heard best on expiration. Bronchovesicular sounds are the combination of these two sounds and are heard best over the hilar area.
- Abnormal respiratory sounds include attenuated sounds and increased, abnormal sounds.

- Attenuated bronchovesicular lung sounds are caused by thoracic masses, pleural effusion, pneumothorax, obesity, pneumonia, shallow breathing, or early consolidation of the pulmonary parenchyma.
- Rhonchi are caused by air passing through partially obstructed airways in the bronchial tubes or smallest airways. Rhonchi from the large bronchi are low pitched, sonorous, and almost continuous. They are heard best on inspiration. Rhonchi from the small bronchi are high pitched, sibilant, or squeaky and are heard best on expiration.
- Crackles are interrupted, crepitant, inspiratory sounds heard in many disease conditions and are not pathognomonic for pulmonary edema. They are caused by the opening of alveoli or airways that are collapsed or partially filled with fluid or bubbles bursting in the airways. They are further defined as fine or coarse in quality.
- Other sounds that can be auscultated include pleural friction rubs. Pleural friction rubs are grating, rubbing sounds heard during inspiration and expiration that are due to the moving of two relatively dry, roughened pleural surfaces against each other. Pericardial friction rubs are short, scratchy noises produced by

pericarditis and heart movement. Pericardial knocks are diastolic sounds that occur in animals with constrictive pericarditis. Wheezes are relatively high-pitched, musical sounds and are often a sign of pulmonary disease.

SUGGESTED READINGS

Bell JS, Cavanagh KE, Tilley LP, Smith FWK Jr: Veterinary medical guide to dog and cat breeds, Jackson, Wyoming, 2012, Teton New Media.

Ferasin L, Crews L, Biller DS, et al: Risk factors for coughing in dogs with naturally acquired myxomatous mitral valve disease, J Vet Intern Med 27:286, 2013.

Keene B, Smith FWK Jr, Tilley LP, Hansen BB: Rapid interpretation of heart sounds, murmurs, arrhythmias, and lung sounds: a guide to cardiac auscultation in dogs and cats, ed 3, Philadelphia, 2015, Elsevier.

Mazzone SB: An overview of the sensory receptors regulating cough, Cough 1:2, 2005.

Rishniw M, Ljungvall I, Porciello F, et al: Sleeping respiratory rates in apparently healthy adult dogs, Res Vet Sci 93:965, 2012.

Schober KE, Hart TM, Stern JA, et al: Detection of congestive heart failure in dogs by Doppler echocardiography, J Vet Intern Med 24:1358, 2010.

Radiology of the Heart 2

Brian A. Poteet

Thoracic radiography is a key component of the cardiovascular evaluation. Careful attention to proper positioning is of primary importance to the use of radiographic guidelines for interpretation. Radiographic interpretation relies heavily on possible disease considerations (i.e., differential diagnosis) derived from signalment, physical examination, and clinical pathology. Radiographic findings are not consistently specific enough to lead to the derivation of a definitive diagnosis without supportive clinical evidence. The radiographic study isolated from clinical information will not provide a diagnosis. The clinician must be aware of certain parameters and guidelines for interpretation to derive information from the radiographic image.

RADIOGRAPHIC TECHNIQUE

EXPOSURE TECHNIQUE AND FILM QUALITY

- Exposure technique will vary depending on equipment and film-screen combinations. The current standard for veterinary radiographic equipment is a 300 mA/125 to 75 kVp machine.
- The current standard for economic film-screen combination imaging systems is the rare earth systems. Because of the motion created by respiration, relatively high-speed (400) film-screen combinations that allow shorter exposure times are best suited for thoracic radiography.
- Use of a grid is imperative for adequate image quality when chest thickness exceeds 10 cm. Table 2.1 is a representative thoracic technique chart with a 400-speed imaging system and 300 mA/125 kVp radiographic equipment.

RADIOGRAPHIC PROJECTIONS

LATERAL PROJECTION

- There are subtle differences in cardiac conformation and position when the right lateral radiographic projection is compared with the left lateral radiographic projection. These differences are not significant enough to warrant further discussion except to note that the same projection

should be used on all serial radiographic examinations when repeated evaluation is required.
- Patient positioning and adequate radiographic exposure are critical to an accurate radiographic interpretation in the lateral projection.

Guidelines for proper exposure and positioning of a lateral thoracic radiograph (Figure 2.1) *include the following:*

- Radiographic exposure should be adequate to define the dorsal spinous process of the cranial thoracic vertebrae superimposed on the scapula.
- For assurance of a lateral projection, the dorsal heads of the ribs should be superimposed.
- The forelimbs should be pulled forward so that they are not superimposed over the cranial thorax or cranial margin of the heart.
- The radiographic exposure is taken during full inspiration, identified as an adequate lung field spacing between the caudal margin of the heart and the cupula of the diagram. Two primary disease considerations for consistent expiratory phase radiographs are the following:
  - Obesity and pickwickian syndrome, where the overabundance of abdominal fat prevents adequate inspiratory distraction of the diaphragm.
  - Upper airway disease, which most commonly causes obstruction during the inspiratory phase of respiration.

DORSOVENTRAL/VENTRODORSAL PROJECTION

- The dorsoventral (DV) radiographic projection is preferred over the ventrodorsal (VD) projection for cardiac evaluation for two reasons:
  1. The anatomic positioning of the heart in the DV projection is less dependent on

Table 2.1 Small Animal Thoracic Radiographic Technique Chart with a 400-Speed Film-Screen System and Standard Radiographic Equipment*

	mA	Time	mAs	Thickness (cm) kVp												
				Tabletop												
Thorax	100	1/60	1.7	3/48	4/50	5/52	6/54	7/56	8/58	9/60	10 cm/62					
				In the Table (Using Grid)												
Thorax	200	1/60	3.3	4/52	5/54	6/56	7/58	8/60	9/62	10/64	11/66	12/68	13/70	14/72	15/74	16 cm/76
	300	1/60	5	17/76	18/78	19/80	20/82	21/84	22/86	23/88	24/90	25/92	26/95	27/98		28 cm/101

*Single-phase fully rectified 300 mA/125 kVp generator focal-film distance = 38 in.
Technique rules of thumb: Change exposure—(1) 10% kVp; (2) two thirds of milliampere-second.

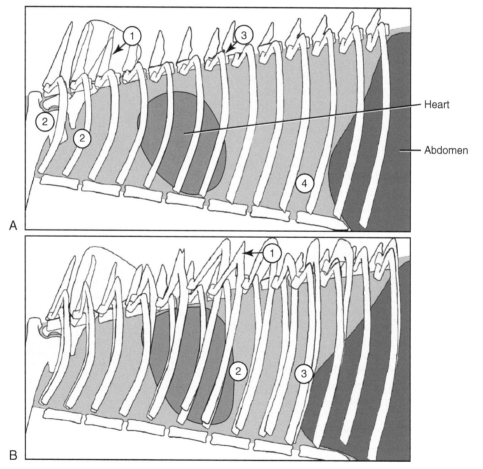

Figure 2.1 A, Guidelines for proper exposure and positioning of a lateral thoracic radiographic projection. (*1*) Exposure should allow delineation of the thoracic vertebral dorsal spinous process superimposed over the scapula. (*2*) The forelimbs should be pulled forward to provide a nonsuperimposed view of the cranial thorax. (*3*) The dorsal rib heads should be superimposed (compare with **B**). (*4*) The exposure should be performed during inspiration, which provides maximum separation between the caudal cardiac margin and diaphragmatic cupula. **B**, Improperly positioned lateral thoracic radiographic projection (compare with **A**). (*1*) Nonsuperimposed left and right rib heads. (*2*) The oblique projection markedly distorts cardiac silhouette conformation and intrathoracic position. (*3*) Expiratory phase radiographic exposure with poor lung volume between caudal cardiac margin and cupula of the diaphragm.

thoracic cavity conformation (deep-chested vs. barrel-chested breeds).

2. The dorsal lung fields are hyperinflated, and the vessels to the caudal lung fields are magnified because of increased object-film distance. This produces an improved radiographic definition of the large pulmonary arteries and veins of the caudal lung fields. The DV projection also allows increased detection of early pulmonary infiltrates (most commonly with cardiac disease in the hilar and caudodorsal lung fields). However, an improperly positioned DV/VD projection is worthless for cardiac radiographic interpretation.

KEY POINT

Although the DV projection is preferred, a straight (symmetric) projection is the ultimate goal, with patient compliance determining which projection (DV or VD) is attainable.

Guidelines for proper exposure and positioning for the DV/VD projections (Figure 2.2) *include the following:*

- Radiographic exposure should be sufficient to define the outline of the thoracic vertebrae superimposed over the cardiac silhouette.
- The kilovolt (peak) should be increased 10% from technique-chart values for obese patients. Examination of the thoracic body wall thickness on the VD view should assist in evaluation of obesity.
- The dorsal spinous processes of the thoracic vertebrae should be centered over the vertebral bodies along the full length of the thoracic spine. The thoracic sternal vertebrae also should be superimposed over the thoracic spine and should be essentially indistinguishable.
- The radiograph is taken during full inspiration and identified as an adequate lung field spacing between the caudal cardiac margin and cupula of the diaphragm.

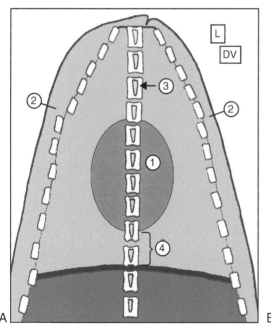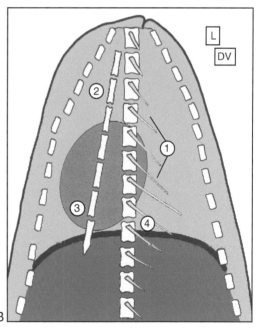

Figure 2.2 **A,** Guidelines for proper exposure and positioning of a dorsoventral (*DV*)/ventrodorsal thoracic radiographic projection. (*1*) The radiographic exposure should provide outline definition of thoracic vertebra superimposed over the cardiac silhouette. (*2*) Exposure should be increased (usually a 10% kVp increase with obesity as suggested by an increase in thoracic body wall thickness). (*3*) The thoracic vertebral dorsal spinous processes should be superimposed over the body portions for the entire length of the thoracic spine. (*4*) Adequate lung volume between the caudal cardiac margin and cupula indicates an inspiratory phase radiographic exposure. **B,** Improperly positioned DV radiographic projection. Thoracic vertebral dorsal spinous processes projected over the left hemithorax (*1*) and the sternal vertebra projected over the right hemithorax (*2*); these projections indicate an oblique thoracic dorsoventral radiographic projection. A lack of lung volume between caudal cardiac margin (*3*) and cupula (*4*) indicates an expiratory phase radiographic exposure. *L,* Lateral.

PROJECTION SELECTION IN CARDIAC-RELATED DISEASE

PULMONARY EDEMA

- The DV projection is preferred over the VD projection for radiographic detection of pulmonary edema. The DV view accentuates disease in the dorsal lung field, which is the most common location for the formation of early cardiogenic pulmonary edema. Adequate exposure is critical to ensure definition of caudal pulmonary vasculature superimposed over the cupula of the diaphragm.
- The radiographic detection of caudodorsal pulmonary vasculature is the best objective parameter for the detection of pulmonary edema. Vessels in healthy lungs are detected by their soft tissue opacity that contrasts with the normal radiolucent gas-filled lung parenchyma that surrounds them. As pulmonary parenchyma (interstitial spaces and alveoli) becomes filled with edema fluid, the normal radiographic soft tissue/gas contrast is lost; and delineation of the vessels diminishes. In other words, the vessels start to "disappear" from radiographic detection with the increased opacity of the surrounding edematous lung parenchyma (Figure 2.3).
- The phase of inspiration is critical when this method is used for interpretation in the DV/VD and the lateral projections. Pulmonary disease can be mimicked when underinflation decreases the parenchymal gas content per unit volume and thus reduces the radiographic contrast between lung parenchyma and associated vasculature. This phenomenon is especially common in older patients, who already have slightly increased pulmonary parenchymal radiographic opacity because of age-related pulmonary degenerative changes (interstitial fibrosis, bronchial mineralization, heterotopic pulmonary bone formation).

PLEURAL EFFUSION

- Pleural effusion is radiographically evident as focal areas of increased soft tissue opacity located within the thoracic cavity. It causes separation of lung lobes from both the thoracic wall and the adjacent lobes. This is seen on the lateral projection as an increase in the soft tissue thickness of the caudodorsal thoracophrenic angle and diaphragm and linear soft tissue opacities (pleural fissures) at anatomic locations comparable with interlobar fissures (Figure 2.4). Pleural effusion also contributes to loss of definition of the cranial and caudal margins of the heart, and this loss produces a radiographic positive-silhouette sign.
- In cases of pleural effusion, the VD projection is much preferred over the DV view for detection and delineation of cardiac size and shape. If intrathoracic fluid volumes are severe enough,

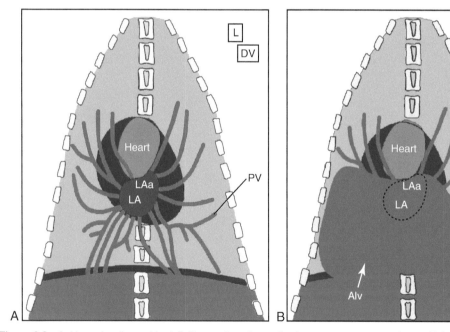

Figure 2.3 **A,** Normal radiographic definition and contrast of pulmonary venous vasculature (*PV*) with surrounding normal radiolucent lung parenchyma. **B,** Radiographic obliteration of PV by alveolar consolidation (*Alv*) of hilar and caudal lung lobes, a characteristic distribution for cardiogenic pulmonary edema. *DV,* Dorsoventral; *L,* lateral; *LA,* left atrium; *LAa,* left atrial auricular appendage.

the heart can effectively disappear on the DV view because of the relative distribution of the fluid and heart in the thoracic cavity. The positive-silhouette phenomenon is accentuated in the DV compared with the VD view (Figure 2.5). However, patient positioning for the DV projection puts less physiologic demand on the patient compromised by

pleural effusion and thus is favored over the VD projection. The patient's physiologic stability and degree of respiratory compromise should always be assessed before thoracic imaging.

- If significant amounts of pleural effusion are suspected, increasing radiographic exposure to abdominal technique-chart levels results

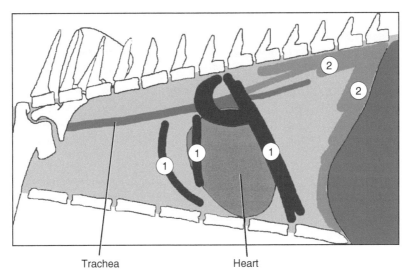

Trachea   Heart

Figure 2.4 Lateral thoracic radiographic projection of pleural effusion. Intrathoracic fluid accumulation causes separation of adjacent lung lobes by (1) linear interlobar opacities, radiographically defined as pleural fissures, and (2) separation of lung lobes from the thoracic wall.

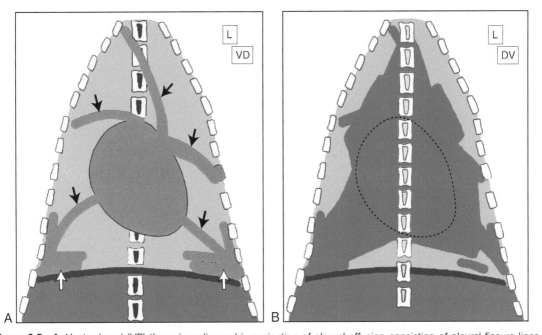

Figure 2.5 **A**, Ventrodorsal (VD) thoracic radiographic projection of pleural effusion consisting of pleural fissure lines (*closed arrows*) with blunting of the thoracophrenic angles (*open arrows*). Note that the cardiac silhouette is still well outlined. **B**, Dorsoventral (DV) thoracic radiographic projection of pleural effusion. The intrathoracic fluid distribution creates a "positive silhouette sign" where a complete loss of the cardiac silhouette has occurred. Thus the VD projection (**A**) is preferred for cardiac silhouette definition in the presence of pleural effusion. *L*, Lateral.

in better intrathoracic radiographic contrast. When possible, thoracocentesis and fluid drainage before radiography are always preferred.

RADIOGRAPHIC ANATOMY

LATERAL THORACIC RADIOGRAPHIC PROJECTION

CARDIAC PARAMETERS

- Even though the lateral radiographic projection defines the cranial-caudal and dorsal-ventral dimensions of the thorax, the anatomy of the heart of the dog and the cat as it resides in the thorax also allows this projection to detail the left and right aspects of the heart. The reason is that in the dog and the cat the heart is slightly rotated along its base-apex axis so that the right-sided cardiac chambers are positioned more cranially, and the left-sided cardiac chambers are positioned more caudally. Thus the cardiac silhouette, as it appears on the lateral projection, defines the right side of the heart along the cranial margin, and the left side is defined by its caudal margin (Figures 2.6 to 2.8).
- The canine and feline heart shape or radiographic silhouette is ovoid, with the apex more pointed in conformation than the broader base.

This base-apex difference in conformation is accentuated in the cat. The heart axis is defined by drawing a line from the tracheal bifurcation (carina) to the apex at an angle approximately 45 degrees to the sternal vertebrae. This angle can decrease in the cat with age and is often called a "lazy" heart. It has been postulated that this may be related to a loss of aortic connective tissue elasticity. This is most often seen in cats older than 7 years. Shallow, barrel-chested dog breeds (e.g., Dachshund, Lhasa Apso, Bulldog) tend to have more globular-shaped hearts, with increased sternal contact of the cranial margin of the heart. The heart chambers can be roughly defined by a line connecting the apex to the tracheal bifurcation and a second line perpendicular to the base-apex axis and positioned at the level of the ventral aspect of the caudal vena cava (see Figure 2.8).

- The dorsal cardiac margin includes both atria, pulmonary arteries and veins, the cranial and caudal vena cavae, and the aortic arch (see Figures 2.6 to 2.8). The cranial border is formed by both the right ventricle and the right atrial appendage, resulting in the radiographically defined "cranial waist" (see Figures 2.6 and 2.8). The caudal margin is formed by the left atrium and left ventricle, with the atrioventricular

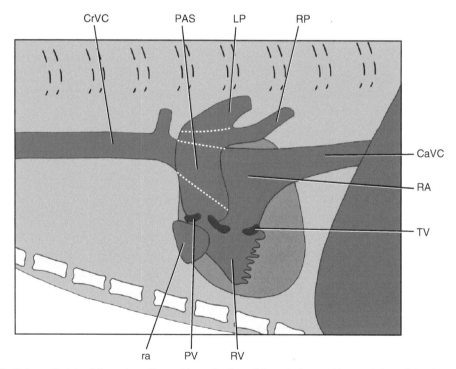

Figure 2.6 Schematic lateral thoracic radiographic projection of the relative position and size of the right-side structures of the heart. Note the more cranial position of the right chambers of the heart. *CaVC,* Caudal vena cava; *CrVC,* cranial vena cava; *LP,* left pulmonary artery; *PAS,* main pulmonary artery segment; *PV,* pulmonic valve; *ra,* right atrial auricular appendage; *RA,* right atrium; *RP,* right pulmonary artery; *RV,* right ventricle; *TV,* tricuspid valve.

junction defined as the radiographic "caudal waist."

- The base-to-apex cardiac dimension or length occupies approximately 70% of the DV distance of the thoracic cavity at its position within the thorax. For objective measurements, thoracic cavity distance between the thoracic spine and the sternum should be measured *at an axis perpendicular to the thoracic spine.*
- The cranial-caudal dimension or width, as it appears on the lateral projection, is measured at its maximum width (which is usually at the level of the ventral aspect of the insertion of the caudal vena cava) and perpendicular to the

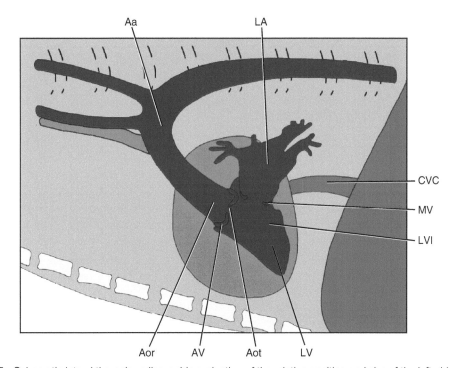

Figure 2.7 Schematic lateral thoracic radiographic projection of the relative position and size of the left-side structures of the heart. Note the more caudal position of the left chambers of the heart. *Aa,* Aortic arch; *Aor,* aorta; *AV,* aortic valve; *Aot,* aortic outflow tract; *CVC,* caudal vena cava; *LA,* left atrium; *LV,* left ventricle; *LVI,* left ventricular inflow tract; *MV,* mitral valve.

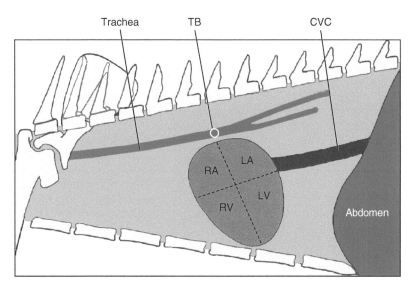

Figure 2.8 Schematic lateral thoracic radiographic projection outlining the approximate location of the four heart chambers. *CVC,* Caudal vena cava; *LA,* left atrium; *LV,* left ventricle; *RA,* right atrium; *RV,* right ventricle; *TB,* tracheal bifurcation.

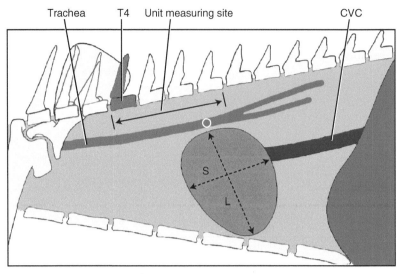

VHS = S + L
Measured in vertebral units beginning at T4

Figure 2.9 Schematic representation parameters for the vertebral scale system of cardiac size. The vertebral heart sum (*VHS*) is the sum of the long axis cardiac dimension (*L*) and the maximal perpendicular short axis dimension (*S*). S and L are measured in vertebral units beginning at T4. *CVC*, Caudal vena cava.

base-apex axis. This has been classically defined as between 2.5 (deep-chested conformation breeds [Setters, Afghans, Collies]) and 3.5 (barrel-chested conformation breeds [Dachshunds, Bulldogs]) intercostal spaces (ICSs) in the dog, and between 2.5 and 3.0 ICSs in the cat. The ICS measurement is made at an axis *perpendicular to the long axis of the ribs*. Thus the cardiac width distance determination may have to be shifted in axis angle before comparison with ICS length.

- A more objective determination of cardiac size has been formulated for the dog and uses a vertebral scale system in which cardiac dimensions are scaled against the length of specific thoracic vertebrae (Figure 2.9). In lateral radiographs the long axis of the heart (L) is measured with a caliper extending from the ventral aspect of the left main stem bronchus (tracheal bifurcation hilus, carina) to the left ventricular apex. The caliper is repositioned along the vertebral column beginning at the cranial edge of the fourth thoracic vertebra. The length of the heart is recorded as the number of vertebrae caudal to that point and estimated to the nearest tenth of a vertebra. The maximum perpendicular short axis (S) is measured in the same manner beginning at the fourth thoracic vertebra. If obvious left atrial enlargement is present, the short axis measurement is made at the ventral juncture of left atrial and caudal vena caval silhouettes.
- The lengths in vertebrae (v) of the long and short axes are then added to obtain a vertebral heart sum (VHS), which provides a single number

representing heart size proportionate to the size of the dog. The average VHS in the dog is 9.7 v (range, 8.5-10.5 v). Caution must be exercised in some breeds that have excessively disproportionate skeletal–body weight conformations. An example is the English Bulldog, which has relatively small thoracic vertebrae and commonly has hemivertebrae as well; thus a normal heart may be interpreted as large with the VHS method. Although the VHS concept is more precise, clinical judgment is still necessary to avoid overdiagnosing or underdiagnosing heart disease.

VESSEL PARAMETERS

- The main pulmonary artery (pulmonary trunk) cannot be seen on the lateral projection because of a positive-silhouette sign with the craniodorsal base of the heart. The left pulmonary artery can sometimes be seen extending dorsal and caudal to the tracheal bifurcation (carina). The right pulmonary artery is frequently seen end on as it leaves the main pulmonary artery immediately ventral to the carina (Figure 2.10). This end-on appearance may be confused with a mass lesion on normal radiographs and is accentuated in cases of pulmonary hypertension such as heartworm disease. The pulmonary veins are best identified as they enter the left atrium caudal to the heart base.
- With the use of the larger, more proximal segments of the mainstem bronchi as a reference, the pulmonary arteries are dorsal to the

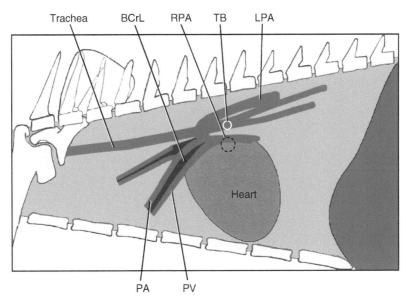

Figure 2.10 Pulmonary vascular anatomy in the lateral thoracic projection. Cranial lung lobe branch of the pulmonary artery (*PA*), cranial lung lobe branch of the pulmonary vein (*PV*), end-on view of the right main pulmonary artery (*RPA*) as it traverses the thorax from left to right, and left main pulmonary artery (*LPA*). *BCrL*, Bronchus to a cranial lung lobe; *TB*, tracheal bifurcation (carina).

bronchus, and the pulmonary veins are ventral to the bronchus (see Figure 2.10).

- The vessels to the cranial lung lobes are usually seen as two pairs of vessels, each with their respective bronchi. The more cranial pair of vessels generally corresponds to the side on which the lateral projection was made. Thus, in the right lateral projection, the right cranial lobar vessels are more cranial than vessels of the left cranial lung lobe. The pulmonary arteries and veins should be equal in size. The width of the vessels where they cross the fourth rib should not exceed the width of the narrowest portion of that rib at its juncture with the rib head (the dorsal aspect of the rib near the thoracic spine). The dorsal section of the rib is used as a reference to adjust for radiographic magnification because of thoracic conformation.

DORSOVENTRAL AND VENTRODORSAL PROJECTIONS

CARDIAC PARAMETERS

- The heart is rotated on its long axis so that the right chambers are oriented to the right and cranially, and the left chambers reside to the left and caudally. The degree of rotation is less in the cat. The cranial-caudal rotation is most significant when the location of the left and right atria is defined.
- The canine heart appears in radiographs as an elliptical opacity with its base-apex axis orientation approximately 30 degrees to the left of the

midline. The width of the heart across its widest point is usually 60% to 65% of the thoracic width at its location within the thorax. In the cat, the cardiac axis is most commonly on or close to midline, and its width does not usually exceed 50% of the width of the thoracic cavity during full inspiration. The cardiac silhouette may be artificially increased in the obese patient because of an excessive amount of pericardial fat. In these cases, the cardiac silhouette margin appears to be less well defined or blurred because the margin of contrast among soft tissue (heart), fat (pericardial), and air is not as distinct as that between soft tissue and air.

- Assessing the obesity of the patient with evaluation of the thickness of the abaxial thoracic wall and width of the mediastinum (as well as with examination of the patient) will assist in the determination of pericardial fat contribution to cardiac size. In deep, narrow-chested breeds, the heart stands more vertical in the thorax and thus produces a smaller and more circular cardiac silhouette conformation. The broad, barrel-chested breeds produce a radiographic silhouette that appears wider than that of standard breeds.
- The margins of the heart that create the cardiac silhouette contain a number of structures that often overlap. A clock face analogy can be used to simplify the location of these structures. The aortic arch extends from the 11 to 1 o'clock position (Figure 2.11). The main pulmonary artery is located from the 1 to 2 o'clock position, with its radiographic designation as

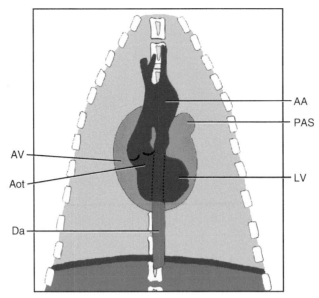

Figure 2.11   Schematic anatomy of the chambers and vasculature of the left ventricular outflow tract of the heart in the dorsoventral radiographic projection. *AA*, Aortic arch; *Aot*, aortic outflow tract; *AV*, aortic valve; *Da*, descending aorta; *LV*, left ventricle; *PAS*, pulmonary artery segment.

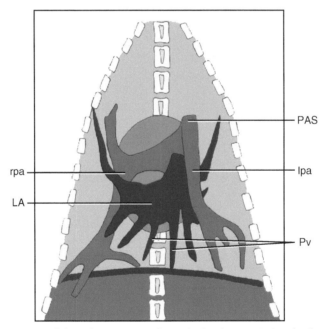

Figure 2.12   Schematic anatomy of the pulmonary vasculature in the dorsoventral projection. *LA*, Left atrium; *lpa*, left pulmonary artery; *PAS*, main pulmonary artery (radiographic description—pulmonary artery segment); *Pv*, pulmonary veins; *rpa*, right pulmonary artery.

the pulmonary artery segment (PAS) (Figures 2.12 and 2.13). In the cat, the body of the left atrium proper forms the 2 to 3 o'clock position of the cardiac silhouette. In the dog, the left atrium is superimposed over the caudal portion of the cardiac silhouette in the DV projection (see Figure 2.12). With severe cases of left atrial enlargement in the dog, the left auricular appendage contributes to the definition and enlargement of the cardiac silhouette at the 2 to 3 o'clock position (see Figure 2.13). The left ventricle forms the left heart margin from the 2 to 6 o'clock position (see Figure 2.11). The right ventricle is located from the 7 to 11 o'clock position (the right ventricle does not extend to the apex of the heart) (Figure 2.14). The right

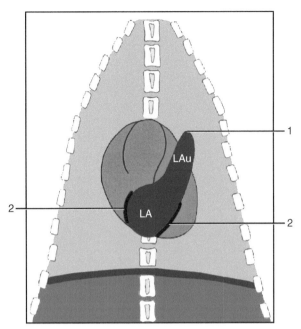

Figure 2.13 Dorsoventral thoracic radiographic projection of a dog with severe left atrial (*LA*) enlargement. The left atrial auricular appendage (*LAu*) contributes to the cardiac silhouette at the 2 to 3 o'clock position (*1*). The body of the left atrium superimposed over the caudal cardiac silhouette produces a radiolucent "mach" line, a radiographic edge effect caused by an acute change in soft tissue thickness (*2*).

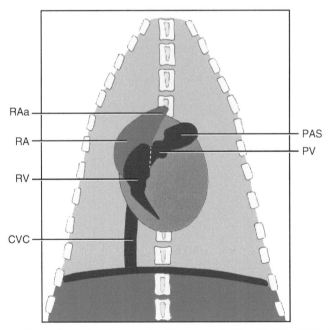

Figure 2.14 Schematic anatomy of the chambers and outflow tract of the right side of the heart in the dorsoventral radiographic projection. *CVC*, Caudal vena cava; *PAS*, main pulmonary artery segment; *PV*, pulmonic valve; *RA*, right atrium; *RAa*, right atrial auricular appendage; *RV*, right ventricle;

atrium is located at the 9 to 11 o'clock position (see Figure 2.14). Pericardial fat in the dog can asymmetrically contribute to cardiac silhouette enlargement at the 4 to 5 o'clock and 8 to 11 o'clock positions.

VESSEL PARAMETERS

- The pulmonary arteries originate from the main pulmonary artery or the PAS with the right branch coursing transversely, superimposed over the cranial portion of the heart silhouette, extending beyond the right heart margin at approximately the 8 o'clock position (see Figure 2.12). The left pulmonary artery branch courses caudally, superimposed over the caudal left ventricular portion of the heart, and extends beyond the left heart margin at approximately the 4 o'clock position. The pulmonary veins are best seen as they enter the left atrium along the caudal margin of the cardiac silhouette (see Figure 2.12). Compared with the pulmonary arteries, they are clustered in a more axial position. Thus the pulmonary arteries extend to both the cranial and caudal lung fields in a more abaxial position relative to the pulmonary veins.

- The aortic arch is within the cranial mediastinum at the cranial heart margin and is normally not visible. The descending aorta is superimposed over the heart and extends caudally, dorsally, and medially. The left lateral margin of the aorta can be seen to the left of the vertebral column on both DV and VD views (see Figure 2.11). The caudal vena cava courses cranially from the diaphragm to the right of midline and into the right caudal margin of the heart (see Figure 2.14). This is one of the most useful landmarks for determination of proper orientation of the DV radiograph on a viewbox.

RADIOGRAPHIC INTERPRETATION

A systematic evaluation of the entire thoracic cavity involves adherence to and inclusion of the following steps with each radiographic interpretation. Abnormalities supportive of disease should be substantiated on multiple radiographic views where applicable.

- Evaluate the radiographs for technical quality, positioning, and proper exposure. *If the study is substandard, then stop right here and repeat the radiographic study.*
- Determine the phase of respiration.
- Review the entire thoracic cavity: spine, sternum, diaphragm, thoracic wall, ribs, cranial and caudal mediastinum, conformation, and position of the diaphragm.
- Review the portion of the cranial abdomen included in the projection. Thoracic radiographic exposure is usually *half* of that required for abdominal imaging, but a cursory evaluation of abdominal contrast, detail, and hepatic size (with gastric axis) can be performed.
- Evaluate the position, course, and diameter of the trachea and mainstem bifurcations.
- Evaluate the position of the cardiac apex and caudal mediastinum.

- Evaluate the size, shape, and course of the main pulmonary artery, and peripheral pulmonary arteries and veins.
- Evaluate the lung fields for hyperinflation or underinflation and for distribution and pattern of increased or decreased opacity.
- Evaluate the cardiac margin (cranial, caudal, right, left "clock position" segmentation) for enlargement, abnormal position, or conformation.

NONCARDIAC-RELATED VARIABLES THAT CAN MIMIC RADIOGRAPHIC SIGNS OF CARDIAC DISEASE

CARDIAC POSITION

- Pulmonary disease (such as lung consolidation, atelectasis, or pleural disease) can cause a mediastinal shift and alter the position and axis of the heart in the thoracic cavity.
- Mediastinal mass lesions can affect the cardiac position and axis and obscure the cranial and cardiac margins when in contact with the heart by producing a radiographic positive-silhouette sign.
- Pneumothorax can produce disproportionate hemithoracic volume changes, altering cardiac position and axis. Pneumothorax commonly produces elevation of the cardiac apex from the sternum. This is supported by other radiographic signs of pneumothorax:
  - Premature termination of lung vasculature into the periphery of the thoracic cavity
  - Lung lobe margin detection as it contrasts with nonparenchymal free intrathoracic gas
- Sternal conformational abnormalities due to congenital defects or previous trauma can alter cardiac position and axis.

CARDIAC SIZE AND LATERAL PROJECTION

- Younger animals appear to have larger hearts relative to their thoracic size than do mature patients.
- The heart appears smaller on inspiration than on expiration. During expiration, increased sternal contact of the right-sided heart margin and dorsal elevation of the trachea occurs, falsely suggesting right-sided heart enlargement.
- Anemic or emaciated patients often have small hearts because of hypovolemia and are hyperinflated to compensate for hypoxemia. In deep-chested conformation breeds, the cardiac apex can be elevated far enough from the sternum to mimic pneumothorax.

CARDIAC POSITION AND DORSOVENTRAL/ VENTRODORSAL PROJECTION

- Malposition of the heart to the right is a normal variant in the cat.

- Uneven lung inflation secondary to disease or previous lobectomy can produce a mediastinal shift and resultant apex shift.
- If radiographs are taken on diseased, recumbent patients or patients during or immediately after the administration of general anesthesia, then hypostatic congestion and atelectasis of the dependent lung fields can produce a mediastinal shift, altering cardiac position.
- Pectus excavatum or "funnel chest" sternal conformation is a result of congenital deformities.

EVALUATION OF HEART CHAMBER ENLARGEMENT

RIGHT ATRIAL ENLARGEMENT

RADIOGRAPHIC SIGNS

- Lateral projection (Figure 2.15):
  - Elevation of the trachea as it courses dorsally over the right atrium.
  - Accentuation of the cranial waist. Preferential enlargement of the more dorsal margin of the cranial margin of the cardiac silhouette defines selective enlargement of the right atrial auricular appendage.
  - Increased soft tissue opacity of the cranial aspect of the cardiac silhouette due to increased soft tissue thickness of the right atrium superimposed over the right ventricle.
- DV projection (Figure 2.16):
  - Enlargement of the cardiac margin at the 9 to 11 o'clock position.

- Enlargement can be dramatic in severe cases (especially in the cat) and can be easily mistaken for a pulmonary hilar mass lesion.

CAUSES OF RIGHT ATRIAL ENLARGEMENT

- Right-sided heart failure
- Tricuspid insufficiency
- Cardiomyopathy
- Right atrial neoplasia (e.g., hemangiosarcoma)

DIFFERENTIAL DIAGNOSIS

- Cranial mediastinal mass
- Heart base neoplasia (most common in brachycephalic breeds)
- Tracheobronchial lymphadenopathy
- Superimposition of the aortic arch or main pulmonary artery
- Right cranial or middle lobar pulmonary alveolar consolidation or mass lesion

RIGHT VENTRICULAR ENLARGEMENT

RADIOGRAPHIC SIGNS

- Lateral projection (see Figure 2.15)
  - Increased sternal contact of cranial cardiac margin
  - Elevation of the cardiac apex from the sternum
  - Rounding of the conformation of the entire cardiac silhouette; increased cardiac width

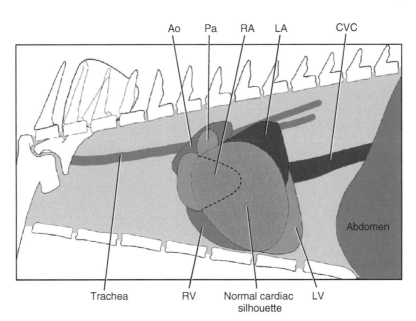

Figure 2.15 Cardiac silhouette changes associated with vessel and chamber enlargement in the lateral thoracic radiographic projection. *Ao*, Aortic arch; *CVC*, caudal vena cava; *LA*, left atrium; *LV*, left ventricle; *Pa*, main pulmonary artery; *RA*, right atrium; *RV*, right ventricle. *Dotted line*, area of right atrial superimposition over the right ventricle.

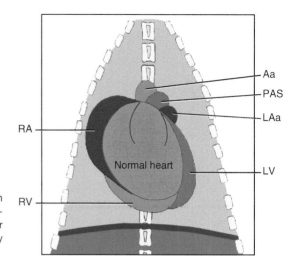

Figure 2.16 Cardiac silhouette changes associated with vessel and chamber enlargement in the dorsoventral radiographic projection. *Aa,* Aortic arch; *LAa,* left atrial auricular appendage; *LV,* left ventricle; *PAS,* main pulmonary artery segment; *RA,* right atrium; *RV,* right ventricle.

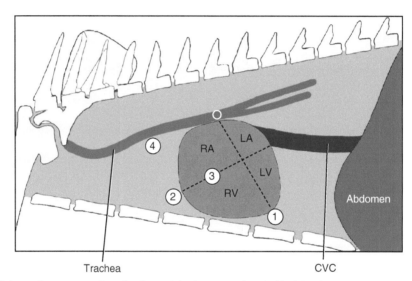

Figure 2.17 Schematic representation of radiographic signs associated with right-sided heart enlargement in the lateral projection. (*1*) Dorsal lifting of apex from sternum. (*2*) Increased sternal contact of cranial cardiac margin. (*3*) Disproportionate enlargement of the cranial portion of the cardiac silhouette when empirically divided into its right and left chambers. (*4*) Elevation of the trachea as it courses dorsally over the right atrium. *CVC,* Caudal vena cava; *LA,* left atrium; *LV,* left ventricle; *RA,* right atrium; *RV,* right ventricle.

- Disproportionate enlargement of the cranial portion of the cardiac silhouette when empirically divided into its right and left chambers (Figure 2.17)
- Dorsal elevation of the caudal vena cava
- DV projection (see Figure 2.16)
  - Cardiac silhouette enlargement at the 6 to 11 o'clock position
  - Given the enlargement and rounded conformation of the right margin, the left margin in comparison assumes a more straightened conformation; an overall "reverse-D" conformational appearance of the cardiac silhouette results
  - Shift of cardiac apex to the left

CAUSES OF RIGHT VENTRICULAR ENLARGEMENT

- Secondary to left-sided heart failure
- Tricuspid insufficiency
- Cardiomyopathy

Trachea

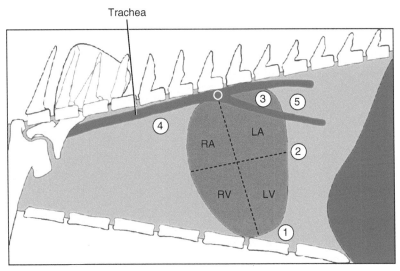

Figure 2.18 Schematic representation of radiographic signs associated with left-sided heart enlargement in the lateral projection. (*1*) Rounding and widening of the cardiac apex conformation. (*2*) Straightening and increased vertical axis of the caudal cardiac margin. (*3*) Left atrial enlargement with characteristic right-angular caudodorsal margin conformation. (*4*) Dorsal elevation of the intrathoracic portion of the trachea, carina, and mainstem bronchi. The angle between the thoracic spine axis and the trachea is diminished to the point of becoming parallel. (*5*) Separation of normally superimposed caudal mainstem bronchi. Left side is more dorsal in position than the right side. *LA*, Left atrium; *LV*, left ventricle; *RA*, right atrium; *RV*, right ventricle.

- Cor pulmonale
- Dirofilariasis
- Congenital heart disease: pulmonic stenosis, patent ductus arteriosus (PDA), ventricular septal defects, tetralogy of Fallot, tricuspid valve dysplasia

LEFT ATRIAL ENLARGEMENT

RADIOGRAPHIC SIGNS

- Lateral projection (see Figure 2.15)
  - Dorsal elevation of the caudal portion of the trachea and carina
  - Disproportionate dorsal elevation of the mainstem bronchi (the two will no longer be superimposed; the left bronchus will appear more dorsal than the right bronchus)
  - Enlargement and straightening of the caudodorsal portion of the cardiac silhouette with almost a right-angle margin conformation (Figure 2.18); straightening of the caudal margin of the heart and loss of the caudal waist (determined by the atrioventricular junction)
- DV projection (see Figure 2.16)
  - The dog
    - Enlargement of the atrial auricular appendage, which now produces a noticeable focal "bulge" enlargement at the 2 to 3 o'clock position (see Figures 2.13 and 2.16)
    - A double opacity of the atrial body over the caudal aspect of the cardiac silhouette; the

body of the left atrium superimposed over the caudal cardiac silhouette produces a radiolucent "Mach" line, a radiographic edge effect caused by an acute change in soft tissue thickness (see Figure 2.13)
  - The cat
    - Enlargement of the cardiac margin at the 2 to 3 o'clock position of the silhouette

CAUSES OF LEFT ATRIAL ENLARGEMENT

- Mitral insufficiency
- Cardiomyopathy
- Congenital heart disease; mitral valve dysplasia, PDA, ventricular septal defects, atrial septal defects
- Left ventricular failure

DIFFERENTIAL DIAGNOSIS

- Hilar lymphadenopathy
- Pulmonary mass adjacent to hilus

LEFT VENTRICULAR ENLARGEMENT

RADIOGRAPHIC SIGNS

- Lateral projection (see Figure 2.15)
  - Loss of the caudal waist
  - Caudal cardiac margin straighter and more vertical than normal
  - Dorsal elevation of the intrathoracic portion of the trachea, carina, and mainstem bronchi;

the angle between the thoracic spine axis and trachea is diminished to the point of becoming parallel
- Disproportionate enlargement of the caudal portion of the cardiac silhouette when empirically divided into its right and left cardiac chambers (see Figure 2.18)
- DV projection (see Figure 2.16)
  - Rounding and enlargement of the left ventricular margin
  - Rounding and broadening of the cardiac apex conformation
  - Shift of the cardiac apex to the right

CAUSES OF LEFT VENTRICULAR ENLARGEMENT

- Mitral insufficiency
- Cardiomyopathy
- Congenital heart disease: PDA, aortic stenosis, ventricular septal defects
- High-output cardiac disease: fluid overload, chronic anemia, peripheral arteriovenous fistula, obesity, chronic renal disease, hyperthyroidism

ENLARGEMENT OF THE AORTIC ARCH AND AORTA
RADIOGRAPHIC SIGNS

- Lateral projection (see Figure 2.15)
  - Widening of the dorsal aspect of the cardiac silhouette
  - Enlargement of the craniodorsal cardiac margin
- DV projection (see Figure 2.16)
  - Widening and increased cranial extensions of the cardiac margin between the 11 and 1 o'clock positions

CAUSES OF AORTIC ARCH ENLARGEMENT

- PDA; enlargement more abaxial (1 o'clock position)
- Aortic stenosis with poststenotic enlargement of the aortic arch; enlargement more axial and cranial (11 o'clock position)
- Aortic aneurysm (very rare)

DIFFERENTIAL DIAGNOSIS

- Normal variation in some dogs
- Very common variant in older cats with "lazy" heart conformation; very prominent on the DV projection
- Cranial mediastinal mass
- Thymus or the "sail-sign" in young dogs
- Cranial mediastinal fat in obese brachycephalic dogs

ENLARGEMENT OF THE PULMONARY ARTERY
RADIOGRAPHIC SIGNS

- Lateral projection (see Figure 2.15)
  - Protrusion of the craniodorsal heart border
- DV projection (Figure 2.16)
  - Lateral bulge of the cardiac margin at the 1 to 2 o'clock position
  - Radiographically defined as PAS

CAUSES OF PULMONARY ARTERY SEGMENT ENLARGEMENT

- Dirofilariasis
- Pulmonary thrombosis and thromboembolism
- Cor pulmonale
- Congenital disease: pulmonic stenosis, PDA, septal defects both ventricular and atrial, with left-to-right shunting

DIFFERENTIAL DIAGNOSIS

- Previous dirofilariasis infection and treatment
- Rotational (oblique) positional artifact (usually on VD projection) most commonly experienced with deep-chested conformation dogs

EVALUATION OF THE PULMONARY CIRCULATION
UNDERCIRCULATION
RADIOGRAPHIC SIGNS

- Lung field more radiolucent than normal because of lack of pulmonary vascular volume
- Hyperinflation caused by hypoxemia or ventilation/perfusion mismatch
- Pulmonary arteries smaller than normal; may be smaller in size when compared with corresponding pulmonary veins

CAUSES OF PULMONARY UNDERCIRCULATION

- Congenital disease: pulmonic stenosis, tetralogy of Fallot, reverse PDA (right-to-left shunting)

DIFFERENTIAL DIAGNOSIS

- Emphysema, chronic obstructive pulmonary disease
- Hyperinflation
- Pneumothorax
- Overexposure
- Pulmonary thromboembolism
- Hypovolemia, shock (the heart will also be smaller than normal)
- Hypoadrenocorticism (Addison's disease); the heart may also be smaller than normal

OVERCIRCULATION

RADIOGRAPHIC SIGNS

- Both the pulmonary arteries and the veins are enlarged
- Arteries are frequently larger than the veins
- Pulmonary thoracic opacity is increased because of larger vascular volume

CAUSES OF PULMONARY OVERCIRCULATION

- Dirofilariasis (arteries are larger than corresponding veins)
- PDA: both arteries and veins enlarged
- Left-to-right shunts (ventricular and atrial septal defects): both arteries and veins enlarged
- Congestive heart failure: veins may be larger than arteries if mainly left sided; both arteries and veins enlarged with concurrent left- and right-sided failure
- Fluid overload

DIFFERENTIAL DIAGNOSIS

- Underexposure
- Expiratory phase of respiration

RADIOGRAPHIC DIAGNOSIS OF HEART FAILURE

The radiographic diagnosis of heart failure is dependent on recognition of imbalances in the blood and fluid distribution within the body. This circulatory imbalance is the result of diminished cardiac output into the pulmonary or systemic vascular systems, or reduced acceptance of blood by the failing ventricle (hypertrophy), or both. Depending on which side of the heart is most severely affected, blood is shifted from the systemic to the pulmonary circulation (left-sided heart failure) or from the pulmonary to the systemic circulation (right-sided heart failure).

RIGHT-SIDED HEART FAILURE

PHYSIOLOGIC PHENOMENON

- In right-sided heart failure, an inadequate right ventricular output into the pulmonary arteries exists concurrently with a reduced acceptance of blood from the systemic veins. The blood volume and pressure in the splanchnic and systemic veins are elevated. The venous congestion causes hepatomegaly.
- With further progression of right-sided heart failure, a progression of systemic hypertension leads to increased amounts of fluid, solutes, and protein escaping from the capillary beds of the major organs. The lymphatic circulation

is overtaxed, and fluid exudes into the serosal cavities, producing ascites, pleural, and even pericardial effusions.
- The extracardiac radiographic signs of progressively worsening right-sided heart failure are hepatomegaly see, ascites, and then pleural effusion.

RADIOGRAPHIC SIGNS

- Right-sided cardiomegaly (see Figures 2.15 through 2.17). Patients with concentric cardiac hypertrophy (e.g., pulmonic stenosis), thin-walled cardiomyopathy, or acute arrhythmias often may not have dramatic radiographic cardiomegaly. Thus subtle cardiac silhouette changes in both the DV and the lateral projections must be considered significant with supportive clinical evidence of cardiac disease.
- Hepatomegaly: rounded liver margin, which extends caudal to last rib; displacement of stomach caudally and to the left.
- Ascites: abdominal distention; diffuse loss of intraabdominal detail.
- Pleural effusion.
- Generalized increase in thoracic opacity.
- Visualization of interlobar pleural fissures (see Figures 2.4 and 2.5, A).
- Obliteration of cardiac silhouette definition (best demonstrated on the DV projection) (see Figure 2.5, B).
- Separation of pulmonary visceral pleural margin away from thoracic wall (see Figures 2.4 and 2.5).

CAUSES OF PLEURAL EFFUSION SECONDARY TO RIGHT-SIDED HEART FAILURE

- Decompensated mitral and tricuspid insufficiency
- Decompensated pulmonic stenosis, tetralogy of Fallot
- Dirofilariasis (caval syndrome)
- Pericardial effusion with tamponade
- Restrictive pericarditis

DIFFERENTIAL DIAGNOSIS

- Pleuritis
- Chylothorax
- Hemothorax
- Pyothorax
- Hypoproteinemia
- Neoplasia (pleural, mediastinal, cardiac, pulmonary, primary, or metastatic)

LEFT-SIDED HEART FAILURE

PHYSIOLOGIC PHENOMENON

- In left-sided heart failure, inadequate left ventricular output into the aorta occurs, and a diminished acceptance of blood from the pulmonary veins entering the left atrium results. This causes pulmonary venous congestion and leakage of fluid into the pulmonary interstitium, with progression to flooding of the alveoli.

- Clinically, this evolves as a progression of physiologic events: pulmonary venous congestion, interstitial pulmonary edema, alveolar edema, and lung consolidation.

RADIOGRAPHIC SIGNS

- Left-sided cardiomegaly (see Figure 2.18). Patients with concentric cardiac hypertrophy (e.g., aortic stenosis), thin-walled cardiomyopathy (large- and giant-breed dogs), or acute arrhythmias often may not have dramatic radiographic cardiomegaly. Thus subtle cardiac silhouette changes in both the DV and lateral projections and noncardiac changes (e.g., pulmonary vascular changes, pulmonary edema) must be evaluated.
- Pulmonary venous congestion
  - Engorgement and distention of the pulmonary veins, especially in the hilar area as they enter the left atrium. On the DV view these are identified as the more axial of the caudal vasculature (see Figure 2.12).
  - The diameter of the pulmonary veins is greater than that of their corresponding pulmonary arteries (best seen on the lateral projection with cranial lobar vessels) (see Figure 2.10).
  - The radiopacity of the lung parenchyma distal and peripheral to the hilus is unchanged.
- Interstitial edema
  - Diffuse increased radiopacity of the lung fields owing to a hazy interstitial opacity is apparent.
  - The margins of the pulmonary veins and arteries are indistinct owing to perivascular edema. As the lung parenchyma surrounding the pulmonary vasculature fills with fluid, the normal pulmonary radiographic contrast between gas (air-filled lung) and soft tissue (blood-filled vessels) is lost. Thus, the pulmonary vasculature becomes indistinct and begins to disappear in the surrounding fluid-filled lung parenchyma.
  - In some patients, fluid accumulates around major bronchi, producing prominent peribronchial markings.
- Alveolar edema
  - Radiographic signs
    - Fluid enters the alveolar air spaces and peripheral bronchioles, causing a coalescent fluffy alveolar infiltrate. Air bronchograms (black tubes in a white radiopaque background) and air alveolograms (lung parenchyma with the radiopacity of *liver* containing no vascular markings) are present. In the cat, cardiogenic alveolar consolidations can appear as a well margined, "cloudlike" conformation area of increased pulmonary radiopacity.
    - The margins of the pulmonary vessels are usually completely obscured (see Figure 2.3, *B*). The alveolar infiltrate is of greatest opacity in the perihilar area, fading peripherally. In the dog, alveolar edema can be asymmetrical, with the right lung fields more severely affected than the left (best seen on the DV projection).
  - Differential diagnosis for pulmonary edema
    - Neurogenic: electrocution, head trauma, postseizure, encephalitis, brain neoplasm
    - Hyperdynamic (excessive negative intrathoracic pressures): choking, strangulation, upper airway obstructions
    - Fluid overload: overhydration
    - Toxicity
    - Systemic shock
    - Hypersensitization
    - Drowning
- Increased bronchial markings in some cases
- Pleural effusion
  - In the dog, this can occur only in progressive or severe forms of left-sided heart failure; this usually indicates early concurrent left- and right-sided heart failure.
  - In the cat, pleural effusion is common with only left-sided heart failure; this can be separated from right-sided heart failure by the absence of accompanying hepatomegaly and ascites.

RADIOGRAPHIC DIAGNOSIS OF PERICARDIAL EFFUSION

- Generalized enlargement of cardiac silhouette in a "basketball" conformation, with elimination of all normal cardiac margin contours on all views
- Increased sternal contact of the cranial margin and convex bulging of the caudal margin without the angular conformation and straightening characteristic for left atrial and ventricular enlargements (Figure 2.19)
- Elevation and enlargement of the caudal vena cava
- Dorsal elevation of the trachea (similar to left-side enlargement)
- Hepatomegaly, ascites, and pleural effusion secondary to cardiac tamponade (see Figures 2.4 and 2.5)

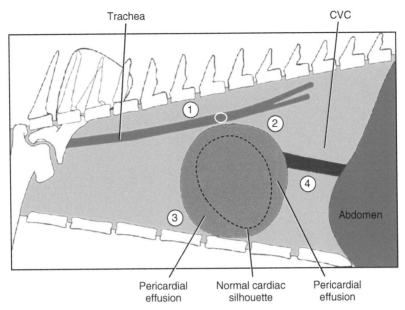

Figure 2.19 Schematic representation of radiographic signs associated with pericardial effusion. (*1*) Dorsal elevation of the intrathoracic portion of the trachea, carina, and mainstem bronchi. The angle between the thoracic spine axis and the trachea is diminished to the point of becoming parallel. (*2*) Convex enlargement of the caudodorsal cardiac margin without a "right-angle" conformation characteristic for left atrial enlargement. (3) Increased sternal contact of cranial margin. (*4*) Dorsal elevation and enlargement of the caudal vena cava (*CVC*). The cardiac silhouette takes on a smoothly contoured circular conformation with obliteration of normal cardiac contour.

SUMMARY OF RADIOGRAPHIC SIGNS

The clinician must be armed with both potential radiographic parameters and a clinically derived differential diagnostic list for cardiac disease before the radiographic image can begin to provide useful information. Table 2.2 summarizes the radiographic signs associated with congenital and acquired heart diseases. Awareness of noncardiac and artifactual conditions that can present with the same radiographic signs is also paramount to a correct diagnosis.

INTRODUCTION TO DIGITAL RADIOGRAPHY

Digital radiography (DR) is a relatively new technology that is becoming commonplace in veterinary medicine. It has been used in human medicine for more than 20 years, and has been thoroughly tested and proven. There are many advantages to DR beyond the excellent image quality (Figure 2.20), which include the following:

- No lost films
- No film degradation over time
- The ability to view images on any networked computer at a clinic or at home
- The ability to easily send images to specialists for consultation

- There are several types of digital acquisition systems, including flat panel radiology, computed radiography (CR), and charge-coupled device (CCD) systems.
- Other devices such as film scanners and digital cameras can be used to digitize conventional x-ray film, which allows the image to be stored on a computer. Once the image is acquired and stored, it can be manipulated by the user to taste.
- There are financial savings over time, including the following:
  - No cost for radiology disposables (film, chemicals).
  - No expense for processor maintenance, film jackets, and storage space.
  - Perhaps the most significant means of recouping revenue pertains to the fact that there will be a significant reduction in the number of retakes because there should be little to no need to retake images caused by underexposure or overexposure.
- Flat panel technology (also known as digital radiography [DR] or direct digital radiography [DDR] [Figure 2.21]) is the most expensive form of DR; however, this technology results in the highest quality image. These systems consist of a DR plate that is physically mounted in the area of the Bucky tray under the x-ray tabletop. The plate is then electronically interfaced to both

Table 2.2   Summary of Radiographic Signs of Congenital and Acquired Cardiac Disease

Lesion	RA	RV	LA	LV	Aorta	MPAs	PAb	PV	CVC	Failure/Side	Failure/Type
Congenital Defects											
Patent ductus arteriosus	N	In	In	In	In	In	In	In	N/In	Left	Volume
Pulmonic stenosis	In	In	N/De	N/De	N	In	N/De	N/De	In	Right	Pressure
Aortic stenosis	N	N/In	N/In	In	In	N	N	N/In	N	Left	Pressure
Ventricular septal defect	N	In	In	In	N	N/In	In	In	N/In	Left	Volume
Tetralogy of Fallot	N/In	In	N/De	N/De	N	De/N/In	De	De	N	Right	Pressure
Atrial septal defect	In	In	N/In	N	N	N/In	N/In	N/In	N/In	Left	Volume
Acquired Heart Disease											
Mitral insufficiency	N	N/In	In	In	N	N	N	In	N	Left	Fluid
Tricuspid insufficiency	In	In	N	N	N	N	N	N	In	Right	Fluid
Aortic insufficiency	N	N	In	In	N/In	N	N	In	N	Left	Fluid
Hypertrophic cardiomyopathy	In	In	In	In	N	N	N/In	N/In	N/In	Left > Right	Myocardial
Dilated cardiomyopathy	In	In	In	In	N	N	N/In	N/In	N/In	Right > Left	Myocardial
Pericardial	In	In	In	In	N	N	N/De	N/De	In	Right	Tamponade

CVC, Caudal vena cava; De, smaller or decreased; In, enlarged or increased; LA, left atrium; LV, left ventricle; MPAs, main pulmonary artery segment; N, normal; PAb, pulmonary artery branches; PV, pulmonary vein; RA, right atrium; RV, right ventricle.

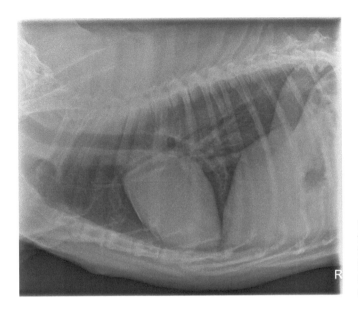

Figure 2.20 Right lateral view of the thorax taken with a flat panel detector system (digital radiography [DR]). Note that all structures (e.g., bone, lung, pulmonary vessels, spine) are visible in the same image. There are no areas of overexposure or underexposure.

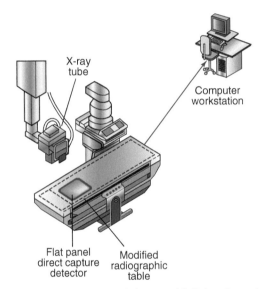

Figure 2.21 A flat panel detector (digital radiography [DR] plate) is mounted out of sight under the x-ray tabletop in the location the Bucky tray. The plate converts x-ray photon energy to an electrical pulse, which is then interfaced with an acquisition station computer. (From Fauber TL: Radiographic imaging & exposure, ed 4, St. Louis, 2013, Mosby.)

the x-ray machine and a dedicated computer (acquisition station). DR systems are extremely forgiving as far as technique (kilovolt [peak] and milliampere settings) is concerned (Figure 2.22). This in turn simplifies a typical technique chart to essentially three or four settings (small, medium, large, and extra large) whether you are imaging bone, thorax, or abdomen. Another advantage of DR systems includes extremely quick image time (3 to 8 seconds before the

image is seen on a computer monitor), which allows the user to either save or delete the image immediately if it is not satisfactory (e.g., rotated, crooked).

- CR systems use imaging plates that resemble traditional x-ray cassettes. The major difference is that the intensifying screen and film within the cassette is replaced by a flexible phosphor plate that has the ability to store a latent image. These storage phosphor plates operate similarly to the screen inside a conventional cassette in that they emit light (scintillate) in response to incident x-ray energy. However, unlike an x-ray screen, a storage phosphor plate retains a portion of the energy as a latent image, which is extracted ("read out") by a CR reader. In general, the image quality from a CR system is very high (similar to that of DR); however, CR is typically less forgiving as to technique (compared with DR), which necessitates a more complicated technique chart. The image time for most CR systems ranges from about 55 to 90 seconds. However, CR systems are less expensive than DR systems.
- CCD systems consist of a phosphor storage plate mounted under the x-ray tabletop that is in turn interfaced with a small light-sensitive chip (CCD chip) similar to that found in digital cameras and video cameras. These CCD chips are commonly about 2 cm in size and may have thousands of individual light-sensitive elements on them. Because of the small size of the chips, the aerial image (e.g., 14 × 17) must be minified down to the size of the CCD chip. This is usually accomplished with a series of mirrors and lenses, which unfortunately results in a significant loss (90%) of the photon data. This loss of data can often make the resultant image appear

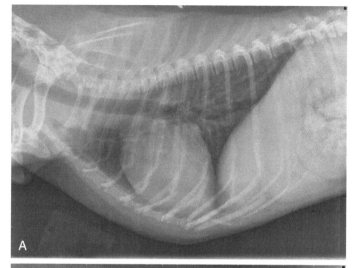

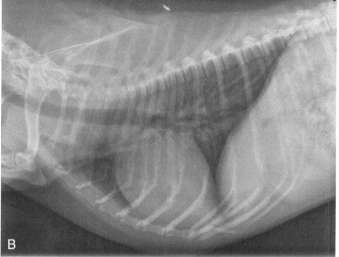

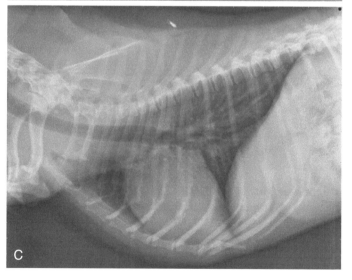

Figure 2.22 Technique independence. These three exposures were made with different milliampere-second (mAs) settings and identical kilovolt potential (KvP) of 90. **A**, 1.8 mAs. **B**, 2.5 mAs. **C**, 5.0 mAs. Note that all three exposures appear similar and are diagnostic. The computer software corrects for underexposure or overexposure automatically. This capability decreases the number of retakes and increases productivity. On the other hand, if image **A** is magnified, it will appear much grainier than the other images.

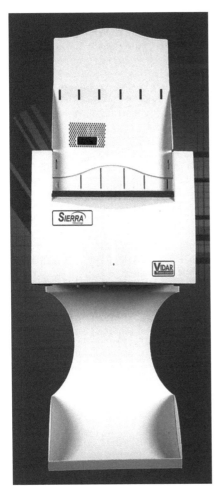

Figure 2.23 Dedicated x-ray film scanner (SIERRA Advantage film digitizer). X-ray film is fed into the machine, and it is converted to a digital image that can be stored on a computer. (Courtesy VIDAR Systems Corp., Herndon, Va.)

- Digital radiography (DR) is extremely fast, is technique independent, has the highest image quality, but is the most expensive method.
- Computed radiography (CR) is slower, is somewhere between conventional film-screen technology and DR as to reliance on x-ray technique, has high image quality, and is moderately expensive.
- Charged-coupled device (CCD) systems are fast, are similar to CR systems as to technical factors, have the poorest image quality, and are the least expensive.
- Film scanners and digital cameras are not forms of DR and have a limited role.

INTRODUCTION TO TELERADIOLOGY

- Teleradiology (telemedicine) offers the practitioner quick access to board-certified specialists for case consultation. Once the radiographic images are in a digital format, they can be sent to any specialist for review via the Internet. There are several methods of accomplishing this, including using dedicated teleradiology companies, e-mailing images directly to specialists, or by using DICOM (digital imaging and communication in medicine).
- At this time, there are four or five companies in the United States that cater to veterinary telemedicine. In general, these companies provide the necessary software that allows the veterinarian to upload digital images to the company's server, and they in turn send those images to affiliated specialists, such as radiologists and internists. The referring practice pays a fee to the teleradiology company, which in turn pays the specialists to read their images. The disadvantage of this type of service is that referring veterinarians often pay a premium fee (more than they would pay if they could send the images directly to the specialist), they may have little or no input on exactly which specialist their images are sent to, and they may have little ability to directly communicate with that specialist.
- Submission of images through standard e-mail can be simple, but it is not recommended. Because of the very large image size of digital radiographs (a 14 × 17 radiograph of the thorax can be 14 megabytes of information), these images must be compressed or saved in a "lossy" format (such as JPG) before they are e-mailed, thus making the transmitted image of poor quality. Also, in my experience, these images are often submitted with a lack of necessary patient information and history.
- DICOM is a proven and worldwide recognized method of transmitting high-quality, lossless,

"grainy" or pixelated on the computer monitor, which is accentuated if the image is electronically magnified. On the other hand, CCD systems have fast image time (similar to DR systems) and are less expensive than DR systems. Because of the nature of these systems, they are usually sold as a complete system that includes the x-ray machine.

- Dedicated x-ray film scanners (Figure 2.23) and digital cameras are not forms of DR. Both of these methods only reproduce the traditional hard copy radiograph and, in general, do a poor job of image reproduction. Even expensive multi-megapixel digital cameras now available do a poor job of converting an analog x-ray image into a digital format without the loss of significant gray scale data. Because of this, the use of film scanners and digital cameras is not recommended as a means of sending images for consultation (teleradiology).

digital radiographs (and other medical images such as ultrasound) from one place to another. DICOM images are embedded with specific information regarding patient data, as well as the type of system that the images were acquired on, and this information cannot be altered. Also, DICOM allows transmission of images without the need for proprietary software that is vendor specific. For example, if you have a GE brand ultrasound machine, the images can be read by any radiologist with a DICOM viewer (which can be found for free), and they do not need to have specific GE software to view the images. DICOM allows the practicing veterinarian to send nonlossy, high-quality images that incorporate patient data directly to any radiologist of his or her choosing. Although DICOM "compliance" initially met with resistance (mostly from vendors), it has become commonplace in veterinary medicine and will continue to flourish.

FREQUENTLY ASKED QUESTIONS

A. A Weimaraner dog is being anesthetized. Because of a murmur and mild coughing episodes, the heart and especially lung fields are of interest. The DV radiograph is not too light, and not too dark. This judgment is determined by the:

1. Inability to see the bony column details (very white) and a light (white) appearance of the lung fields.
2. Ability to see the outline of the heart clearly against the lungs.
3. Ability to see the thoracic vertebrae in the area where they overlap the cardiac silhouette.
4. The appearance of the lungs as a dark air density and full visualization of the bony structures.

The most correct answer is #3. This indicates the appropriate technique. The first option indicates that this is too light a technique. This is common where the technique has not been adjusted in obese patients. In #2, seeing the outline of the heart clearly against the lungs is not necessarily associated with technique but may be due to disease in the area. The #4 answer is burning through the soft tissues and is not appropriate for heart and lung studies.

B. A new DR system has just been installed. The practice has opted for the flat panel technology. It does not appear that the image is different even when thin, obese, or barrel-shaped dogs undergo imaging with the same settings. This means:

1. Further staff training is needed.
2. This is normal—only four basic settings will be needed with DR, and that is why the system was chosen!
3. The chart needs to be evolved further because something must be wrong if the same setting works for a large range of animals.
4. The equipment is working better than promised.

Answer #2 is most correct. Answer #1 is probably not an issue because this is the most forgiving of the imaging systems, digital or traditional. Answer #3 is not relevant because only three or four settings will capture all dog breeds and body condition scores. Answer #4 is normal for this system. Although most expensive, this DR system is known to be the most forgiving and is known to produce the highest quality images.

C. The thoracic radiographs for this patient are not easily interpreted so the plan is to:

1. Take another view and use foam supports to help stabilize the body in a fully vertical position; ensuring that the sternum and spine are superimposed provides a better image. This still does not provide a clear answer, so "no significant findings" is placed on the medical record, assuming that the standard of care has been met caused by acquisition of the best possible radiographs.
2. Follow the steps in answer #1 and send a JPG to the telemedicine group for a radiologist's opinion.
3. Follow the steps in answer #1 and send a DICOM image to the telemedicine group for a radiologist's opinion.

Answer #3 is the best option as a lossless format, and an expert opinion will provide best practices here. Answer #2 is going to degrade the image; if an important detail is lost during image compression, it could compromise patient care. Answer #1 is a good first step, but if the attending clinician does not have a confident interpretation, then use of a specialist will provide the gold standard for care. General practitioners cannot be the master of all trades, and with the ability to transmit high-quality images of reasonable size, questionable interpretations for radiographs should always be referred for a specialist evaluation by telemedicine.

SUGGESTED READINGS

Animal Insides. Retrieved from www.animalinsides.com (accessed October, 2006).

Buchanan JW, Bucheler J: Vertebral scale system to measure canine heart size in radiographs, J Am Vet Med Assoc 206:194–199, 1995.

Bushberg JT, Seibert JA, Leidholdt EM, Boone JM: The essential physics of medical imaging, Philadelphia, 2002, Lippincott, Williams & Wilkins.

Kittleson MD, Kienle RD: Small animal cardiovascular medicine, St. Louis, 1998, Mosby.

Lord PF, Suter PF: Radiology. In Fox PR, Sisson D, Moiuse NS, eds: Textbook of canine and feline cardiology, ed 2, Philadelphia, 1999, WB Saunders.

Matton JS: Digital radiography, Vet Comp Orthop Traumatol 19:123–132, 2006.

Owens JM: Radiographic interpretation for the small animal clinician, St Louis, 1982, Ralston Purina Co.

Electrocardiography 3

Larry P. Tilley | Francis W. K. Smith, Jr.

Electrocardiography in clinical practice is the recording at the body surface of electrical fields generated by the heart. Specific waveforms represent stages of myocardial depolarization and repolarization. The electrocardiogram (ECG) is a basic and valuable diagnostic test in veterinary medicine and is relatively easy to acquire. It is the initial test of choice in the diagnosis of cardiac arrhythmias and may also yield information regarding chamber dilation and hypertrophy.

INDICATIONS AND ROLE OF THE ELECTROCARDIOGRAM IN CLINICAL PRACTICE

DOCUMENTATION OF CARDIAC ARRHYTHMIAS

- An ECG should be recorded when an arrhythmia is detected during physical examination. This may include bradycardia, tachycardia, or irregularity in rhythm that is not secondary to respiratory sinus arrhythmia.
- Animals with a history of syncope or episodic weakness may have cardiac arrhythmias, and an ECG is indicated in these cases. Arrhythmias in such cases may be transient—a normal ECG result does not rule out transient arrhythmias. In some cases, long-term electrocardiographic monitoring (Holter monitor or cardiac event recorder) is warranted.
- Arrhythmias often accompany significant heart disease and may significantly affect the clinical status of the patient. An ECG should be recorded in animals with significant heart disease.
- The ECG is also used to monitor efficacy of antiarrhythmic therapy and to determine whether arrhythmias may have developed secondary to cardiac medications (e.g., digoxin).
- Significant arrhythmias may also occur in animals with systemic disease, including those diseases associated with electrolyte abnormalities (hyperkalemia, hyponatremia, hypercalcemia, and hypocalcemia), neoplasia (particularly splenic neoplasia), gastric dilatation-volvulus, and sepsis.

ASSESSMENT OF CHAMBER ENLARGEMENT PATTERNS

- Changes in waveforms may provide indirect evidence of cardiac chamber enlargement. The ECG result may be normal, however, in cases with chamber enlargement. Right ventricular hypertrophy most consistently results in waveform changes.
- As heart disease progresses, waveform changes may indicate progressive chamber enlargement.
- Thoracic radiography and, ideally, echocardiography should be performed for definitive assessment of chamber enlargement.

MISCELLANEOUS INDICATIONS FOR ELECTROCARDIOGRAPHY

- The ECG may provide evidence of pericardial effusion (electrical alternans, low-amplitude complexes).
- Electrocardiographic abnormalities are often present with hypothyroidism and hyperthyroidism.
- A pronounced sinus arrhythmia may be present in animals with elevated vagal tone (often seen with diseases affecting the respiratory tract, central nervous system [CNS], and gastrointestinal tract).

PRINCIPLES OF ELECTROCARDIOGRAPHY

PLACEMENT OF SURFACE ELECTRODES IN A DESIGNATED FASHION TO OBTAIN STANDARD ELECTROCARDIOGRAPHIC LEADS

- A lead consists of the electrical activity measured between a positive electrode and a negative electrode.
- Electrical impulses with a net direction toward the positive electrode will generate a positive waveform or deflection. Electrical impulses with a net direction away from the positive electrode will generate a negative waveform or deflection. Electrical impulses with a net direction perpendicular to the positive electrode will not generate a waveform or deflection (isoelectric).

- Standard electrocardiographic lead systems are used to create several angles of assessment. A single lead would provide information on only one dimension of the current (e.g., left compared with right). Two leads would allow two-dimensional information (e.g., left compared with right and cranial compared with caudal). As many as 12 leads may be acquired simultaneously.

STANDARD LEAD SYSTEMS

- The standard leads are I, II, III, aVR, aVL, and aVF (Figure 3.1, Box 3.1). Placement of electrodes to generate each lead is illustrated in Figure 3.2.
- Leads I, II, and III are bipolar limb leads. These are termed *bipolar* because the ECG is recorded from two specific electrodes.
- Leads aVR, aVL, and aVF are augmented unipolar leads. For these leads to be generated,

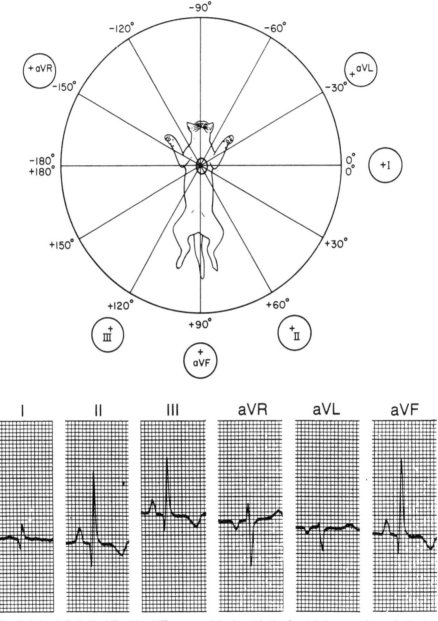

Figure 3.1   The limb leads (I, II, III, aVR, aVL, aVF) surround the heart in the frontal plane as shown in the top part of the figure (feline). The circled limb lead names indicate the direction of electrical activity if the QRS is positive in that lead. The mean electrical axis in this canine electrocardiogram (*bottom part of the figure*) is +90. Lead I is isoelectric. The lead perpendicular to lead I is aVF (see axis chart on top). Lead aVF is positive, making the axis +90. If lead aVF had been negative, the axis would have been −90. (From Tilley LP: Essentials of canine and feline electrocardiography: interpretation and treatment, ed 3, Malvern, Penn, 1992, Lea & Febiger.)

two electrodes are electrically connected (as a negative electrode) and compared with the single electrode (positive).

- Precordial chest leads are obtained with an exploring unipolar positive electrode at specific locations on the chest. These leads may provide additional information or supportive evidence of cardiac chamber enlargement. They are also useful in the evaluation of the P wave when limb leads are equivocal.
- The base-apex lead is often used in equine electrocardiography and may also be used in small-animal practice for rhythm assessment. A positive electrode is placed on the left side of the chest, over the heart, and the negative electrode is placed in the area of the right shoulder or neck.
- The esophageal ECG electrode lead for surgical monitoring is useful because recorded complexes are increased in size, providing increased accuracy for diagnosing an arrhythmia during surgery (Figure 3.3).
- Handheld, wireless ECG and ECG real-time computer display represents new technology for recording ECGs (Figures 3.4 and 3.5.)

RECORDING THE ELECTROCARDIOGRAM

- The ECG should be recorded in an area as quiet and as free of distraction as possible. Noises from clinical activity and other animals may significantly affect rate and rhythm. Any use of electrically operated equipment, such as clippers, may cause interference and should be minimized during the ECG. In some cases, fluorescent lighting may result in electrical interference.
- The patient should ideally be placed in right lateral recumbency.
  - Electrocardiographic reference values were obtained from animals in right lateral recumbency.
  - Limbs should be held perpendicular to the body. Each pair of limbs should be held parallel, and limbs should not be allowed to contact one another.
  - The animal should be held as still as possible during the ECG. When possible, panting should be prevented.
  - When dyspnea or other factors prevent standard positioning, the ECG may be recorded while the animal is standing or, less ideally, sitting.
- Electrode placement
  - Alligator clips or adhesive electrodes may be used. For reduction of discomfort, teeth of alligator clips should be blunted, and the spring should be relaxed.
  - Limb electrodes are placed either distal or proximal to the elbow (caudal surface) and over the stifle. Electrodes placed proximal to the elbow may increase respiratory artifact.
  - Each electrode should be wetted with 70% isopropyl alcohol to ensure electrical contact.
- Recording the ECG
  - Approximately three to four complete complexes should be recorded from each lead at 50 mm/sec.
  - A lead II rhythm strip should then be recorded at 25 mm/sec or 50 mm/sec.

Box 3.1   Lead Systems Used in Canine and Feline Electrocardiography

Bipolar Limb Leads

I: Right thoracic limb (–) compared with left thoracic limb (+)

II: Right thoracic limb (–) compared with left pelvic limb (+)

III: Left thoracic limb (–) compared with left pelvic limb (+)

Augmented Unipolar Limb Leads

aVR: Right thoracic limb (+) compared with average voltage of left thoracic limb and left pelvic limb (–)

aVL: Left thoracic limb (+) compared with average voltage of right thoracic limb and left pelvic limb (–)

aVF: Left pelvic limb (+) compared with average voltage of right thoracic limb and left thoracic limb (–)

Unipolar Precordial Chest Leads and Exploring Electrode

CV_5RL (rV_2): Right fifth intercostal space near the sternum

CV_6LL (V_2): Left sixth intercostal space near the sternum

CV_6LU (V_4): Left sixth intercostal space near the costochondral junction

V_{10}: Over the dorsal process of the seventh thoracic vertebra

Base-Apex Bipolar Lead

Record in lead I position on ECG machine with leads placed as follows: LA electrode over left sixth intercostal space at costosternal junction; RA electrode over spine of right scapula near the vertebra.

KEY POINT

The 1-mV standardization marker should be recorded at the onset of the ECG and any time the sensitivity is changed.

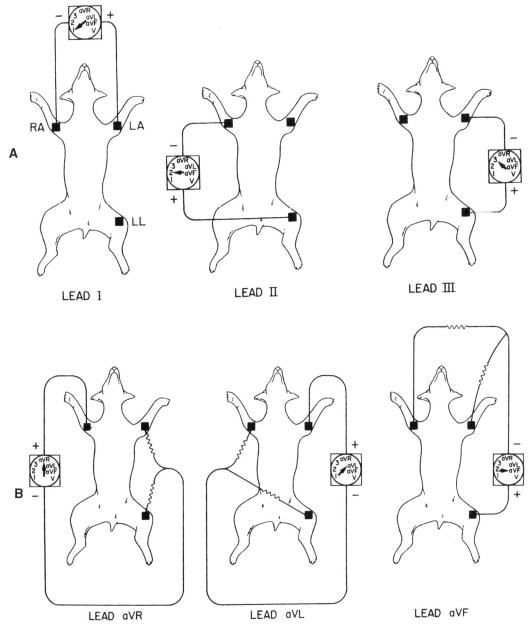

Figure 3.2   A, Three bipolar standard leads. By means of a switch incorporated in the instrument, the galvanometer can be connected across any pair of several electrodes. Each pair of electrodes is called a lead. The leads illustrated here are identified as I, II, and III. **B,** Augmented unipolar limb leads aVR, aVL, and aVF. (From Tilley LP: Essentials of canine and feline electrocardiography: interpretation and treatment, ed 3, Malvern, Penn, 1992, Lea & Febiger.)

CARDIAC CONDUCTION AND GENESIS OF WAVEFORMS

• The function of the cardiac conduction system is to coordinate the contraction and relaxation of the four cardiac chambers (Figures 3.6 and 3.7).

• For each cardiac cycle, the initial impulse originates in the sinoatrial (SA) node located in the wall of the right atrium near the entrance of the cranial vena cava. This impulse is rapidly propagated through the atrial myocardium, with a resulting depolarization of the atria. Depolarization of the atria results in the P wave and atrial contraction. The initial S-A nodal impulse is small and does not produce an electrocardiographic change on the body's surface.

• Immediately after atrial depolarization, the impulse travels through the atrioventricular (AV) node, located near the base of the right atrium. Conduction is slow here, which allows atrial contraction to be completed before

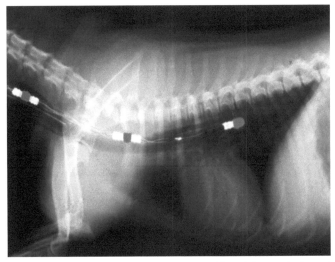

Figure 3.3 Esophageal ECG electrode and temperature probe positioned for surgical monitoring. This technique is useful as complexes recorded are increased in size, providing increased accuracy for diagnosing an arrhythmia during surgery.

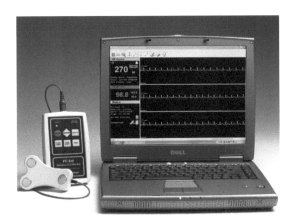

Figure 3.4 Handheld, wireless electrocardiogram (ECG) and ECG real-time computer display. (Courtesy Vmed Technology, Redmond, Wash. www.vmedtech.com.)

ventricular depolarization occurs. As the impulse travels through the AV node, there is no electrocardiographic activity on the body's surface—rather, the PR interval is generated.

- On leaving the AV node, conduction velocity increases significantly, and the impulse is rapidly spread through the bundle of His, bundle branches, and Purkinje system. This results in rapid and nearly simultaneous depolarization of the ventricles. Depolarization of the ventricles results in the prominent QRS complex and causes ventricular contraction.
- The Q wave represents initial depolarization of the interventricular septum and is defined as the first *negative* deflection following the P wave and occurring before the R wave. A Q wave may not be identified in all animals.

- The R wave represents depolarization of the ventricular myocardium from the endocardial surface to the epicardial surface. The R wave is the first *positive* deflection following the P wave and is usually the most prominent waveform.
- The S wave represents depolarization of the basal sections of the ventricular posterior wall and interventricular septum. The S wave is defined as the first negative deflection following the R wave in the QRS complex.
- Ventricular repolarization quickly follows ventricular depolarization and results in the T wave. The delay in repolarization results in the ST segment on the surface ECG.

EVALUATION OF THE ELECTROCARDIOGRAM

- The ECG should be evaluated from left to right.
- Areas of artifact should be identified and avoided in the evaluation.
- Calculate the heart rate (HR).
  - Determine the number of R waves (or R-R intervals) within 3 seconds and multiply by 20 to obtain beats per minute (beats/min) (for an ECG recorded at 50 mm/sec, vertical timing marks above the gridlines occur every 1.5 seconds).
  - If the rhythm is regular, the HR may be derived by determining the number of small boxes in one R-R interval and dividing 3000 by that number (for paper speed of 25 mm/sec, use 1500). The method is also useful for determining the rate of paroxysmal ventricular tachycardia and other arrhythmias lasting less than 3 seconds.

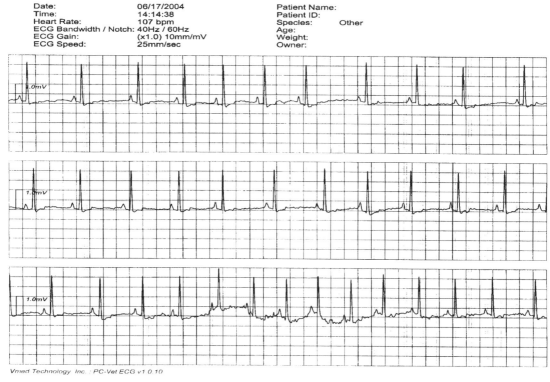

Date: 06/17/2004
Time: 14:14:38
Heart Rate: 107 bpm
ECG Bandwidth / Notch: 40Hz / 60Hz
ECG Gain: (x1.0) 10mm/mV
ECG Speed: 25mm/sec
Patient Name:
Patient ID:
Species: Other
Age:
Weight:
Owner:

Vmed Technology Inc. : PC-Vet ECG v1.0.10

Figure 3.5 Wireless electrocardiogram (ECG) printout report from laptop computer software system in Figure 3.4. (Courtesy Vmed Technology, Redmond, Wash. www.vmedtech.com.)

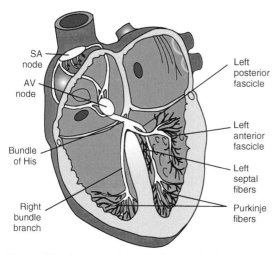

Figure 3.6 Anatomy of the cardiac conduction system. *AV,* Atrioventricular, *SA,* sinoatrial. (Modified from Tilley LP: Essentials of canine and feline electrocardiography: interpretation and treatment, ed 2, Philadelphia, 1985, Lea & Febiger.)

- Obtain measurements for the waveforms and intervals (Figure 3.8).
  - P wave height and width
  - Duration of PR interval
  - Duration of QRS complex and height of R wave
  - Duration of QT segment

- Determine the approximate mean electrical axis (MEA).
  - The MEA refers to the direction of the net ventricular depolarization and refers solely to the QRS complex. If there is significant right ventricular hypertrophy, then the MEA will shift to the right. Because the left ventricle is normally the dominant ventricle, the normal MEA is to the left. A degree system is used: if the MEA is directly to the left, then it is said to be 0 degrees; if the MEA is directly downward, then it is 90 degrees; and if it is directly to the right, then it is 180 degrees. The MEA of the normal dog is 40 to 100 degrees. For the cat, the MEA is more variable, ranging from 0 to 160 degrees.
  - The MEA may be determined with the six standard leads and the Bailey axis system (see Figure 3.1). If there is a lead with isoelectric QRS complexes, then the MEA equates to the lead on the Bailey axis perpendicular to the isoelectric lead.
  - The MEA may also be determined by plotting the net amplitude of a lead I QRS complex (horizontal axis) and the net amplitude of a lead aVF QRS (vertical axis). The intersection will provide the vector equal to the MEA (see Figure 3.1).
  - The MEA may be approximated by inspecting leads I and aVF.

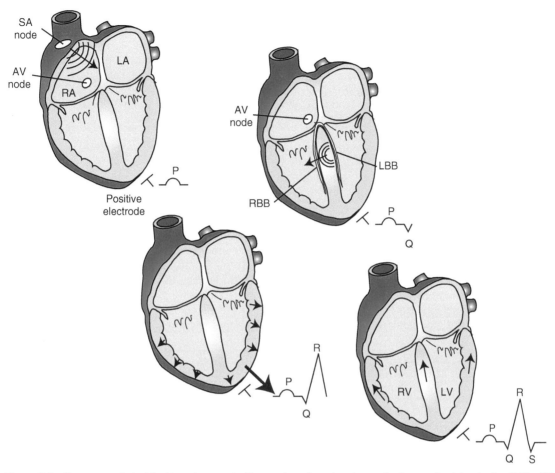

Figure 3.7 Sequence of electrical impulse conduction and cardiac chamber activation as it relates to the ECG. *AV,* Atrioventricular; *LA,* left atrium; *LBB,* left bundle branch; *LV,* left ventricle; *RA,* right atrium; *RBB,* right bundle branch; *RV,* right ventricle; *SA,* sinoatrial. (Modified from Tilley LP: Essentials of canine and feline electrocardiography: interpretation and treatment, ed 3, Philadelphia, 1992, Lea & Febiger.)

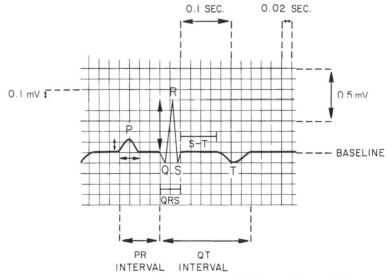

Figure 3.8 Close-up of a normal feline lead II P-QRS-T complex with labels and intervals. Measurements for amplitude (millivolts) are indicated by positive (+) and negative (–) movement; time intervals (hundredths of a second) are indicated from left to right. Paper speed, 50 mm/sec; sensitivity, 1 cm = 1 mV. (From Tilley LP: Essentials of canine and feline electro-cardiography: interpretation and treatment, ed 2, Philadelphia, 1985, Lea & Febiger.)

- If the net direction of the lead I QRS is positive, then the MEA is to the left. If the net deflection of the lead I QRS is negative, then the MEA is to the right.
- If the net direction of the lead aVF QRS is positive, then the MEA is downward or caudal. If the net deflection of the lead aVF QRS is negative, then the MEA is upward or cranial.
- The approximate angle can be estimated by examining the relative amplitudes of leads I and aVF.
- Determine the rhythm.
- Compare patient values with reference values (Table 3.1).

EVALUATION OF WAVEFORMS

P WAVE

- Atrial enlargement patterns (Figure 3.9)
  - The P wave is generated by atrial depolarization. Atrial enlargement may result in an increase in width or height of the P waves recorded in lead II.
- Enlargement of the right atrium may result in an increased P wave height. This is referred to as P pulmonale. The height of the P wave should not exceed 0.4 mV (dog) or 0.2 mV (cat). Chronic pulmonary disease may result in P pulmonale in the absence of heart disease.
- Enlargement of the left atrium may result in an increased P wave width or duration. This is referred to as P mitrale. The duration of the P wave should not exceed 0.04 second (dog or cat). Left atrial enlargement may also result in notching of the P wave.
- Presence or absence of P waves
  - There is no minimum height or duration for the P wave. In some cases, P waves may be indistinct. In this situation, carefully evaluate all leads for P wave activity. If P waves cannot be discerned in any of the limb leads, evaluation of chest leads is recommended.

Table 3.1   Normal Canine and Feline Electrocardiogram Values*

	Canine	Feline
HR	Puppy: 70220 beats/min Toy breeds: 70180 beats/min Standard: 70160 beats/min Giant breeds: 60140 beats/min	120240 beats/min
Rhythm	Sinus rhythm Sinus arrhythmia Wandering pacemaker	Sinus rhythm
P wave		
Height	Maximum: 0.4 mV	Maximum: 0.2 mV
Width	Maximum: 0.04 sec (Giant breeds, 0.05 sec)	Maximum: 0.04 sec
PR interval	0.06-0.13 sec	0.05-0.09 sec
QRS		
Height	Large breeds: 3.0 mV maximum[†] Small breeds: 2.5 mV maximum	Maximum: 0.9 mV
Width	Large breeds: 0.06 sec maximum Small breeds: 0.05 sec maximum	Maximum: 0.04 sec
ST segment		
Depression	No more than 0.2 mV	None
Elevation	No more than 0.15 mV	None
QT interval	0.15-0.25 sec at normal HR	0.12-0.18 sec at normal HR
T waves	May be positive, negative, or biphasic Amplitude range ± 0.05-1.0 mV in any lead Not more than ¼ of R wave amplitude	Usually positive and <0.3 mV
Electrical axis	+40 to + 100	0 ± 160
Chest leads		
CV$_5$RL (rV$_2$)	T positive; R <3.0 mV	
CV$_6$LL (V$_2$)	S <0.8 mV; R <3.0 mV	R <1.0 mV
CV$_6$LU (V$_4$)	S <0.7 mV; R <3.0 mV	R <1.0 mV
V$_{10}$	QRS negative; T negative except in Chihuahua	T negative; R wave/Q wave <1

*Measurements are made in lead II unless otherwise stated.
†Not valid for thin, deep-chested dogs younger than 2 years.
HR, Heart rate; *S,* Second.

- P waves may be absent in several arrhythmias, including atrial fibrillation and atrial standstill. P waves may be superimposed on other waveforms in ventricular tachycardia and supraventricular tachycardia (SVT).
- Variation of P wave height is a normal finding in the dog and a manifestation of alterations in vagal tone.

PR INTERVAL

- The PR interval reflects the slowed conduction through the AV node. The normal PR interval is 0.06 to 0.13 second for dogs and 0.05 to 0.09 second for cats.
- A significantly shortened PR interval may occur when an accessory pathway allows conduction to bypass the AV node.
- Prolongation of the PR interval represents first-degree AV block.
- Variation of the PR interval may occur with alterations in vagal tone or secondary to the presence of ectopic beats, causing dissociation of atrial and ventricular activity.

QRS COMPLEX

- The QRS complex is generated by ventricular depolarization (left ventricle, interventricular septum, and right ventricle). Ventricular enlargement may result in changes in the QRS complex.
- Left ventricular enlargement pattern
  - Increased amplitude of the R wave
    - Dog
      - Amplitude of R wave greater than 3.0 mV (2.5 mV in small-breed dogs) in lead II, lead aVF, and the precordial chest leads CV_6LU, CV_6LL, and CV_5RL
      - Amplitude of R wave greater than 1.5 mV in lead I
      - Sum of R wave amplitudes in leads I and aVF greater than 4.0 mV
    - Cat
    - Amplitude of R wave greater than 0.9 mV in lead II
    - Amplitude of R wave greater than 1.0 mV in CV_6LU and CV_6LL
    - R wave/Q wave greater than 1.0 in lead V_{10}
  - QRS duration greater than 0.06 second (large dogs), 0.05 second (small dogs), or 0.04 second (cats)
  - ST slurring or coving
  - Shift in the MEA to the left (less than 40 degrees for dog, less than 0 degrees for cat)
- Right ventricular enlargement pattern (Figure 3.10)
  - Increased amplitude of S waves
    - Dog
      - Presence of S waves in leads I, II, III, and aVF
      - S wave in lead I greater than 0.05 mV
      - S wave in lead II greater than 0.35 mV
      - S wave in lead CV_6LL greater than 0.8 mV
      - S wave in lead CV_6LU greater than 0.7 mV
    - Cat
      - Presence of S waves in leads I, II, III, and aVF
      - Prominent S waves in CV_6LU and CV_6LL
      - T wave positive in lead V_{10} (except Chihuahua)
      - W-shaped QRS complex in V_{10} (dog)
    - R/S ratio less than 0.87 in CV_6LU
    - Shift in the MEA to the right (more than 100 degrees for the dog or more than 160 degrees for the cat)
- Widening of the QRS complexes may occur with left ventricular enlargement, right or left bundle

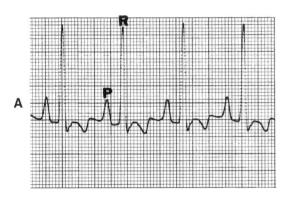

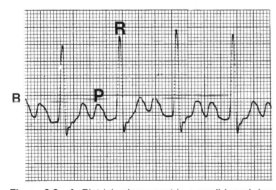

Figure 3.9 A, Biatrial enlargement in a small-breed dog with a collapsed trachea and compensated mitral regurgitation. The P wave is 0.5 mV tall (P pulmonale) and 0.05 second wide (P mitrale). **B,** Left atrial enlargement in a geriatric, small-breed dog with chronic acquired valvular disease (mitral insufficiency). P waves are wide (0.075 second), notched, and equivocally tall. (From Fox PR, Sisson D, Moise NS, eds: Textbook of canine and feline cardiology, Philadelphia, 1999, Saunders.)

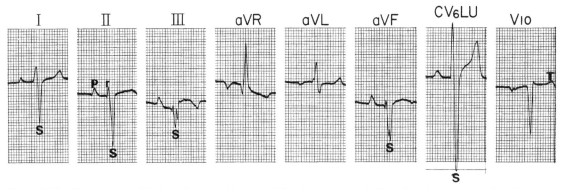

Figure 3.10   Severe right ventricular enlargement in a dog with pulmonic stenosis. There is a right axis deviation of approximately 110 degrees. Note the deep S waves in leads I, II, III, aVF, and CV$_6$LU. The T wave is positive in V$_{10}$. (From Tilley LP: Essentials of canine and feline electrocardiography: interpretation and treatment, ed 3, Philadelphia, 1992, Lea & Febiger.)

branch block (LBBB), and complexes of ventricular origin (ventricular premature complexes [VPCs] or ventricular escape complexes).

- Electrical alternans (Figure 3.11, *A*)
  - In electrical alternans, there is a pattern of regular variation in the amplitude of normal electrocardiographic complexes (excluding ventricular ectopy). This is usually manifested by an alteration in R wave height, although variation in other waveforms may be seen. The amplitude may change significantly with every complex and alternate in height.
  - Electrical alternans is most often associated with pericardial effusion. A severe pleural effusion may cause electrical alternans.
  - SVT may result in an electrical alternans pattern.
- Low-amplitude QRS complexes
  - The minimum height for the normal R wave in the dog is 0.05 mV to 1.0 mV.
  - Low-amplitude R waves may occur when transmission of the cardiac electrical impulse to the skin is hindered. This may occur with pericardial effusion, pleural effusion, obesity, or subcutaneous edema. Pneumothorax and pulmonary edema may also decrease R wave height.
  - Hypothyroidism may result in low-amplitude R waves (usually with accompanying slow rate).

ST SEGMENT

- ST segment elevation (Figure 3.11, *B*)
  - Elevation of the ST segment greater than 0.15 mV in leads II, III, or aVF is abnormal in the dog. Any ST segment elevation in the cat is abnormal.
  - ST segment elevation may be caused by myocardial hypoxia, transmural myocardial infarction, or pericardial effusion. In

cats, digoxin toxicity may cause ST segment elevation.

- ST segment depression (Figure 3.11, *C*)
  - Depression of the ST segment greater than 0.2 mV in leads II, III, or aVF is abnormal in the dog. Any ST segment depression in the cat is abnormal.
  - ST segment depression may be caused by myocardial hypoxia, hyperkalemia, hypokalemia, subendocardial myocardial infarction, or digoxin toxicity.
  - Pseudodepression due to prominent T$_a$ waves (atrial repolarization) caused by atrial disease or tachycardia also causes ST segment depression.
- Miscellaneous ST segment changes
  - ST segment changes may occur as a result of bundle branch blocks, myocardial hypertrophy, or VPCs. The changes in the ST segment are in the opposite direction from the main QRS deflection.

KEY POINT

Baseline artifact may mimic changes with the ST segment.

QT INTERVAL

- The normal QT interval is 0.15 to 0.25 second (dog) and 0.12 to 0.18 second (cat). The QT interval tends to increase with slow HRs and decrease with rapid rates. In general, the QT interval should be less than half of the preceding R-R interval.
- The length of the QT interval is chiefly determined by an interplay of autonomic influences. HR and QT interval are governed separately by different sympathetic neurons that may or may not be activated together. Corrections of the

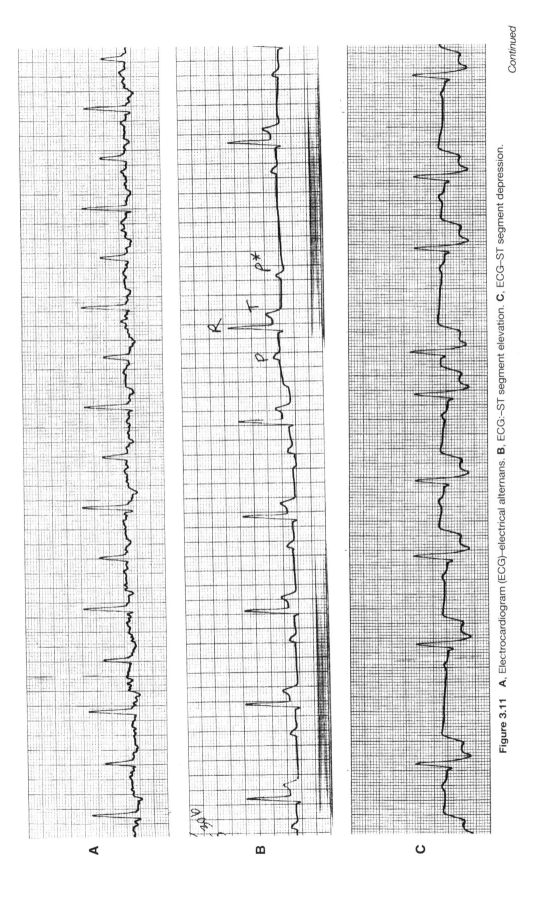

Figure 3.11   A, Electrocardiogram (ECG)–electrical alternans. **B,** ECG:–ST segment elevation. **C,** ECG–ST segment depression.

Continued

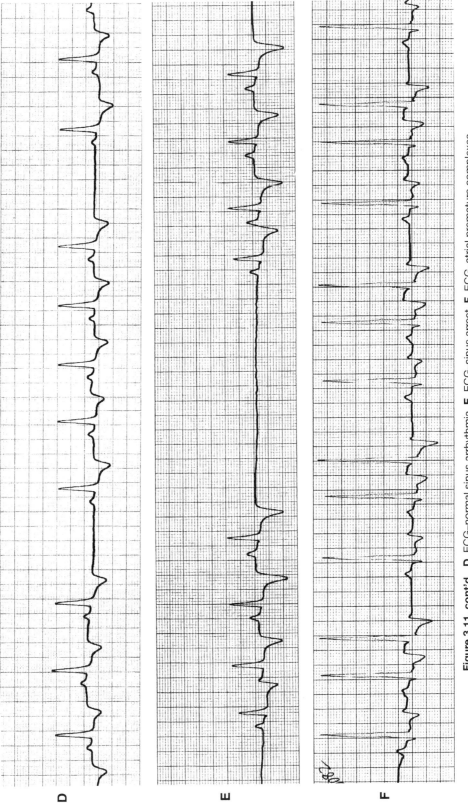

Figure 3.11, cont'd   D, ECG–normal sinus arrhythmia. **E,** ECG–sinus arrest. **F,** ECG–atrial premature complexes.

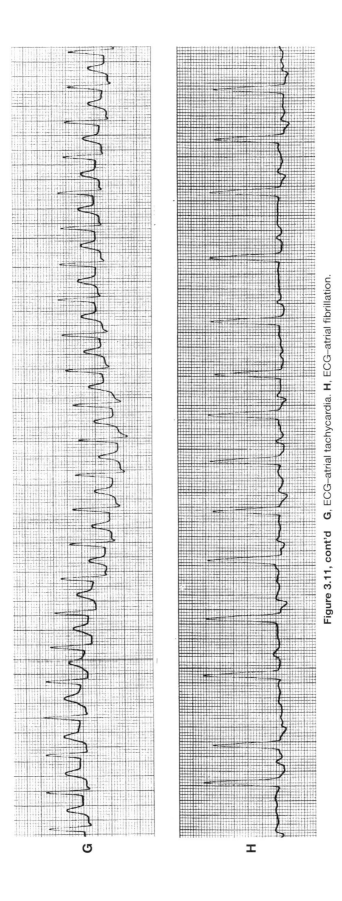

Figure 3.11, cont'd **G**, ECG–atrial tachycardia. **H**, ECG–atrial fibrillation.

QT interval (QT_c) for HR appear to be applicable under circumstances such as exercise.

- Within the past two decades, the overall ventricular repolarization and its relationship to the QT_c interval has led to studies in which the QT_c interval is used as a prognostic marker of ventricular tachyarrhythmias and death. Class IA or class III antiarrhythmic drugs, such as quinidine and sotalol, are known to prolong myocardial repolarization. This may either provide a protective effect against arrhythmias or lead to an increased occurrence of QT_c interval-related arrhythmias, including torsades de pointes ventricular tachycardia.
- Torsades de pointes (turning about a point) is a rare arrhythmia in the dog. It is a form of polymorphic ventricular tachycardia or flutter in which the amplitude of the complexes increases and decreases in size so that it appears to twist around the baseline. Humans with torsades de pointes are at risk for sudden death.

POSSIBLE FORMULAS FOR CORRECTED QT INTERVALS

- Many formulas and methods exist for correcting the QT interval for the effects of HR, including logarithmic, hyperbolic, and exponential functions, but they also have limitations. These limitations result from both physiologic and computational problems. The Bazett formula, for example, predicts an ever-increasing increment in the QT interval as the HR slows and an ever-decreasing increment as the rate rises, both of which are physiologically improbable. In addition, these formulas do not account for the effects of autonomic tone on the QT interval independent of the effects on rate. They also do not account for the relatively slow adaptation of repolarization to changes in rate. The Fridericia formula (QT divided by the cube root of the R-R interval) is a modification of the Bazett formula. This modification is important because the Bazett formula will overcorrect for rates higher than 60 beats/min. The Van de Water formula (based on a study in dogs) involves regression analysis yielding the following equation: QT_c = Van de Water formula = $QT - 87(60/HR - 1)$. Recent publications have recommended the use of the log-log formula for correcting the QT interval for HR (linear regression with $\log_e HR$ as the covariate: $QT = a + b [\log_e HR]$; a and b are constants).
- Prolongation of the QT interval may occur with interventricular conduction disturbances that are associated with prolongation of the QRS complexes, bradycardia, ethylene glycol toxicity, strenuous activity, or CNS disturbances. QT prolongation has been reported with many drugs and electrolyte imbalances. These include hypokalemia, hypocalcemia, quinidine, procainamide, bretylium, tricyclic antidepressants, and many anesthetics.
- Shortening of the QT interval may occur with hypercalcemia, hyperkalemia, or digoxin therapy.

T WAVE

- The T wave is quite variable in the dog and cat. In most leads, the T wave may be positive, negative, or biphasic. The height of the T wave should not exceed one fourth the height of the R wave, one fourth the height of the Q wave (if Q wave is greater than R wave), or 0.5 to 1.0 mV in any lead.
- The T wave should be positive in CV_5RL in dogs aged 2 months and should be negative in V_{10}, except in the Chihuahua.
- Prominent T waves may occur with myocardial hypoxia, with interventricular conduction with disturbances, with ventricular enlargement, and in some animals with heart disease and bradycardia.
- Prominent and peaked T waves are associated with hyperkalemia.
- Small, biphasic T waves may occur with hypokalemia.
- Nonspecific T wave changes may occur with metabolic disturbances (hypoglycemia, anemia, shock, fever), drug toxicity (digoxin, quinidine, procainamide), and neurologic disease.
- T wave alternans has been reported as a result of hypocalcemia, increased circulating catecholamines, and sudden increases in sympathetic tone.

ARRHYTHMIAS AND CONDUCTION DISTURBANCES

- An arrhythmia (or dysrhythmia) refers to an irregularity in the cardiac rhythm. In general, an arrhythmia denotes an abnormality of the cardiac rhythm, although in the dog the term *normal sinus arrhythmia* is used to describe the normal variation in HR associated with respiration (Box 3.2).
  - Arrhythmias may be classified according to their **origin.**
    - Supraventricular arrhythmias arise from the atria or AV node.
    - Ventricular arrhythmias arise from the ventricles.
  - Arrhythmias may be classified according to their **rates.**

Box 3.2 Classification of Cardiac Arrhythmias

Normal sinus impulse formation
  Normal sinus rhythm
  Sinus arrhythmia
  Wandering sinus pacemaker
Disturbances of sinus impulse formation
  Sinus arrest
  Sinus bradycardia
  Sinus tachycardia
Disturbances of supraventricular impulse formation
  Atrial premature complexes
  Atrial tachycardia
  Atrial flutter
  Atrial fibrillation
  Atrioventricular junctional rhythm
Disturbances of ventricular impulse formation
  Ventricular premature complexes
  Ventricular tachycardia
  Ventricular asystole
  Ventricular fibrillation
Disturbances of impulse conduction
  Sinoatrial block
  Persistent atrial standstill ("silent" atrium)
  Atrial standstill (hyperkalemia)
  Ventricular pre-excitation
  First-degree AV block
  Second-degree AV block
  Complete AV block (third degree)
  Bundle branch blocks
Disturbances of both impulse formation and impulse conduction
  Sick sinus syndrome
  Ventricular pre-excitation and the Wolff-Parkinson-White (WPW) syndrome
  Atrial premature complexes with aberrant ventricular conduction
  Escape rhythms
  Junctional escape rhythms
  Ventricular escape rhythms (idioventricular rhythm)

- Arrhythmias with slow rates are referred to as bradyarrhythmias.
- Arrhythmias with rapid rates are referred to as tachyarrhythmias.
- Arrhythmias may be classified according to their **regularity.**
  - Fibrillation is an irregular, chaotic rhythm.
  - Tachycardia is a regular (nonirregular) rhythm.
- Examples: Atrial fibrillation is an irregular, chaotic arrhythmia originating from the atria; ventricular tachycardia is a regular arrhythmia originating from the ventricles.
- There are several pathophysiologic causes of arrhythmias.
  - Abnormal automaticity of normal pacemaker cells

- Shift of the pacemaker from the SA node to other areas of the heart
- Conduction blocks that terminate or slow normal conduction through the heart
- Abnormal pathways of impulse conduction through the heart
- Spontaneous impulse formation in any area of the heart
- Systemic approach to arrhythmia recognition and evaluation
  - Any lead may be used for arrhythmia evaluation; lead II is generally used because waveforms are usually best defined in this lead. A significant duration of artifact-free lead II should be carefully evaluated.
  - Determine if P waves are present. Examine all leads: P waves may be small or isoelectric in several leads. You must distinguish baseline motion (artifact) from P waves. P waves are generally consistent in size and distance from associated QRS complex. The presence of P waves indicates a sinus (originating from SA node) rhythm.
  - Determine if an atrial (P wave) and ventricular (QRS complex) association exists. There should be a P wave for every QRS complex. If there are a greater number of P waves or QRS complexes, then an arrhythmia exists.
    - P waves should slightly precede QRS complexes.
    - If P waves follow the QRS complex, then AV dissociation exists, and the rhythm is ventricular or junctional rather than sinus.
    - There should be a QRS complex following each P wave. If not, then a conduction disturbance is present.
  - Determine the regularity of the rhythm.
    - Normal sinus rhythm—insignificant (less than 10%) variation in the P-P or R-R intervals.
    - Normal sinus arrhythmia—significant (more than 10%) variation in the P-P or R-R intervals.
      - A pattern of irregularity is usually noted; the HR increases during inspiration and decreases during expiration in a cyclical pattern.
      - This may be referred to as a respiratory sinus arrhythmia.
    - Check for pauses in the rhythm—periods of inactivity greater than two R-R intervals.
    - Check for P waves occurring prematurely (occurring earlier than expected)—distinguish from normal sinus arrhythmia, where P wave rate increases during inspiration. Premature P waves will noticeably

break the rhythm. Premature P waves indicate the presence of atrial premature complexes (APCs).

- Check for QRS complexes occurring prematurely. These may occur without preceding P wave, may be superimposed on P wave, or may follow P wave with shortened PR interval. Premature QRS complexes indicate presence of VPCs.

KEY POINT

Remember, a ventricular *premature* complex is *premature*. A ventricular complex occurring after a pause is *not* premature–it is a ventricular escape complex.

- Evaluation of PR interval
  - PR interval may vary slightly with changes in vagal tone—this would also result in a sinus arrhythmia.
  - Progressive prolongation of the PR interval signals first-degree AV block.
  - P waves without associated QRS complexes are usually indicative of second-degree AV block.
  - Shortened PR interval may be seen with increased sympathetic tone and pre-excitation syndromes (presence of an accessory pathway bypassing AV node).
- Evaluation of QRS complexes
  - Height of R wave and duration of QRS complex
  - Presence of prominent S waves
  - Shape of QRS complexes should not vary significantly. Variation may be caused by the following:
    - VPCs or ventricular escape complexes
    - Fusion beats—simultaneous occurrence of VPC and normal QRS
    - Electrical alternans
    - Intermittent bundle branch block
    - Artifact
  - Premature QRS complexes suggest VPCs; QRS complexes without P waves and occurring after a pause suggest ventricular escape complexes.
- Note shape of any premature complexes: APCs have a QRS of normal shape; VPCs have a QRS that is significantly different from the normal QRS.

KEY POINT

QRS complexes should not vary in their shape in a normal animal.

NORMAL RHYTHMS

NORMAL SINUS RHYTHM

- Normal rhythm in the dog and cat.
- P wave for every QRS complex, regular rhythm.
- Rate between 60 beats/min and 180 beats/min for the dog, depending on size of dog and degree of anxiousness.
- Rate between 140 beats/min and 240 beats/min for the cat, depending on degree of anxiousness.
- Rate and rhythm dependent on SA nodal discharge. This is highly influenced by changes in autonomic tone. An elevated sympathetic tone will increase rate of SA nodal discharge; an elevated parasympathetic (vagal) tone will decrease rate of SA nodal discharge.

NORMAL SINUS ARRHYTHMIA

- Sinus arrhythmia is usually normal in the dog and generally abnormal in the cat.
- A pattern of irregularity is present—the HR increases during inspiration and decreases during expiration in a cyclical pattern (Figure 3.11, *D*).
- Irregularity is secondary to fluctuations in vagal tone associated with the respiratory cycle.
- When respiratory effort is increased (brachycephalic breeds, animals with respiratory disease), fluctuations in vagal tone may be dramatic, producing a pronounced sinus arrhythmia.
- Normal sinus arrhythmia is a rhythm of high vagal tone and low sympathetic tone; this situation is rare in dogs with congestive heart failure. The presence of a sinus arrhythmia in a dog with severe cough is more supportive of primary respiratory disease than of congestive heart failure.

WANDERING SINUS PACEMAKER

- The origin of SA nodal discharge may change as a consequence of alterations in vagal tone. This is noted on the ECG as a cyclical change in the height of the P wave. At times, the P wave may become isoelectric and not detectable.
- Often associated with normal sinus arrhythmia or pronounced sinus arrhythmia.

KEY POINT

Sinus arrhythmia is *not* expected in the cat but is normal and is the result of variations in vagal tone in dogs.

DISTURBANCES OF SINUS IMPULSE FORMATION

SINUS ARREST

- When the SA node fails to discharge as expected, a pause in the rhythm will occur. The duration of the pause is at least twice the preceding R-R interval. When severe, pause duration may be 5 to 12 seconds (Figure 3.11, *E*).
- For survival, the pause is ended by a ventricular escape complex, junctional escape complex, or normal complex.
- Causes include fibrosis of the SA nodal tissue, greatly increased vagal stimulation, drug influences (digoxin, beta-blockers), and, rarely, neoplasia.
- If severe and frequent, intermittent weakness or syncope may occur.

SINUS BRADYCARDIA

- A sinus rhythm with an abnormally slow rate.
- May be physiologic: during sleep, the HR of many dogs drops to 30 to 40 beats/min. Calm animals or athletic animals at rest may have a physiologic sinus bradycardia.
- Elevated vagal tone may result in a sinus bradycardia.
- Drug-induced: anesthetics and sedatives, digoxin, calcium channel blockers, beta-blockers.
- Pathologic: hypothermia, hypothyroidism, sick sinus syndrome (SSS).
- Specific therapy for sinus bradycardia is not warranted unless clinical signs (weakness, reduced cardiac output) have developed as a result of the arrhythmia.

SINUS TACHYCARDIA

- A sinus rhythm with an abnormally rapid rate.
- May be physiologic—associated with exercise, stress, anxiousness, pain.
- Drug-induced: atropine or glycopyrrolate, methylxanthines (theophylline), excessive thyroid supplementation, catecholamines (epinephrine, dobutamine).
- Pathologic: fever, shock, hyperthyroidism, anemia, hypoxia, and congestive heart failure.
- Specific therapy for sinus tachycardia is usually indicated for rate control in congestive heart failure patients.

KEY POINT

The underlying cause of the sinus tachycardia should be identified and addressed if necessary.

DISTURBANCES OF SUPRAVENTRICULAR IMPULSE FORMATION

ATRIAL PREMATURE COMPLEXES

- An APC is an abnormal beat occurring prematurely and originating in atrial tissue.
- Electrocardiographic features in the following (Figure 3.11, *F*):
  - Presence or absence of ectopic P wave; P wave is usually of normal shape.
  - Ectopic P wave may be superimposed on preceding T wave.
  - Premature QRS may have identical or nearly identical appearance to normal QRS.
  - A compensatory pause may follow the APC.
  - If the APC occurs when the ventricles are refractory, then an isolated ectopic P wave will be noted; it is nonconducted because of the refractoriness of the ventricles.
- Causes generally include any disease associated with atrial enlargement, such as degenerative valve disease, congenital heart disease, or cardiomyopathy. Other causes include hypoxia, atrial neoplasia, and chronic obstructive pulmonary disease.
- Therapy is not generally warranted for infrequent APCs. Antiarrhythmic therapy may be needed if APCs are frequent and thought to be compromising cardiac output or if there is a concern of impending atrial tachycardia or atrial fibrillation.

ATRIAL TACHYCARDIA

- A paroxysmal tachycardia originating from atrial tissue (other than SA node)
- Electrocardiographic features (Figure 3.11, *G*)
  - There is a rapid rate—from 200 to 350 beats/min.
  - There is usually a regular rhythm. If originating from multiple atrial sites, then an irregular rhythm may occur.
  - P waves may be difficult to discern. QRS complexes are generally normal but may widen, or electrical alternans may develop.
  - The onset and termination of arrhythmia is sudden.
  - It may occur as a reentrant arrhythmia within the AV node.
- Same causes as for APCs
- May be clinically significant depending on rate, frequency of runs, and length of runs

ATRIAL FLUTTER

- An uncommon arrhythmia characterized by a rapid atrial rate (greater than 250 beats/min) and altered atrial depolarization resulting in bidirectional saw-toothed atrial complexes

(F waves). Ventricular rate varies depending on refractoriness of AV node.
- It is usually a result of severe structural heart disease.
- Clinical significance depends on ventricular rate. If excessive, then cardiac output is reduced.

ATRIAL FIBRILLATION

- A common arrhythmia in the dog characterized by lack of P waves, rapid ventricular rate, and irregularity of ventricular depolarizations. In atrial fibrillation, there are numerous sites of ectopic atrial depolarization and varying AV nodal refractoriness (Figure 3.11, *H*). Atrial fibrillation is uncommon in the cat.
- Baseline may be flat or may exhibit fine fibrillation potentials.
- Causes include the following:
  - Structural heart disease (advanced degenerative valve disease, dilated cardiomyopathy, atrial neoplasia, congenital heart disease)
  - Lone atrial fibrillation, which occurs in large- to giant-breed dogs without structural heart disease
  - May occur as a complication of noncardiac disease, such as gastric dilatation-volvulus or other disorders altering vagal tone
  - May be drug-induced (e.g., digoxin)
- Clinical significance depends on ventricular rate in most cases. With atrial fibrillation there is also loss of atrial contraction (atrial kick), which may reduce ventricular performance. If the rate is not controlled, then lone atrial fibrillation may cause myocardial deterioration and secondary dilated cardiomyopathy.

JUNCTIONAL PREMATURE COMPLEXES

- A junctional premature complex is an abnormal beat occurring prematurely and originating in the AV nodal area.
- Electrocardiographic characteristics include abnormal-appearing P wave (often inverted), which may precede QRS, be superimposed on QRS, or follow QRS complexes. The QRS complex is usually unaffected.
- Causes are the same as for APCs.
- Clinical significance is the same as APCs.

ATRIOVENTRICULAR JUNCTIONAL TACHYCARDIA

- A paroxysmal or sustained rhythm originates from AV nodal tissue.
- Electrocardiographic features.
  - Rate is greater than 60 beats/min (inherent rate of AV nodal tissue is approximately 40 to 60 beats/min).
  - There is a regular rhythm.

- Abnormal-appearing P wave (often inverted in lead II) may precede QRS, be superimposed on QRS, or follow QRS complexes.
  - QRS complexes may be normal or may be widened as a result of aberrant conduction.
- Causes include digoxin toxicity and structural heart disease.
- It may be clinically significant depending on ventricular rate.

> **KEY POINT**
>
> AV junctional tachycardia may be difficult to distinguish from atrial tachycardia.

SUPRAVENTRICULAR TACHYCARDIA

- SVT refers to a rapid arrhythmia originating from supraventricular tissue but in which the exact site of origin cannot be determined. Atrial tachycardia and AV junctional tachycardia are often indistinguishable, so the term *SVT* may be more precise in these cases.

DISTURBANCES OF IMPULSE CONDUCTION

SINUS BLOCK

- The SA node discharges normally, but the impulse is blocked by neighboring tissue.
- It produces a pause equal to twice the preceding R-R interval, with immediate restoration of rhythm.
- Causes are the same as for sinus arrest.
- Sinus block is usually not clinically significant.

ATRIAL STANDSTILL

- Atrial standstill is characterized by an absence of P waves and can be temporary in nature or persistent. The most common cause of temporary atrial standstill is hyperkalemia. Persistent atrial standstill is caused by an atrial muscular dystrophy, most commonly occurring in English Springer Spaniels.
- In atrial standstill caused by hyperkalemia, SA nodal discharge occurs, but atrial depolarization is blocked by the effects of hyperkalemia. Because there is no atrial depolarization, P waves are absent. The impulse originating from the SA node reaches the AV node by way of internodal fibers. Hyperkalemia also slows the rate of SA nodal discharge and affects ventricular depolarization and repolarization.
- Electrocardiographic characteristics of persistent atrial standstill include the following:
  - Absence of P waves
  - HR usually slow (<60 beats/min)
  - Rhythm regular with supraventricular-appearing QRS complexes

- No increase of HR with atropine administration
- The following are electrocardiographic characteristics of atrial standstill caused by hyperkalemia (Figure 3.12, *A*):
  - As serum potassium increases, P wave amplitude diminishes. Absence of P waves occurs when the potassium approaches 8.0 mEq/L.
  - The ventricular rate is slow: the rhythm is termed *sinoventricular,* and the rate is approximately 20 to 40 beats/min.
  - As serum potassium increases, T wave amplitude increases and becomes peaked.
  - QRS duration progressively increases, and R wave height decreases as serum potassium levels increase.
  - HR may increase slightly with atropine administration.
- Causes of hyperkalemia include hypoadrenocorticism, anuric or oliguric renal failure, uncontrolled diabetic ketoacidosis, metabolic acidosis, urethral obstruction, and rupture of the urinary bladder.

KEY POINT

Atrial standstill caused by hyperkalemia is usually life-threatening.

VENTRICULAR PRE-EXCITATION SYNDROME

- In these syndromes, an abnormal accessory pathway exists, which bypasses the AV node. This results in a shortening or loss of the PR interval due to premature activation of the ventricles. With an accessory pathway, there are two electrical connections between the atria and the ventricles, and both may simultaneously be relaying impulses. There also exists the potential for reentry because the impulse may leave the atria through one pathway and immediately reenter through the other. The accessory pathway may connect the atria to the distal AV node, to the bundle of His, or directly to ventricular tissue.
- Electrocardiographic features include the following (Table 3.2 and Figure 3.13):
  - The PR interval is shortened.
  - If the accessory pathway terminates in ventricular tissue, then initial slurring of the QRS complex (delta wave) occurs.
  - There is paroxysmal reentrant tachycardia in some cases.
- Causes include congenital anomalies, feline hypertrophic cardiomyopathy, and other structural heart diseases.
- Clinical significance depends on the frequency and severity of secondary tachycardia resulting from the accessory pathway.

FIRST-DEGREE ATRIOVENTRICULAR BLOCK

- Conduction through the AV node is delayed.
- Produces prolongation of the PR interval (more than 0.13 second for the dog, more than 0.09 second for the cat) (see Figure 3.12, *B*).
- Causes include fibrosis of the AV node, vagal stimulation, and drug-induced (digoxin) and electrolyte imbalance.
- Isolated first-degree AV block is not clinically significant but may be an early indicator of progressive AV nodal dysfunction.

SECOND-DEGREE ATRIOVENTRICULAR BLOCK

- There is intermittent blockage of conduction through the AV node.
- After discharge of the SA node and atrial depolarization, there is no associated ventricular depolarization.
- Electrocardiographic features include absence of QRS-T complexes following P wave (see Figure 3.12, *C*).
  - In Mobitz type I (Wenckebach) block, there is progressive prolongation of the PR interval, followed by occurrence of second-degree AV block.
  - In Mobitz type II block, there is second-degree AV block without preceding prolongation of the PR interval.
  - A pattern of block may exist; a 2:1 AV block would refer to the presence of two P waves for every QRS complex.
  - Advanced or high-grade AV block consists of more than two consecutive blocked atrial depolarizations.
- Causes are identical to those of first-degree AV block.
- High-grade AV block may reduce cardiac output and result in clinical signs.

KEY POINT

Second-degree block may progress to complete AV block. This is more common with Mobitz type II AV block.

THIRD-DEGREE ATRIOVENTRICULAR BLOCK (COMPLETE HEART BLOCK)

- All conduction through the AV node is blocked. Atrial and ventricular depolarizations are no longer coordinated and occur independently of one another. Ventricular depolarization is initiated by discharge of a ventricular escape focus.
- Electrocardiographic features (see Figure 3.12, *D*) include the following:

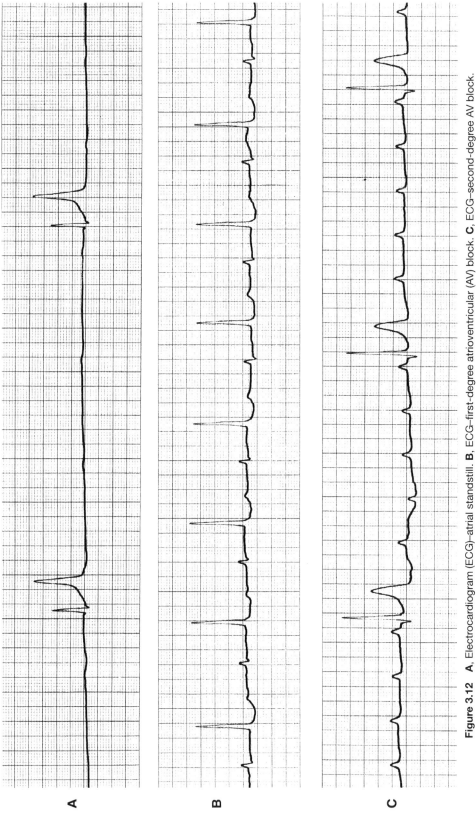

Figure 3.12 **A**, Electrocardiogram (ECG)–atrial standstill. **B**, ECG–first-degree atrioventricular (AV) block. **C**, ECG–second-degree AV block.

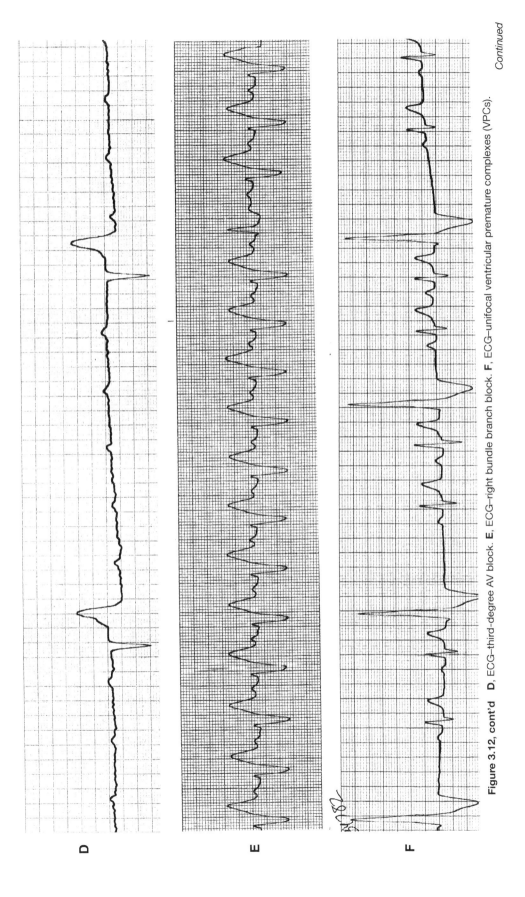

Figure 3.12, cont'd   D, ECG–third-degree AV block. **E**, ECG–right bundle branch block. **F**, ECG–unifocal ventricular premature complexes (VPCs).

Continued

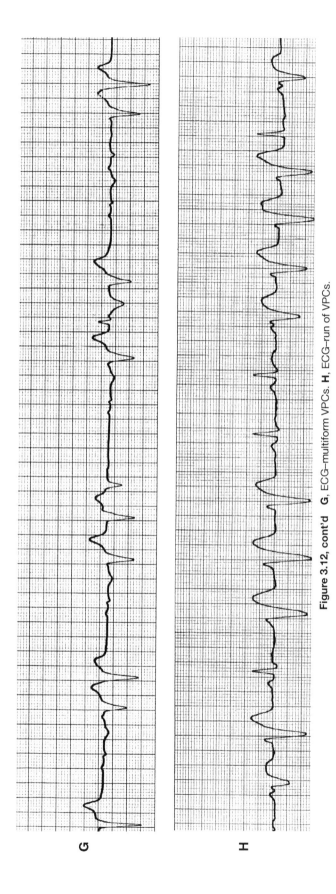

Figure 3.12, cont'd   G, ECG—multiform VPCs. **H,** ECG—run of VPCs.

Table 3.2   Summary of Pre-Excitation Syndrome

Cardiac Sequence	Mechanism	Electrocardiogram
Sinus impulse	Normal	—
Atrial depolarization	Normal	Normal P wave
AV node accessory pathways	Relatively rapid conduction, skirting the A-V nodal system	Short PR interval
Early ventricular depolarization	One ventricle activated early	Initial QRS slurred (delta wave) (widened QRS)
Retrograde conduction from ventricles to atria	Atrial reentry impulse	Tendency to supraventricular paroxysmal arrhythmias
Late ventricular depolarization	Fusion between normal and anomalous ventricular activation	Delay, often with altered direction, of terminal QRS

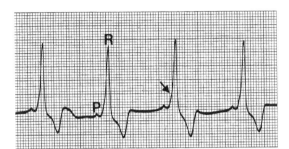

Figure 3.13   Ventricular pre-excitation in a dog. A short P-R interval and a widened QRS complex with slurring or notching (*arrow*) of the upstroke ("delta" wave) are present. (From Fox PR, Sisson D, Moise NS, eds: Textbook of canine and feline cardiology, St Louis, 1999, Elsevier.)

- There is no association between P waves and QRS-T complexes.
- P waves are of normal shape and usually occur at a normal rate.
- QRS complexes are of ventricular origin shape.
- Ventricular rate is typically 30 to 50 beats/min.
- Causes include fibrosis of the AV node, drug-induced (digoxin), infiltrative disease, Rickettsial myocarditis, and hyperkalemia.
- Usually associated with clinical signs of weakness or collapse. Complete AV block warrants implantation of a permanent pacemaker in most cases.

LEFT BUNDLE BRANCH BLOCK

- A conduction delay or block in both the left posterior and the left anterior fascicles of the left bundle. A supraventricular impulse activates the right ventricle first through the right bundle branch. Left ventricular depolarization is delayed.
- Electrocardiographic features include the following (Figure 3.14):
  - QRS duration is prolonged (>0.08 second for the dog; > 0.06 second for the cat)

- QRS is wide and positive in leads I, II, III, and aVF.
- Unlike VPCs, the QRS complex is associated with a preceding P wave.
- It may be difficult to distinguish from left ventricular enlargement pattern.
- Causes include structural heart disease (cardiomyopathy, congenital anomalies, neoplasia, trauma, fibrosis).
- The presence of an LBBB does not impair cardiac performance directly but is a marker of significant heart disease.

KEY POINT

Complete heart block will occur if right bundle branch block (RBBB) develops in an animal with LBBB.

LEFT ANTERIOR FASCICULAR BLOCK

- There is a block in the left anterior fascicle of the left bundle branch slowing depolarization of the left ventricle.
- Electrocardiographic features include the following:
  - QRS duration within normal limits
  - Left axis deviation (dog, less than 40 degrees; cat, less than 0 degrees)
  - Small Q wave and tall R wave in leads I and aVL (small Q wave not consistent)
  - Deep S waves in leads II, III, and aVF (exceeding R wave)
  - Associated with feline hypertrophic cardiomyopathy, other diseases associated with left ventricular hypertrophy, hyperkalemia, ischemia, and postcardiac surgery

KEY POINT

Left anterior fascicular block (LAFB) does not directly impair cardiac function, but if present, one should look for underlying causes.

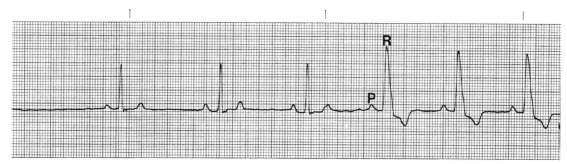

Figure 3.14 Intermittent left bundle branch block in a dog. The QRS complexes are wider and taller than normal in the fourth, fifth, and sixth complexes. (From Fox PR, Sisson D, Moise NS, eds: Textbook of canine and feline cardiology, St Louis, 1999, Elsevier.)

RIGHT BUNDLE BRANCH BLOCK

- There is a block of the right bundle branch, delaying depolarization of the right ventricle.
- Electrocardiographic features include the following (see Figure 3.12, *E*):
  - Increase of QRS duration
  - Prominent S waves in leads I, II, III, and aVF
  - Right axis shift
- It is associated with structural heart disease, Chagas disease, heartworm disease, acute pulmonary thromboembolism, and hypokalemia.

KEY POINT

As in the case of LAFB, RBBB does not significantly impair cardiac function, but one should look for underlying causes.

DISTURBANCES OF VENTRICULAR IMPULSE FORMATION

VENTRICULAR PREMATURE COMPLEXES

- An abnormal beat originates in the ventricles and occurs earlier than expected in relation to the existing rhythm. A compensatory pause often follows a VPC.
  - Unifocal VPCs occur from one ventricular site and have identical shapes (see Figure 3.12, *F*).
  - Multifocal VPCs usually occur from more than one ventricular site and have differing shapes. Electrophysiologic studies have demonstrated that a single ventricular site may produce VPCs of differing shape; this is due to altered conduction of the VPCs rather than multiple ectopic sites. It is more precise, therefore, to use the term *multiform* rather than *multifocal* (see Figure 3.12, *G*).
  - When the VPC does not alter the underlying normal rhythm, it is considered to be interpolated.
  - When normal ventricular depolarization is interrupted by a VPC, a fusion beat occurs;

this is essentially the electrocardiographic merging of a normal QRS and VPC.
- Electrocardiographic features include the following (see Figures 3.12, *F* to *H*):
  - As the site of depolarization is ventricular, there is no AV association. P waves are not associated with the QRS complexes of the VPCs.
  - QRS complexes are wide and bizarre, consistent with ventricular origin.
  - T wave polarity is often reversed.
  - Compensatory pause following VPC is typical.
  - The following are patterns of VPCs:
    - Two consecutive VPCs are referred to as a couplet.
    - Three or more consecutive VPCs are a salvo or run (see Figure 3.12, *H*).
    - When every other complex is a VPC, ventricular bigeminy exists.
    - When every third complex is a VPC, ventricular trigeminy exists.
    - R-on-T phenomenon occurs when the VPC occurs immediately following a normal beat within the T wave. This may predispose to development of ventricular tachycardia.
- Causes are numerous and include structural heart disease, inheritance in young German Shepherds, arrhythmogenic right ventricular cardiomyopathy (Boxer cardiomyopathy), hypoxia, anemia, uremia, gastric dilatation-volvulus, splenic torsion and splenic neoplasia, pancreatitis, myocarditis, and use of drugs (digoxin, anesthesia).
- Clinical significance depends on the frequency of VPCs, pattern of ectopy, and cause of the arrhythmia.
  - Isolated VPCs usually pose no significant problems but may signal the presence of progressive disease and potential for more serious arrhythmia.
  - Runs of VPCs do suggest the potential for ventricular tachycardia and possibly ventricular fibrillation.

KEY POINT

The finding of isolated VPCs in a young to middle-aged Doberman Pinscher or Boxer is highly suggestive of occult dilated cardiomyopathy or arrhythmogenic right ventricular cardiomyopathy, respectively.

VENTRICULAR TACHYCARDIA

- These are runs of VPCs occurring in succession at a rate usually greater than 100 beats/min. The inherent discharge rate of the ventricle is approximately 40 to 50 beats/min (seen with complete heart block). In normal animals, this is overdriven by the sinus rhythm. An accelerated idioventricular rhythm refers to a ventricular rhythm at a rate of 60 to 100 beats/min. Ventricular tachycardia may be sustained or paroxysmal.
- Electrocardiographic features include the following (Figure 3.15, A):
  - P waves not associated with QRS complexes
  - QRS complexes wide and bizarre, consistent with ventricular origin
  - Regular rhythm, as contrasted with atrial fibrillation and RBBB
- Causes are the same as for VPCs.
- Ventricular tachycardia indicates significant heart disease or systemic disease. Cardiac output may be significantly impaired, and the arrhythmia predisposes to ventricular fibrillation.

VENTRICULAR FIBRILLATION

- Completely irregular, chaotic variable fibrillation potentials, indicating lack of organized ventricular depolarization and impending death
- Electrocardiographic features (Figure 3.15, B)
  - No evidence of organized cardiac depolarization (absence of P-QRS-T waves)
  - Wavy, undulating baseline
  - Coarse ventricular fibrillation that is characterized by large wavelets
  - Fine ventricular fibrillation that is characterized by small wavelets

KEY POINT

Ventricular fibrillation indicates cardiopulmonary arrest, and immediate restoration of rhythm is required to preserve life.

VENTRICULAR ASYSTOLE

- There is lack of any significant ventricular electrical activity.

- ECG demonstrates flat baseline; occasional ventricular escape complexes may occur.
- A terminal rhythm requires immediate restoration of rhythm to preserve life.

DISTURBANCES OF BOTH IMPULSE FORMATION AND IMPULSE CONDUCTION

SICK SINUS SYNDROME

- SSS is a progressive heart disease characterized by a variety of arrhythmias, including sinus bradycardia, sinus arrest, paroxysmal atrial tachycardia (bradycardia-tachycardia syndrome), intermittent AV nodal block, and lack of ventricular escape complexes (Figure 3.15, C).
- Breeds predisposed include Miniature Schnauzers, Cocker Spaniels, Dachshunds, Pugs, and West Highland White Terriers. SSS is most common in older female dogs.
- The cause is unknown but likely involves idiopathic degeneration of the conduction system.
- Most patients have a history of intermittent weakness and collapse.
- Medical therapy may be successful in some cases; many require pacemaker implantation.

ATRIAL PREMATURE COMPLEXES WITH ABERRANT CONDUCTION

- When the impulse of an APC encounters an area of refractoriness (AV node, bundle of His, or ventricular myocardium), it may terminate or continue with aberrant conduction. The latter may result in a wide and bizarre QRS configuration resembling a beat of ventricular origin.
- Most often occur at slow HRs.
- QRS may take the form of RBBB.

ESCAPE RHYTHMS

JUNCTIONAL ESCAPE BEAT

- When not activated by atrial depolarization, the junctional AV nodal area may spontaneously discharge. This impulse results in ventricular depolarization in a normal fashion. Junctional escape beats may occur when there is a significant pause in the sinus rhythm.
- Electrocardiographic features include the following:
  - Inverted P wave, occurring before, during, or just after QRS complex
  - Normal or relatively normal QRS complex
  - Occurrence after significant pause in sinus rhythm
- Clinical significance—this complex is adaptive and helps to maintain cardiac output in the face of a slow rate or sinus arrest.

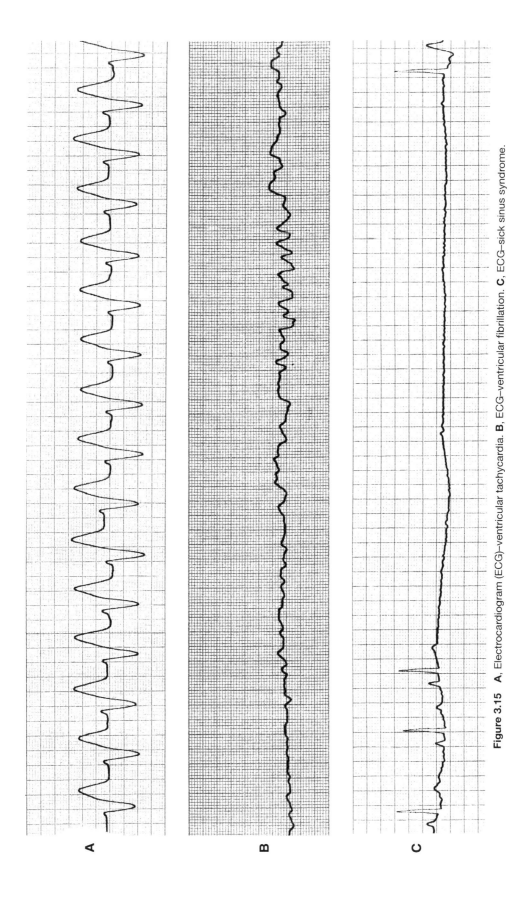

Figure 3.15 **A**, Electrocardiogram (ECG)–ventricular tachycardia. **B**, ECG–ventricular fibrillation. **C**, ECG–sick sinus syndrome.

Junctional escape beats should not be suppressed.

JUNCTIONAL RHYTHM

- This rhythm is a succession of junctional escape beats in absence of adequate sinus node function.
- Rate of junctional escape rhythm is typically 40 to 60 beats/min.
- This rhythm is adaptive and should not be suppressed. Correction of the cause of sinus node dysfunction is warranted.

VENTRICULAR ESCAPE BEAT

- When not activated by atrial depolarization, a ventricular focus may spontaneously discharge. This impulse results in an abnormal ventricular depolarization, but contraction is not affected. Ventricular escape beats may occur when there is a significant pause in the sinus rhythm and lack of junctional escape complexes.
- Electrocardiographic features include the following:
  - Occurrence of ventricular escape beat after a pause in the rhythm
  - QRS wide and bizarre, consistent with ventricular origin
- Clinical significance—this complex is adaptive and helps to maintain cardiac output in the face of a slow rate or sinus arrest.

These ventricular escape beats should not be suppressed.

VENTRICULAR ESCAPE RHYTHM

- This rhythm is a succession of ventricular escape beats in absence of adequate sinus node function.
- Rate of ventricular escape rhythm is typically 30 to 40 beats/min.
- This rhythm is adaptive and should not be suppressed. Correction of the cause of sinus node dysfunction is warranted.

MISCELLANEOUS

ARTIFICIAL PACEMAKER

- A permanent pacemaker is used to control bradyarrhythmias that caused clinical signs and were unresponsive to medical therapy.
- Transvenous implantation with an endocardial lead is the preferred means and is much less invasive than abdominal surgery and epicardial lead implantation.
- Most pacemakers used in dogs are set at 100 beats/min.
- Electrocardiographic features include the following:
  - If the sinus node is functioning and the HR is greater than 100 beats/min (or the pacemaker's discharge rate), then there will be no electrocardiographic changes.
  - Once the HR decreases below the pacemaker's minimum rate, a pacing spike will appear, followed by a wide and bizarre QRS (ventricular origin of impulse).

The beats generated by the pacemaker are not of normal shape; this is expected.

PARASYSTOLE

- In parasystole, there is an independent focus discharging spontaneously. There is an entrance block, so the focus is not overdriven by the normal cardiac impulse. The parasystolic focus will discharge at a regular rate and may cause complete depolarization of the atria or ventricles.
- Atrial parasystole focus is located within atrial myocardium and produces small P waves, usually unassociated with QRS complexes.
- Ventricular parasystole focus is located within ventricular myocardium and produces regularly spaced QRS complexes. When the focus discharges during the ventricle's refractory period, a QRS will not be created.

ASHMAN'S PHENOMENON

- Tendency of premature supraventricular beats to have aberrant ventricular conduction when a short cycle follows a long one

Ashman's aberrance may mimic a VPC.

FREQUENTLY ASKED QUESTIONS

If a veterinarian auscults an abnormality that comes and goes and the ECG does not show an arrhythmia, what should be done?

Repeat ECGs may be required to pick up changes in heart activity occurring only in a paroxysmal pattern. In some cases, a Holter monitor must be used for a 24-hour recording so that the pattern and frequency of abnormality can be properly tracked.

Interference is occurring on an ECG tracing; it appears to be 60 cycle (small waveforms) and is not improved when the fluorescent bulbs and all electrical equipment in the room are turned off. What could cause this ongoing interference?

Sometimes interference may travel through the walls from the adjacent room, and proximity to power supply in the wall could also send off interference. Electrical supply to the facility must be properly grounded, so if the problem persists when all of those factors have been controlled, an electrician should examine the electrical system of the building.

We must do a surgery that requires an unusual position for the dog. Will abnormal relative and absolute positioning of the clips interfere with our routine intraoperative monitoring?

Position is not critical for routine intraoperative electrocardiography, as opposed to position required for a primary ECG with multiple leads for diagnostic purposes, and a useful capture can be done despite unorthodox limb or animal position. Any position for the recording will still always give an analysis of an arrhythmia, conduction abnormality, or both. Watching that the extreme positioning required will not lead to the lead wires or clips touching a metal surgical table is important because such contact can cause interference.

SUGGESTED READINGS

Davis AS, Middleton BJ: Relationship between QT interval and heart rate in Alderley Park beagles, Vet Rec 145:248–250, 1999.

Detweiler DK: The dog electrocardiogram: a critical review. In MacFarlane PW, Lawrie TDV, eds: Comprehensive electrocardiography: theory and practice in health and disease, New York, 1998, Pergamon Press.

Finley MR, Lillich JD, Gilmour RF, Freeman LC: Structural and functional basis for the long QT syndrome: relevance to veterinary patients, J Vet Med 17:473–488, 2003.

Kittleson MD: Electrocardiography. In Kittleson MD, Kienle RD, eds: Small animal cardiovascular medicine, St Louis, 1998, Mosby.

Miller MS, Tilley LP, Detweiler DK: Cardiac electrophysiology. In: Duke's physiology of domestic animals, ed 11, Ithaca, NY, 1993, Cornell.

Miller MS, Tilley LP, Smith Jr FWK, Fox PR: Electrocardiography. In Fox PR, Sisson D, Moise NS, eds: Textbook of canine and feline cardiology, St Louis, 1999, Elsevier.

Orvalho JS: Electrocardiographic techniques. In Ettinger SJ, Feldman EC, eds: Textbook of veterinary internal medicine, ed 7, St Louis, 2010, Saunders.

Redfern WS, Carlsson L, Davis AS, et al.: Relationships between preclinical cardiac electrophysiology, clinical QT interval prolongation and torsade de pointes for a broad range of drugs: evidence for a provisional safety margin in drug development, Cardiovasc Res 58:32–45, 2003.

Smith FWK, Tilley LP, Miller MS: Disorders of cardiac rhythm. In Brichard SJ, Sherding RG, eds: Manual of small animal practice, ed 3, St Louis, 2007, Saunders.

Smith FWK, Tilley LP, Miller MS: Electrocardiography. In Brichard SJ, Sherding RG, eds: Manual of small animal practice, ed 3, St Louis, 2007, Saunders.

Tilley LP: Essentials of canine and feline electrocardiography, ed 3, Ames, Iowa, 1992, Wiley Blackwell.

Tilley LP: Electrocardiography. In Knoll J, Vaden S, Smith FWK, Tilley LP, eds: Lab tests and diagnostic procedures—the 5 minute veterinary consult, Ames, Iowa, 2009, Wiley Blackwell.

Echocardiography and Doppler Ultrasound

4

Virginia Luis Fuentes

Echocardiography remains the most important diagnostic technique for the diagnosis of canine and feline heart disease. Cardiac shape, motion, and blood flow can all be displayed as a result of the interaction between the heart and ultrahigh frequency sound waves. Echocardiography is complementary to physical examination, radiography, and electrocardiography (ECG) and has replaced invasive techniques such as cardiac catheterization for all but a few specific indications.

TYPES OF IMAGING

TWO-DIMENSIONAL ECHOCARDIOGRAPHY

- A sector-shaped beam of ultrasound waves is reflected by the interfaces of cardiac tissue to provide a two-dimensional (2D) cross-sectional (tomographic) image in real time (Figure 4.1).

APPLICATIONS OF TWO-DIMENSIONAL ECHOCARDIOGRAPHY

- Demonstrating cardiac lesions
- Demonstrating abnormal cardiac chamber geometry
- Demonstrating abnormal cardiac wall motion
- Demonstrating pleural and pericardial effusions

M-MODE ECHOCARDIOGRAPHY

- M-mode echocardiography uses a single narrow beam of ultrasound but displays the resulting echoes as a distance-time graph (Figure 4.2). The only advantage over 2D echocardiography is superior time resolution.

APPLICATIONS OF M-MODE ECHOCARDIOGRAPHY

- Time-dependent measurements (chamber dimensions, wall motion)

DOPPLER ECHOCARDIOGRAPHY

- Doppler echocardiography uses the Doppler principle to estimate the *velocity* and *direction* of blood flow or myocardial motion.

- The change in frequency (or Doppler shift) when an ultrasound wave is reflected by a moving red blood cell depends on the transmitted frequency and the direction and velocity of the red blood cell, allowing the blood flow velocity to be calculated if the transmitted frequency and change in frequency are known.
- Aligning the beam parallel with flow (or at least within 20 degrees of flow) is critical to avoid underestimation of blood flow velocity.
- There are several types of Doppler echocardiography, with the direction and velocity of motion displayed in different formats or modes.

SPECTRAL DOPPLER ECHOCARDIOGRAPHY

- With spectral Doppler, the velocity of blood flow is calculated in a region of interest selected by aligning a cursor parallel with flow on a 2D echocardiographic image and then plotted as a graph of blood flow velocity against time (Figure 4.3).
- Blood flow velocities toward the transducer are displayed as positive (above the baseline), and blood flow velocities away from the transducer are displayed as negative (below the baseline).
- The Doppler shift can also be represented by an audible sound because the shift in frequency is usually small and within the audible range (around 10 kHz) so that most machines will show a visual spectral display with a simultaneous audible signal.
- Spectral Doppler is usually recorded with guidance from 2D echocardiographic images (2D Doppler, or duplex Doppler). This allows a cursor to be superimposed over a 2D image, showing the angle of interrogation of the Doppler beam in two dimensions.
- Spectral Doppler can be further subdivided into pulsed wave, continuous wave, and high-pulse repetition frequency.

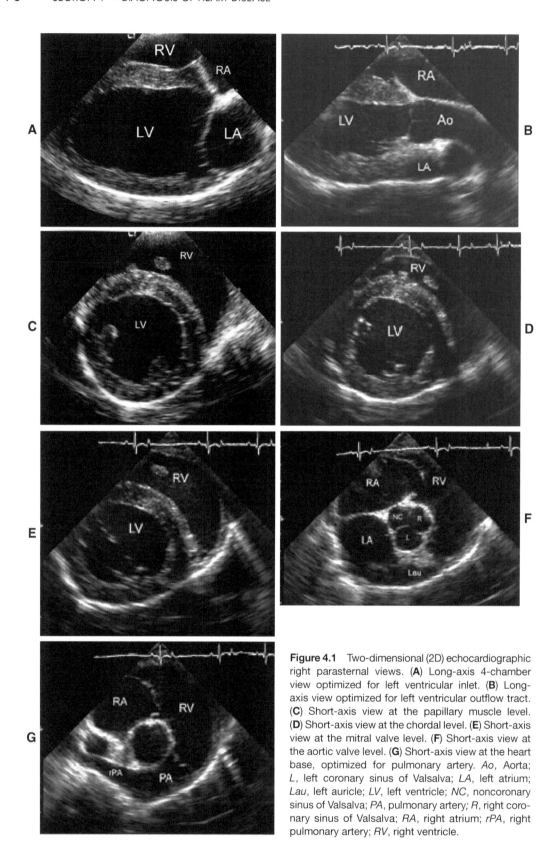

Figure 4.1 Two-dimensional (2D) echocardiographic right parasternal views. (**A**) Long-axis 4-chamber view optimized for left ventricular inlet. (**B**) Long-axis view optimized for left ventricular outflow tract. (**C**) Short-axis view at the papillary muscle level. (**D**) Short-axis view at the chordal level. (**E**) Short-axis view at the mitral valve level. (**F**) Short-axis view at the aortic valve level. (**G**) Short-axis view at the heart base, optimized for pulmonary artery. *Ao*, Aorta; *L*, left coronary sinus of Valsalva; *LA*, left atrium; *Lau*, left auricle; *LV*, left ventricle; *NC*, noncoronary sinus of Valsalva; *PA*, pulmonary artery; *R*, right coronary sinus of Valsalva; *RA*, right atrium; *rPA*, right pulmonary artery; *RV*, right ventricle.

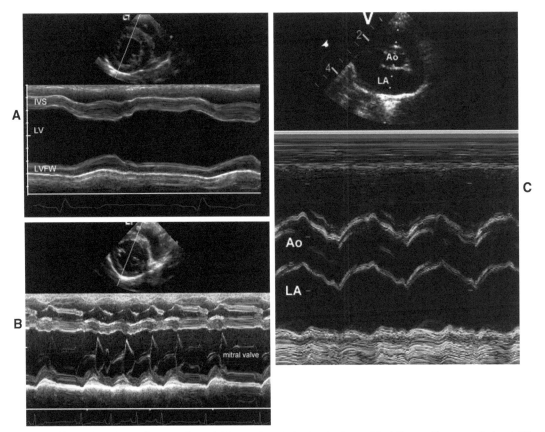

Figure 4.2 M-mode echocardiograms from right parasternal short-axis views: (**A**) at the papillary muscle level; (**B**) at the mitral valve level; (**C**) at the aortic (*Ao*) and left atrial (*LA*) level in a cat. *IVS,* Intraventricular septum; *LV,* left ventricle; *LVFW,* left ventricular free wall.

PULSED WAVE DOPPLER

- The ultrasound waves are transmitted as pulses of waves, with the transducer acting at different times as a receiver or transmitter of ultrasound waves, allowing the interrogation of blood flow velocities within a specific region of interest.
- This region of interest is represented as a *sample volume* on the cursor.
- Pulsed wave Doppler has limitations in the maximum velocities that it can display without ambiguity: high velocities result in "aliasing," where blood flow will be displayed as both positive and negative velocities (i.e., signal wraps around the baseline).
- The velocity at which aliasing will occur depends on the *Nyquist limit* (half the pulse repetition frequency), with higher velocities less likely to alias with the use of lower transducer frequencies and with reduced depth from the transducer.

CONTINUOUS WAVE DOPPLER

- In contrast, with continuous wave (CW) Doppler echocardiography, ultrasound waves can be transmitted and received simultaneously. This allows much higher velocities to be displayed, but it is

not possible to draw any conclusions about the depth along the cursor from where these velocities are originating (i.e., there is *range ambiguity*).

HIGH-PULSE REPETITION FREQUENCY DOPPLER ECHOCARDIOGRAPHY

- High-pulse repetition frequency Doppler echocardiography is a form of pulsed Doppler echocardiography that shares some similarities with CW Doppler echocardiography. Frequent pulses of ultrasound waves are produced so that a number of sample volumes will be superimposed on the 2D image. This not only allows the display of higher velocities without aliasing, but also increases the number of possible sites from which the velocities are being recorded.

COLOR FLOW DOPPLER ECHOCARDIOGRAPHY

- Color flow Doppler echocardiography represents the velocity and direction of blood flow in color, superimposed on a black-and-white 2D image (Figure 4.4). In effect, the color is displayed within a very large sample volume superimposed on the 2D image. Blood flow

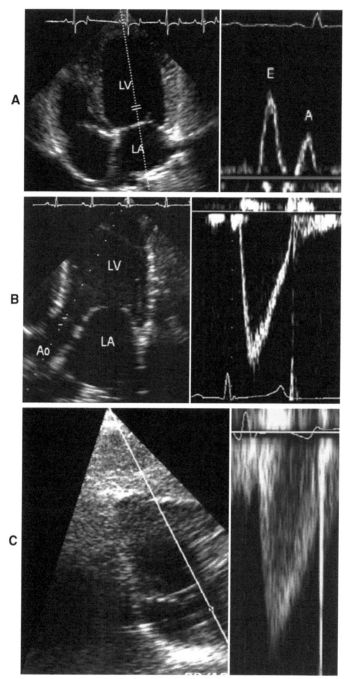

Figure 4.3 Doppler echocardiographic studies. **(A)** Mitral inflow obtained from the left caudal parasternal (apical) 4-chamber view, with the cursor placed parallel with mitral inflow, and a small sample volume placed at the tips of the mitral valve leaflets when the mitral valve is open. The typical spectral Doppler waveform of mitral inflow displays an early diastolic (*E*) wave and an atrial contraction (*A*) wave of filling. **(B)** Aortic flow obtained from the left caudal parasternal (apical) "5-chamber" view, showing left ventricular outflow tract and placement of pulsed wave sample volume in ascending aorta. The typical spectral Doppler waveform of aortic flow is displayed. **(C)** Aortic flow obtained from the subcostal view, showing continuous wave (CW) cursor positioned in ascending aorta. The typical spectral Doppler waveform of aortic flow is displayed.

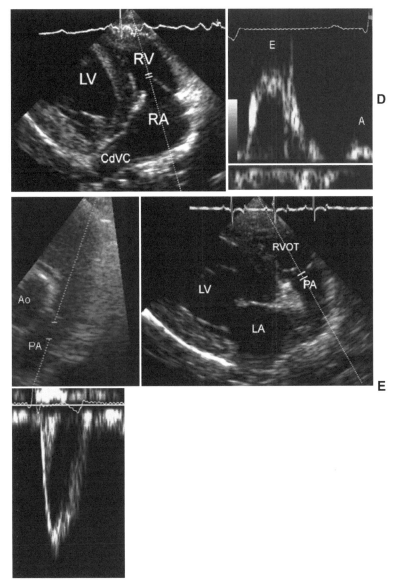

Figure 4.3, cont'd   (**D**) Tricuspid valve flow obtained the left cranial parasternal view optimized for right ventricular inflow. The pulsed wave sample volume is placed at the tricuspid leaflet tips, with the probe in a cranial position. The spectral waveform is similar to that of mitral inflow, although sometimes an additional systolic forward flow wave is recorded. (**E**) Pulmonary artery flow from the right parasternal short axis view and from the left cranial parasternal view optimized for the pulmonary artery. The typical spectral Doppler waveform of pulmonary artery flow is displayed. *Ao,* Aorta; *CdCV,* caudal vena cava; *LA,* left atrium; *LV,* left ventricle; *PA,* pulmonary artery; *RA,* right atrium; *RV,* right ventricle; *RVOT,* right ventricular outflow tract.

away from the transducer is shown in blue, and blood flow toward the transducer is displayed in red ("BART": *b*lue *a*way, *r*ed *t*oward). Disturbed or turbulent flow may be displayed in green or yellow. Aliasing may also occur in color flow Doppler echocardiography.

TISSUE DOPPLER IMAGING

• More sophisticated machines may include facilities for recording the velocity of myocardial motion. The signals reflected by the moving myocardium are high amplitude but low velocity. These myocardial velocities can be displayed in spectral format, as a color display, or as color M-mode (Figure 4.5, *E*). It is thought that tissue Doppler imaging (TDI) indices may have advantages over conventional echocardiographic indices because they may be less influenced by loading conditions.

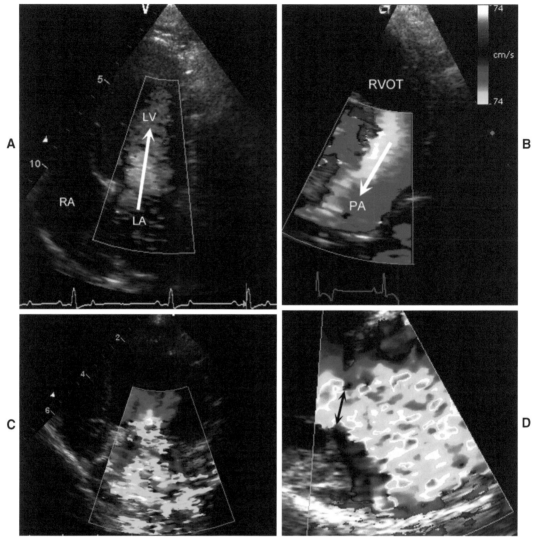

Figure 4.4   Color flow Doppler echocardiographic images. (**A**) Normal mitral inflow in a left caudal parasternal view, showing blood flow toward the transducer in red. (**B**) Normal pulmonary artery flow in a right parasternal short axis view, with blood flow away from the transducer shown in blue (a few pixels are coded as yellow because of "aliasing" when blood flow velocity exceeds the Nyquist limit; in this case, at >74 cm/sec). (**C**) Severe mitral regurgitation in a left apical four chamber, with a large color jet filling the left atrium. (**D**) Right parasternal long-axis view of a dog with severe mitral regurgitation, showing a large vena contracta diameter (*black arrow*). *LA,* Left atrium; *LV,* left ventricle; *PA,* pulmonary artery; *RA,* right atrium; *RVOT,* right ventricular outflow tract.

APPLICATIONS OF DOPPLER ECHOCARDIOGRAPHY

- Doppler echocardiography is used to characterize abnormal direction or velocity of blood flow, or to indicate the origin of turbulent blood flow. Doppler echocardiography can also be used to estimate differences in intracardiac pressures between chambers and to assess systolic and diastolic function.
- *Abnormal blood flow direction* may be noted with conditions such as valvular insufficiency.
- *Abnormal blood flow velocity* can be used to deduce abnormal chamber pressures because the velocity of blood flow across an orifice is chiefly determined by the difference in pressure. If there is a large difference in the pressures of the chambers on each side of a valve, then the velocity of flow across the valve will be high. For example, during systole the pressure in the left ventricle is very high, and the pressure in the left atrium is very low. If the mitral valve is incompetent and regurgitation occurs,

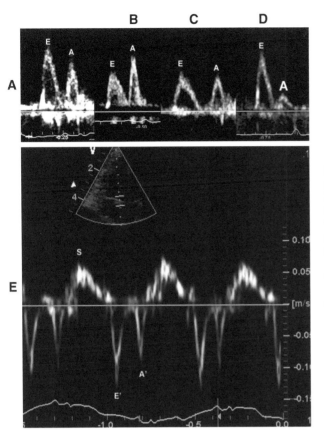

Figure 4.5 Spectral Doppler transmitral flow showing different diastolic filling patterns. (**A**) Normal transmitral flow pattern demonstrating an early filling wave (*E*) with higher velocity than the atrial contraction wave (*A*). (**B**) Delayed relaxation transmitral flow pattern demonstrating reduced amplitude and prolonged duration of the E wave. (**C**) Pseudonormal transmitral flow pattern demonstrating a normal E:A velocity ratio, but this is the result of the combined effects of delayed relaxation, increased left atrium (LA) pressures, and increased left ventricle (LV) stiffness. (**D**) Restrictive transmitral flow pattern. High LA pressures result in increased E wave amplitude despite delayed relaxation. Decreased LV compliance (sometimes with atrial systolic dysfunction) results in a diminished A wave. (**E**) Pulsed wave tissue Doppler imaging (TDI) of mitral annulus velocity, displaying a systolic wave (*S*), early diastolic wave (*E'*), and atrial wave (*A'*).

then the velocity of the regurgitant jet traveling from the left ventricle to the left atrium will be very high, reflecting the large difference in pressures. Conversely, for much of diastole, the pressure in the left atrium is only slightly higher than the pressure in the left ventricle so that the velocity of the early filling (E) wave is fairly low. This velocity information can therefore be used to derive information about intracardiac pressures.

- *Turbulent blood flow* is relatively uncommon in the normal heart, but when present, it most likely occurs where velocity is highest (i.e., within the aorta). Even in a normal heart, vigorous ejection into the aorta can sometimes result in signal aliasing on color Doppler echocardiography. Blood flow will be turbulent whenever velocity is high, and valvular insufficiency or stenosis almost inevitably results in turbulent blood flow. Turbulent blood flow may be displayed in a different color (green/yellow) or color distribution (mosaic pattern); this is termed *variance*. In most cases, turbulent flow will be present when a murmur is audible, making Doppler echocardiography particularly useful in conditions where a murmur is present.

- *Assessment of pressure gradients* (PGs) is possible with the modified Bernoulli equation, where [4 × (blood flow velocity)^2] gives the difference in pressure across a valve or between chambers.
- *Diastolic dysfunction* can also be assessed with Doppler echocardiography, although many measurements are influenced by loading conditions. Evaluation of transmitral and pulmonary venous flow in conjunction with TDI indices can suggest abnormal left ventricular (LV) relaxation and filling pressures.

ECHOCARDIOGRAPHIC TECHNIQUE

EQUIPMENT

ECHOCARDIOGRAPHIC MACHINES

- Almost all echocardiography machines have appropriate software for cardiac measurements and will be capable of 2D and M-mode imaging, and higher specification machines will also have the facility for Doppler echocardiography. Image quality remains the most important feature, and appropriate transducer choice is also essential. High-specification machines may have additional options such as TDI or even three-dimensional (3D) echocardiography.

TRANSDUCERS

- Linear scanners are unsuitable for echocardiography because of the limited acoustic window available between ribs.
- Sector probes produce a fan-shaped arc of ultrasound waves, so they will provide a wide image of the far field from a small acoustic window. These are ideal for cardiac applications.
- Types of sector probes include the following:
  - *Curvilinear* probes which are similar to linear probes but have a rounded surface. They tend to produce good images when the footprint is placed between ribs, but rib shadows are a problem when they are rotated through 90 degrees.
  - *Phased array* transducers are also available and have an array of crystals that are electronically fired in sequence to produce the fan-shaped wavefront. They are more expensive, but they have better beam focusing.
- Low frequency transducers have high penetrating power but poor resolution, whereas high frequency transducers have low penetrating power but high resolution.
- Most transducers have a wide frequency bandwidth that allows a single probe to operate at more than one frequency, but ideal results are not usually obtained across the entire bandwidth.
- Higher-end machines may have *harmonic imaging*, which results in a better signal-to-noise ratio.

KEY POINT

Although the information that can be obtained from echocardiography is greatly affected by the ultrasound machine and transducer, the echocardiographer's level of skill and training have the greatest impact.

ECHO TABLE

- Most echocardiographers position animals in lateral recumbency and approach from underneath, with the probe on the dependent chest wall. This minimizes air artifact in the lung tissue between the probe and the heart. The ideal table will have a wedge-shaped cut-out rather than a circular hole, and it should be covered with a comfortable but hygienic surface.

PATIENT PREPARATION

CLIPPING

- Most dogs will need to be clipped for echocardiography. In some short-coated breeds and cats, good acoustic contact may be obtained with liberal use of alcohol and acoustic gel (but check first that the transducer in use is not damaged by alcohol).

SEDATION

- The ideal is to perform echocardiography on patients without sedation, but a sedated patient may be better than a restless one because it can be impossible to obtain the necessary images without adequate patient cooperation. A reasonable compromise for most canine and feline patients is either butorphanol alone or butorphanol with low-dose acepromazine. General anesthesia and alpha-2 agonists will affect systolic function and may affect ventricular dimensions. Sometimes offering treats can work as well as sedation to distract the patient and prevent movement.

ELECTROCARDIOGRAPHY

- An ECG should be obtained simultaneously to allow accurate timing of measurements. Adhesive ECG electrodes are more comfortable than traditional alligator clips and can be attached with tape or bandage, and electrical contact can be maintained with additional alcohol, if necessary.

KEY POINT

Recording a concurrent ECG allows a much longer period of screening for arrhythmias than would normally be practical with an ECG machine and a paper trace.

ECHOCARDIOGRAPHIC VIEWS

TWO-DIMENSIONAL IMAGING

- A consistent technique should be adopted so that the same views are obtained in the same sequence with each study. Some views may be more difficult to obtain in some patients. The most commonly used imaging planes are obtained with the transducer on the right side of the chest (right parasternal views; see Figure 4.1). Views obtained from the left apical windows (caudal and cranial left parasternal views; see Figure 4.3) are mainly used for Doppler echocardiography applications, but as with radiography, it is helpful to confirm lesions in more than one view.

DOPPLER IMAGING

- Most Doppler recordings can be made from the left parasternal view, with the subcostal view preferred for aortic velocities. Color Doppler echocardiography used in the right parasternal views can be used for screening for mitral and aortic insufficiency. The features of blood flow across each valve are listed in the following sections. Normal values for blood flow velocity are derived from several studies (see the Suggested Readings) and are summarized in the following sections.

PULMONARY ARTERY FLOW

- Pulmonary artery flow is recorded from the right parasternal short-axis view or the left cranial parasternal position (see Figure 4.3, E). Both should be recorded in an attempt to record the highest velocity. A large sample volume should be used to minimize aliasing.
- There is usually one single systolic envelope, away from the transducer, with peak velocities <1.5 m/sec.
- There may be some positive flow (toward the transducer) during diastole associated with pulmonic insufficiency. A small amount of pulmonic insufficiency is common in healthy dogs and *is usually considered a normal finding*.

AORTIC FLOW

- Aortic flow is recorded from the left caudal parasternal (apical) 5-chamber (see Figure 4.3, B) or from the subcostal position (see Figure 4.3, C). The subcostal view usually allows the best alignment with flow. A large sample volume should be used to minimize aliasing.
- There should be one single systolic envelope, away from the transducer, with peak velocities <1.7 m/sec (left caudal parasternal view) or <2.0 m/sec (subcostal).

MITRAL INFLOW

- Mitral inflow is recorded from the apical four- or two-chamber view (see Figure 4.3, A). As small a sample volume as possible should be used, with the sample volume placed at the leaflet tips during diastole.
- Two peaks of flow are generally recorded, corresponding to early passive filling at the start of diastole (the E wave: 0.5 to 1.0 m/sec) and filling across the mitral valve during atrial contraction (the A wave: 0.3 to 0.6 m/sec).

TRICUSPID FLOW

- Tricuspid flow is recorded one or two intercostal spaces cranial to the position for mitral inflow (see Figure 4.3, D). As small a sample volume as possible should be used.
- Two peaks of flow are recorded, corresponding to early passive filling at the start of diastole (the E wave: 0.3 to 0.9 m/sec) and filling

across the tricuspid valve during atrial contraction (the A wave: 0.3 to 0.6 m/sec). In addition, a systolic forward wave is sometimes recorded, corresponding to vena caval inflow.

ECHOCARDIOGRAPHIC MEASUREMENTS

- Echocardiography is ideally suited to identification of structural lesions, but quantitative assessment of cardiac dimensions and function is also important. Echocardiography allows quantification of chamber dimensions, systolic and diastolic performance, valve function, and hemodynamic estimates (e.g., intracardiac pressures).
- Measurements should be repeated in three to five cardiac cycles (or more, with atrial fibrillation) to obtain an average. Ectopic beats and postectopic beats should be avoided for measurements.

LEFT VENTRICULAR DIAMETER

- LV diameter is typically measured from M-mode images (Figure 4.6, A).

M-MODE MEASUREMENT TECHNIQUE

- Measure from "leading edge" to "leading edge."
- Diastolic measurements are made at onset of QRS (LVDd).
- Systolic measurements are made at peak excursion (LVDs).
- Average several beats, particularly if the rhythm is irregular.

PROBLEMS WITH LEFT VENTRICULAR DIAMETER MEASUREMENTS

- Poor alignment may result in diameter inaccuracies.
- Because of difficulties in the establishment of normal reference intervals for a widely varying canine population, various strategies are used to take into account size variation:
  - Allometric scaling, where LVDd is divided by [body weight]$^{0.294}$ (95% prediction intervals <1.73)
  - Ratio indices, with LVDd divided by aortic diameter
  - Breed-specific reference intervals

INDEX OF SPHERICITY

- One solution to the problem of identifying LV dilation (eccentric hypertrophy) in a wide range of breeds is to measure the long axis from a 2D image and divide by the M-mode LV diameter because LV dilation usually results in a more spherical chamber (caused by a bigger increase in diameter than length). Normal values >1.65 have been reported but only in limited breeds.

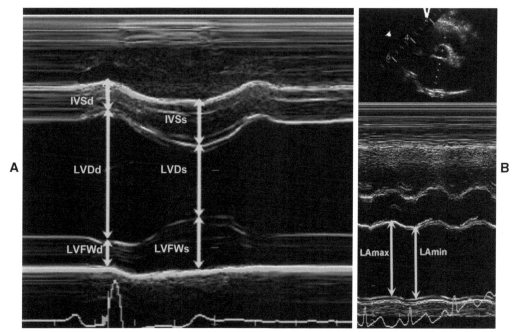

Figure 4.6 M-mode measurements. **(A)** M-mode at papillary muscle level, showing measurements at end-diastole (onset of QRS) and end-systole (peak septal motion). **(B)** M-mode at the aortic level, showing measurement of left atrial fractional shortening (LAFS%). *IVSd*, Septal thickness in diastole; *IVSs*, septal thickness in systole; *LAmax*, maximal left atrial diameter; *LAmin*, minimal left atrial diameter; *LVDd*, left ventricular diameter in diastole; *LVDs*, left ventricular diameter in systole; *LVFWd*, left ventricular free wall in diastole; *LVFWs*, left ventricular free wall in systole.

LEFT VENTRICULAR WALL THICKNESS

- Detection of LV hypertrophy is more important in cats than in dogs because hypertrophic cardiomyopathy (HCM) is so important in cats. M-mode imaging planes may miss localized areas of hypertrophy or erroneously include papillary muscles so that wall thickness is best measured from 2D images if the frame rate is adequate. 2D echocardiography has the advantage of allowing measurements irrespective of the location of hypertrophy.
- Measurements *must* be made at end-diastole, when the walls are at their thinnest. There is a risk of overestimating wall thickness from 2D images with machines with slow frame rates.
- LV septal and free wall thickness should be measured in several 2D views, taking care to avoid linear endocardial structures ("false tendons").
- LV hypertrophy is usually defined in cats as an end-diastolic septal or free wall thickness ≥6 mm, and LV walls of most normal cats will be <5 mm, with a "gray zone" of uncertainty between these values. There is some increase in LV wall thickness with increasing body weight.

LEFT ATRIAL DIAMETER

- Left atrial (LA) size is measured from a 2D short-axis view or a 2D long-axis view.

- ***Right parasternal short-axis view:*** The LA diameter/aortic diameter ratio (LA/Ao) should be <1.6. Measurements are usually made in early diastole, in the first frame where the aortic leaflets are visible. Pulmonary veins are often present in this view, complicating identification of the far LA wall (Figure 4.7, *A*).
- ***Right parasternal long-axis views:*** The LA/Ao ratio should be <2.5, where the aortic diameter is measured from a right parasternal long-axis five-chamber view at the valve level during systole, and the LA diameter is measured in a four-chamber view perpendicular to the long axis (Figure 4.7, *B*).
- In cats, there is no need to normalize the LA diameter to the aortic diameter; absolute diameter should be <1.6 cm (note, however, that this is a technically difficult view to achieve in cats).

KEY POINT

LA size is one of the most important echocardiographic measurements, particularly in chronic valve disease and feline cardiomyopathy, where it is essential for staging and assessing prognosis. It is also a key measurement in the assessment of patients with respiratory distress, where the presence of LA enlargement suggests an increased risk of congestive heart failure.

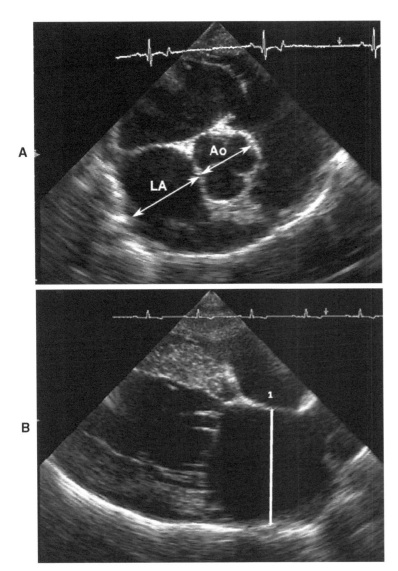

Figure 4.7 Measurement of the left atrial (*LA*) and aortic (*Ao*) diameters from the right parasternal short-axis view (**A**) and LA diameter from the right long-axis view optimized for the left ventricular inlet (**B**).

LEFT ATRIAL FUNCTION

- LA function is also an important prognostic indicator in cats, and it can be evaluated with M-mode images at the level of the aortic valve in a right parasternal short-axis view (see Figure 4.6, *B*).
- LA fractional shortening (LAFS%) is the percentage change in LA diameter, measured from the maximal LA diameter (LAmax) and the minimal LA diameter (LAmin). It is calculated as the following:

  LAFS % = [(LAmax − LAmin)/LAmax] × 100.

- Normal LAFS% values in cats are reported to be between 18% and 38%.

LEFT VENTRICULAR SYSTOLIC FUNCTION

- Many different echocardiographic measurements can be made to assess systolic performance, but virtually all are affected by ventricular loading conditions.
- Loading conditions include the degree of LV end-diastolic stretch (preload) and the forces opposing LV ejection (afterload).

FRACTIONAL SHORTENING

- LV fractional shortening (FS%) is the most commonly used echo index of systolic function (Figure 4.8, *A*) and is calculated as the following formula:

  FS % = [(LVDd − LVDs)/LVDd] × 100.

- FS% will increase with improved contractility, increased preload, or decreased afterload, and it only assesses ventricular shortening in the minor axis dimension.
- Normal reported *mean* values range from 25% to 40%, with lower values in larger dogs

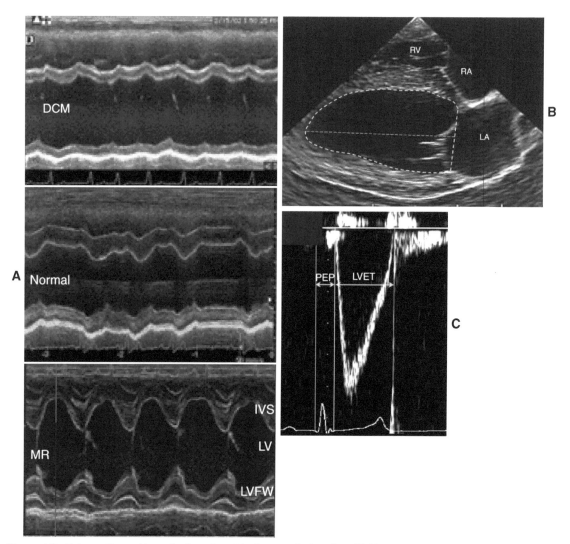

Figure 4.8 Echocardiographic evaluation of ventricular systolic function. **(A)** M-mode of ventricular hypokinesis from a dog with dilated cardiomyopathy (*DCM*) (*top panel*), normal ventricular motion from a healthy dog (*middle panel*), and ventricular hyperkinesis from a dog with mitral regurgitation (*MR*) (*bottom panel*). *IVS,* Intraventricular septum; *LV,* left ventricle; *LVFW,* left ventricular free wall. **(B)** Measurement of left ventricular volume from a right parasternal long-axis view. The endocardial borders are traced, with the left ventricular length measured from a line drawn across the mitral annulus to the apex. *LA,* Left atrium; *RA,* right atrium; *RV,* right ventricle. **(C)** Spectral Doppler aortic blood flow velocity, showing pre-ejection period (*PEP*) and left ventricular ejection time (*LVET*).

and possibly athletic dogs. Note that individual normal dogs may have values less than 25%.

END-SYSTOLIC VOLUME INDEX

- End-systolic volume index (ESVI) is end-systolic volume divided by body surface area; it is thought to be a measure of LV systolic function.
- LV volumes should be measured from 2D images, *not* from indices derived from M-mode such as with the Teichholz formula.

- Endocardial borders of the LV are traced in a right parasternal long-axis or left caudal parasternal view, and an area-length formula or modified Simpson rule is generally used to calculate LV end-diastolic volume (EDV) and LV end-systolic volume (ESV) (see Figure 4.8, *B*).
- Normal ESVI is often quoted as 30 mL/m², although this value has been extrapolated from human reference ranges and may not be accurate for dogs. The relationship with body weight may not be linear.

EJECTION FRACTION

- Calculation of LV volumes allows calculation of ejection fraction (EF%):

$$EF\% = [(EDV - ESV)/EDV] \times 100.$$

- Normal EF% in dogs is 50% to 65%.

SYSTOLIC TIME INTERVALS

- The ratio of preejection period (PEP) and LV ejection time (LVET) is another global index of systolic function, and it can be measured from the spectral Doppler aortic velocity waveform (see Figure 4.8, *C*). Normal PEP/LVET should be <0.40.

VALVE FUNCTION

- Color Doppler can be used as a quick screen for valve function, but caution should be used in determining severity of valvular regurgitation by regurgitant jet size or in relying on the presence of turbulent signals to identify valvular stenosis.

MITRAL INSUFFICIENCY

- 2D echocardiography is very important in the assessment of mitral insufficiency. It should be used to determine whether structural valve disease is responsible or whether the mitral insufficiency is secondary to an increase in LV dimensions.
- Mitral insufficiency can be assumed to be severe when the following criteria are present:
  - Large regurgitant jet area compared with LA area
  - Increased width of the vena contracta (see Figure 4.4, *D*)
  - Presence of a large proximal flow convergence region
  - High-intensity CW spectral Doppler signal
  - Increased mitral E wave velocity
  - Dilated left atrium or left ventricle (in chronic mitral valve disease)
- Similar criteria apply to tricuspid regurgitation on the right side of the heart.

AORTIC INSUFFICIENCY

Less common than mitral insufficiency, aortic insufficiency is considered severe when the following criteria are present:

- Large aortic insufficiency jet diameter compared with aortic valve area in a short-axis view
- Increased width of vena contracta
- Rapid deceleration of aortic insufficiency noted on spectral Doppler signal

AORTIC AND PULMONIC STENOSIS

- The severity of aortic or pulmonic stenosis is generally assessed in terms of the magnitude of the PG across the stenosis.

KEY POINT

PGs across a valve or between chambers can be estimated with the modified *Bernoulli equation:*
PG (pressure gradient, mm Hg) = 4 × (V²)
where V = velocity of blood flow distal to the orifice (m/sec). For example, if the velocity in the aorta is 5 m/sec, then the PG can be estimated as 4 × (5²), or 4 × 25 = 100 mm Hg. This means that the LV systolic pressure is 100 mm Hg greater than the aortic systolic pressure (or absolute LV pressure is around 240 mm Hg if systemic blood pressure is 140 mm Hg in systole).

DIASTOLIC FUNCTION

- Diastolic function is complex: clinically relevant aspects of diastolic function include LV relaxation, LV compliance, LA pressures, LA systolic function, and heart rate and rhythm. Clearly, no single echocardiographic measurement will provide a complete overview of diastolic function, although the presence of LA enlargement indicates hemodynamic disturbances that result in increased LA pressures. A range of Doppler measurements can be used to give a composite assessment of diastolic function or highlight specific aspects.

TRANSMITRAL FLOW

- Transmitral flow reflects the instantaneous pressure gradient across the mitral valve. There is a progressive change in the ventricular filling pattern with advancing disease across a range of underlying cardiac diseases (see Figure 4.5, *A* through *D*). The principal difficulty with use of transmitral flow patterns is the confounding effect of a "pseudonormal" phase, where the transmitral flow pattern is similar to that seen in the normal animal. Transmitral flow patterns should therefore be interpreted in the context of other clinical and echocardiographic findings. Pulmonary venous flow patterns and TDI of mitral annular velocities (see Figure 4.5, *E*) have been used to distinguish pseudonormal filling from normal.

COMMON ACQUIRED CARDIAC CONDITIONS

DEGENERATIVE (MYXOMATOUS) MITRAL VALVE DISEASE

- Degenerative mitral valve disease (endocardiosis) is relatively straightforward to diagnose in older small-breed dogs, although echocardiography is the principal technique for confirming a diagnosis.

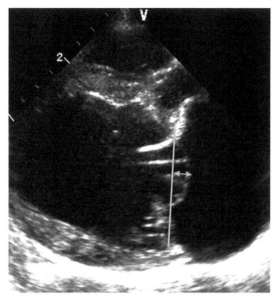

Figure 4.9 Myxomatous mitral valve disease. Right parasternal long-axis view showing thickened, distorted mitral leaflets with prolapse of the anterior leaflet (*green arrow,* extending beyond line drawn across mitral annulus).

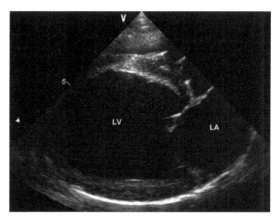

Figure 4.10 Dilated cardiomyopathy (DCM) in a dog. Right parasternal long-axis view, showing a rounded left ventricle (*LV*) with normal mitral valve appearance (and no mitral valve prolapse). *LA,* Left atrium.

ROLE OF ECHOCARDIOGRAPHY

- Diagnosis
  - Prolapse of thickened mitral leaflets (Figure 4.9)
  - Color Doppler jet of mitral insufficiency (often eccentric)
  - Hyperdynamic LV wall motion with severe mitral insufficiency (see Figure 4.8, *A*)
  - In severe cases, a flail leaflet following rupture of a chordae tendineae
- Staging preclinical mitral valve disease
  - Dogs with normal left heart dimensions (stage B1) remain free of clinical signs for longer than dogs with increased diastolic LV diameter or LA dilation (stage B2).
- Identifying pulmonary hypertension
  - Dogs with high-velocity tricuspid regurgitation associated with pulmonary hypertension may benefit from treatment with sildenafil.

DILATED CARDIOMYOPATHY

- In the presence of clinical signs of congestive heart failure, dilated cardiomyopathy (DCM) is a relatively easy diagnosis to make, with global hypokinesis of a dilated heart in the absence of any other lesions (Figure 4.10). Occult DCM is more difficult, and caution is advised when diagnosing DCM in asymptomatic dogs. DCM should not be diagnosed on the basis of a low

fractional shortening value alone (especially in dogs of nonpredisposed breeds).

ROLE OF ECHOCARDIOGRAPHY

- Diagnosis
  - Dilation of LA and LV
  - ± Dilation of right atrium (RA) and right ventricle (RV)
  - LV hypokinesis (decreased FS%, EF%) (see Figure 4.8)
  - Increased E point-septal separation (EPSS)

HYPERTROPHIC CARDIOMYOPATHY

- HCM is very common in cats, with a wide spectrum of disease. It can be difficult to differentiate cats with mild HCM from normal cats, but it is fortunately easier to identify cats at high risk of congestive heart failure or aortic thromboembolism (Figure 4.11).

ROLE OF ECHOCARDIOGRAPHY

- Diagnosis:
  - End-diastolic septal or LV free wall thickness is >6.0 mm on 2D echocardiography or M-mode.
  - Systolic anterior motion of the mitral valve is common in cats with HCM and causes dynamic LV outflow tract obstruction.
- Prognosis
  - The most important indicators of a poor prognosis are poor LA function, LA dilation, LV systolic dysfunction, and extreme LV hypertrophy (>9 mm).
  - Additional markers of increased congestive heart failure or thromboembolic risk include presence of spontaneous echocontrast

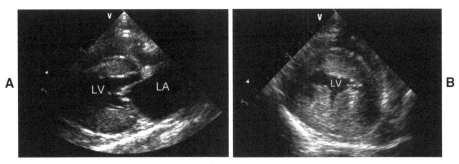

Figure 4.11 Hypertrophic cardiomyopathy (HCM) in a cat. Right parasternal long-axis view (**A**) and short-axis view at the papillary muscle level (**B**), showing marked left ventricular (*LV*) hypertrophy and left atrial (*LA*) enlargement.

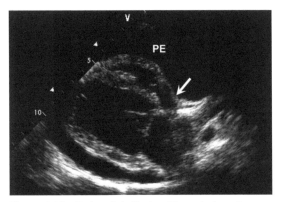

Figure 4.12 Pericardial effusion. The echolucent space around the heart is a pericardial effusion (*PE*), which is causing collapse of the right atrium (RA) (cardiac tamponade, *arrow*).

("smoke") and a restrictive diastolic filling pattern.

PERICARDIAL DISEASE

- *Pericardial effusions* can be identified as an echo-free space around the heart, although they may be confused with pleural effusions. Tamponade is suggested by collapse of the right atrial wall (Figure 4.12). The heart may be affected by a number of different neoplasms that can result in pericardial effusions, and these are most easily imaged while some pericardial fluid is present. Some pericardial effusions are considered idiopathic, although failure to identify a mass lesion does not rule out a neoplastic cause (mesotheliomas are extremely difficult to diagnose with echocardiography).
- *Chemodectomas* generally involve the heart base and may be imaged as homogeneous soft tissue densities encircling the aortic and pulmonary artery roots.
- *Hemangiosarcomas* frequently affect the RA, although they can be difficult to image at this site. They may also infiltrate other areas of the heart (such as the septum and ventricular walls) where they may have an irregular echotexture compared with surrounding myocardium.

FREQUENTLY ASKED QUESTIONS

Can any ultrasound machine be used for echocardiography?

A. Most ultrasound machines in small animal practices can be applied to imaging the heart, although a sector probe will be required. The echocardiographer's level of training and experience is usually a bigger issue. For novice echocardiographers, identification of pleural effusions is achievable with relatively little practice. Assessment of LA size is much more challenging, but time and effort spent on obtaining (and interpreting) a short-axis view at the LA level is very worthwhile, as this is such useful information.

How important is it to measure cardiac chamber dimensions?

A. Measurements are not helpful unless the recorded image is of high quality and the measurer uses a consistent technique. For this reason, for less experienced echocardiographers, it may be more reliable to make a qualitative echocardiographic assessment than to base a clinical decision on suboptimal measurements.

How does one interpret a low value for fractional shortening in an otherwise healthy dog?

A. Caution should be used when making a diagnosis of DCM in an asymptomatic dog based on a fractional shortening value <25%. Multiple other variables should be assessed, including evidence of chamber dilation, any increase in ESVI, whether the EF% is also subnormal, and systolic time intervals (PEP/LVET). Guidelines have been proposed for a scoring scheme for diagnosis of DCM in asymptomatic dogs (see Dukes-McEwan J, et al. in Suggested Readings).

SUGGESTED READINGS

Bonagura J, Luis Fuentes V: Echocardiography. In Mattoon JS, Nyland TG, eds: Small animal diagnostic ultrasound, ed 3, St. Louis, 2015, Saunders.

Boon JA: Veterinary echocardiography, ed 2, Chichester, West Sussex, 2011, Wiley-Blackwell.

Borgarelli M, Crosara S, Lamb K, et al.: Survival character-istics and prognostic variables of dogs with preclinical chronic degenerative mitral valve disease attributable to myxomatous degeneration, J Vet Intern Med 26:69, 2012.

Cornell CC, Kittleson MD, Della Torre P, et al.: Allome-tric scaling of M-mode cardiac measurements in normal adult dogs, J Vet Intern Med 18:311, 2004.

Dukes-McEwan J, Borgarelli M, Tidholm A, et al.: Proposed guidelines for the diagnosis of canine idiopathic dilated cardiomyopathy, J Vet Cardiol 5:7, 2003.

Reynolds CA, Brown DC, Rush JE, et al.: Prediction of first onset of congestive heart failure in dogs with degenera-tive mitral valve disease: the PREDICT cohort study, J Vet Cardiol 14:193, 2012.

Thomas WP, Gaber CE, Jacobs G, et al.: Recommendations for standards in transthoracic two-dimensional echocar-diography in the dog and cat, J Vet Intern Med 7:247, 1993.

Wess G, Mäurer J, Simak J, et al.: Use of Simpson's method of disc to detect early echocardiographic changes in Doberman pinschers with dilated cardiomyopathy, J Vet Intern Med 24:1069, 2010.

Special Diagnostic Techniques for Evaluation of Cardiac Disease

5

Meg M. Sleeper

Many special diagnostic techniques are available for evaluation of animals with cardiovascular disease. Ambulatory electrocardiographic (ECG) equipment is available through commercial services, continuous in-hospital ECG monitoring equipment is widely available, and several large diagnostic laboratories provide specialized clinical pathology services specific to the heart. Additionally, veterinary cardiology referral centers are increasingly available for special diagnostic techniques such as cardiac catheterization.

CONTINUOUS IN-HOSPITAL ELECTROCARDIOGRAPHIC MONITORING

Continuous ECG monitoring is recommended for hospitalized patients at risk of heart rate or rhythm disturbances. These patients include the following:

- Patients with congestive heart failure
- Patients hospitalized with clinical signs (e.g., syncope) secondary to arrhythmia
- Patients with systemic disease that puts them at risk for arrhythmias (e.g., shock, sepsis, gastric dilation-volvulus, etc.)

TECHNIQUE

- Continuous ECG monitoring requires an ECG unit with an oscilloscope or light-emitting diode (LED) display.
- Use of a chest lead configuration with adhesive electrode patches will minimize artifacts on the tracing while allowing the patient the most freedom for mobility.
- Clip two 2- to 3-cm square areas at the left apex and the heart base (where the apex beat is palpable on the left chest and at the heart base caudal to the right or left scapula).
- Clean and de-fat the area with 70% isopropyl alcohol. Allow to dry.

- Place the positive electrode patch at the left apical site and the negative electrode at the heart base site. A ground electrode may be placed at either site (Figure 5.1).
- Apply a light chest wrap to secure the electrodes and wires.
- If a multiple-lead ECG unit is being used, then use the left arm electrode for the positive electrode, the right arm electrode for the negative electrode lead, and lead I for display/recording.
- If the patient is recumbent and unlikely to move, leads attached directly to the patient limbs can be used.
- Depending on the unit available, the signal is transmitted to the machine by cables or by radiotelemetry.
- Many ECG units will print out an ECG strip, which can be added to the permanent patient record.

LIMITATIONS

- Excessive patient motion may result in displacement of electrodes or motion artifact on the ECG.
- Adhesive patches may occasionally result in contact dermatitis.
- Electrical interference can occur from other monitoring or therapeutic machinery (i.e., fluid pumps, heating pads, blood pressure measurement equipment).

PROVOCATIVE ELECTROCARDIOGRAPHIC TECHNIQUES

In some patients, the history or baseline ECG is suggestive of pathologic arrhythmias, but a definitive diagnosis is elusive. In these cases, vagal stimulation or abolition may be informative. A provocative vagal maneuver will transiently elevate parasympathetic tone. In normal animals, the technique typically slows the heart rate or

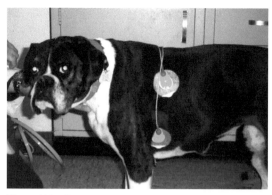

Figure 5.1 Chest lead preparation in a Boxer. The negative lead should be placed in the upper patch behind the scapula, and the positive lead should be placed at the left apex (behind the elbow). This configuration can be used for in-hospital continuous electrocardiographic (ECG) monitoring or ambulatory monitoring.

has no effect. However, when there is sinoatrial or atrioventricular (AV) nodal dysfunction, or an abnormal sensitivity to parasympathetic tone, transient sinus arrest or significant AV block may occur. Similarly, a vagal maneuver may be diagnostic or therapeutic for an ectopic supraventricular tachycardia (SVT). A sinus tachycardia typically slows over several seconds, whereas an ectopic SVT may terminate abruptly (see Frequently Asked Questions).

An ECG recorded immediately after exercise may demonstrate cardiac arrhythmias associated with increased sympathetic tone or abolition of arrhythmias caused by high resting vagal tone. Likewise, an atropine response test can also be used to determine if a slow heart rate is associated with elevated vagal tone, as can occur with respiratory disease, gastrointestinal disease, or neurologic disease, or is associated with primary cardiac conduction system disease. If the bradycardia is due to elevated vagal influence, then atropine administration or exercise will result in its abolition.

VAGAL MANEUVER

- The following techniques can be used for elevating vagal tone. The patient should be restrained and calm so that a good quality lead II ECG is obtained before and during the technique.

OCULAR PRESSURE

- Moderately firm digital pressure is applied over the closed eyelid to one or both eyes for a period of 5 to 10 seconds or until significant slowing of the heart rate occurs.

CAROTID BODY MASSAGE

- The carotid bodies are located in the area behind the larynx. Apply moderate digital pressure around the larynx while monitoring the ECG. Initiation of a gag response or a cough yields similar results and suggests adequate pressure has been applied.

INHIBITION OF VAGAL TONE

- Two techniques are possible for abolishing vagal tone and are useful if the patient is suspected of having a vagally mediated bradycardia. With either technique, it is important to first obtain a baseline ECG.

POSTEXERCISE ELECTROCARDIOGRAPHY

- Typically, strenuous leash running is used; however, the duration of exercise is not standardized. Evidence of exertion, such as panting, is sufficient to stop exercise, and an immediate postexercise ECG is obtained. A delay of as little as 30 seconds may alter results, and heavy panting can result in artifacts making the ECG difficult to interpret.

ATROPINE RESPONSE TEST

- Atropine (0.04 mg/kg intravenously or intramuscularly) will result in abolition of vagal influence. An ECG should be obtained 10 to 15 minutes after administration of the drug for comparison with the baseline ECG.

CLINICAL UTILITY

VAGAL MANEUVER

The vagal maneuver is clinically useful in two scenarios:

- In the evaluation of dogs with a history of syncope, a vagal maneuver may demonstrate sinus arrest or AV block, suggestive of parasympathetic hypersensitivity or primary nodal disease.
- In dogs with tachycardia, abrupt termination of the arrhythmia with a vagal maneuver suggests an ectopic supraventricular origin because ventricular tachycardias are not usually sensitive to vagal tone; however, lack of response is not helpful in differentiating the origin of the tachycardia. The maneuver can also be useful to differentiate sinus tachycardia (no response or gradual slowing of heart rate) from pathologic ectopic SVT (no response or abrupt termination of tachycardia).

POSTEXERCISE ELECTROCARDIOGRAPHY

- This test can be performed in the evaluation of dogs with subaortic stenosis or occult cardiomyopathy. In affected dogs, the combination of exercise, myocardial disease, and left ventricular hypertrophy may result in ECG indicators of myocardial ischemia (e.g., ST segment depression or ventricular ectopy). Lack of response does not necessarily rule out heart disease. In dogs with bradycardia, abolition of the arrhythmia after exercise suggests a vagally mediated etiology. The increased availability of ambulatory ECG recordings has markedly reduced the use of postexercise ECGs in clinical practice.

ATROPINE RESPONSE TEST

- Sinus tachycardia with a heart rate greater than 135 beats/min suggests normal sinus node function in the dog. In addition, this response suggests that medical management with vagolytic therapy may be effective if the bradycardia is associated with clinical signs, such as syncope or collapse, and implantation of a pacemaker is not possible. Atropine administration commonly induces transient type I or II AV block. Parasympathomimetic effects occur most rapidly and parasympatholytic effect is greatest after intravenous administration.

KEY POINT

Provocative ECG techniques are easily performed, relatively inexpensive, and can be very helpful for diagnostic and therapeutic purposes in animals with bradycardias and/or tachycardias.

AMBULATORY ELECTROCARDIOGRAPHY (HOLTER MONITORING AND CARDIAC EVENT RECORDING)

INDICATIONS

Routine in-hospital electrocardiograms provide only a glimpse of daily ECG activity. Moreover, arrhythmia detection may be confounded by iatrogenic changes in the autonomic nervous system activity. A 24-hour ambulatory (Holter) recording of the ECG increases the sensitivity of arrhythmia detection. Major indications include the following:

- Detection of transient arrhythmias associated with syncope or periodic weakness
- Screening of breeds at high risk for cardiomyopathy (e.g., Boxers, Doberman Pinschers)
- Evaluation of frequency, severity, and significance of arrhythmias detected on in-hospital ECGs
- Monitoring efficacy of antiarrhythmic therapy (e.g., control of heart rate in patients with chronic atrial fibrillation)
- Determining the true incidence and type of arrhythmia in patients with heart disease

TECHNIQUE

Holter monitors use a high-fidelity digital recorder to capture and store the cardiac electrical activity for 24 hours. Some digital recorders are capable of monitoring the patient for up to 7 days. Two to three simultaneous ECG chest leads are typically recorded.

- Electrode sites are prepared by clipping, shaving, cleaning, and drying the chest.
- Adhesive patches are firmly adhered to the skin (see Figure 5.1).
- A chest wrap is essential for securing electrodes, wires, and the recorder. A vest or harness can also be used (Figure 5.2).
- Once the monitor has been applied, the animal returns home to resume normal activity. Very small dogs and cats that find it cumbersome to ambulate with the monitor in place may respond better to hospitalization with cage restraint during the 24-hour recording session.
- Owners or caretakers should maintain a diary of significant changes in activity, such as sleeping, exercising, and so on. Any clinical signs such as syncopal events must be noted.
- At least 24 hours should be evaluated to assess a full circadian cycle.
- At the conclusion of the recording period, the components are removed, and the monitor is analyzed with the aid of automated computer-based software. Operator interaction and editing are essential for diagnostically accurate results.
- Consultation with a veterinary cardiologist is recommended regarding the significance of any identified arrhythmias and the need for therapy. Many normal dogs will have infrequent ventricular premature complexes or

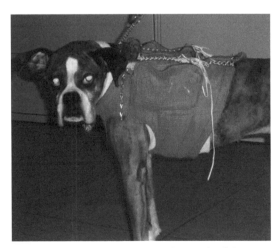

Figure 5.2 A vest can be placed over the light wrap, which secures Holter or cardiac event recorder (CER) monitor electrodes in place. The vest has pockets to hold the monitor and helps keep the device in place.

sinus pauses noted during a 24-hour period. Assessment of an arrhythmia's significance and the risk/benefit ratio of antiarrhythmic medications is essential.

CARDIAC EVENT RECORDERS

The cardiac event recorder (CER) is an ambulatory microprocessor with a solid-state memory loop capable of storing portions of ECG tracings when activated. The CER is lightweight, activated by a person witnessing an event (e.g., weakness or syncope), and can be worn by small dogs and cats without restricting activity. Unlike most 24-hour Holter monitors, which are worn for only 1 day, the CER can be worn for up to a week, increasing the diagnostic yield in animals with infrequent clinical signs.

- CERs can be programmed to store up to five separate, 1-minute duration, single-channel ECGs, or fewer ECGs of longer duration.
- Recording is activated by pressing the event button on the device. The CER uses a memory loop to store the ECG (most commonly 30 seconds before activation to 30 seconds after activation); however, these times may be changed as indicated for the individual patient.
- After one or more events, the CER is detached, and the stored ECG is transmitted and downloaded to a receiving station for computer-based analysis and interpretation.

APPLICATION

- The CER uses two adhesive electrodes in a base-apex configuration and is relatively easy to apply.
- A light chest wrap is used to secure the unit over the dorsum. As with Holter monitoring, the patient may be discharged to resume routine activity.

USE OF CARDIAC EVENT RECORDERS

- The CER will not store an ECG unless the activation button is pressed; therefore the event must be witnessed by the owner. If an event does not occur during the time the unit is worn, a definitive diagnosis is not possible.
- CERs may be rented from a commercial service, or the patient may be referred to a specialty practice offering this service.

IMPLANTABLE CARDIAC EVENT RECORDERS

- Implantable loop recorders are available for those unusual cases in which syncope is very rare and difficult to capture with a 7-day CER. These devices are small enough to implant subcutaneously in most dogs or cats. They are capable of monitoring the ECG for longer than 18 months and can be activated to store the ECG by a person observing an episode or can be programmed to store the ECG if the heart rate is slower or faster than the programmed limits (set at the time of implantation). The device is interrogated by a radiotelemetry device (similar to those used for pacemakers) to determine if unobserved episodes occurred. The devices require specialized programming and telemetry equipment, similar to that used in pacemaker implantation; they can be very helpful in cases with rare clinical signs (syncope).

> **KEY POINT**
>
> If syncope is very infrequent, then a CER, rather than a 24-hour Holter recording, is much more likely to result in definitive diagnosis.

NONSELECTIVE ANGIOGRAPHY

INDICATIONS

- Nonselective angiography is occasionally helpful to identify congenital or acquired abnormalities of intracardiac or intravascular blood flow. Abnormalities of the right side of the heart (e.g., right atrium, right ventricle, pulmonary arteries) are most readily identified by this technique. Echocardiography and ultrasound have superseded the need for this technique at most facilities.

TECHNIQUE

- Sedation or a light plane of anesthesia is usually necessary.
- A large-bore catheter (18 gauge or larger) is placed intravenously (preferably in the jugular vein).
- The animal is placed in the most appropriate position for opacification of the structures of interest (i.e., lateral recumbency for most cardiac defects, sternal recumbency to visualize pulmonary arteries).
- A large bolus of contrast is rapidly injected intravenously. Typically, 1 mL of radiopaque contrast per kilogram of body weight is used for the injection. Alternatively, the dose of iodine to be injected can be calculated, with 400 mg iodine per kilogram body weight as the desirable dose.
- A fluoroscopy unit allows continuous assessment. If fluoroscopy is not available, radiographic exposures are obtained 2 to 8 seconds after the injection is initiated (depending on

the structures of interest and cardiovascular performance). Shorter times should be used for evaluation of the right heart and pulmonary arteries and longer times for evaluation of structures on the left side of the heart or in animals with heart failure and slow circulation.

CLINICAL UTILITY

- Nonselective angiography is an alternative technique primarily used to evaluate lesions that involve the right side of the heart, particularly when echocardiography or cardiac catheterization either is not an option or is inconclusive.

LIMITATIONS, RISKS, AND COSTS

- Dilution of contrast material occurs as it moves through the circulation. Thus, nonselective angiography results in poor opacification of structures that are very distal to the site of injection (e.g., left side of the heart and systemic arteries).
- Timing of radiographs is difficult to predict, and several attempts are often required unless fluoroscopy is available.
- Intravenous contrast agents may result in transient hypotension, cardiac arrhythmias, nephrotoxicity (especially in patients with preexisting renal dysfunction), and allergic reactions.

KEY POINT

Nonselective angiography is significantly limited, particularly in the assessment of left-sided heart structures. Echocardiography, ultrasound, or both are preferred, and if the results remain inconclusive, cardiac catheterization and angiography are more likely to be diagnostic than nonselective angiography.

CARDIAC CATHETERIZATION

INDICATIONS

- In general, cardiac catheterization is defined as a combined angiographic and hemodynamic study undertaken for therapeutic or diagnostic purposes. The standard cardiac catheterization procedure for evaluation of congenital or acquired cardiac diseases typically includes measurement of intracardiac pressures, blood oximetry, and selective angiocardiography. The most common indication for cardiac catheterization in veterinary species is to ameliorate congenital heart disease (e.g., pulmonic stenosis or patent ductus arteriosus). For the purposes of diagnosis, advances in echocardiography have markedly reduced the need for routine cardiac catheterization.

TECHNIQUE

- Anesthesia is usually required.
- Surgical preparation of the neck (carotid artery or jugular vein) or inguinal area (femoral vein or artery) is required.
- Vascular access can be obtained by dissecting down to the vessel or with a percutaneous catheter introducer system with a modified Seldinger technique.
- Catheter advancement to the chamber of interest is performed under fluoroscopic or pressure waveform guidance (Figure 5.3).

OXIMETRY

- Blood samples are obtained from various cardiac or great vessel locations to measure oxygen saturation and to calculate shunt fraction in animals with congenital shunting defects.

ANGIOCARDIOGRAPHY

- Radiopaque contrast material is injected through the catheter(s) located at the appropriate areas of interest, and the image is recorded on videotape, radiographic film, or cineangiography; it can also be digitally stored (Figure 5.4). Postprocessing can be performed on digital images with digital subtraction techniques. The primary advantage over nonselective angiography involves superior opacification of structures of interest.

HEMODYNAMICS

- Cardiac output may be determined with thermodilution or indicator dye techniques.
- Intravascular or intracardiac pressures are recorded from chambers of interest. Pressures are typically recorded before and after therapeutic interventions (e.g., balloon valvuloplasty) to assess procedure efficacy.
- Additional procedures such as balloon valvuloplasty, patent ductus arteriosus coil occlusion, endomyocardial biopsy, heartworm retrieval, and cardiac pacing can be performed.

CLINICAL UTILITY

- Angiocardiography is valuable to diagnose cases of complex heart disease and to guide therapeutic interventions such as balloon valvuloplasty or patent ductus arteriosus occlusion. The approach provides useful morphologic and physiologic information regarding interventional responses to therapy.

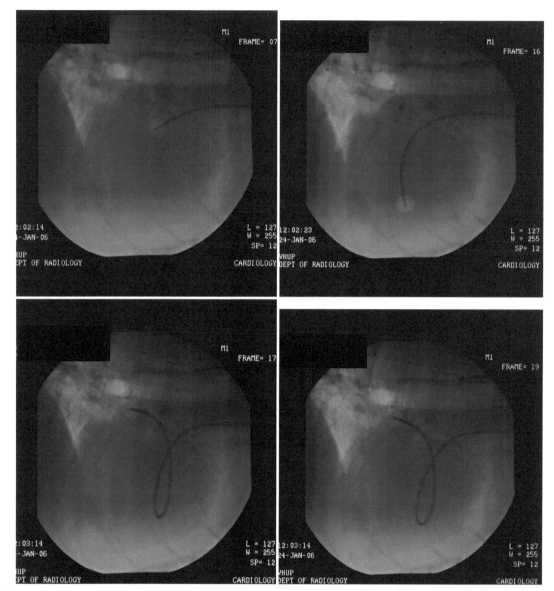

Figure 5.3   Fluoroscopically obtained images of a balloon-tipped cardiac catheter being placed into the right side of the heart. The catheter is advanced to the heart via the jugular vein. The balloon on the tip of the catheter facilitates traversing the tricuspid valve because it will tend to follow blood flow.

LIMITATIONS, RISKS, AND COSTS

- Cardiac catheterization requires specialized equipment and training and is typically limited to tertiary care facilities.
- The technique can be time consuming.
- Contrast solutions can result in hemodynamic abnormalities. Patients with severe heart disease or renal disease are at a relatively higher risk.
- Infection, cardiac arrhythmias, air embolism, vascular thromboembolism, or perforation are possible complications. With appropriate experience and case selection, mortality rate is low.

SEROLOGIC TESTING

INDICATIONS

Animals with clinical signs suggestive of myocardial dysfunction resulting from infectious or immune-mediated causes and animals at risk of myocardial toxicity from chemotherapeutic agents are candidates.

- Trypanosoma titer. Animals from Mexico, southern Texas, or other regions where Chagas disease is endemic, with right-heart failure.

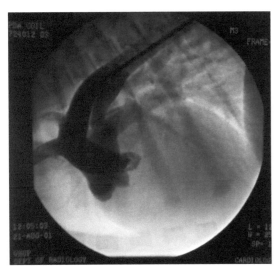

Figure 5.4 Selective aortogram demonstrating a patent ductus arteriosus with radiographic contrast material crossing the ductus and entering the pulmonary artery (left to right flow).

- Antinuclear antibody titer. Animals with heart failure or arrhythmias in addition to other clinical signs suggestive of immune-mediated disease.
- Toxoplasmosis titer. Cats with myocardial dysfunction, fever, pneumonia, neurologic disease, chorioretinitis, or other signs compatible with toxoplasmosis.

TECHNIQUE

- Serum or plasma should be submitted to a laboratory that has the appropriate facilities to perform the indicated serologic testing.

CLINICAL UTILITY

- In selected cases, these tests can be useful in establishing an etiologic agent and in monitoring patients at risk for myocardial toxicity. Results must be interpreted in concert with the patient's clinical signs.

LIMITATIONS, RISKS, AND COSTS

- These tests are limited only by correct interpretation. Otherwise, there are no particular risks. Costs are dependent on the laboratory.

NEWER CARDIAC IMAGING TECHNIQUES

- These techniques are becoming more widely available, and familiarity with their potential applications is helpful to identify referral candidates. Computed tomography (CT) and magnetic resonance imaging (MRI) are useful adjunctive techniques that are less invasive than angiocardiography and may be advantageous

over echocardiography for certain diseases such as cardiac neoplasia and pericardial disease. Nuclear scintigraphy is particularly useful for quantitative assessment of intracardiac shunts.

COMPUTED TOMOGRAPHY

- CT is an x-ray technique that displays cross-sectional images of the body.
- Assessment of cardiac function and precise definition of intracardiac anatomy requires either ECG gating or a millisecond CT scanner.
- An intravenous injection of contrast agent (iodinated or noniodinated) is used to define the blood pool.
- Multiple veterinary case reports have demonstrated the utility of cardiac CT for identifying or confirming less common structural heart diseases such as aortic coarctation, intrathoracic vascular abnormalities, and vascular ring anomalies.
- CT is becoming widely available for use in veterinary patients.

MAGNETIC RESONANCE IMAGING

- With MRI, a high natural contrast exists between blood and cardiovascular structures; therefore contrast medium is not required to discriminate the blood pool.
- Physiologic gating of the imaging sequence is necessary for cardiac imaging, and this capability may not be available at all facilities that offer MRI.
- Despite this limitation, as MRI has become more available, reports have demonstrated that it can add useful information regarding complex congenital heart disease and acquired diseases such as cardiac neoplasia.
- MRI gives useful information on cardiovascular morphology, function, and tissue character without ionizing radiation.

NUCLEAR CARDIOLOGY

- Gamma ray–emitting radiopharmaceuticals (radionuclides) are injected intravenously and either are extracted by the myocardium or remain in the blood pool. A scintillation (gamma) camera interfaced with a computer analyzes and stores the data.
- The direction and severity of congenital intracardiac shunts can be determined. Regional distribution of myocardial perfusion can also be visualized.

LIMITATIONS

The required technical expertise and expense of equipment limit use in general veterinary cardiology.

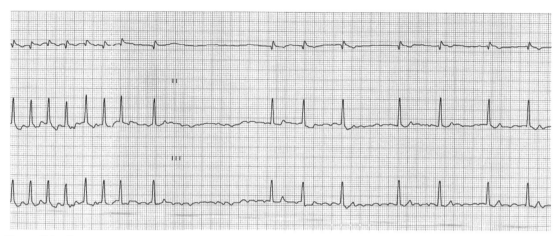

Figure 5.5 Simultaneous lead I, II, and III electrocardiographic (ECG) showing the effect of a vagal maneuver on a supraventricular tachycardia (SVT) (atrial fibrillation in this example). Note the dramatic slowing of the heart rate, which results in clearer demonstration of the hallmarks of atrial fibrillation (irregularly irregular rhythm, lack of P waves and fibrillation waves). 50 mm/sec; 10 mm/mV.

FREQUENTLY ASKED QUESTIONS

How is a vagal maneuver helpful when a dog with a suspected SVT is assessed?

An effective vagal maneuver will transiently increase vagal tone. The technique can be helpful to differentiate between sinus tachycardia, as during a normal physiologic response to pain, fever, and so on, and a pathologic ectopic SVT, such as paroxysmal atrial tachycardia. A gradual slowing of the heart rate (over several seconds) suggests the focus is sinus because the sinus node accelerates and decelerates gradually. An abrupt cessation of the tachycardia is suggestive of a pathologic focus (i.e., SVT). Lack of response to a vagal maneuver can occur with either condition and is nondiagnostic. Occasionally an SVT will respond to a vagal maneuver with slowed AV nodal conduction, resulting in second-degree AV block with an underlying rapid P-wave rate (Figure 5.5).

SUGGESTED READINGS

Gilbert SH, McConnell FJ, Holden AV, et al.: The potential role of MRI in veterinary clinical cardiology, Vet J 183:124–134, 2010.

Kittleson MD: Syncope. In Kittleson MD, Kienle RD, eds: Small animal cardiovascular medicine, St Louis, 1999, Mosby.

Miller MS, Calvert CA: Special methods for analyzing arrhythmias, In Tilley LP, ed: Essentials of canine and feline electrocardiography, ed 3. Malvern, Penn, 1992, Lea & Febiger.

Rishniw M, Kittleson MD, Jaffe RS, Kass PH: Characterization of parasympatholytic chronotropic responses following intravenous administration of atropine to clinically normal dogs, Am J Vet Res 60:1000–1003, 1999.

Rush JE: Syncope and episodic weakness. In Fox PR, Sisson DD, Moise NS, eds: Textbook of canine and feline cardiology, Philadelphia, 1999, Saunders.

Thomas WP, Sisson D: Cardiac catheterization and angiography. In Fox PR, Sisson DD, Moise NS, eds: Textbook of canine and feline cardiology, Philadelphia, 1999, Saunders.

Genetic and Biomarker Testing of Cardiovascular Diseases

6

Mark A. Oyama

Laboratory testing for cardiovascular disease is an attractive proposition because of the relative ease, availability, and low cost of blood-based testing. Laboratory testing can involve genetic testing for mutations associated with specific cardiac diseases or testing for circulating substances indicative of heart disease or injury. This chapter describes both forms of laboratory testing; however, the testing for genetic markers is very different from testing for the more general "biomarkers" of heart disease, and the indications for, and interpretation of, the two types of tests are considered separately. Genetic testing can be performed for hypertrophic cardiomyopathy (HCM) in the Maine Coon and Ragdoll cat, dilated cardiomyopathy (DCM) in the Doberman Pinscher, arrhythmogenic right ventricular cardiomyopathy (ARVC) in the Boxer, and subaortic stenosis (SAS) in the Newfoundland Retriever. Genetic testing helps identify young animals at risk for development of disease in adulthood and helps guide choice of breeding stock. Genetic testing might also help predict future morbidity and mortality in animals that have clinical disease.

A second type of laboratory testing involves substances released by the heart in proportion to presence and severity of disease. The two main types of cardiac substances that can be tested for in the dog and cat are markers of cardiomyocyte damage and natriuretic peptides that provide unique information about cardiac injury or hemodynamic stress, respectively. The most established indication for laboratory testing of cardiovascular disease is to help differentiate between cardiac and noncardiac causes of respiratory signs in dogs and cats. Other indications include diagnosis of occult cardiomyopathy, prediction of morbidity and mortality in dogs with myxomatous mitral valve disease, and diagnosis of myocarditis. As with any diagnostic test, the value of blood-based testing for cardiovascular disease depends on proper utilization and interpretation. The remainder of this chapter discusses the indications, techniques, clinical utility, and limitations of laboratory diagnosis in the assessment of heart disease.

GENETIC TESTING

INDICATIONS

- Genetic testing involves analysis of a patient's DNA for genetic abnormalities or mutations known to be associated with a specific disease entity. For mutations involving genes in the somatic (autosomal) chromosomes, results are reported as to whether the mutation is present in neither (negative), one (heterozygous), or both (homozygous) alleles.
- In many instances, the influence of one or more copies of the mutation is "incomplete," so that presence of the mutation does not automatically induce the disease. This "incomplete penetrance" means that many individuals, although carriers of genetic mutation, will not experience the disease during their lifetime. This is an important fact when considering the use of genetic testing for diagnosis of disease. The presence of the mutation does not equate to clinical disease. Conversely the most common acquired heart diseases of dogs and cats, including valvular and myocardial disease, most likely have more than one genetic association. In human beings, there are several hundred different mutations associated with HCM or DCM, and absence of any one single mutation does not ensure that the individual will remain disease free.
- In general, individuals that are homozygous for a mutation are at greater risk for developing disease and will produce offspring that have at least one abnormal copy of the gene. Thus, individuals that are homozygous for the mutation should not be bred. If animals that are heterozygous for the mutation are bred, they should only be bred to individuals that are negative for the mutation.

Genetic testing is mostly performed for the following reasons:

- Confirm a suspected diagnosis. In a patient with clinical findings suggestive of disease, the finding of an associated genetic abnormality can increase the likelihood of a positive diagnosis. The scenario in which this relationship is most reliable is one in which there is a single known genetic mutation that causes disease, and the disease is not caused by anything other than the mutation. In small animal cardiology, this is not the case for any of the known mutations or diseases.

- Detect individuals that are carriers of the mutation.
- Predict likelihood of future disease.
- Predict response to medication or therapy.

I use the veterinary genetics service at North Carolina State University (www.ncstatevets.org/genetics) to perform genetic testing for cardiac disease in the dog and cat. The veterinary genetics service at the University of California at Davis performs genetic testing for cardiac disease in the cat only (www.vgl.ucdavis.edu/services/cat/). Genetic tests are available for the following cardiac conditions:

- HCM in the Maine Coon cat
  - Test for a mutation in the autosomal gene that encodes for cardiac myosin-binding protein C (MBPC). This mutation, called A31P, affects the production of normal MBPC and is associated with idiopathic left ventricular concentric hypertrophy or HCM. The A31P mutation is highly prevalent in Maine Coons, with as many as 30% of individuals being heterozygous for the mutation. Cats that have the A31P mutation in one or both alleles are approximately twofold and eighteenfold more likely to develop HCM than are cats without the mutation, respectively. As heterozygous and homozygous cats reach adulthood, particular attention to screening for the development of clinical disease that involves physical examination, detection of heart murmurs or gallops, electrocardiography (ECG), cardiac biomarkers, or echocardiography should be considered. The A31P test can be used to help select breeding stock and hopefully reduce the prevalence of the mutation over successive generations. Homozygous cats should not be bred, and heterozygous cats should only be bred to negative cats.
- HCM in the Ragdoll
  - Test for a mutation in the autosomal gene that encodes for cardiac MBPC. This mutation, called R820W, affects the production of normal MBPC and is associated with idiopathic left ventricular concentric hypertrophy or HCM, much in the same way as the A31P mutation in Maine Coon cats. The R820W mutation is highly prevalent in Ragdolls, with as many as 30% of individuals being heterozygous for the

mutation. Cats that have the R820W mutation in one or both alleles are more likely to develop HCM than are cats without the mutation, respectively. As heterozygous and homozygous cats reach adulthood, particular attention to screening for development of clinical disease that involves physical examination, detection of heart murmurs or gallops, ECG, cardiac biomarkers, or echocardiography should be considered. The R820W test can be used to help select breeding stock and hopefully reduce the prevalence of the mutation over successive generations. Homozygous cats should not be bred, and heterozygous cats should only be bred to cats that are negative for the mutation.

- DCM in the Doberman Pinscher
  - Test for a mutation, the autosomal gene that encodes for pyruvate dehydrogenase kinase 4 (PDK4). This mutation likely affects glucose oxidation within myocardial cells and high-energy phosphate production. In one study, 68% of Doberman Pinschers with the mutation demonstrated clinical disease. The PDK4 mutation is not the only cause of DCM in Doberman Pinschers, and as many as 18% of Doberman Pinschers with DCM are negative for the mutation. Diagnosis of occult or preclinical DCM in adult Doberman Pinschers can be challenging (see Chapter 8) and is based on a combination of ECG, Holter recording, and echocardiographic findings. In adult dogs with equivocal findings, the presence of either a heterozygous or homozygous PDK4 mutation might sway one toward a positive diagnosis. In young dogs that are found to be heterozygous or homozygous, particular attention to annual screening for DCM starting at 4 years of age is recommended. The PDK4 test can be used to help select breeding stock and hopefully reduce the prevalence of the mutation over successive generations. Homozygous dogs should not be bred, and heterozygous dogs should only be bred to individuals that are negative for the mutation.
- ARVC in the Boxer
  - Test for a mutation in the autosomal gene that encodes for the protein striatin. Striatin is a desmosomal protein involved in the cell-to-cell junctions. Mutations in a variety of other desmosomal proteins are associated with ARVC in human beings. In one study, 59 of 62 Boxers (95%) with ARVC possessed the striatin mutation. Dogs that were homozygous were more likely to possess not only ventricular arrhythmias but also left ventricular myocardial failure (i.e., decreased contractility). Three dogs with ARVC were negative for the mutation, indicating that there are other still unidentified

causes of ARVC. There might be important geographic differences in the prevalence of the mutation because reports suggest that affected Boxer dogs from Europe are much less likely to be positive for the striatin mutation compared with dogs in the United States. In adult Boxers with equivocal findings, the presence of either heterozygous or homozygous striatin mutation might sway one toward a positive diagnosis. In young dogs that are found to be heterozygous or homozygous, particular attention to annual screening for ARVC starting at 4 years of age is recommended. The striatin test can be used to help select breeding stock and hopefully reduce the prevalence of the mutation over successive generations. Homozygous dogs should not be bred, and heterozygous dogs should only be bred to individuals that are negative for the mutation.

- SAS in the Newfoundland Retriever
  - Test for a mutation in the autosomal gene that encodes for PICALM (phosphatidylinositol-binding clathrin assembly protein), a protein involved in the development of the fetal heart and cell membrane vesicle formation. In one study, 25 of 26 Newfoundland Retrievers with SAS were found to possess the mutation. The presence of the mutation, however, does not automatically ensure presence of SAS because 6 of 23 healthy Newfoundland Retrievers had the mutation. In young dogs found to possess the mutation, particular attention to auscultation during the first year of life is recommended. SAS usually develops as puppies grow to their adult size, and if no murmur is detected beyond a year of age, the likelihood of developing disease during adulthood is low. The PICALM test can be used to help select breeding stock and hopefully reduce the prevalence of the mutation over successive generations. Homozygous dogs should not be bred, and heterozygous dogs should only be bred to individuals that are negative for the mutation.

TECHNIQUE

- DNA testing can be performed on a variety of sample types including a buccal mucosal (cheek) swab and whole blood.
- Cheek swabs are obtained with a special kit consisting of a sterile cotton or brush-tipped swab and a shipping package. The dog's or cat's mouth should be inspected before swabbing to ensure that no food particles are present in the cheek or lip folds. The swab is inserted into the animal's mouth between the cheek and gum line and external manual pressure is applied so that the tip is in contact with both the cheek and gum line as it is rotated along the inside of the animal's cheek for 10 to 15 seconds. The swab is withdrawn from the animal's mouth and allowed to air dry for 30 seconds before being inserted into the shipping package. It is important that nothing other than the animal's cheek touches the tip of the swab and that the collector does not blow on the tip to dry it before shipping. DNA is particularly hardy and resistant to degradation under most normal environmental situations. The main concern regarding the swab is overgrowth of bacterial contaminants. Thus the swabs should be completely dry before being sealed in the shipping envelope, and the swabs should not be stored in the refrigerator or shipped with cold packs because this can cause moisture to form within the packages. Two swabs should be collected from each animal to maximize the chances of successful DNA recovery.
- Two to 5 mL of whole blood collected in EDTA (ethylenediamine tetraacetic acid) can be used for genetic testing. The blood tubes should be adequately sealed and protected against breakage or leakage during shipping. The blood does not need to be refrigerated or shipped with cold packs.

KEY POINTS

- Genetic testing can be performed for HCM in Maine Coon and Ragdoll cats, for DCM in Doberman Pinschers, for ARVC in Boxer dogs, and for SAS in Newfoundland Retrievers.
- Genetic testing identifies mutations associated with disease and can help select individuals best suited for breeding. Individuals that are homozygous for the mutation should not be bred.
- The results of the genetic test, whether positive or negative, do not provide information about the presence or absence of cardiac disease or about cardiac function at the time of testing. Echocardiography and other diagnostics are required to determine cardiac function.
- A genetic test with a positive result increases the likelihood of disease development in the future, but because there are likely many other unknown mutations that are associated with disease, a genetic test with a negative result does not preclude the chance of the disease.

BIOMARKER TESTING

- Biomarkers are substances specific to a particular organ or tissue and are released in proportion to the presence and severity of injury or disease. Biomarkers are clinically useful if they provide information that is not readily available from other forms of diagnostic testing. Biomarkers, although a relatively new area of study in veterinary cardiology, are familiar in the setting of other organ systems such as the kidney (e.g., blood urea nitrogen and creatinine) or liver (e.g., GGT [gamma-glutamyl transferase]). Recommendations regarding biomarker testing at the time of this writing are relatively new and evolving. The interested reader is referred to more detailed discussion provided by the articles listed in the Suggested Readings section at the end of this chapter.

- Two main classes of cardiac biomarkers are currently evaluated in dogs and cats with heart disease: markers of myocardial tissue injury or necrosis, such as cardiac troponin-I (cTnI), and markers of neurohormonal activation and cardiac wall stress, such as the natriuretic peptides, B-type natriuretic peptide (BNP), N-terminal pro-B-type natriuretic peptide (NT-proBNP), and N-terminal pro-atrial natriuretic peptide (NT-proANP). Differences among BNP, NT-proANP, and NT-proBNP exist, but clinical utility among the different forms of the natriuretic peptides is likely to be similar. The vast majority of published studies involve assays for NT-proBNP.

- cTnI is a component of the actin-myosin contractile apparatus of the myocyte. Cell injury due to ischemia, inflammation, trauma, or other insults to the myocardium causes release of cTnI into the circulation, where it can be detected in plasma or serum samples.

BIOMARKERS ARE ELEVATED IN CARDIAC DISEASE

- Both the natriuretic peptides and cTnI tend to be elevated in the presence of cardiac disease. The most studied diseases include myxomatous mitral valve disease (MMVD), HCM, and DCM. Cardiac biomarkers also appear elevated in cases of restrictive cardiomyopathy (RCM) and congenital heart disease such as patent ductus arteriosus, although the amount of information regarding these diseases is relatively limited. Increased cardiac wall stress, ischemia, and neurohormonal activation trigger increased cardiac production of natriuretic peptides, although ischemia and myocardial cell injury result in the release of cTnI.

- Both biomarker types tend to be elevated in proportion to the severity of disease. Biomarker concentrations are correlated to radiographic heart size and the presence of congestive heart failure (CHF), and to echocardiographic indices of disease severity including left atrial (MMVD, DCM, HCM) and ventricular chamber dimensions (MMVD, DCM), contractility (DCM), and left ventricular wall thickness (HCM).

INDICATIONS FOR TESTING

The primary indications for cardiac biomarker testing include the following:

- Diagnosis or detection of occult cardiomyopathy in a cat suspected to be at high risk for disease
- Differentiation of cardiac compared with noncardiac causes of respiratory signs in the dog and cat
- Prognostic tool in dogs with MMVD or DCM

In many instances where biomarker testing is used to help achieve a diagnosis, testing helps clarify the need for additional diagnostics, such as thoracic radiography or echocardiography, rather than being the sole tool on which a diagnosis or clinical judgment is made.

Routine biomarker testing is *not* recommended for the following:

- Diagnosis or staging of MMVD in dogs
- Routine prescreening of anesthetic cases, particularly young healthy animals undergoing spay or neuter
- Routine screening of dogs or cats at low risk of cardiac disease

USE OF BIOMARKER TESTING FOR THE DETECTION OF OCCULT CARDIOMYOPATHY IN THE CAT

HCM and RCM are relatively common cardiac diseases in the adult and geriatric cat. Cardiomyopathy is characterized by an often long preclinical (occult) phase in which clinical signs of disease are absent or undetected despite the presence of underlying cardiac dysfunction. Cats at risk for occult cardiomyopathy include those with a heart murmur or gallop, arrhythmias, or radiographic cardiomegaly. The Maine Coon and Ragdoll breeds are especially predisposed to HCM. The utility of NT-proBNP in the detection of occult cardiomyopathy has been evaluated in multiple studies. Elevated NT-proBNP (>100 pmol/L) signifies an approximately fourfold increase in the risk of occult cardiomyopathy compared with cats with normal values. Studies involving cTnI reveal that most healthy cats have cTnI concentrations at or below the lowest limit of detection (<0.03 ng/mL) of the most sensitive assays, although cats with either occult or symptomatic HCM have a median cTnI of 0.66 ng/mL. NT-proBNP and cTnI values can overlap between cohorts of healthy and affected cats, and no single diagnostic value ensures either the presence of absence of disease. Incorporation of biomarker testing is best done in the early stages of assessment, and positive results are used to encourage pet owners to pursue further diagnostic testing such as echocardiography. Both cardiac biomarkers have high negative predictive values so that negative results indicate a very low likelihood of substantial cardiac disease. Accordingly, testing is most useful to help rule out the presence of cardiac disease (Table 6-1). False positives can occur with both NT-proBNP and cTnI, and clinicians are discouraged from indiscriminate testing of populations with low likelihood of disease, such as young healthy animals undergoing spay or neuter.

DIFFERENTIATION OF CARDIAC COMPARED WITH NONCARDIAC CAUSES OF RESPIRATORY SIGNS

Dogs and cats that have respiratory signs such as dyspnea, tachypnea, or coughing often represent a diagnostic dilemma with respect to the etiology of their signs. In the geriatric dog with coughing, the most common cause is either chronic airway disease or CHF due to MMVD. Because NT-proBNP is produced in response to cardiac volume overload, normal NT-proBNP values make the presence of CHF less likely than in animals with elevated values. As a result of the potential for symptomatic airway disease and subclinical MMVD or HCM (i.e., a dog with coughing as a result of a collapsing trachea and with concurrent mild MMVD, or a cat with asthma and occult HCM), the positive predictive value of NT-proBNP testing to identify cases of CHF is generally lower than the negative predictive value of the assay to rule out CHF. This is similar to the situation in human medicine wherein low natriuretic peptide results are used as a way to rule out CHF. In all instances, the decision to perform NT-proBNP testing and any subsequent results should be integrated into the results of the physical examination, medical history, and other diagnostics such as thoracic radiographs or echocardiography. For instance, in a small breed dog with coughing and without a heart murmur, biomarker testing is unnecessary as the likelihood of significant MMVD is low. In general, cTnI is less useful than NT-proBNP for differentiation of respiratory signs. cTnI is released secondary to cardiomyocyte injury, including ischemia that results from severe primary respiratory disease and hypoxemia. Thus, similar to NT-proBNP assay, positive cTnI results should be interpreted with caution (see Table 6-1).

PREDICTION OF MORBIDITY AND MORTALITY IN DOGS WITH MYXOMATOUS MITRAL VALVE DISEASE

One of the most intriguing applications for biomarker testing involves the potential of biomarkers

---

Table 6-1   Diagnostic Indications and Values for Use of NT-proBNP and cTnI Assay in Dogs and Cats*

Indication	Cutoff Assay Value and Interpretation
Detection of occult cardiomyopathy in cats	NT-proBNP: <49 pmol/L, disease unlikely NT-proBNP: >100 pmol/L, disease likely, echocardiography recommended cTnI: <0.03 ng/mL, disease unlikely cTnI: >0.16 ng/mL, disease likely, echocardiography recommended
Differentiation of respiratory signs in cats	NT-proBNP: >260 pmol/L, CHF is more likely NT-proBNP: <49 pmol/L, CHF is unlikely cTnI: >0.94 ng/mL, CHF is more likely cTnI: <0.94 ng/mL, CHF is less likely
Differentiation of respiratory signs in dogs	NT-proBNP: >1400 pmol/L, CHF is more likely NT-proBNP: <900 pmol/L, CHF is unlikely cTnI: assay hindered by high degree of overlap between causes
Prediction of morbidity and mortality in dogs with MMVD	NT-proBNP: >1500 pmol/L: future CHF is more likely NT-proBNP: <1500 pmol/L: future CHF is less likely NT-proBNP: >1500 pmol/L: future mortality is more likely NT-proBNP: >524 pmol/L and cTnI: >0.025 ng/mL: future mortality is more likely

*Cutoff values should be interpreted with caution as overlap between groups exists. Biomarker testing should be integrated with results of the physical examination, medical history, and other diagnostic tests as available.
CHF, Congestive heart failure; *cTnI,* Cardiac troponin-I; *MMVD,* myxomatous mitral valve disease; *NT-proBNP,* N-terminal pro-B-type natriuretic peptide.

to predict first-onset CHF and mortality in dogs with MMVD. A common clinical scenario involves assessment of risk of future CHF in a dog with asymptomatic MMVD. Typically, radiographic or echocardiographic left-sided heart and pulmonary vein size are used to assess disease severity and determine risk for development of pulmonary edema. Many cardiologists choose to start angiotensin-converting enzyme (ACE) inhibitors, increase frequency of rechecks, or counsel owners to monitor resting or sleeping respiratory rates in patients deemed at high risk. Study has indicated that elevated NT-proBNP in dogs with preclinical MMVD increases risk of CHF by almost sixfold compared with dogs with lower values (NT-proBNP >1500 pmol/L; 5.8-fold risk over dogs with lower values). This heightened risk is in addition to the risk due to radiographic cardiomegaly (vertebral heart size >12, 15.8-fold risk over dogs with smaller heart size) or echocardiographic left ventricular enlargement (left ventricular to aortic root dimension ratio >3.0; 6.1-fold higher risk than dogs with smaller left ventricular dimensions). Thus the dogs at highest risk for CHF are those with elevated NT-proBNP, large radiographic heart size, and increased left ventricular echocardiographic dimensions. Both NT-proBNP and cTnI are associated with increased risk of mortality. In one study, dogs with the highest NT-proBNP and cTnI values experienced significantly shorter survival than those with lower values. Currently, there is no substantial evidence indicating that therapy can be guided by or modified on the basis of cardiac biomarker values and lead to improved outcome. Thus I regard dogs with elevated cardiac biomarkers as candidates for closer monitoring, reexamination, or other testing rather than prescribed therapy. Note that diagnosis or routine staging of MMVD does not automatically include biomarker testing. Diagnosis and initial staging is easily accomplished by auscultation of the typical left-sided apical systolic murmur and thoracic radiography, respectively. In cases of MMVD, biomarker testing should be considered adjunctive to the physical, radiographic, electrocardiographic, and echocardiographic exam (see Table 6-1).

EFFECT OF EXTRACARDIAC DISEASE ON CARDIAC BIOMARKER TESTING

Both NT-proBNP and cTnI elimination is partly dependent on renal excretion, and values can be elevated in both dogs and cats with renal insufficiency. Both biomarkers can be elevated because of cardiac disease or injury as a result of primary extracardiac disease such as systemic hypertension, hyperthyroidism, or pulmonary hypertension. In animals with these conditions, elevated biomarker values can be difficult to interpret, and caution should be exercised.

TECHNIQUE

- Natriuretic testing is performed on serum or EDTA plasma. An in-house pet-side NT-proBNP assay that uses serum is available for detection of occult cardiomyopathy in cats.
- Proper sampling and handling of samples is required to obtain accurate results. Users should consult the guidelines and instructions that accompany each assay.

KEY POINTS

- Testing should be used in conjunction with the medical history, physical examination, and other diagnostics.
- Testing can be performed to help detect occult cardiomyopathy in cats, rule out CHF in dogs and cats with respiratory signs, and predict morbidity and mortality in dogs with MMVD.
- Elevated natriuretic peptide or cTnI in cats with heart murmurs, gallops, arrhythmias, or cardiomegaly indicates a high likelihood of underlying disease, and further diagnostics such as echocardiography should be pursued. Cats with low natriuretic or cTnI values are unlikely to have clinically meaningful heart disease.
- Normal natriuretic peptide or cTnI values in dogs and cats with respiratory signs indicate a low likelihood of CHF, and primary respiratory causes of the signs should be considered.
- Dogs with MMVD that have elevated natriuretic peptides and cTnI and radiographic or echocardiographic left-sided heart enlargement are at higher risk for CHF and mortality than dogs with lower values and smaller hearts. Dogs at high risk might benefit from greater scrutiny, reexaminations, reevaluation of treatment decisions, or closer monitoring at home.
- The potential of cardiac biomarkers to guide therapy and improve outcome is highly intriguing and is currently the subject of ongoing study.

SUGGESTED READINGS

Connolly DJ: Natriuretic peptides: the feline experience, Vet Clin North Am Small Anim Pract 40:559–570, 2010.

Connolly DJ, Brodbelt DC, Copeland H, et al: Assessment of the diagnostic accuracy of circulating troponin I concentration to distinguish between cats with cardiac and non-cardiac causes of respiratory distress, J Vet Cardiol 11:71–78, 2009.

Fox PR, Rush JE, Reynolds CA, et al: Multicenter evaluation of plasma N-terminal probrain natriuretic peptide (NT-pro BNP) as a biochemical screening test for asymptomatic (occult) cardiomyopathy in cats, J Vet Intern Med 25:1010–1016, 2011.

Herndon WE, Kittleson MD, Sanderson K, et al: Cardiac troponin I in feline hypertrophic cardiomyopathy, J Vet Intern Med 16:558–564, 2002.

Hezzell MJ, Boswood A, Chang YM, et al: The combined prognostic potential of serum high-sensitivity cardiac troponin I and N-terminal pro-B-type natriuretic peptide concentrations in dogs with degenerative mitral valve disease, J Vet Intern Med 26:302–311, 2012.

Oyama MA, Boswood A, Connolly DJ, et al: Clinical usefulness of an assay for measurement of circulating N-terminal pro-B-type natriuretic peptide concentration in dogs and cats with heart disease, J Am Vet Med Assoc 243:71–82, 2013.

Payne EE, Roberts BK, Schroeder N, et al: Assessment of a point-of-care cardiac troponin I test to differentiate cardiac from non-cardiac causes of respiratory distress in dogs, J Vet Emerg Crit Care (San Antonio) 21:217–225, 2011.

SECTION 2

CARDIOVASCULAR DISEASE

Acquired Valvular Disease

7

Jonathan A. Abbott

Acquired primary valvular disease in dogs and cats generally is degenerative or, less commonly, infective. Other pathologic processes, such as neoplasia, rarely affect the cardiac valves. Myxomatous degeneration of the mitral valve is the most common cardiac disease in the dog. Mitral valve incompetence caused by valvular degeneration can result in progressive cardiac enlargement and, in some cases, heart failure (HF). Clinical signs, including cough that might be caused by compression of the mainstem bronchi by an enlarged left atrium, may precede the development of cardiogenic pulmonary edema. The clinical consequences of degenerative valvular disease are observed primarily in elderly, small-breed dogs.

Infective endocarditis (IE) is an uncommon form of acquired valvular disease that is observed occasionally in dogs and rarely in cats. Middle-aged, medium- and large-breed dogs are affected most often. The clinical signs of IE relate to sepsis, thromboembolism, and HF.

DEGENERATIVE MITRAL VALVE DISEASE

Numerous designations for degenerative mitral valve disease (MVD) have been proposed on the basis of its clinical and pathologic features. The terms *myxomatous valvular degeneration, myxomatous transformation, mucoid degeneration, endocardiosis, chronic valvular disease,* and *degenerative valvular disease* all refer to the same disorder.

KEY POINT

Degenerative MVD is the most common cardiac disease in the dog; it is an acquired disease, and the prevalence is greatest in the geriatric population.

PREVALENCE AND INCIDENCE

- Degenerative MVD is the most common cardiac disease in the dog; it is an acquired disease, and the prevalence is greatest in the geriatric population.

- Clinical evidence of degenerative valvular disease is detected in approximately 30% of dogs aged 13 years and older.
- MVD is a progressive disease, and subtle changes in valve structure precede the development of clinically evident valvular dysfunction. Consequently, the prevalence of MVD detected by postmortem examination is higher than that reported in clinical studies.
- Postmortem evidence of advanced degenerative valvular disease was found in 58% of dogs older than 9 years; when mild degenerative changes are included, the postmortem prevalence exceeds 90% in dogs older than 13 years.
- MVD may affect any breed of dog, but clinical consequences of MVD are observed most often in small-breed dogs. Miniature Poodles, Pomeranians, Yorkshire Terriers, Chihuahuas, and other small dogs are commonly affected. The prevalence of MVD in Cavalier King Charles Spaniels is particularly high, and in dogs of this breed, the disease is sometimes clinically evident at a young age.
- Male dogs are affected somewhat more often than female dogs.
- Degenerative valvular disease is uncommon in cats, and when it occurs, it seldom results in clinical consequences.

PATHOLOGY

- MVD is grossly characterized by nodular distortion of the valve leaflets, as well as by thickening and, sometimes, lengthening of the chordae tendineae. The appearance of a small number of nodules at the free edge of the valve leaflet is the initial disease. As the disease progresses, these nodules increase in number and size and coalesce. In severe cases, the leaflets are contracted, and the free edge of the leaflet rolls inward toward the ventricular endocardium (Figure 7.1). When severe, these abnormalities prevent coaptation of the valve leaflets, resulting in mitral valve incompetence.
- MVD is histologically characterized by the deposition of mucopolysaccharides primarily

111

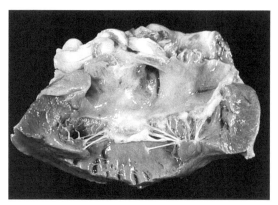

Figure 7.1 A specimen that demonstrates the gross features of severe mitral valve degeneration. The mitral valve leaflets are abnormally thick and nodular. (The author acknowledges the Department of Veterinary Pathology, Western College of Veterinary Medicine, University of Saskatchewan, Saskatoon, Canada, for providing this photograph.)

within the spongiosa layer of the valve leaflet. Fibrosis of the valve is also present but is not the dominant histologic feature. Inflammatory infiltrates are absent; MVD is a sterile, degenerative disease that bears no known relationship to endocarditis.

ETIOPATHOGENESIS

KEY POINT

The prevalence of endocarditis is no greater in dogs affected by MVD than in other, nonaffected dogs.

- The cause of MVD is unknown.
- MVD is often observed in chondrodysplastic dog breeds. Because MVD has been associated with concurrent disorders such as bronchomalacia and intervertebral disc disease, it has been suggested that MVD is one expression of a systemic connective tissue disease, although support for this supposition is lacking.
- Recent investigations of the molecular biology and biomechanics of MVD suggest that a complex interaction of mechanical stresses and signaling pathways leads to altered gene expression and induction of growth factors. A unified explanation for myxomatous transformation has not been established. However, an inductive effect of tensile and shear strains, conversion of valvular interstitial cells to a myofibroblastic phenotype, enzymes, and signaling molecules, including metalloproteinases, serotonin, and transforming growth factor, may all play a role.

- Because distinct breed predispositions are recognized, it is likely that there is a genetic predisposition for the development of MVD. Available evidence suggests that the tendency to develop MVD is not subject to simple Mendelian inheritance but is a polygenic trait or, if monogenic, subject to genetic or environmental comodification.
- In Cavalier King Charles Spaniels, parental status with respect to age and murmur intensity is an important determinant of the prevalence of murmurs in 5-year-old offspring.
- Recent genome-wide analyses of Cavalier King Charles Spaniels disclosed two chromosomal regions that are associated with MVD, but specific causative genes have not been identified.

PATHOPHYSIOLOGY

KEY POINT

The cause of MVD is unknown, but genetic factors are likely important.

- The mitral valve apparatus consists of the mitral valve leaflets, the fibrous valve annulus, the chordae tendineae, and the left ventricular papillary muscles.
- The two mitral leaflets are known as the septal (anterior) and the caudal (posterior) leaflets. In health, the mitral leaflets are thin, translucent structures that are tethered to the left ventricular papillary muscles by the chordae tendineae. The two left ventricular papillary muscles arise from the caudal (free) wall of the left ventricle. The basilar attachment of the mitral leaflets is to the fibrous left atrioventricular valve ring, known as the mitral annulus.
- The initiation of valve closure is a passive process; in early systole, when left ventricular pressure exceeds left atrial pressure, the mitral valve leaflets are forced into apposition. In normal individuals, the tethering effect of the chordae tendineae prevents prolapse, or bowing, of the leaflets into the left atrium.
- Coaptation of the normal mitral leaflets is complete, and there is little or no regurgitation through the valve orifice. The normal mitral valve ensures that the entirety of the left ventricular stroke volume is ejected through the aorta. When the mitral valve is incompetent, a fraction of the left ventricular stroke volume (regurgitant fraction) is ejected through the mitral valve orifice into the left atrium.
- Mitral regurgitation (MR) may be mild and have minimal consequences, or it can be severe.

The severity of MR is determined principally by the size of the regurgitant orifice and the relationship between left atrial and left ventricular systolic pressure. Potentially, both of these determinants can be pharmacologically manipulated by administration of vasodilators.

- MR increases left atrial pressure, which potentially results in left atrial dilation. When the mitral valve leaks, the pulmonary venous return is augmented by the regurgitant volume; in consequence, the ventricle is filled in diastole not only by blood that has returned from the lungs but also by blood that has been regurgitated into the atrium. Therefore MR imposes a volume load on the left ventricle and the left atrium.
- High end-diastolic pressures and volumes result in ventricular dilation and hypertrophy. Hypertrophy of this type, in which the ratio of wall thickness and chamber size remains roughly unchanged, is known as eccentric hypertrophy.
- Severe MR may increase left ventricular filling pressures. High filling pressures are reflected backward, raising pulmonary vein pressure and potentially initiating the development of pulmonary edema.
- The syndrome of clinical signs and neuroendocrine activation that results from cardiac dysfunction is known as HF. Because veterinary patients cannot offer subjective observations—for example, the perception of breathlessness during exertion—the presence of congestive signs is generally used as an objective criterion for the diagnosis.
- Congestive heart failure (CHF) is the syndrome of clinical signs caused by venous pressure elevations that result from cardiac dysfunction. Left-sided CHF is defined by the presence of cardiogenic pulmonary edema. Right-sided CHF refers to clinical signs that result from systemic congestion; in dogs, ascites is the most common manifestation of right-sided CHF.
- Because of maladaptive neuroendocrine responses associated with HF, cardiac dysfunction tends to be progressive. Because of this, the elimination of congestive signs does not signify resolution of the HF state. When the responsible disorder cannot be definitively corrected, HF is a terminal syndrome.
- The imposition of a chronic volume load on the heart can result in deterioration of systolic myocardial function, a state sometimes known as cardiomyopathy of overload. In general, MR is relatively well tolerated by the myocardium because the left atrium represents a low-pressure reservoir into which the ventricle can eject blood. In fact, dogs that have CHF caused by MR often do so at a time when systolic myocardial function (contractility) is, according to echocardiographic indices, normal or only mildly diminished.
- MR may remain clinically silent until it is advanced. When HF results from MR, clinical signs may include weakness, syncope, cough, and dyspnea.
- Cough is a centrally mediated reflex, and most cough receptors are located in the large airways. The cause of cough associated with MR in small-breed dogs may result from the following:
  - Pulmonary edema, when fluid floods the alveoli.
  - Reflexes mediated through stimulation of the juxtapulmonary (J) receptors; these receptors are associated with the pulmonary capillaries and are sensitive to increases in pulmonary venous pressure.
  - Compression of the mainstem bronchi by an enlarged left atrium.
  - Recent findings suggest that the pathogenesis of cough in patients with MVD is complex. For example, bronchoscopic evaluation of dogs with MVD that have a history of cough often reveals airway collapse, but this finding is not statistically associated with the presence of an enlarged left atrium. In spite of that, a recent retrospective investigation identified left atrial enlargement, but not radiographic pulmonary edema, as a risk factor for cough in patients with MVD.
- It is likely that the cause of cough observed in patients with MVD is multifactorial. Pulmonary congestion or edema, cardiac enlargement, and the presence of concurrent airway disease may all contribute.

CLINICAL PRESENTATION

HEART FAILURE

The number of distinct, extant definitions of "heart failure" is evidence of the semantic difficulty the term presents. It is now generally accepted that HF is a clinical syndrome characterized by congestive signs, exercise intolerance, or both that result from diseases that impair filling or emptying of the heart. In 2009, a working group of the American College of Veterinary Internal Medicine (ACVIM), Specialty of Cardiology, developed Guidelines for the Diagnosis and Treatment of Canine Chronic Valvular Heart Disease. A schema for classification of patients, modified from one proposed for the description of humans with HF, was presented. Traditionally, patients with HF have been categorized according to the degree of functional limitation that results from cardiac disease. Examples include the New York Heart Association Functional Classification and a similar system proposed by the International Small Animal Cardiac Health

Council. However, a classification of patients that is based on functional limitation is imperfect; such systems are poorly suited to the development of therapeutic guidelines partly because they do not reflect the progressive nature of the HF state. Furthermore, they do not take into account that the outcome of patients that have *never* had pulmonary edema is superior to those that have a *history* of edema that has resolved because of treatment.

In the ACVIM Guidelines, patients with MVD were classified as follows:

- Stage A: patients predisposed to the development of MVD/HF
- Stage B: patients with subclinical MVD
  - B1—without cardiac remodeling
  - B2—with cardiac remodeling
- Stage C: patients with MVD that have current *or prior* clinical signs
- Stage D: patients with refractory HF

HISTORY

KEY POINT

It is important to recognize that cough can be associated with MVD in the absence of pulmonary edema. When this is the case, the cough may be a sign of heart disease but not a sign of pulmonary edema; this distinction is important because a diagnosis of pulmonary edema carries important prognostic and therapeutic implications.

- MVD exhibits a broad spectrum of severity. In most affected dogs, MVD does not cause clinical signs, and the disease is detected when a cardiac murmur is incidentally identified in patients presented for routine health care or for management of noncardiac disease.
- In cases in which MVD does become clinically apparent, cough is usually the clinical sign that is first observed by the dog owner. Coughing associated with bronchial compression is often dry and harsh. When coughing is caused by pulmonary edema or congestion, other signs, such as exercise intolerance and tachypnea, are usually present. The cough associated with pulmonary edema may be moist and productive. The expectoration of pink froth is sometimes observed in patients with fulminant pulmonary edema.
- Occasionally, syncope is the clinical sign that is seen first in dogs with MVD. Syncope is a transient loss of consciousness caused by a sudden and precipitous decline in cerebral perfusion. MVD can be responsible for syncope when cardiac enlargement predisposes to arrhythmias. In addition, exertional syncope may result when

MR limits stroke volume so that cardiac output does not adequately increase to meet the physiologic demands of exercise. Alternatively, syncope on exercise or excitement or associated with paroxysmal cough can result from sudden onset of reflex-mediated bradycardia.
- Other clinical signs related to reduced cardiac performance, including tachypnea, exercise intolerance, and abdominal distention caused by ascites, occasionally prompt owners of affected dogs to seek veterinary attention.

PHYSICAL FINDINGS

- The most notable feature of the physical examination is a systolic murmur that is usually heard best over the left cardiac apex. The murmur of MVD is indistinguishable from the murmur caused by other disorders, such as IE or dilated cardiomyopathy (DCM), which also can result in MR. Importantly, however, an acquired, left apical, systolic murmur in an older, small-breed dog is almost always caused by MVD. The intensity of the murmur depends on a number of factors, but severe MR usually causes a loud murmur. Severe MR associated with a nonrestrictive regurgitant orifice can result in a soft murmur, but this is extremely uncommon in MVD. Phonocardiographically, the murmur of MR typically has a plateau-shaped configuration, meaning that the murmur has a similar intensity throughout systole; when the murmur is loud, the second heart sound (S_2) may be obscured (Figure 7.2).

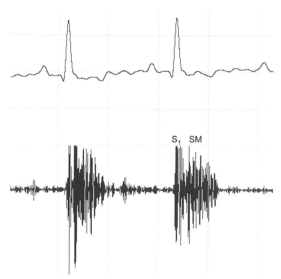

Figure 7.2 A phonocardiogram recorded from a 13-year-old female spayed mixed-breed dog with a grade 4/6 systolic murmur (*SM*). The SM begins at the first heart sound (S_1), is evident throughout systole and obscures the second heart sound (S_2).

- An exaggerated apical impulse is often evident on precordial palpation of patients with moderate or severe MR. By definition, a precordial thrill is present when the murmur intensity is grade 5/6 or greater.
- A high-frequency, midsystolic click (Figure 7.3) is sometimes heard in older, small-breed dogs. These clicks may be associated with mitral valve prolapse. In many dogs, clicks are a precursor of MR. Often, a soft systolic murmur of MR can also be heard in patients that have systolic clicks.
- When MR is severe, the third heart sound (S₃) is sometimes audible and results in an S₃ gallop. Care must be taken to distinguish a midsystolic click from a gallop. In general, a systolic click is louder than the S₃, and in patients with MVD, a click typically is heard in association with findings that suggest mild MR. In contrast, an S₃ gallop usually reflects severe MR and generally is heard in patients with loud murmurs. Note that S₃ is sometimes audible in patients with DCM. However, DCM is typically a disorder of large and giant-dog breeds.
- The femoral arterial pulse is usually of normal strength when MR is present, but the pulse may have a rapid rise. Very severe MR can be associated with diminished pulse strength.

- Crackles may be heard in patients with pulmonary edema. It should be recognized that the prevalence of primary respiratory diseases such as chronic bronchitis in the patients most often affected by MVD is relatively high. Primary respiratory tract diseases can explain adventitious pulmonary sounds, such as crackles, in the absence of pulmonary edema.
- Abdominal palpation is usually normal in patients with MVD, but hepatic enlargement or even ascites may be present when there is severe tricuspid valve disease or when pulmonary hypertension complicates the presentation of MVD.

PATIENTS WITH MITRAL REGURGITATION AND CONCURRENT RESPIRATORY TRACT DISEASE

- Primary diseases of the respiratory tract, such as collapsing trachea and chronic bronchitis, are common in the patient group that is affected by MVD. In an individual patient, it can be difficult to determine whether cardiac disease or respiratory disease bears the greatest responsibility for the development of clinical signs.
- In general, patients with severe MR are more likely than patients with respiratory disease to have poor body condition.

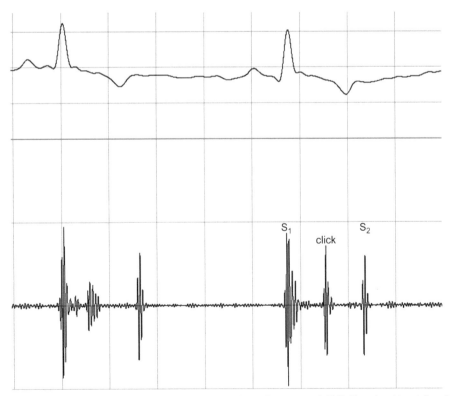

Figure 7.3 A phonocardiogram recorded from an 11-year-old male castrated Shih-Tzu. A midsystolic click (*click*) is shown. S₁, first heart sound; S₂, second heart sound.

- Although loud murmurs of MR are sometimes clinically inconsequential, it is extremely uncommon for soft murmurs to indicate severe MR with cardiac enlargement.
- The presence of respiratory sinus arrhythmia (RSA) can also be of diagnostic value. Much of the moment-to-moment heart rate variability observed in healthy dogs is due to the effect of vagal discharge. In patients with severe cardiac disease, there is little vagal influence on heart rate and rhythm, and as a result, RSA is not prominent. In contrast, sinus arrhythmia is often preserved or even accentuated when primary respiratory tract disease is responsible for clinical signs. The physical finding of RSA is virtually incompatible with the presence of cardiogenic pulmonary edema.
- Although exceptions occur, clinical signs are usually related to respiratory tract disease in patients that are overweight and have sinus arrhythmia and a soft cardiac murmur.
- In contrast, the clinical signs of thin patients with loud murmurs and tachycardia are more likely to result from cardiac disease or CHF.
- Coughing in elderly, small-breed dogs that do not have cardiac murmurs is almost always due to primary respiratory tract disease (Table 7.1).

LARGE-BREED DOGS WITH MITRAL VALVE DISEASE

- A syndrome of severe MR and concurrent myocardial dysfunction is recognized in medium- and large-breed dogs. The fact that this observation was made relatively recently is probably explained by the increasing availability of echocardiography and not by a change in the epidemiology of MVD. Before widespread availability of this technology, large-breed dogs with HF generally were assumed to have primary myocardial disease.
- For reasons that are unknown but may relate to the geometry or pattern of contraction of inherently larger ventricles, large dogs breeds with MR are more apt to have echocardiographically evident myocardial dysfunction than are small dog breeds.
- The gross appearance of valvular lesions in large dogs tends to be less impressive than it is in small dogs.
- Perhaps because myocardial dysfunction complicates MVD in large dogs more often than it does in small dogs, the prognosis may be worse than in smaller dogs.

DIAGNOSTIC FINDINGS
THORACIC RADIOGRAPHY

In most cases, thoracic radiography is the most important element of the diagnostic approach to MVD. MVD is extremely common but progresses at a rate that varies greatly among individuals. Many patients with MVD are subclinical ("asymptomatic") and never have clinical signs related to MR. Early in the course of MVD, the cardiac silhouette is normal. If clinically consequential MR develops, then there is enlargement of the cardiac silhouette. It should be recognized that the ability of thoracic radiographs to delineate specific cardiac chambers is limited. In general, the left atrium can be assessed with the greatest certainty. This is fortunate because, in the overwhelming majority of cases, left atrial enlargement precedes the development of edema. A diagnosis of left-sided cardiogenic pulmonary edema secondary to MVD can rarely be supported in the absence of radiographic left atrial enlargement.

RADIOGRAPHIC APPEARANCE OF LEFT ATRIAL ENLARGEMENT

- The left atrium is left of, and caudal to, the right atrium. Radiographically, it occupies the caudodorsal area of the cardiac silhouette in the lateral projection.
- In the absence of left atrial enlargement, the caudal portion of the trachea curves ventrally over the caudal aspect of the cardiac silhouette.

Table 7.1	Guidelines for Clinical Assessment of Elderly Small-Breed Dogs With Cough and Cardiac Murmur*	
	Cardiac Disease	**Respiratory Disease**
Body condition	Thin	Obese
Cardiac murmur	Loud	Often soft, occasionally loud
Heart rate	Rapid	Normal or slow
Rhythm	Regular, unless pathologic arrhythmias are present	Exaggerated respiratory arrhythmia may be present

*It is important to recognize that exceptions to these generalities occur. However, when a patient exhibits all of the findings in the left-side column, it is likely that cardiac disease or perhaps congestive heart failure is responsible for the cough. It must be recognized that some patients have both respiratory tract and cardiac disease. Ultimately, the distinction between respiratory tract and cardiac disease is made through diagnostic imaging; thoracic radiographs are indispensable, and echocardiography often provides useful complementary data.

- When the left atrium is enlarged, the caudal border of the cardiac silhouette straightens, and the trachea is forced dorsally to varying degrees. With marked left atrial enlargement, the left mainstem bronchus is narrowed, and the trachea adopts a path that is parallel to the thoracic vertebrae. Occasionally, severe left atrial enlargement has the appearance of a mass that splits the mainstem bronchi.
- In the ventrodorsal projection, the left atrium is located near the center of the cardiac silhouette. When enlarged, the left atrium splits the mainstem bronchi to varying degrees. This is apparent in well-penetrated radiographs and results in an appearance that is sometimes known as the "crab sign" or the "bowlegged cowboy" (Figures 7.4 and 7.5).
- In addition, in the ventrodorsal view, enlargement of the left atrium may cause a bulge that represents the atrial appendage at the 3 o'clock position.

RADIOGRAPHIC FINDINGS OF PULMONARY CONGESTION AND EDEMA

- The radiographic finding of pulmonary venous distention reflects increases in pulmonary venous pressure. Pulmonary venous distention suggests pulmonary congestion and may precede the development of pulmonary edema.
- A central, or perihilar, distribution often characterizes cardiogenic pulmonary edema in dogs, but cardiogenic edema is commonly asymmetric and focal; there is a predilection for the right caudal lung lobe.
- The development of interstitial pulmonary edema precedes the appearance of alveolar edema.

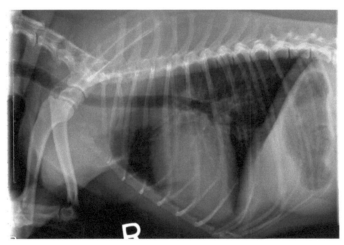

Figure 7.4 Lateral thoracic radiograph obtained from an 11-year-old mixed-breed dog with degenerative mitral valve disease (MVD). There is relatively mild but distinct left atrial enlargement, as evidenced by elevation of the trachea and straightening of the caudal border of the cardiac silhouette.

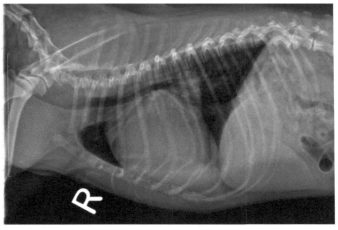

Figure 7.5 A lateral thoracic radiograph obtained from an 8-year-old male castrated Pomeranian dog with severe mitral valve incompetence caused by degenerative disease. The left atrium is markedly enlarged, and the mainstem bronchi are compressed. The appearance of the trachea suggests concurrent tracheal collapse.

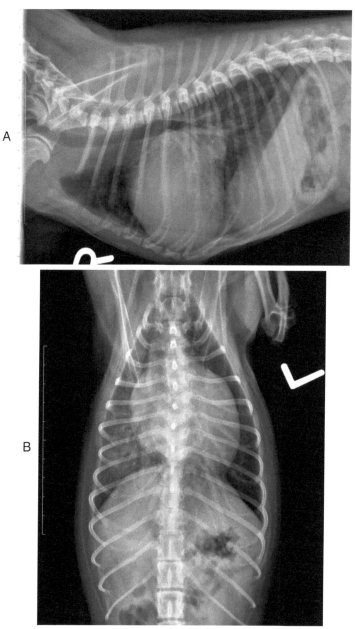

Figure 7.6   Lateral (**A**) and ventrodorsal (**B**) thoracic radiographs obtained from a 10-year-old male castrated Chihuahua with degenerative mitral valve disease (MVD). The cardiac silhouette is markedly enlarged, and there is evidence of left atrial enlargement. Pulmonary opacities compatible with edema are distributed throughout the lung; the edema most noticeably affects the right caudal lung lobe.

- Blurring of vascular detail in the presence of left atrial enlargement and, sometimes, concurrent pulmonary venous distention characterizes the radiographic appearance of interstitial pulmonary edema.
- When tissue fluid weeps into the pulmonary alveoli, it provides contrast with air-filled structures such as the bronchi, resulting in air bronchograms. Alveolar pulmonary opacities, together with radiographic evidence of left atrial enlargement, are diagnostic of left-sided CHF (Figure 7.6). The presence of alveolar pulmonary edema indicates severe HF that is almost invariably associated with noticeable respiratory distress.

ECHOCARDIOGRAPHY

- Echocardiographic examination of patients with MVD demonstrates variable degrees of left

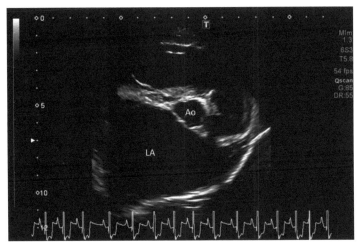

Figure 7.7 A right parasternal short-axis echocardiogram obtained from a 13-year-old female spayed mixed-breed dog with severe mitral valve regurgitation (MR). The left atrium (*LA*) is markedly enlarged; the dimension of the body of the atrium is more than twice the diameter of the aorta (*Ao*).

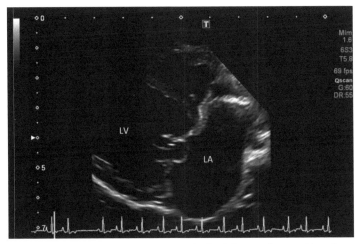

Figure 7.8 A right parasternal long-axis echocardiogram obtained from a 9-year-old male castrated Cavalier King Charles Spaniel with mitral regurgitation caused by degenerative disease. The image was obtained during systole. The left atrium (*LA*) is enlarged, and there is distinct prolapse of the mitral valve leaflets. *LV*, Left ventricle.

atrial (Figure 7.7) and left ventricular dilation. Hypertrophy is usually adequate to preserve a near-normal relationship between the diastolic luminal dimension and wall thickness.
- The mitral leaflets may be noticeably thicker than normal, and prolapse of the leaflets into the left atrium in systole is commonly observed (Figure 7.8).
- The echogenicity of affected leaflets is generally uniform, and nodular thickening is diffuse. In contrast, infective vegetations typically are localized, may exhibit motion that is independent of the valve leaflet, and are more, or less, echogenic than the valve leaflet.
- Often, the tricuspid leaflets are affected, although seldom as markedly as the mitral valve.

- Evaluation of myocardial function in patients with MR is difficult. When MR is moderate or severe, loading conditions imposed on the left ventricle are altered, and left ventricular performance is hyperdynamic (Figure 7.9), provided myocardial function (contractility) is preserved.
- Ejection phase indices of systolic performance such as fractional shortening are elevated because these variables are highly load dependent. When MR is present, impedance to ventricular emptying is reduced because the ventricle is able to eject blood into the low-pressure reservoir of the left atrium. In addition, end-diastolic ventricular stretch associated with MR increases the force of contraction and contributes to the finding of hyperdynamic ventricular

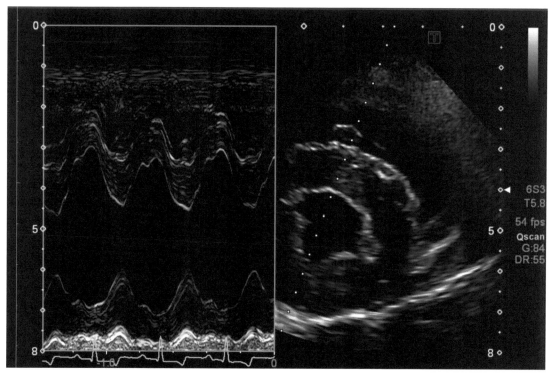

Figure 7.9 M-mode echocardiogram obtained at the level of the left ventricular papillary muscles from a 9-year-old male castrated Cavalier King Charles Spaniel. Left ventricular dilation and hypertrophy are evident. Left ventricular systolic performance is hyperdynamic; the fractional shortening exceeds 50%.

performance. A normal or subnormal fractional shortening in the setting of MR that has resulted in left ventricular dilation suggests systolic myocardial dysfunction (Figures 7.10 and 7.11).

- Because the end-systolic left ventricular dimension is determined by relatively few factors, it is a better index of myocardial function; however, because cardiac dimensions are related to body size, end-systolic left ventricular dimension must be interpreted in the context of body weight or, perhaps more appropriately, the cube root of body weight. Recently a method of echocardiographic mensuration in which cardiac dimensions are indexed to aortic diameter or the aortic diameter predicted based on body weight was proposed. Both allometric scaling, in which linear echocardiographic dimensions are related to the cube root of body weight, and the use of aorta-based ratio indices overcome some of the theoretic and practical limitations of comparing cardiac dimensions to body weight.

- The end-systolic volume index, which is calculated as $LVIDs^3/BSA$, where *LVIDs* is the end-systolic left ventricular dimension and *BSA* is body surface area, has been used in the assessment of myocardial function in dogs with MR. An index greater than 30 mL/m² suggests myocardial dysfunction.

- Doppler echocardiography is used to evaluate velocity, direction, and character of blood flow.

- Doppler evidence of disturbed flow within the left atrium during systole is noninvasive confirmation of the presence of MR (see Figure 7.8). When stroke volume is severely affected by MR or systolic failure, reductions in aortic outflow velocities may be apparent.

- Assessment of the severity of MR can be evaluated quantitatively or, more often, semiquantitatively by Doppler echocardiography.

- Quantitative methods include evaluation of the radius of color Doppler proximal flow convergence and the calculation of regurgitant fractions through volumetric flow analysis; however, these methods are time consuming and have not found widespread clinical application.

- The area of the color Doppler regurgitant jet relative to that of the receiving chamber is one means of semiquantitatively evaluating the severity of valvular regurgitation; however, many physiologic and technical factors influence the size of the jet, and this simple and intuitive method has limitations. The *width* of the regurgitant jet at its origin is another, perhaps more accurate, means of evaluating the severity of regurgitation; a greater width indicates a larger orifice and more severe regurgitation

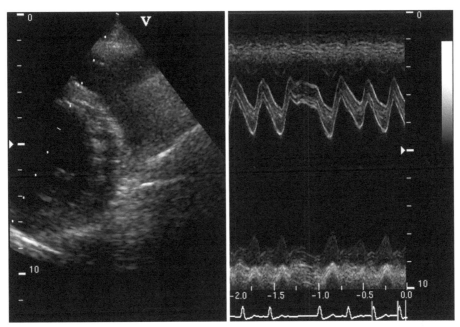

Figure 7.10 M-mode echocardiogram obtained at the level of the left ventricular papillary muscles from 12-year-old male castrated Keeshond weighing 18 kg. There was Doppler evidence of severe mitral regurgitation (MR) caused by degenerative valve disease. Left ventricular systolic performance evaluated by fractional shortening is normal (38%), but the end-systolic left ventricular dimension is markedly enlarged, which provides evidence of systolic myocardial dysfunction. The cardiac rhythm is atrial fibrillation.

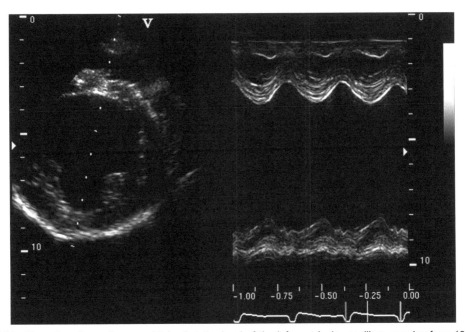

Figure 7.11 M-mode echocardiogram obtained at the level of the left ventricular papillary muscles from 12-year-old male castrated Dalmatian. There was Doppler evidence of severe mitral regurgitation (MR) caused by degenerative valve disease. Left ventricular systolic performance evaluated by fractional shortening is subnormal (22%), and the end-systolic left ventricular dimension is markedly enlarged. These findings provide evidence of systolic myocardial dysfunction. An examination 3 years previously demonstrated MR and mildly hyperdynamic systolic performance. In the interim, the end-diastolic and end-systolic left ventricular dimensions had enlarged. Large dogs are more apt to have systolic myocardial dysfunction as a consequence of mitral valve disease (MVD) than are small dogs.

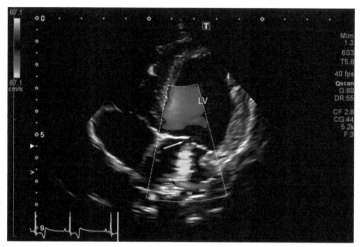

Figure 7.12   An apical echocardiographic image obtained from a 9-year-old male castrated Miniature Schnauzer with mitral regurgitation (MR) caused by early degenerative disease. Color-flow Doppler mapping demonstrates mild MR. The color mosaic occupies less than 50% of the area of the left atrium, and the jet is relatively narrow at its origin (*arrow*). *LV*, Left ventricle.

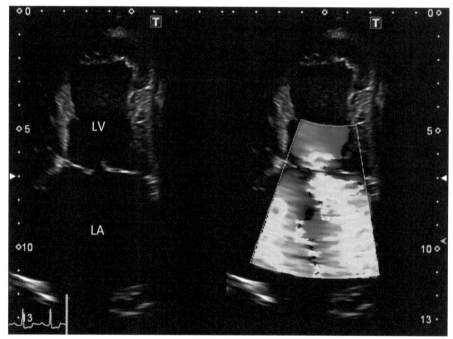

Figure 7.13   Apical echocardiographic image obtained from a 13-year-old female spayed mixed breed dog with (*right*) and without (*left*) superimposed color Doppler map. There is marked MR caused by valvular degeneration. The color mosaic nearly fills the enlarged left atrium (*LA*), and more important, with respect to evaluation of the severity of regurgitation, the jet is very broad at its origin. *LV*, Left ventricle.

(Figures 7.12 and 7.13). The appearance of proximal flow convergence—the color Doppler appearance of acceleration through the regurgitant orifice—suggests that MR is at least moderate in severity (Figure 7.14).
- The density of the regurgitant continuous-wave spectral Doppler signal is roughly proportional to the number of cells that move into the receiving chamber and is an alternative means of

semiquantitatively evaluating regurgitant severity (Figure 7.15).
- Ultimately, it is important that the echocardiographic assessment is clinically relevant. In veterinary patients in whom valvular repair is seldom performed, the effect of valvular regurgitation might be of greater importance than its magnitude. Information regarding chamber size and myocardial function is essential in

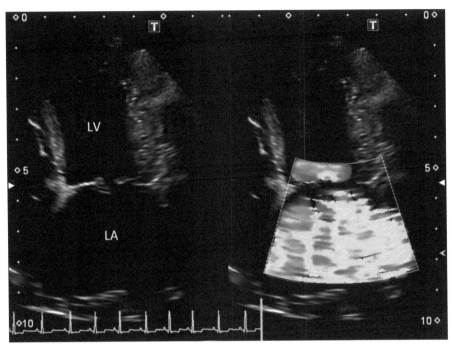

Figure 7.14 Apical echocardiographic images obtained from a 14-year-old male castrated Chinese Crested dog with (*right*) and without (*left*) superimposed color Doppler map. Color-flow Doppler mapping demonstrates marked mitral valve regurgitation (MR). The region of proximal flow acceleration (*arrow*) is evident within the left ventricle (*LV*). *LA,* Left atrium.

placing Doppler findings in the appropriate clinical context.

- Technologically advanced echocardiographic methods have recently been investigated in the setting of MVD. Tissue Doppler imaging, for example, which defines the velocity of the myocardium, provides potentially useful information regarding diastolic and systolic myocardial function. Determinations of myocardial strain and strain rate—measurements of the deformation of the heart muscle—also have been investigated in MVD. These modalities may have promise in the evaluation of myocardial function because they are, relative to conventional measures of cardiac dimensions, less dependent on ventricular loading conditions. The potential of real-time three-dimensional echocardiography has also been explored.

RELATIVE MERITS OF RADIOGRAPHY AND ECHOCARDIOGRAPHY IN MITRAL VALVE REGURGITATION

It should be emphasized that MVD exhibits a broad spectrum of severity. Often, the presence of MR is incidental to the presentation, and clinical signs such as cough are not the result of HF or even heart disease but, rather, of primary respiratory disease. Therefore, in most cases, the thoracic radiograph provides the most useful diagnostic and prognostic information in patients with

MVD. Thoracic radiography not only provides an assessment of cardiac size but also allows visualization of the pulmonary vessels and parenchyma. Thus thoracic radiography provides an indirect assessment of cardiac performance, and currently it is the only widely available noninvasive route to a diagnosis of cardiogenic pulmonary edema.

Echocardiography provides a noninvasive means by which to evaluate valvular structure, assess cardiac dimensions, evaluate left ventricular systolic performance, and, with Doppler studies, confirm the clinical diagnosis of MR. However, echocardiography cannot provide a diagnosis of HF; it can only demonstrate that cardiac disease is sufficiently severe that a diagnosis of HF is plausible. Although the clinical signs associated with MVD may have a sudden onset, the disease process itself is chronic. Therefore left atrial dilation and, usually, concurrent left ventricular dilation are expected before the onset of clinical signs. Echocardiographic evidence of MR in the absence of left atrial and left ventricular dilation is seldom of clinical importance. In many cases, echocardiography is not essential for the clinical management of patients with MR. In patients with suspected MR, echocardiography is likely to provide clinically useful information in the following scenarios:

- When the cause of a cardiac murmur is uncertain (for example, patients in which the signalment is atypical, when the murmur may possibly

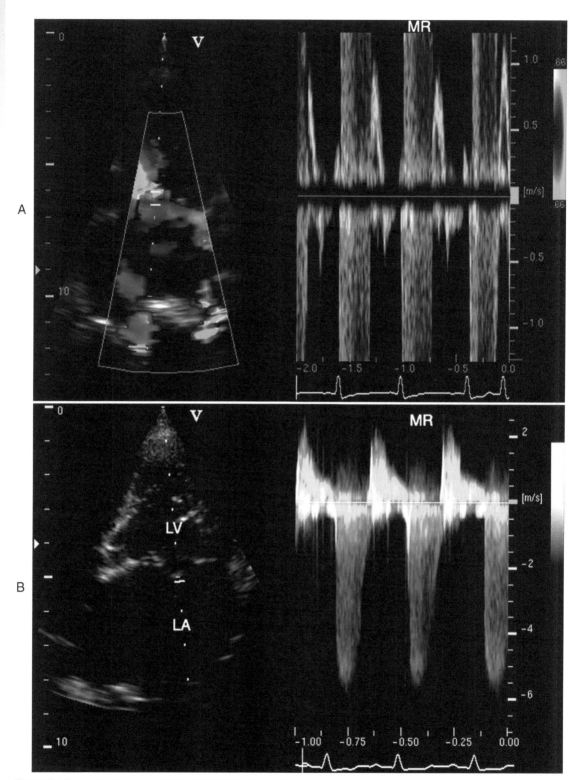

Figure 7.15   A, Pulsed-wave Doppler echocardiogram obtained from a dog with mitral valve incompetence caused by degenerative mitral valve disease (MVD). The pulsed-wave sample volume was placed within the left atrium (*LA*); during systole there is a dense, aliasing multifrequency signal. **B**, Continuous-wave Doppler study of the LA of a dog with severe mitral valve incompetence caused by degenerative MVD. The signal is quite dense, suggesting severe regurgitation. *LV,* Left ventricle; *MR,* mitral valve regurgitation.

be congenital, or when the murmur is louder over the right, rather than left, hemithorax).

- When it is difficult to discern from thoracic radiographs whether the left atrium is enlarged.
- When sudden deterioration has occurred and rupture of the chordae tendineae or left atrium is suspected.
- When it is important to evaluate systolic myocardial function.
- When pulmonary hypertension is suspected.
- The ACVIM guidelines include a consensus recommendation for echocardiographic examination of dogs with stage B MVD; for these patients, echocardiography is suggested when clinical questions persist after physical examination and radiography. For large dog breeds with MVD, echocardiography is thought to be "generally indicated" because of the prevalence of myocardial dysfunction in this patient population. For dogs with stage C MVD, echocardiography is suggested as one component of the optimal diagnostic approach.

ELECTROCARDIOGRAPHY

- Electrocardiography is primarily useful for the diagnosis of arrhythmias, but it also can provide indirect evidence of chamber enlargement.
- The electrocardiogram is an insensitive gauge of cardiac chamber size. Nevertheless, it is likely that findings such as P mitrale are relatively specific; that is, when P waves in the caudal frontal leads (II, III, and aVF) are wide, the left atrium is usually enlarged (Figure 7.16).
- Arrhythmias can complicate the presentation of MVD. Most often, arrhythmias in MVD take the form of supraventricular tachyarrhythmias that reflect atrial stretch. Atrial premature complexes and paroxysms of atrial tachycardia are relatively common in patients with MVD. Atrial fibrillation develops occasionally and generally

indicates advanced disease with marked atrial dilation. Ventricular arrhythmias (ventricular premature complexes) may develop in association with left ventricular dilation and myocardial fibrosis.

BLOODBORNE BIOMARKERS

- Biomarkers are objectively determined characteristics that potentially have a role in diagnosis, risk stratification, evaluation of disease progression, and assessment of response to therapy. A number of bloodborne biomarkers, including endothelin, troponin I, atrial natriuretic peptide, and B-type natriuretic peptide (BNP), have been investigated in the settings of MVD and canine HF. BNP is released by atrial and ventricular cardiomyocytes in response to increases in ventricular filling pressures and therefore is a potential bloodborne diagnostic marker of the HF state.
- BNP concentration is associated with the severity of canine degenerative MVD, and statistically significant differences between BNP concentrations from healthy dogs and dogs with MVD have been identified. It is relevant, however, that the finding of statistically significant intergroup differences does not necessarily imply that a variable, in this case BNP, usefully discriminates between groups. Elevated BNP concentrations do distinguish patients with respiratory distress caused by HF from those with distress caused by respiratory tract disease with sensitivity and specificity that exceed 80%.
- The prognostic potential of BNP determination has also been evaluated in canine cardiac disease. Not only is BNP concentration related to severity of disease, but also, longitudinal investigations have disclosed a relationship between mortality and NT-ProBNP (N-terminal pro–B-type natriuretic peptide) concentration

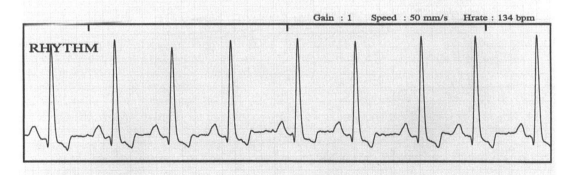

Figure 7.16 An electrocardiogram recorded from a 13-year-old Beagle with physical findings of mitral valve regurgitation (MR). There is P mitrale, and the R amplitude exceeds 3 mV, suggesting left atrial enlargement and left ventricular hypertrophy, respectively. (Lead II, 50 mm/sec, 1 mV = 1 cm.)

in dogs with MVD. Furthermore, a decrease in BNP concentration in association with medical therapy for MVD is predictive of outcome. An assay for canine NT-proBNP is offered by a commercial laboratory.

- Troponin I is a myocardial regulatory protein that is released from damaged cardiomyocytes; a rise in blood troponin concentration generally reflects cardiac necrosis, and this variable, considered together with BNP, may provide additional prognostic information. A cage-side assay for troponin I is commercially available.

THERAPY
STAGE B MITRAL VALVE DISEASE

- Definitive published evidence that medical therapy slows the progression of subclinical ("asymptomatic") MVD is lacking.
- A theoretic ideal treatment for MVD could be used to prevent or reverse myxomatous degeneration. Unfortunately, drug therapy that affects this pathologic process has not been identified.
- In the absence of evidence that medical therapy can alter the progression of valvular degeneration, interest has been directed toward the possibility that drug therapy might improve prognosis in subclinical MVD by decreasing MR or by modifying the process of ventricular remodeling.
- Unfortunately, despite evidence that angiotensin-converting enzyme (ACE) inhibitors favorably affect prognosis in humans with asymptomatic ventricular dysfunction, only limited efficacy of ACE inhibitors in subclinical canine MVD has been demonstrated.
- The possibility that enalapril might delay the onset of HF in subclinical MVD has been addressed by two separate clinical trials. In both the Scandinavian Veterinary Enalapril Prevention (SVEP) trial and the Veterinary Enalapril Trial to Prove Reduction in Onset of Heart Failure (VETPROOF), dogs with subclinical MR were randomized to receive placebo or **enalapril.** Neither trial demonstrated a statistically significant effect of enalapril on time to development of CHF. Although the result of the VETPROOF was not statistically significant with respect to the primary end point, the data did show a tendency toward a favorable treatment effect. Atrial enlargement was an inclusion criterion for VETPROOF but not for the SVEP trial; however, it is worthy of consideration that both trials included patients with relatively mild MR. Patients with mild and slowly progressive disease tend to experience few events of interest (e.g., death or

occurrence of HF) even during relatively long periods of follow-up. The inclusion of mildly affected patients in a clinical trial might mask a treatment effect that is evident only for patients with severe disease. It is therefore possible that a subpopulation of preclinical patients with severe MR and cardiomegaly would benefit from ACE inhibition. Although this hypothesis has not been specifically tested, it is partly refuted by the results of the SVEP trial, in which a treatment effect was not observed in the subset of dogs that had radiographic cardiomegaly at study entry.

- The reason that ACE inhibitors do not appear to improve prognosis in subclinical MVD is not known; however, it should be recognized that the widely cited clinical trials of ACE inhibition in humans with heart disease generally have enrolled humans with past myocardial infarction or idiopathic DCM. MVD in humans is generally treated surgically, and, indeed, medical therapy is not recommended for asymptomatic humans with MR.
- Pathophysiologic differences between humans with ventricular myocardial dysfunction and dogs with MVD might also be relevant. In contrast to the effect of renin-angiotensin-aldosterone system (RAS) suppression in dogs with experimentally induced primary myocardial disease, neither ACE inhibitors nor angiotensin II antagonists favorably affect ventricular remodeling in dogs with experimentally induced MR. However, the syndrome that results from acute disruption of the mitral valve in the laboratory may differ markedly from spontaneous valvular degeneration associated with chronic, progressive MR. Therefore the clinical relevance of these research findings is uncertain.
- Theoretic considerations aside, definitive evidence that ACE inhibitors improve prognosis in subclinical MVD is lacking. Although it might be argued that trials to date have had inadequate statistical power, it is likely that a favorable effect of ACE inhibition, if one exists, is modest; the results of VETPROOF suggest that 2 years of therapy with enalapril may delay the onset of pulmonary edema by approximately 4 months. On the basis of available data, I generally do not treat dogs with subclinical MVD. On a pragmatic level, the practitioner is sometimes presented with subclinical patients for which radiographic findings suggest that the development of frank HF is imminent. In cases where there is marked left atrial enlargement and pulmonary venous distension, I prescribe an ACE inhibitor. It is noteworthy that long-term ACE inhibition has not been associated with detrimental effects. Furthermore, it is possible that these drugs have benefits that relate to effects

on other geriatric disorders such as hypertension or renal disease. On the basis of this and the suggestion of a favorable effect in the VET-PROOF, ACE inhibition may be a therapeutic consideration for some patients with cardiac enlargement and subclinical MR; however, the evidence to support this approach is neither direct nor strong.

COUGH CAUSED BY AIRWAY COMPRESSION

- Some dogs with MVD have a cough that is apparently associated with compression of the mainstem bronchi by an enlarged left atrium. This type of cough can develop before the development of pulmonary edema.
- Radiographically, there is an enlarged cardiac silhouette with distinct evidence of left atrial enlargement. The mainstem bronchi may be noticeably narrowed. The pulmonary veins are sometimes distended, but the pulmonary interstitium and parenchyma have a normal appearance.
- It is important to recognize that primary respiratory tract diseases such as tracheal collapse and chronic bronchitis are common in the same patient group that has MVD. With very few exceptions, clinical signs related to MVD do not occur in the absence of radiographic left atrial enlargement.
- When radiographic findings suggest that the cause of cough is airway compression but not pulmonary edema, the use of an antitussive such as **hydrocodone** or **butorphanol** is rational.
- Vasodilation causes a decrease in systemic vascular resistance and, in the setting of MR, can increase stroke volume through a decrease in the regurgitant fraction. Potentially these effects can decrease left atrial and pulmonary venous pressures and perhaps reduce left atrial size.
- Cough caused by compression of the airways is generally associated with considerable chamber enlargement, and this latter finding is a risk factor for the ultimate development of HF. Because of the proven favorable effect of ACE inhibition in patients with HF caused by MVD, it is reasonable to administer an ACE inhibitor in addition to an antitussive when cough appears to result from bronchial compression.
- Some of the benefits of ACE inhibition likely relate to their neuroendocrine effects. Because of this and because ACE inhibitors are not potent vasodilators, a case might be made for the use of **hydralazine** or perhaps **amlodipine** for dogs with MVD and cough caused by bronchial compression. Caution must be exercised if these drugs are used, and patients should be monitored for the development of systemic hypotension.

- Diuretic administration effectively reduces cardiac volumes and may also be efficacious. The argument can be advanced that this may result in harmful activation of the renin-angiotensin axis. Therefore, in this clinical situation, furosemide should be added only when ACE inhibition in combination with an antitussive fails to result in clinical improvement.
- When cough fails to respond to ACE inhibition and modest diuresis, it is important to consider the possibility that the cough results not from heart disease but rather from primary respiratory tract disease.

STAGE C MITRAL VALVE DISEASE

- When MR causes clinical signs in humans, it is treated surgically. Mitral valve repair with preservation of chordal attachments is generally preferred to replacement of the valve with a prosthesis. Surgical treatment of dogs with MVD has been reported. However, the expense and the need for expertise in open-heart surgery performed during cardiopulmonary bypass have limited its availability.
- In general, HF caused by MVD is treated medically (Table 7.2). Unless the cause can be definitively treated, HF is a terminal syndrome. Therefore medical management is intended to alleviate clinical signs and prolong life. Drug therapy for HF consists primarily of interventions that manipulate the determinants of cardiac output and blunt the maladaptive neuroendocrine response to cardiac dysfunction.
- In CHF caused by MR, left ventricular filling pressure (preload) is excessive, and the consequent increase in venous pressures causes tissue fluid to weep into the pulmonary interstitium and alveoli. Drugs that reduce intravascular volume, such as diuretics, or that increase venous capacitance, such as nitroglycerin, are therefore mainstays of therapy.
- **Nitroglycerin** is usually administered transdermally and is used most often as short-term therapy in patients with fulminant edema or occasionally as adjunctive therapy in patients with advanced disease. The efficacy of transdermal nitroglycerin is uncertain, and in dogs with experimentally induced MR, the effect of nitroglycerin on filling pressure did not differ from that of placebo.
- **Furosemide**, a potent agent that acts on the loop of Henle, is the diuretic that is used most often in veterinary practice. It can be administered orally or parenterally; the route of administration is based on the patient's clinical status. The resultant decrease in intravascular volume reduces left ventricular filling pressures and

Table 7.2   Suggested Strategies for Diagnostic and Therapeutic Management of Canine Degenerative Valvular Disease

	Stage B MVD	Cough Caused by Airway Compression	Stage C MVD	Stage D MVD
Diagnostic approach	Radiographs as indicated by clinical circumstances (i.e., before elective anesthesia, loud murmurs particularly if associated with tachycardia) ECG when auscultation suggests pathologic arrhythmia	Radiographs Echocardiography recommended when radiographic evidence of left atrial enlargement is equivocal ECG when auscultation suggests pathologic arrhythmia	Radiographs Echocardiography not usually necessary but provides potentially useful ancillary information in most cases ECG when auscultation suggests pathologic arrhythmia	Radiographs Echocardiography ECG when auscultation suggests pathologic arrhythmia
Therapeutic approach	Generally none indicated, although in some circumstances, the use of an ACE inhibitor might be considered for patients with distinct cardiac enlargement (see text)	Antitussive agent and an ACE inhibitor. Short-term antiinflammatory dose of corticosteroids, or therapeutic diuretic trial considered for refractory cases	Standard therapy for HF caused by MR consists of furosemide, an ACE inhibitor, pimobendan, and moderate dietary salt restriction	The following can be considered in addition to standard therapy; treatment should be tailored to the individual • Triple diuretic therapy • Amlodipine • Spironolactone

ACE, Angiotensin-converting enzyme; *ECG,* electrocardiogram; *HF,* heart failure; *MR,* mitral valve regurgitation; *MVD,* mitral valve disease.

allows lymphatic drainage of tissue fluid and resolution of edema.

- It should be recognized that diuretics reduce preload; this decrease in ventricular filling pressures is generally well tolerated by patients with ventricular dilation and has obvious benefits when edema is present. However, excessive diuresis can result in hypotension related to low cardiac output, prerenal azotemia, and electrolyte disturbances. It is generally thought that the optimal dose of furosemide is the lowest one that controls signs of congestion.
- More important, many dogs with clinically evident MVD cough in the absence of pulmonary edema, and many of these patients have concurrent primary respiratory tract disease. Therefore aggressive diuresis following radiographically demonstrated resolution of pulmonary edema is to be avoided. In most cases of HF caused by MVD, the administration of furosemide rapidly and effectively resolves signs. Failure of patients with MR and respiratory distress to respond promptly to diuretic administration should cause the practitioner to question the diagnosis of HF.
- Most patients that have radiographic pulmonary edema caused by MR require lifelong diuretic therapy. Early in the course of the

syndrome, an oral dose of 1 mg/kg q12h may be adequate, although the inevitable progression of MR and HF and renal tubular adaptations ultimately necessitate higher doses.
- Moderate dietary salt restriction is suggested for patients with CHF caused by MVD.
- The benefits of ACE inhibition in HF caused by MR have been demonstrated. Thus the use of an ACE inhibitor together with furosemide has become standard therapy for stage C HF caused by MVD.
- **Pimobendan** is an "inodilator" that has complex pharmacologic properties. It inhibits phosphodiesterase and therefore causes vasodilation and an increase in the inotropic state. In addition, pimobendan increases the sensitivity of the contractile apparatus to available calcium, which also contributes to the inotropic effect. This latter property may be favorable because an increased inotropic state is associated with relatively low cost in terms of myocardial oxygen consumption.
- A randomized clinical trial (QUEST) compared pimobendan with benazepril against a background of conventional therapy that consisted of furosemide, digoxin, or both in dogs with stage C MVD. With respect to survival, pimobendan was superior to benazepril. Recent post

hoc analyses of the data from this trial provide evidence that, relative to benazepril, pimobendan delayed intensification of cardiac therapy.

- The effect of pimobendan, when used together with an ACE inhibitor in dogs with valvular disease, has not been addressed in published trials to date. Therefore the stage of disease at which pimobendan is most appropriately added to conventional therapy can be debated, but concurrent use of pimobendan, an ACE inhibitor, and furosemide as initial therapy can be justified in stage C MVD. Indeed, this "triple therapy" has become standard and is consistent with the consensus recommendation included in the ACVIM guidelines. When pet owners are constrained financially and only pimobendan or an ACE inhibitor can be prescribed, the available data suggest that either drug is appropriate but that pimobendan is superior.
- In Beagles with mild MVD, chronic oral administration of pimobendan was associated with histologic valvular lesions that were more severe than those in a similar group of Beagles that received benazepril. These data and a clinical case report suggest that in some circumstances, pimobendan might accelerate the development of degenerative valvular lesions. Pimobendan is not indicated for the management of subclinical MVD.
- When atrial tachyarrhythmias, particularly atrial fibrillation, complicate MVD, the use of digoxin (0.22 mg/m^2 PO q12h) is generally accepted. However, the role of digoxin in the management of patients with HF who are in normal sinus rhythm remains a point of controversy.
- **Digoxin** has two principal effects: it acts as a positive inotrope and as a negative chronotrope. The latter property is related to the autonomic effects of the drug, which include a central vagomimetic effect and effects that may serve to normalize the baroreceptor dysfunction associated with HF. There is evidence to suggest that chronic activation of the adrenergic nervous system is detrimental and that this abnormality may be partly reversed by digoxin.
- The need for digoxin in the patient with HF caused by MVD is difficult to assess. Because the commonly used echocardiographic indices of contractility depend on preload and afterload, as well as myocardial function, they are difficult to interpret when MR is severe. Furthermore, the results of clinical trials that enrolled people with HF cast doubt on the intuitive notion that chronic inotropic therapy is beneficial.
- The effect of digoxin on dogs with HF and sinus rhythm has not been evaluated. However, on the basis of the results of a clinical trial that addressed the role of digoxin in humans with

HF, it seems likely that the magnitude of effect in dogs—whether positive or negative—is probably small.

NEUROENDOCRINE MODULATION

- ACE inhibitors are part of the standard therapeutic approach to HF caused by MR. It is likely that the favorable effect of ACE inhibition is not simply the result of vasodilation. In addition to this mechanical effect, ACE inhibition serves to protect the heart from the apparently detrimental effects of RAS activation.
- Pharmacologic ACE inhibition generally is not complete, and because aldosterone may contribute to the development of myocardial fibrosis, more complete suppression of the RAS may yield positive results. Accordingly, the use of **spironolactone,** a weak diuretic that antagonizes the effect of aldosterone, is considered adjunctive therapy for patients with severe HF caused by MVD. In humans with HF, the use of subdiuretic doses of spironolactone prolongs survival.
- A placebo-controlled clinical trial provided evidence that administration of spironolactone to dogs receiving an ACE inhibitor with or without furosemide or digoxin for HF caused by MVD improved outcome. The publication of the trial results provoked some controversy, and the use of spironolactone was not a consensus recommendation of the ACVIM guidelines.
- Beta blockers decrease mortality in humans with HF. Because these drugs have a potent negative inotropic effect, the mechanism by which beta blockers improve survival is not intuitively obvious. However, it is now recognized that seemingly compensatory activation of the adrenergic nervous system and RAS is ultimately maladaptive and contributes to the progressive nature of HF. The use of beta blockers in this setting is consistent with this paradigm.
- Acutely, beta blockers have a negative effect on cardiac performance and should be used in canines with HF only with caution. Beta blockers must be initiated at very low doses and titrated to effect or target dose over the course of weeks.
- The use of beta blockers in patients with systolic failure is predicated on the belief that they preserve myocardial function. Although invasive measures may disclose myocardial function in dogs with MR, the primary cause of clinical signs in patients with MVD is likely the mechanical effect of the volume load. Nevertheless, studies of dogs with experimentally induced

MR suggest that beta blockade may have a role in the management of MVD.
- **Carvedilol** is a third-generation beta blocker that is also an alpha-adrenergic antagonist. Because of this latter property, carvedilol is a weak vasodilator, which might make it particularly well suited to the management of MVD.
- I consider the use of carvedilol when echocardiographic findings suggest incipient or patent myocardial dysfunction.

THERAPY OF SEVERE CONGESTIVE HEART FAILURE CAUSED BY ADVANCED MITRAL VALVE REGURGITATION

- The use of triple diuretic therapy—the combination of **furosemide** with a **thiazide** and a potassium-sparing diuretic such as **spironolactone**—can be considered for patients that require high doses of furosemide to remain free of congestive signs. The use of three different diuretic agents interferes with nephron function at anatomically and functionally distinct sites; together, the drugs may have synergistic effects, allowing the use of lower doses of the individual agents. In addition, the use of a potassium-sparing agent such as spironolactone serves to limit some of the adverse effects that are associated with the use of high doses of loop diuretics such as furosemide.
- Despite proved efficacy in the management of HF caused by MVD, the ACE inhibitors are not potent vasodilators. In some patients with HF caused by severe MVD, the use of the vasoselective calcium channel blocker **amlodipine,** in addition to an ACE inhibitor, may be helpful. When vasodilators are used in addition to ACE inhibitors, the initial dose should be low; ideally, the dose is titrated to effect based on serial blood pressure determinations.

COMPLICATIONS OF MITRAL VALVE DISEASE AND ITS TREATMENT

CARDIORENAL SYNDROME

- The cardiorenal syndrome has been defined in different ways, but the term is generally used to describe worsening renal function in patients with cardiac disease. A decrease in stroke volume related to declining cardiac performance likely contributes to the development of azotemia in the setting of HF. However, the relationship between cardiac dysfunction and worsening renal function is complex; invasively acquired data from humans demonstrate that increases in cardiac output do not prevent worsening of renal function or necessarily improve long-term outcome.

- Monitoring of renal function is particularly important for patients with stage C or D HF that generally are receiving diuretics and ACE inhibitors. ACE inhibitors are not generally thought to be directly nephrotoxic; however, ACE inhibition results in relatively selective dilation of the efferent arteriole of the nephron, a hemodynamic effect that can predispose to the development of prerenal azotemia. Those patients with pre-existing renal disease and those receiving overly aggressive doses of diuretics seem most likely to have azotemia. In addition, patients with severe cardiac dysfunction that are critically dependent on the effects of angiotensin II to maintain glomerular filtration fraction may also have azotemia when ACE inhibitors are administered.
- There are few circumstances under which diuretic therapy can increase stroke volume and renal blood flow; in general, diuretics decrease filling pressures and potentially decrease cardiac performance. In contrast, judicious vasodilation in the setting of MR may increase stroke volume. Thus the development of azotemia is usually managed first by a cautious reduction in the diuretic dose. Should creatinine values fail to decrease, the diuretic can be discontinued; the patient's respiratory rate and character should be carefully monitored. If azotemia persists after discontinuation of diuretic therapy, the ACE inhibitor can be discontinued, and cautious intravenous infusion of fluid can be initiated.

RUPTURE OF CHORDAE TENDINEAE

- Rupture of chordae tendineae is a relatively common complication of MVD. When a primary chorda ruptures, the attached mitral leaflet becomes suddenly flail (Figure 7.17), potentially resulting in catastrophic MR, marked elevations in ventricular filling pressures, and fulminant pulmonary edema. Rupture of minor chordae may result in less impressive clinical signs or be subclinical.
- Rupture of a primary chordae tendineae may occur in patients with substantial preexisting MR and cardiac enlargement and result in clinical decompensation, with varying degrees of severity. However, the development of acute pulmonary edema in patients with normal cardiac dimensions is uncommon.
- Acute CHF caused by chordal rupture is treated similarly to acute or decompensated HF caused by other disorders; however, there may be a particular role for the intravenous administration of nitroprusside in addition to parenteral diuretic administration.
- Prognosis depends on numerous factors; the most important is probably response to therapy.

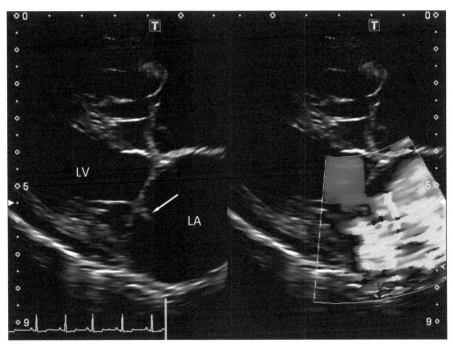

Figure 7.17   Right parasternal long-axis echocardiographic images obtained from a 14-year-old male castrated Chinese Crested dog with (*right*) and without (*left*) superimposed color Doppler map. The anterior mitral valve leaflet (*arrow*) is partially flail—a segment of the leaflet is perpendicular to the plane of the mitral annulus—because of past rupture of a chordae tendineae. *LA,* Left atrium; *LV,* left ventricle.

LEFT ATRIAL RUPTURE

- Left atrial rupture is an uncommon complication of advanced MVD that generally is associated with marked left atrial dilation. Cocker Spaniels and Dachshunds may be predisposed to left atrial rupture. Unsurprisingly, a complete and full thickness tear of the atrial wall can be lethal. However, compressive pericardial effusions and structures in the pericardial space assumed to represent thrombi are occasionally evident when patients with severe MR are subject to echocardiographic examination. These findings provide indirect evidence of past partial left atrial rupture.
- The clinical consequences of left atrial rupture are variable; marked clinical deterioration or sudden death can be observed, but a few patients seemingly have a subclinical left atrial rupture. A recent publication described a series of 11 dogs with presumed left atrial rupture for which the median survival was 203 days. Rupture of the interatrial septum resulting in an atrial septal defect also has been reported as a complication of MVD.

PULMONARY HYPERTENSION

- Pulmonary hypertension occasionally complicates the clinical presentation of MVD in the dog. Doppler studies can provide noninvasive estimates of pulmonary artery pressure. Doppler echocardiographic evidence of tricuspid valve regurgitation (TR) is commonly observed in patients with MVD. The velocity of the TR jet is related to the systolic pressure difference between the right atrium and the right ventricle by the modified Bernoulli equation ($\Delta P = 4v^2$, where ΔP is the pressure difference and v is the velocity of the regurgitant jet). The right atrial pressure is approximated on the basis of clinical findings; in the absence of cardiogenic ascites, the right atrial pressure is likely less than 10 mm Hg. Provided pulmonary stenosis is excluded by Doppler evaluation of the right ventricular outflow tract, right ventricular and pulmonary artery pressures are equal during systole. Thus measurement of the velocity of the TR jet can provide noninvasive estimates of systolic pulmonary artery pressure (Figure 7.18).
- The cause of pulmonary hypertension associated with MVD is probably multifactorial. The primary function of the right ventricle is to propel the stroke volume through the pulmonary vascular tree to the left atrium. Elevations in left atrial pressure cause commensurate increases in right ventricular systolic pressure; if mean pulmonary artery pressure does not exceed mean left atrial pressure, there is no impetus

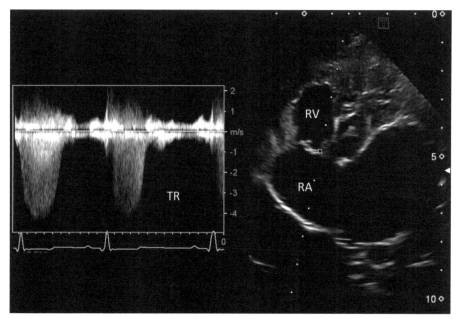

Figure 7.18 Continuous-wave Doppler study performed with the Doppler cursor through the right atrium of a 14-year-old male castrated Chinese Crested dog with severe mitral regurgitation (MR) caused by valvular degeneration. There is tricuspid valve regurgitation (*TR*); the peak velocity of the TR jet is nearly 5 m/sec. This corresponds to a systolic right atrial–right ventricular pressure difference that is close to 100 mm Hg and provides evidence of severe pulmonary hypertension. In this case, elevated left atrial pressure was partly responsible for pulmonary hypertension, but the predicted pulmonary artery pressure was out of proportion to any credible estimate of left atrial pressure. Reactive vasoconstriction of the pulmonary arterioles may have contributed to the development of pulmonary hypertension. *RA,* Right atrium; *RV,* right ventricle.

for forward flow. The tendency for left atrial hypertension to cause pulmonary hypertension is probably the primary explanation for high pulmonary artery pressures in most cases; however, in some patients, the increase in estimated pulmonary artery pressure is disproportionate to any credible estimate of left atrial pressure. In these cases, pulmonary arterial constriction—sometimes known as "reactive vasoconstriction"—probably contributes. Alternatively, pulmonary hypertension may be also related to the presence of concurrent pulmonary or airway disease.

- There is no established therapy for patients with pulmonary hypertension associated with MVD. Most vasodilators have a relatively predictable effect on the systemic vasculature; however, the pulmonary arterioles respond inconsistently to the commonly used vasodilator agents. Consequently, it should be recognized that the use of vasodilators in patients with pulmonary hypertension caused by severe pulmonary vascular disease is not without risk. If a vasodilator with potent peripheral effects fails to decrease pulmonary vascular resistance, systemic hypotension or detrimental increases in right ventricular pressure and myocardial oxygen demand may result.

- As initial therapy, interventions that reduce left atrial pressure are reasonable. Diuretic therapy should be tailored to rid the patient of radiographic evidence of pulmonary congestion or edema. Alveolar hypoxia is a stimulus for constriction of the pulmonary arterioles. If bronchoconstriction associated with primary respiratory disease has contributed to the development of pulmonary hypertension, bronchodilators may be helpful.

- When pulmonary congestion is effectively controlled yet therapy for primary respiratory tract disease fails to lower pulmonary artery pressure and clinical signs such as weakness can plausibly be related to pulmonary hypertension, the use of sildenafil, in addition to an ACE inhibitor, can be considered. Sildenafil is an inhibitor of phosphodiesterase-5 that appears to have a relatively selective effect on pulmonary arterioles. When possible, systemic blood pressure should be monitored when therapy with this drug is initiated (see Chapter 15).

- The prognosis associated with the development of MVD depends on numerous factors. Most patients with MR caused by MVD succumb to noncardiac disease. In fact, in two retrospective investigations in which observation periods were generally longer than 2 years, it was not possible to calculate median survival of patients with subclinical MVD because so few patients died during follow-up. Clinical trial data suggest that the median time for progression from stage B2 to stage C MVD is approximately 2 years. Stage C MVD is generally terminal, and the median survival of patients receiving furosemide and pimobendan is close to 9 months. Echocardiographically determined left atrial enlargement and increased levels of BNP and troponin I are associated with poor outcome.

INFECTIVE ENDOCARDITIS

Infective endocarditis (IE) occurs occasionally in dogs and rarely in cats. The prognosis is generally grave, and most cases are terminal even with aggressive medical therapy. This latter point emphasizes the importance of detecting IE, a disease that sometimes poses a considerable diagnostic challenge.

PREVALENCE AND INCIDENCE

- IE is a relatively uncommon disease that is observed occasionally in dogs but rarely in cats. Mural endocarditis and infection of the tricuspid valve are observed occasionally, as is infection of endocardial pacing leads; however, bacterial infection of the aortic or mitral valve leaflets is most common.
- Male, middle-aged, large dog breeds, including German Shepherds and Boxers, are affected most often.
- In humans, the presence of a congenital cardiac malformation is a risk factor for the development of IE. An association between congenital subvalvular aortic stenosis and IE of the aortic valve has been demonstrated, and it is likely that subvalvular aortic stenosis and, perhaps, other congenital malformations are important factors in the epidemiology of IE in dogs.

ETIOPATHOGENESIS

- On the basis of experimental studies, it is likely that the following factors are important in the pathogenesis of infective valvular endocarditis:
  - Endocardial damage (which may result from valvular insufficiency, stenosis, or a shunting lesion)
  - Activation of clotting factors
  - Bacteremia and colonization of a noninfective thrombus
- The development of a noninfective thrombus precedes valvular infection. Episodes of bacteremia can result in infection of the thrombus and in the initiation of a variably aggressive inflammatory process that results in distortion and destruction of the valve leaflets and their associated structures.
- In clinical cases of canine IE, a congenital cardiac malformation may represent a predisposition for the development of the disease. Prostatitis, pyelonephritis, or even dental disease can be a source for the development of bacteremia; often, however, the site of bacterial entry into the bloodstream remains undiscovered.
- Degenerative valvular disease has no known association with IE. Despite the prevalence of dental disease in patients with MR caused by MVD, IE is extremely uncommon in this group. Indeed, the possibility that there is an association between canine periodontal disease and IE has been systematically investigated. A large retrospective cohort study identified a relationship between IE and periodontal disease. However, the absence of echocardiographic corroboration of diagnoses, together with the improbable incidence data reported for specific cardiac diseases, makes the conclusion that periodontal disease predisposes to IE dubious. A smaller case-control study in which cases were rigorously defined and documented found no such relationship.
- Gram-positive bacteria such as streptococci and staphylococci are most often implicated in the development of IE. Valvular infection with gram-negative organisms such as *Escherichia coli* is less common.
- With regard to the etiology of IE, there has been recent interest in the fastidious, intracellular organisms of the genus *Bartonella*. Four species of *Bartonella* have been documented to cause canine IE. Although geographic distribution of *Bartonella* IE may not be uniform, *Bartonella* is an important cause of IE in northern California and probably elsewhere. Patients with *Bartonella* infection are often concomitantly seropositive for tick-borne diseases, and *Bartonella* itself may be arthropod borne. *Bartonella* species are difficult to culture with standard microbiological techniques. The diagnosis depends on documentation of serum antibodies to *Bartonella*, or, more specifically, demonstration of *Bartonella* antigens through polymerase chain reaction testing performed on bacterial isolates or valve tissue.

PATHOPHYSIOLOGY

- The clinical signs of IE relate to sepsis, thromboembolism, and cardiac dysfunction. IE results in intermittent shedding of bacterial organisms into the bloodstream, resulting in episodes of bacteremia. Signs of sepsis, including pyrexia and rarely circulatory collapse, may be observed.

- Sequelae of sepsis related to chronic antigenic stimulation and consequent development of immune complex disease are observed fairly commonly in IE. Polyarthritis is observed often, and glomerulonephritis can also develop.
- In canine IE, it is often the destruction of the valve leaflets and associated structures that is of greatest clinical importance. The development of infected thrombi results in failure of the valve leaflets to coapt. Occasionally, perforation of the valve leaflets contributes to valvular incompetence. The hemodynamic consequences of MR have been discussed previously.
- IE of the aortic valve typically results in aortic valve incompetence, which is a potentially catastrophic hemodynamic lesion. When the aortic valve becomes incompetent, the left ventricle is filled during diastole by the pulmonary venous return and by the blood that enters through the regurgitant orifice. When severe, the increase in ventricular filling pressures (diastolic ventricular pressures) is reflected back on the pulmonary venous circulation, resulting in pulmonary congestion and edema. In contrast to MR, aortic valve insufficiency (AI) causes a substantial increase in left ventricular afterload and therefore myocardial oxygen demand. As a result, myocardial dysfunction (cardiomyopathy of overload) is observed commonly and early in the course of aortic valve IE.
- Embolization of fragments from the endocarditis lesion occurs commonly. Sites where infected thrombi lodge include the spleen, the kidney, and occasionally the brain. Most often, embolization of the spleen is clinically silent; infarction of the kidneys or central nervous system can be catastrophic, resulting in renal failure and nervous system signs such as head tilt. Embolization of joints, resulting in bacterial arthritis, can also occur.

CLINICAL PRESENTATION
HISTORY

- IE in dogs is observed most commonly in a subacute form. In these cases, historical evidence of prior illness or infectious disease may be lacking. A congenital cardiac murmur may or may not have been detected. IE is also observed in an acute form.
- Clinical signs in subacute IE are often vague; lameness, inappetence, dyspnea, syncope, and exercise intolerance are observed most commonly. The lameness is often mild and may be difficult to localize. The embolization of infected thrombi to joints contributes to lameness, although immune complex arthropathy may be of equal etiologic importance.

- Clinical signs of sepsis may be more prominent in patients that have acute IE. The sudden onset of fever and the development of a new cardiac murmur in the critically ill suggest the presence of IE.

PHYSICAL FINDINGS

- Fever is a common but not necessarily a consistent finding in patients with IE. Published cases series of canine IE reflect the experience of referral centers and are therefore biased. At some point in the natural history of the disease it is likely that most patients are pyrexic; however, fever associated with IE can be intermittent and may resolve before clinical presentation.
- The pulse rate is often elevated because some degree of cardiac dysfunction is commonly present at time of presentation.
- The respiratory rate is elevated, and respiratory distress is usually apparent in patients that have pulmonary edema.
- A cardiac murmur is present in most patients with established valvular infection. MR results in a systolic murmur that is most easily heard over the left cardiac apex. Aortic valve IE usually results in a diastolic decrescendo murmur that is typically heard most easily over the left cardiac base. A concurrent systolic murmur related to the increase in left ventricular stroke volume associated with AI results in a murmur known as a "to-and-fro" or "bellows" murmur.
- Diastolic murmurs are uncommon in veterinary patients and are usually soft; consequently, they may escape detection. Despite this, they are of considerable diagnostic and prognostic importance; acquired diastolic murmurs in dogs most often result from aortic valve IE.
- When moderate or severe AI is present, the arterial pulses are hyperkinetic or bounding; this physical finding should prompt consideration of IE whenever signalment and other clinical findings are suggestive.

DIAGNOSTIC FINDINGS
THORACIC RADIOGRAPHY

- Radiographic findings in IE are variable. Cardiac enlargement is apparent when valvular lesions have imposed a chronic volume overload on the heart. Pulmonary congestion or edema is commonly observed (Figure 7.19). Occasionally, IE results in severe and acute AI; this is one of the few clinical scenarios in which cardiogenic pulmonary edema is observed in association with a normal or minimally enlarged cardiac silhouette.

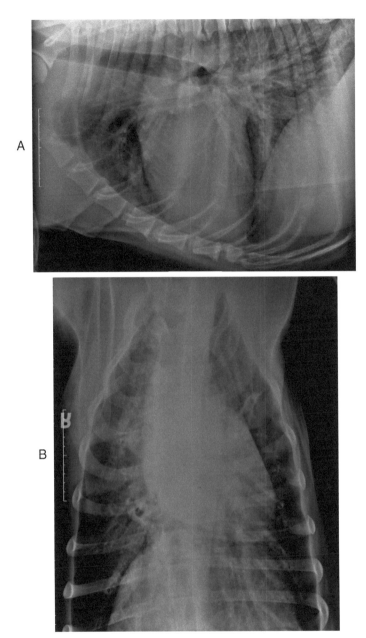

Figure 7.19 Lateral (**A**) and ventrodorsal (**B**) thoracic radiographs obtained from a 7-year-old male castrated Great Dane with mitral valve endocarditis. The cardiac silhouette is enlarged, and there is evidence of left atrial enlargement. Pulmonary opacities indicate the presence of pulmonary edema.

ELECTROCARDIOGRAPHY

- There are no electrocardiographic findings that are diagnostic of IE. However, all manner of cardiac arrhythmias can be observed in association with this disease. Ventricular tachyarrhythmias, including ventricular tachycardia, are relatively common, and supraventricular tachyarrhythmias, including atrial fibrillation, are also observed.
- The association of third-degree atrioventricular block with IE deserves mention. Occasionally an

aggressive aortic lesion will invade the interventricular septum or, alternatively, embolize the nodal coronary artery, resulting in destruction of the atrioventricular node or bundle. This catastrophic complication is relatively uncommon, but lesser degrees of atrioventricular block or intraventricular conduction delays, such as left bundle branch block, are observed fairly often.
- Electrocardiographic evidence of cardiac chamber enlargement is observed in patients that survive long enough for the volume overload

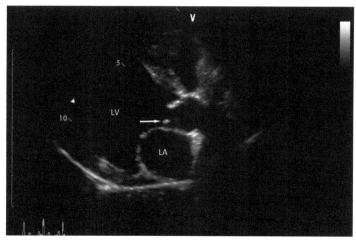

Figure 7.20 Two-dimensional echocardiographic image obtained from a Boxer with aortic valve endocarditis. This right parasternal long-axis view demonstrates the presence of highly echogenic nodules attached to the aortic valve leaflets; one of these lesions (*arrow*) oscillated independently of valve motion. *LA*, Left atrium; *LV*, left ventricle.

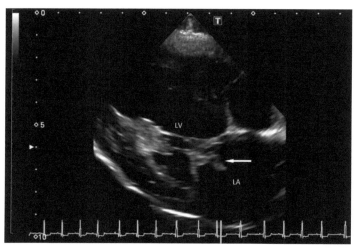

Figure 7.21 Two-dimensional echocardiographic long-axis image obtained from a 2-year-old male-castrated mixed-breed dog with mitral valve endocarditis. A lesion that oscillated independently of valve motion is attached to ventricular surface of the tip of the anterior mitral valve leaflet (*arrow*). *LA*, Left atrium; *LV*, left ventricle.

associated with IE to result in chamber dilation and hypertrophy.

ECHOCARDIOGRAPHIC FINDINGS

- The term *vegetative endocarditis* is generally used to refer to cases in which there is a macroscopic infected thrombus associated with a valve leaflet.
- The echocardiographic findings in vegetative IE are distinctive. In most cases, nodular distortion of the valve leaflets is readily apparent (Figure 7.20). Often the valvular abnormality is discrete, and the lesion may oscillate independently of valve motion.
- When these abnormalities are associated with the aortic valve leaflets, the diagnosis is usually assured.

- Nodules affecting the mitral valve leaflets are of lesser diagnostic specificity (Figure 7.21) because it can be difficult to distinguish severe MVD from infection of the mitral valve leaflets. To some extent, this distinction is made based on the patient's signalment. As stated previously, IE is very uncommon in elderly small dog breeds, which are of course the patients most likely to have severe MVD.
- The interpretation of subtle valvular abnormalities detected by echocardiography poses a difficult clinical problem, and other, ancillary clinical data, including the results of blood cultures, must be considered.
- The absence of a readily detectable valvular nodule on echocardiographic examination does not eliminate IE from the differential diagnosis.

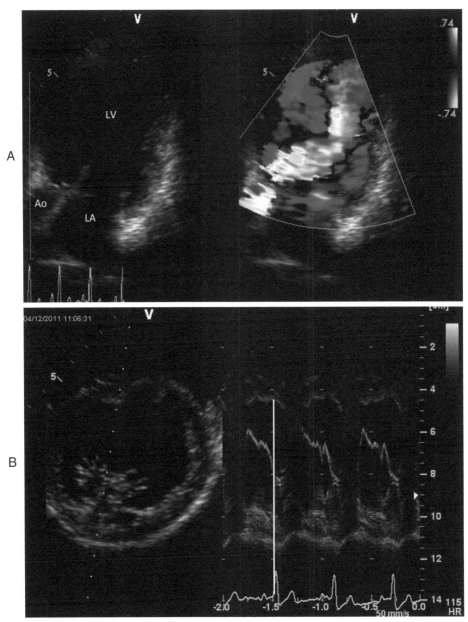

Figure 7.22   Echocardiographic images obtained from a Boxer with severe aortic valve incompetence caused by bacterial endocarditis. **A,** A diastolic apical image with (*right*) and without (*left*) superimposed color Doppler map; severe aortic valve regurgitation is evident. **B,** A short-axis image of the mitral valve and accompanying M-mode image from the same patient. There is diastolic flutter of the anterior mitral valve leaflet and premature closure of the mitral valve (*line*)—indirect echocardiographic evidence of severe aortic valve incompetence. *Ao*, Aorta; *LA*, left atrium; *LV*, left ventricle.

- When vegetative IE of the aortic or mitral valve is present, there is often echocardiographic evidence of left atrial and left ventricular enlargement. Premature diastolic closure of the mitral valve and diastolic flutter of the anterior mitral valve leaflet indicate severe AI (Figure 7.22). Some degree of systolic myocardial dysfunction is typically present when cardiac enlargement results from AI. Doppler echocardiography is used to confirm the presence of valvular incompetence.

LABORATORY DATA

- In many cases of IE, the hemogram reveals leukocytosis, but this finding is not consistently present. In subacute cases of IE, the leukocytosis is relatively mild, and evidence of acute inflammation may or may not be present.
- Abnormalities in the serum chemistries are not specific and, when present, are secondary to the disease process. Azotemia is relatively common and can be prerenal, as a result of poor renal

perfusion, or it can result from renal infarction. Hypoalbuminemia, hyperglobulinemia, and elevations in serum alkaline phosphatase may also be observed.

- Bacteria are cultivated from whole blood samples in 60% to 80% of IE cases. When possible, three whole-blood samples are obtained over a 12- to 24-hour period from a central vein after aseptic preparation of the overlying skin. When clinical circumstances allow, blood samples are obtained before the institution of antibacterial therapy, and the results are used to guide treatment. Taking samples over a shorter time period, say 1 to 3 hours, is reasonable when the clinical findings suggest that initiation of antibiotic therapy should not be delayed. Recent evidence suggests that a polymerase chain reaction test for bacterial nucleic acid may be a useful diagnostic adjunct to conventional blood cultures.

THERAPY

- Therapy of IE is directed toward control of sepsis, prevention of thromboembolism, and management of cardiac dysfunction that results from valvular incompetence.
- Antibacterial therapy is best guided by the results of bacterial culture and sensitivity testing of whole blood samples. When culture results are unavailable or when attempts to isolate bacteria from blood are unsuccessful, antibiotics are chosen on an empiric basis.
- Most often, IE in dogs results from gram-positive organisms, and agents such as the clavulanate-potentiated penicillins or the cephalosporins are appropriate. **Azithromycin** may have a role in the management of IE caused by *Bartonella* species. In general, bactericidal agents are preferred. A long course of therapy, 6 to 8 weeks, is generally recommended. There may be some advantage to initiating antibiotic therapy with the intravenous route because high serum drug levels are achieved quickly and with certainty.
- When clinical signs of sepsis are prominent and blood culture results are negative, initial therapy with a combination of intravenous **gentamicin** (or **amikacin**) and **ampicillin** (or a **cephalosporin**) is justified. When patients are free of gastrointestinal signs such as vomiting or diarrhea, oral antibiotic therapy is probably appropriate.
- Cardioactive agents are chosen on the basis of the results of radiographic and echocardiographic examinations. When there is left atrial and left ventricular enlargement caused by AI, ACE inhibitors are generally used. **Furosemide** (1 to 2 mg/kg PO q12h) is used with an ACE inhibitor in cases where there is radiographic evidence of pulmonary edema. Digoxin may have a role in the management of patients with severe HF. Careful attention to renal function must be paid when digoxin is used in patients with IE. In addition to the presence of HF and the use of ACE inhibitors, which are themselves risk factors for the development of azotemia, patients with IE may have renal dysfunction related to renal infarction.

MONITORING OF THERAPY

- As with other patients with HF, it is prudent to monitor serum electrolytes and renal function. Further monitoring of patients with IE may include serial blood cultures and follow-up echocardiograms.
- It is tempting to think that appropriate antibiotic therapy will result in resolution of echocardiographically detected valvular lesions. The valvular lesions of dogs with the more common form of IE, in which the presentation is subacute and there is echocardiographic evidence of severe valvular incompetence, do not generally resolve. Serial echocardiograms in these cases usually demonstrate progressive valvular incompetence and myocardial dysfunction.

PROPHYLAXIS OF INFECTIVE ENDOCARDITIS

- It is accepted that bacteremia is a requisite for the development of IE. However, although bacteremia results from dental procedures, transient bacteremia occurs in humans associated with normal day-to-day activities. Furthermore, the efficacy of antibiotic prophylaxis is uncertain. Accordingly, guidelines for antibiotic prophylaxis in humans have evolved, and antibiotics are no longer recommended before dental procedures for human patients with MVD.
- Relevant data that relate to canine patients are not available. It is reasonable to provide antibiotic prophylaxis for patients with congenital cardiac disease when they will undergo procedures in which bacteremia can be anticipated. Antibiotic administration intended to treat oral infection is also reasonable, but the value of antibiotic prophylaxis for patients with MVD subject to dental procedures is unknown. It is reasonable to perform dental procedures to improve dental health, but prevention of IE is not a justification with evidentiary basis.

PROGNOSIS

- The long-term prognosis for patients with echocardiographic evidence of vegetative subacute IE is grave. By the time the disease is detected, most cases of IE have progressed to the extent that there is irreversible damage to the valve. Failing surgical valve replacement, which is rarely practical in veterinary patients, the clinical picture is of progressive cardiac dysfunction, although patients with mitral valve involvement generally fare better than those with aortic valve disease. A few dogs die of renal failure related to renal infarction or are euthanized after septic thrombi have embolized to the central nervous system. However, in most cases, death occurs as a result of medically refractory HF or suddenly from malignant arrhythmia, even when antibiotic therapy is successful in controlling signs related to sepsis. In general, when an echocardiographic diagnosis of IE is made in a dog, survival is usually measured in weeks or months. With aggressive medical therapy, survival of 4 to 8 months is occasionally observed. Prognosis associated with more acute forms of IE that are treated early and aggressively is likely better.

FREQUENTLY ASKED QUESTIONS

Subjective evaluation of cardiac size from thoracic radiographs is difficult. Are there objective criteria that define radiographic cardiac enlargement?

Thoracic radiographs are indispensable in the diagnostic evaluation of dogs with MVD, but the accuracy of subjective evaluation of radiographic cardiac size is likely dependent on observer experience. It is relevant that the patients that most often have clinically important MVD are small dogs that have roughly cylindrical thoraces. In the lateral projection particularly, patients with this conformation tend to have a large cardiothoracic ratio even when the heart is, in fact, normal.

One method that can be used to overcome some of the limitations inherent in the subjective evaluation of radiographic cardiac size is the use of the vertebral heart scale. Beginning at the fourth thoracic vertebra and using the vertebral bodies as a scale,

the craniocaudal and dorsoventral dimensions of the cardiac silhouette are summed (Figure 7.23). This index of cardiac size is less than 10.5 in most healthy dogs. Higher values suggest cardiac enlargement.

There is current interest in the use of spironolactone as adjunctive therapy for HF in dogs. What are the indications for spironolactone in MVD?

Spironolactone is an antagonist of the mineralocorticoid aldosterone. It is not a potent diuretic, and interest in its use primarily relates to its presumed extrarenal effects. Cardiac dysfunction is associated with neuroendocrine responses that result in supraphysiologic aldosterone activity. Aldosterone is a ligand for specific renal receptors that mediate retention of sodium and excretion of potassium. In addition, there are data that support a role for aldosterone in the development of myocardial fibrosis in animals with experimentally induced cardiovascular disease. Inhibition of aldosterone activity by spironolactone reduced mortality in humans with severe HF, and this effect was evident at a dose that did not have a diuretic effect. Although invasive studies may disclose systolic myocardial dysfunction in dogs with mild but experimentally induced MR, contractility is apparently preserved until late in the natural history of MVD. On the basis of this, it seems reasonable to reserve spironolactone for patients with HF caused by MVD. In addition, the use of spironolactone is apparently safe but not entirely benign. Because it is generally used in conjunction with ACE inhibitors, there is a potential danger of hyperkalemia resulting from excessively diminished aldosterone activity. Indeed, after publication of a major study documenting the favorable effect of spironolactone in humans, reports of adverse effects appeared in the literature. On the basis of retrospective evaluation of clinicopathologic data, the use of spironolactone, together with ACE inhibitors and furosemide, is apparently safe in dogs; however, it is prudent to monitor serum electrolytes and renal function.

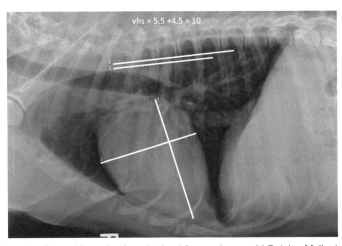

Figure 7.23 Normal lateral radiographic projection obtained from a 4-year-old Belgian Malinois. The dimensions used to calculate the vertebral heart sum (*vhs*) are shown. The vertebral bodies, beginning at the fourth thoracic vertebra, are used as a scale.

SUGGESTED READINGS

Anderson CA, Dubielzig RR: Vegetative endocarditis in dogs, J Am Anim Hosp Assoc 20:149, 1984.

Atkins CD, Keene BW, Brown WA, et al: Results of the veterinary enalapril trial to prove reduction in onset of heart failure in dogs chronically treated with enalapril alone for compensated, naturally occurring mitral valve insufficiency, J Am Vet Med Assoc 231:1061–1069, 2007.

Buchanan JW: Chronic valvular disease (endocardiosis) in dogs, Adv Vet Med 21:75, 1979.

Buchanan JW, Bucheler J: Vertebral scale system to measure canine heart size in radiographs, J Am Vet Med Assoc 206:194, 1995.

Bulmer BJ, Sisson DD: Therapy of heart failure. In Ettinger SJ, Feldman EC, eds: Textbook of veterinary internal medicine, ed 6, Philadelphia, 2005, Saunders.

Calvert CA: Valvular bacterial endocarditis in the dog, J Am Vet Med Assoc 180:1080–1084, 1982.

Chetboul V, Lefebvre HP, Sampedrano CC, et al.: Comparative adverse cardiac effects of pimobendan and benazepril monotherapy in dogs with mild degenerative mitral valve disease: a prospective, controlled, blinded, and randomized study, J Vet Intern Med 21:742–753, 2007.

Dell'Italia LJ: The renin-angiotensin system in mitral regurgitation: a typical example of tissue activation, Curr Cardiol Rep 4:97–103, 2002.

Ettinger SJ, Benitz AM, Ericsson GF, et al: Effects of enalapril maleate on survival of dogs with naturally acquired heart failure, J Am Vet Med Assoc 213:1573–1577, 1998.

Griffiths LG, Orton EC, Boon JA: Evaluation of techniques and outcomes of mitral valve repair in dogs, J Am Vet Med Assoc 224:1941–1945, 2004.

Haggstrom J, Hansson K, Kvart C, Swenson L: Chronic valvular disease in the cavalier King Charles Spaniel in Sweden, Vet Rec 131:549–553, 1992.

Haggstrom J, Kvart C, Pedersen HD: Acquired valvular disease, In Ettinger SJ, Feldman EC, eds: Textbook of veterinary internal medicine, ed 6, Philadelphia, 2005, Saunders.

Haggstrom J, Duelund Pedersen H, Kvart C: New insights into degenerative valve disease in dogs, Vet Clin North Am Small Anim Pract 34:1209–1226, 2004.

Kvart C, Haggstrom J, Pedersen HD, et al: Efficacy of enalapril for prevention of congestive heart failure in dogs with myxomatous valve disease and asymptomatic mitral regurgitation, J Vet Intern Med 16:80–88, 2002.

MacDonald KA, Chomel BB, Kittleson MD, et al: A prospective study of canine infective endocarditis in northern California (1999-2001): emergence of Bartonella as a prevalent etiologic agent, J Vet Intern Med 18.56–64, 2004.

Nakamura RK, Tompkins E, Russell NJ, et al: Left atrial rupture secondary to myxomatous mitral valve disease in 11 dogs, J Am Anim Hosp Assoc 50:405–408, 2014.

Rush JR, Cunningham SM: Chronic valvular heart disease in dogs. In Bonagura JD, Twedt DC, eds: Current veterinary therapy XV, Philadelphia, 2014, Elsevier Saunders.

Sisson D, Thomas WP: Endocarditis of the aortic valve in the dog, J Am Vet Med Assoc 184:570–577, 1984.

Sisson D, Kvart C, Darke PG: Acquired valvular heart disease in dogs and cats. In Fox PR, Sisson D, Moise NS, eds: Textbook of canine and feline cardiology: principles and clinical practice, ed 2, Philadelphia, 1999, Saunders.

Canine Cardiomyopathy

8

Mark A. Oyama

Cardiomyopathy is defined as a primary disease of the heart muscle of unknown etiology. Disease of the heart muscle secondary to toxins, nutritional deficiencies, endocrinopathies, and infectious agents is often regarded as "secondary cardiomyopathy." The most common form of canine cardiomyopathy is dilated cardiomyopathy (DCM), which is characterized by progressive ventricular dilation and loss of myocardial contractility. Other forms of cardiomyopathy, such as hypertrophic cardiomyopathy (HCM), are rare in dogs. DCM is most common in adult large-breed dogs, in particular, the Doberman Pinscher, Irish Wolfhound, Scottish Deerhound, and Great Dane. The important features of canine DCM include the presence of an asymptomatic or occult phase during which diagnosis is difficult, the high prevalence of congestive heart failure (CHF) and sudden death in severely affected dogs, and the need for aggressive and comprehensive medical therapy to help alleviate clinical signs. Boxers with cardiomyopathy possess a unique pathophysiology, clinical presentation, and natural history so that the disease is best described as arrhythmogenic right ventricular cardiomyopathy (ARVC). Sudden death from ventricular arrhythmias is very common in Boxers with ARVC, much more so than death from chronic CHF. Secondary cardiomyopathies caused by nutritional deficiencies appear in small- and medium-size breeds, most notably the American Cocker Spaniel. A highly fatal juvenile form of DCM is seen in the Portuguese Water Dog.

DILATED CARDIOMYOPATHY

PREVALENCE AND SIGNALMENT

Surveys indicate that between two and six dogs are diagnosed with DCM per 600 case referrals. In certain breeds, the prevalence of DCM is remarkably high. Approximately 25% of Irish Wolfhounds, 33% of female Doberman Pinschers, and 50% of male Doberman Pinschers contract DCM. The typical age at diagnosis is between 6 and 8 years; however, it is not uncommon to diagnose DCM

in dogs as young as 3 years and as old as 12 years. Male dogs appear to be more frequently affected, especially in the Doberman Pinscher breed.

NATURAL HISTORY

The clinical progression of DCM is best described as occurring in two distinct phases.

ASYMPTOMATIC OCCULT PHASE

- No clinical signs are evident; however, myocardial or electrical abnormalities are present and may include the following:
  - Increased left ventricular (LV) and atrial dimensions
  - Decreased myocardial contractility
  - Ventricular premature beats
- The duration of the occult phase is highly variable and may possibly last for months to years.
- During this phase, progressive heart enlargement and worsening arrhythmias occur.
- The occult phase ends with the appearance of the first clinical signs of disease.
  - Approximately 40% of Doberman Pinschers experience sudden cardiac death as the first clinical sign.

OVERT CLINICAL PHASE

- Clinical signs develop
  - CHF
  - Syncope
  - Exercise and activity intolerance
- Arrhythmias in the form of ventricular premature beats, ventricular tachycardia, and atrial fibrillation are common.
- Death is due either to advanced CHF that is refractory to medical therapy or sudden death.
  - A total of 30% to 50% of Doberman Pinschers die suddenly.
  - Many dogs with advanced heart failure are euthanized because of chronic respiratory distress, severe activity intolerance, anorexia, and weight loss.

41

HISTORY AND PHYSICAL EXAMINATION FINDINGS

ASYMPTOMATIC OCCULT PHASE

- Common findings include the following:
  - Soft systolic heart murmur
  - Irregular heart rhythm with pulse deficits
- Occasional findings include the following:
  - Diastolic gallop rhythm
  - Decreased intensity of heart sounds
  - Weak femoral pulse quality
  - Jugular vein distension or pulses

OVERT CLINICAL PHASE

- History may include exercise intolerance, syncope, lethargy, anorexia, difficulty breathing, coughing, and abdominal distension.
- Common findings include the following:
  - Moderate-intensity systolic heart murmur
  - Irregular heart rhythm with pulse deficits
  - Increased respiratory rate and effort
  - Increased bronchovesicular sounds
  - Decreased intensity of heart sounds
  - Weakness
- Occasional findings include the following:
  - Jugular vein distension or pulses
  - Hepatomegaly
  - Ascites
  - Pale mucous membranes
  - Hypothermia
  - Pulmonary crackles
  - Depressed mentation

DIAGNOSTIC TESTS

Ideally, all dogs should be evaluated with an electrocardiogram (ECG), chest radiographs, echocardiogram, urinalysis, and serum chemistry. In many cases, additional diagnostics, such as 24-hour ambulatory ECG (Holter) monitoring, are performed.

ELECTROCARDIOGRAPHY

- The ECG is the test of choice for detecting arrhythmias and may provide evidence of heart enlargement; however, a normal ECG does not rule out the presence of cardiomyopathy.
- Asymptomatic occult phase
  - Arrhythmias are often the first indication of disease, and screening is recommended in breeds at high risk for DCM.
  - Routine ECG detects frequent arrhythmias but may have limited sensitivity in dogs with infrequent or intermittent arrhythmias.
  - Detection of the following ECG signs is associated with a high index of suspicion for occult cardiomyopathy:
    - One or more ventricular premature complexes (VPCs) in a Doberman Pinscher or Boxer. In Boxers, VPCs with a left bundle branch block morphology (upright QRS complex in lead II) are highly suggestive of ARVC (Figure 8.1).
    - Criteria for LV (QRS duration >0.06 seconds, R wave amplitude >3.0 mV) or atrial enlargement (P wave duration >0.04 seconds)
    - In Irish Wolfhounds, atrial fibrillation is often an early sign of disease as opposed to other breeds, where atrial fibrillation is associated with advanced stages of disease.
  - Holter monitoring detects arrhythmias with greater sensitivity and is recommended in dogs at high risk (i.e., dogs with a familial history of disease).
    - More than 100 VPCs in a 24-hour period is highly suggestive of occult DCM or ARVC.
    - 50 to 100 VPCs in a 24-hour period is suspicious for disease and should be followed by another Holter examination in 2 to 6 months.
    - Day-to-day variability in the frequency of arrhythmia can produce false-negative results, and if the initial Holter examination is inconclusive, multiple Holter examinations may be indicated, especially in dogs with a family history of disease or in those that have experienced syncope.

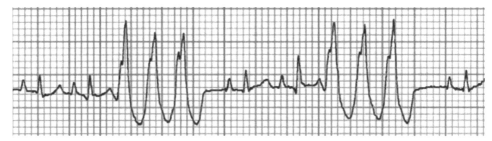

Figure 8.1 Lead II electrocardiogram (ECG) tracing from a 7-year-old male castrated Boxer with arrhythmogenic right ventricular cardiomyopathy (ARVC). Ventricular premature beats with left bundle branch block morphology are a common finding in dogs with this condition. 25 mm/sec; 0.5 cm/mV.

- During the overt clinical phase, the following may be detected:
  - Occasional to frequent ventricular or supraventricular premature beats
  - Ventricular tachycardia
  - Criteria for LV or atrial enlargement (see previous section)
  - Left bundle branch block
  - Atrial fibrillation (Figure 8.2)

CHEST RADIOGRAPHY

- Chest radiographs are relatively insensitive to mild increases in heart size. A single set performed in the asymptomatic occult phase contributes relatively little to the immediate diagnosis; however, serial radiographs are well suited to monitor progressive heart enlargement and progression of disease. In the overt clinical phase, radiographs are invaluable in helping to diagnose CHF and to monitor response to treatment.
  - The chest radiographs in Doberman Pinschers are often misleading in that heart enlargement is less striking than in other breeds with similar clinical signs. In these instances, cardiac ultrasound helps to determine the magnitude of left-sided heart enlargement and systolic dysfunction.
  - The chest radiographs in Boxers with ARVC are usually normal.

ECHOCARDIOGRAPHY

- Echocardiography is widely used to quantify heart enlargement and systolic function. Routine echocardiography is not particularly sensitive in detecting early changes in occult disease, nor is it particularly helpful after a diagnosis of end-stage disease is made. As such, the utility of echocardiography increases as the disease moves from the occult to the overt clinical phase; it then declines again as the patient advances to end-stage disease. Early in the course of disease, many dogs have echocardiograms with normal findings, despite having a significant number of ventricular arrhythmias. Echocardiographic values from any individual dog are compared with weight-based reference ranges or are scaled to body size with allometric techniques. Allometric techniques (Chapter 4) are being increasingly used as they account for the nonlinear relationship between echocardiographic dimensions, such as the left ventricular end-diastolic diameter (LVIDd) and body weight.
- Echocardiographic criteria are used to help diagnose occult DCM. The greater number of indices that are abnormal, the higher the likelihood that occult DCM is present.
- In Doberman Pinschers, a left ventricular end-diastolic diameter (LVIDd) >49 mm or a left ventricular end-systolic diameter (LVIDs) >40 mm is highly suggestive of occult disease. In Doberman Pinschers, fractional shortening is an unreliable index for occult DCM because this breed typically has fractional shortening values in the mid or low 20% range. Similarly, large-breed dogs with athletic lifestyles commonly display fractional shortening values in the mid 20% range, and longitudinal echocardiographic studies or Holter monitoring is required to determine if disease is truly present.
- In Doberman Pinschers, LV volume measurements (Chapter 4) are superior to LV

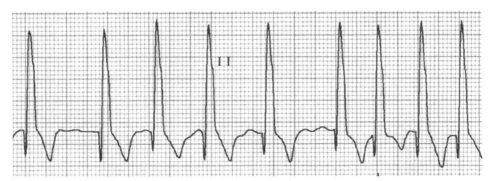

Figure 8.2 Lead II electrocardiogram (ECG) tracing from a dog indicating atrial fibrillation and left ventricular (LV) enlargement. Note the irregular rhythm, lack of P waves, and widened QRS complex. 50 mm/sec; 10 mm/mV.

dimension measurements in detecting occult DCM. Left ventricular end-diastolic volume (LVEDV) to body surface area ratio >95 mL/m^2 or left ventricular end-systolic volume (LVESV) to body surface area ratio >55 mL/m^2 were indicators of occult disease.

- In Doberman Pinschers, blood testing for pro-N-terminal B-type natriuretic peptide (NT-proBNP) can help identify dogs with high probability of abnormal echocardiographic findings. High NT-proBNP values should prompt follow-up echocardiograms.
- In Irish Wolfhounds, occult disease is defined as LVIDd >61.2 mm, LVIDs >41 mm, fractional shortening <25%, end-systolic volume index >41 mL/m^2, or E-point to septal separation >10 mm.
- In Great Danes, occult disease is defined as LVIDd >58.7 mm (males) or >56.1 mm (females), LVIDs >42.5 mm (males) or >41.9 mm (females), fractional shortening <20%, ejection fraction <42.1%, allometric-LVIDd >1.64, and/or allometric-LVIDs >1.11.
- Newer ultrasound modalities such as Doppler tissue imaging may be more sensitive than conventional echocardiography in detecting early abnormalities of myocardial contractility.
- As disease progresses from occult to overt, echocardiography helps monitor heart enlargement, assess contractility, and evaluate secondary mitral regurgitation. Echocardiography is used in conjunction with chest radiographs to help decide when to initiate therapy.
- Common echocardiographic findings in dogs with advanced occult or overt clinical disease include the following:
  - Moderate to severe LV and atrial enlargement (Figure 8.3).
  - Reduced systolic motion of the LV wall and interventricular septum (Figure 8.4).
  - Mild to moderate mitral regurgitation secondary to mitral annulus dilation.
  - Incomplete systolic opening of the aortic valves.
  - Decreased aortic blood flow velocity.
  - Increased mitral valve E-point to septal separation (normal <6 mm)
  - Decreased systolic thickening of the LV wall and interventricular septum.
  - The echocardiogram in Boxer dogs with ARVC is usually normal. Subtle right ventricular

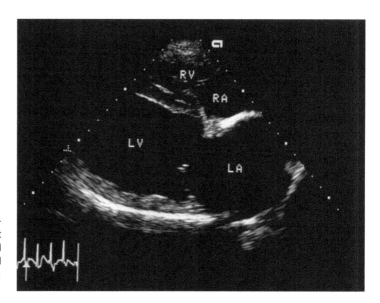

Figure 8.3 Two-dimensional echocardiogram of the left ventricle (*LV*) and left atrium (*LA*) of a Great Dane with dilated cardiomyopathy (DCM). Note the dilated ventricular and atrial chambers. *RA,* Right atrium; *RV,* right ventricle.

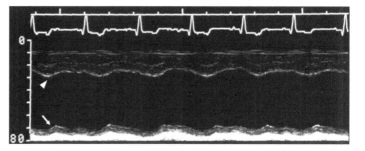

Figure 8.4 M-mode echocardiogram of the left ventricle of a Cocker Spaniel with dilated cardiomyopathy (DCM). Note the decreased systolic motion of the interventricular septum *(arrow)* and left ventricular (LV) free wall *(arrowhead)*.

dilation or wall motion abnormalities may be noted.

GENETIC TESTS

- Genetic mutations involving two different genes, *PDK4* and *striatin,* have been associated with DCM in Doberman Pinschers and ARVC in Boxers, respectively. These two mutations are not the only ones associated with DCM or ARVC because some affected Doberman Pinschers and Boxers do not carry the mutation. There might also be important geographic differences in the prevalence of the mutations based on country of origin and lineage. Importantly, being negative for the mutation at an early age does not ensure that the dog will be free of DCM or ARVC in later years.
- Genetic testing is recommended before use of Doberman Pinschers or Boxers for breeding, and dogs that are homozygous for the mutations are strongly discouraged from breeding. Genetic testing is not recommended in place of ECG and echocardiography as a diagnostic tool to detect the presence of clinical disease.

CONCOMITANT ABNORMALITIES IN MODERATE OR SEVERE DILATED CARDIOMYOPATHY

- Azotemia is commonly detected in dogs that are receiving diuretic therapy and is typically prerenal in nature.
- Mild azotemia (BUN <60 mg/dL and creatinine <2.5 mg/dL) usually does not require specific treatment or cessation or reduction of diuretic therapy.
- More severe azotemia (BUN >80 mg/dL and creatinine >3.0 mg/dL) can contribute to morbidity and may require reduction of an angiotensin-converting enzyme (ACE) inhibitor (e.g., enalapril) and diuretic dose or parenteral fluid supplementation.
  - If fluids are administered, then administering half-strength saline or Ringer solution will reduce the sodium load to the patient.
  - ACE inhibitor therapy can be temporarily discontinued or the dosage reduced. Initiation of the ACE inhibitor therapy should be delayed or done with caution.
  - Aggressive parenteral fluid therapy can aggravate CHF and should be used with caution.
  - Many instances can be treated by reducing diuretics and allowing patients to drink enough water to reestablish hydration on their own.
  - Azotemia reduces renal clearance of digoxin and predisposes to toxicity. Serum digoxin

levels should be determined especially if the patient displays anorexia, vomiting, diarrhea, or frequent arrhythmias.
- Electrolyte abnormalities are common in dogs with CHF because of DCM. Most changes are mild and do not require specific treatment.
- Potassium levels may be high or low. Mild hypokalemia (K^+ 2.5 to 3.0 mEq/L) is commonly associated with high doses of diuretics and usually does not require specific treatment. Severe hypokalemia (K^+ <2.5 mEq/L) can cause cardiac arrhythmias and contribute to muscle weakness. Reduction of potassium-wasting diuretics (e.g., furosemide) or initiation of potassium-sparing agents (e.g., ACE inhibitors, spironolactone) is undertaken. Clinically important *hyper*kalemia is uncommon and usually associated with reduced cardiac output, poor renal perfusion, and renal failure.
- Mild hyponatremia is common and dilutional in nature. Serum concentration of sodium is decreased secondary to water retention and expansion of the plasma volume despite elevated total body sodium content. Mild hyponatremia does not require specific treatment. In my experience, profound hyponatremia (Na^+ <130 mEq/L) signals a poor prognosis. Treatment requires reduction of diuretic dose, water restriction, and dietary sodium supplementation.
- Hypothyroidism is a common concurrent disease in middle-aged to older dogs, especially Doberman Pinschers. A causal relationship between hypothyroidism and DCM is doubtful. Supplementation does not improve survival.
- Natriuretic peptides are produced by the atrial and ventricular tissues in response to increased wall stress. Their biologic actions counter those of the renin-angiotensin-aldosterone system. Atrial natriuretic peptide and NT-proBNP are elevated in dogs with symptomatic DCM and reflect disease severity. Both peptides are able to distinguish between cardiogenic and noncardiogenic causes of dyspnea in dogs. In humans, natriuretic peptides provide information regarding diagnosis, prognosis, and efficacy of treatment. A similar utility is likely to exist for dogs.
- Cardiac troponin I forms part of the actin-myosin contractile apparatus and is released into circulation following myocyte injury or necrosis. Cardiac troponin I is elevated in dogs with DCM and modestly correlates with degree of LV hypertrophy. One study indicated that dogs with plasma cardiac troponin I >0.20 ng/mL have shorter survival times than those with lower values.

NUTRITIONAL DEFICIENCIES

- Taurine deficiency is a contributing cause of DCM in the American Cocker Spaniel and a potential contributing factor in Dalmatians, Labrador Retrievers, and Golden Retrievers. In contrast, the incidence of taurine-responsive disease is virtually nonexistent in the traditional breeds of dogs with DCM. Recognition of taurine deficiency is important in that heart function may be substantially improved following supplementation. In any nontraditional breed of dog—that is, in any dog that is *not* a Doberman Pinscher, Boxer, Great Dane, Irish Wolfhound, or Scottish Deerhound—I recommend plasma taurine assay. Interestingly, most taurine-deficient dogs are receiving an adequate meat-based diet, and abnormalities of taurine absorption, metabolism, or excretion are the likely cause of disease.
- Most dogs with taurine-deficient DCM have plasma taurine <25 nmol/mL.
- L-Carnitine deficiency is not a well-defined cause of canine DCM; however, some dogs that are taurine deficient require both L-carnitine and taurine to improve.
- Plasma L-carnitine concentration is not reflective of myocardial tissue concentration, and plasma assays are of little clinical utility. As such, diagnosis of L-carnitine deficiency requires myocardial biopsy. A presumptive diagnosis of deficiency is often considered when dogs are concurrently taurine deficient.

TREATMENT

Standard treatment involves the use of diuretics, positive inotropes, and ACE inhibitors. Ventricular arrhythmias and atrial fibrillation require the use of specific antiarrhythmics. More recently, beta-adrenergic blocking agents and combined positive inotropic-vasodilator drugs have been used. Treatment depends on the breed, stage of disease, and presence of CHF or arrhythmias.

DRUG CLASSES USED FOR TREATMENT

- **Diuretic** therapy alleviates signs of congestion. As disease worsens, use of multiple diuretics helps achieve increased diuresis. Diuretic monotherapy increases activity of the renin-angiotensin-aldosterone system, and concomitant ACE inhibition should be used. Diuretic therapy is commonly accompanied by mild azotemia and hypokalemia. The potent loop diuretic furosemide is routinely used in patients with symptoms. Thiazide diuretics, though less potent, have a longer half-life, act at a site separate from furosemide, and provide

additional diuresis in patients already receiving high doses of furosemide. Spironolactone is a weak potassium-sparing diuretic that is typically administered in conjunction with a thiazide. Spironolactone's beneficial effects are probably caused by its antiproliferative actions and subsequent reduction of ventricular remodeling and fibrosis, rather than its very weak diuretic action.
- **Positive inotropic** therapy is used to improve contractility. Drugs include digoxin, beta-adrenergic agonists (e.g., dopamine, dobutamine), phosphodiesterase inhibitors (e.g., milrinone), and calcium sensitizers (e.g., pimobendan). As a positive inotrope, digoxin is relatively weak and not useful in the emergency setting; however, it is useful in controlling the ventricular rate in patients with atrial fibrillation. The beta-adrenergic agonists and phosphodiesterase inhibitors are administered with constant rate infusion (CRI) and are useful in the emergency setting. Pimobendan is a unique drug because of its combined inotropic and vasodilatory properties. Survival and quality of life are likely improved by its use.
- **Venous vasodilators** reduce preload and **arterial vasodilators** reduce afterload.
  - ACE inhibitors blunt activity of the renin-angiotensin-aldosterone system, reduce salt and water retention, and elicit mild arterial vasodilation. ACE inhibitors improve survival and quality of life in dogs with DCM. Dogs with severe heart failure and poor renal perfusion may become uremic while taking ACE inhibitors, especially when high doses of diuretics are being given concurrently.
  - Sodium nitroprusside elicits potent arterial and venous vasodilation and is very effective in cases of life-threatening heart failure. Because of the risk for hypotension, arterial blood pressure monitoring is required during its use. Sodium nitroprusside is administered as a CRI.
  - Topical nitroglycerin produces minimal venous vasodilation in dogs because of poor absorption and low plasma concentrations.
- **Antiarrhythmic agents** suppress life-threatening ventricular arrhythmias and control the ventricular rate during atrial fibrillation. For ventricular arrhythmias, drugs in classes I (e.g., lidocaine and mexiletine), II (beta blockers), and III (e.g., sotalol) can be used alone or in certain combinations. Drugs in class II and IV (calcium channel blockers) and digoxin are used for atrial fibrillation.
- **Beta-adrenergic blocking agents** are extensively used in humans with DCM. In dogs, little clinical data exist. Beta-blocking agents blunt the

effects of chronic sympathetic nervous system activity (i.e., tachycardia, arrhythmias, myocyte death, ventricular remodeling, and elevated activity of the renin-angiotensin-aldosterone system). Overly aggressive use may exacerbate CHF, and patients should be clinically stable before being titrated onto this class of drug.

- **Inodilators** are drugs that improve cardiac contractility and elicit vasodilation. Pimobendan is a calcium-sensitizing inodilator that increases the myocardial response to calcium. Pimobendan should be used in dogs with symptomatic disease that are already receiving conventional therapy. Pimobendan improves quality of life and likely survival.

TREATMENT OF ASYMPTOMATIC OCCULT DISEASE

Treatment in the occult phase represents both an opportunity and a challenge. Clearly, treatments that slow progression in this phase would help delay or prevent symptomatic disease, yet the discovery of effective drugs is hindered by the difficulty in performing large-scale prospective clinical trials with sufficient statistical power. There are no known treatments that definitively slow progression of disease in the occult state. Insofar as gradual derangement of neurohormonal activity is associated with worsening cardiac function, use of ACE inhibitors, beta blockers, and spironolactone has been suggested. Current recommendations are based on small veterinary trials and extrapolation from human medicine. Pimobendan, beta blockers, and ACE inhibitors are typically considered during the occult phase.

- Use of pimobendan is scientifically supported in Doberman Pinschers with echocardiographic evidence of occult DCM. In this population, pimobendan delayed the time to CHF or sudden death by 63%. The safety and efficacy of pimobendan in Doberman Pinschers with severe ventricular arrhythmias, such as ventricular tachycardia, or in dogs without echocardiographic changes are unproven (see Frequently Asked Questions).
- Use of beta blockade is scientifically supported in virtually all human patients with LV systolic dysfunction with current or prior symptoms, and consensus opinion extends this recommendation to use in symptom-free patients. In dogs, sympathetic tone is increased during the occult phase, thus providing a rationale for use of beta blockers in dogs with early disease.
- Use of ACE inhibition is scientifically supported in virtually all human patients with LV systolic dysfunction regardless of symptoms. In dogs, the time course of ACE activation is uncertain.

Although several studies indicate that heightened activity of the renin-angiotensin-aldosterone is not present in early disease, there is a need to distinguish between circulating and local ACE activity. Although circulating ACE activity is not upregulated until later in the disease, evidence suggests that a locally contained myocardial ACE system contributes much earlier in the disease. Thus, tissue-penetrating ACE inhibitors, such as benazepril or ramipril, may be beneficial.

- Spironolactone is primarily used in humans with symptomatic DCM; however, the benefit in preventing aldosterone-mediated remodeling may begin in earlier stages of disease.
- Because of the high incidence of sudden death in Boxers with ARVC and Doberman Pinschers with DCM, antiarrhythmic therapy is often initiated in symptom-free dogs according to Holter monitor findings. Dogs with runs of ventricular tachycardia or R-on-T phenomenon are started on sotalol (1.5 to 2.0 mg/kg q12h) or the combination of mexiletine (5 to 8 mg/kg q8h) and atenolol (0.3 to 0.4 mg/kg q12h). The efficacy of this treatment in preventing sudden death is unproven.

KEY POINTS

The natural history of cardiomyopathy is substantially influenced by breed. Large- or giant-breed dogs commonly have atrial fibrillation and CHF, although Doberman Pinschers with DCM and Boxers with ARVC commonly exhibit syncope, ventricular arrhythmias, and sudden death. Thus, in Great Danes, Irish Wolfhounds, and similarly affected breeds, treatment should focus on resolution of heart failure, whereas in Doberman Pinschers and Boxers, antiarrhythmic therapy is commonly prescribed.

TREATMENT OF OVERT CLINICAL DISEASE

TREATMENT OF SEVERE LIFE-THREATENING CONGESTIVE HEART FAILURE

CHF is relieved through aggressive diuretic, vasodilator, and positive inotropic therapy.

- Manual removal of heart failure fluid should be performed in all patients with clinically significant pleural or abdominal effusion because this will rapidly improve respiratory effort and alleviate distress.
- Intravenous or intramuscular furosemide (2 to 6 mg/kg) is administered. When given parenterally, duration of effect is approximately 2 hours; therefore additional doses should be

administered if the patient's respiratory rate and effort have not improved within this time period. Patient recovery can be significantly hindered because of insufficient dosing of furosemide during the first 12 hours of treatment.

- Efficacy of diuretic therapy is assessed by monitoring patient respiratory rate and effort, urine output, and body weight. For confirmation of the resolution of pulmonary edema or for reassessment of patients that are not responding to therapy, chest radiographs are performed 12 to 24 hours after initiation of therapy.
- The presence of severe underlying renal dysfunction may necessitate lower doses and less frequent dosing.
- Sodium nitroprusside (2.0 to 5.0 µg/kg/min CRI) is a very effective vasodilator. Nitroprusside can produce profound hypotension, and arterial blood pressure monitoring is required when it is used. The infusion rate is adjusted to elicit a 15 mm Hg decrease in mean blood pressure as long as the mean value does not fall below 70 mm Hg.
- Intravenous positive inotropes such as dopamine (2 to 10 µg/kg/min CRI) or dobutamine (5 to 15 µg/kg/min CRI) help improve cardiac output. High doses may aggravate ventricular arrhythmias or cause sinus tachycardia.
- Milrinone is a potent positive inotrope that acts downstream of the myocardial beta-adrenergic receptor. It increases contractility in patients receiving beta blockers or in patients that are not responding to dopamine or dobutamine therapy. Milrinone is administered as a 30 to 50 µg/kg loading bolus given intravenously over 10 minutes and then as a CRI of 1 to 8 µg/kg/min.
- Oral pimobendan (0.25 mg/kg q12h) may be useful if intravenous positive inotrope therapy is not available.
- When given orally, digoxin requires several days to reach an effective concentration and, as such, has little role as an emergency positive inotrope. Intravenous digoxin commonly produces toxicity and is not recommended.
- Supplemental oxygen therapy is administered either in an oxygen cage (fraction of inspired oxygen = 40%) or given nasally (50 to 100 mL/kg/min).
- One of the most difficult clinical decisions is whether to specifically treat ventricular arrhythmias. Overly aggressive treatment may cause hypotension or predispose to even more malignant arrhythmias.
  - VPCs and short runs of ventricular tachycardia that occur at relatively slow heart rates

(<160 beats/min) typically do not require treatment. Often, resolution occurs spontaneously once CHF and hypoxia are successfully treated.
- Rapid ventricular arrhythmias that are life-threatening are accompanied by clinical signs (i.e., weakness, syncope, hypotension, blanching of mucous membranes). Intravenous lidocaine (2 mg/kg bolus followed by CRI of 40 to 80 µg/kg/min) or procainamide (6 to 8 mg/kg bolus followed by CRI of 20 to 40 µg/kg/min) are often effective.
- Because of the high incidence of sudden death in Boxers and Doberman Pinschers, aggressive antiarrhythmic therapy in these species is more commonly warranted, especially in dogs that have previously had syncope. Once stabilized, either oral sotalol or a combination of mexiletine and atenolol is prescribed (see next section).

TRANSITIONING THE IMPROVED EMERGENCY PATIENT TO CHRONIC ORAL TREATMENT

Aggressive emergency therapy successfully resolves acute heart failure in approximately 75% of dogs. In most dogs, significant improvement in clinical signs will be apparent within 48 hours. Patients refractory to therapy beyond this point have a grave prognosis. As the patient becomes increasingly stable, intravenous medications are gradually reduced and replaced with oral medications. During this time, patient hydration status, body weight, appetite, respiratory effort, electrolytes, and renal function continue to be monitored.

- Once the patient's respiratory rate and effort has improved, parenteral furosemide is discontinued in favor of oral furosemide (typical oral dose for first time CHF is 2 to 4 mg/kg/day usually divided q12h). Nitroprusside and dopamine or dobutamine are gradually reduced over 12 to 24 hours and replaced by an ACE inhibitor (enalapril 0.5 mg/kg q12h or benazepril 0.5 mg/kg q24h) and pimobendan (0.25 mg/kg q12h). Because of the potential for adverse effects (e.g., anorexia, vomiting), some clinicians stagger the initiation of diuretic and ACE inhibitor therapy. In these cases, the ACE inhibitor is withheld for 3 to 5 days until the patient is tolerating the diuretics. In patients with atrial fibrillation, the urgency for digoxin treatment is more acute, and digoxin (0.003 mg/kg q12h) is started.
- Lidocaine or procainamide is gradually reduced over 12 to 24 hours and replaced by oral drugs: sotalol (1.5 to 2.5 mg/kg q12h) or a combination of sotalol (1 to 2 mg/kg q12h)

and mexiletine (5 mg/kg q8h) or atenolol (0.3 to 0.4 mg/kg q12h) and mexiletine (5 mg/kg q8h).

- Aggressive use of beta-adrenergic blocking antiarrhythmics, such as sotalol or atenolol, may exacerbate heart failure (see next section). Gradual titration of these agents may be required.
- Dietary sodium restriction (40 to 70 mg Na/100 kcal).

TREATMENT OF REFRACTORY HEART FAILURE

- Patients that are already receiving high doses of loop diuretics (e.g., furosemide) may benefit from additional diuretics that target areas of the nephron other than the loop of Henle.
  - Oral hydrochlorothiazide (1 to 4 mg/kg q12 to 48h) is a moderately potent diuretic that acts in the distal convoluted tubule and has a longer half-life than furosemide. Initially, it is given in conjunction with furosemide and gradually increased as needed to control congestion. Hydrochlorothiazide is also available in combination with equal amounts of spironolactone (hydrochlorothiazide spironolactone, 2 to 4 mg/kg q12 to 24h).
- In patients with right-sided heart failure or severely decreased cardiac output, absorption and renal delivery of oral furosemide may be decreased. In these cases, substituting subcutaneous injections of furosemide often restores effectiveness. Usually, the total daily dose of furosemide can be modestly decreased when it is administered in this fashion.
  - End-stage DCM is often accompanied by inappetence and weight loss and requires attention to adequate caloric and protein intake.

TREATMENT OF DILATED CARDIOMYOPATHY ACCOMPANIED BY ATRIAL FIBRILLATION

Atrial fibrillation commonly occurs in dogs with advanced DCM. The incidence of atrial fibrillation is higher in giant-breed dogs (e.g., Great Danes, Irish Wolfhounds) than in Doberman Pinschers and Boxers. Atrial fibrillation with rapid ventricular rates (>180 beats/min) exacerbates CHF and low cardiac output. Conversion of atrial fibrillation back to normal sinus rhythm is usually futile, and management is targeted at slowing the ventricular rate. One of three drugs can be administered orally for this purpose:

- Digoxin (0.003 mg/kg q12h)
- Diltiazem (0.5 to 2.0 mg/kg q8h) or diltiazem XR (1.5 to 4.0 mg/kg q12 to 24h)
- Atenolol (0.25 to 1.0 mg/kg q12h)

In most instances, digoxin is preferred because of its concomitant positive inotropic effects. If rate control is not achieved by digoxin alone, then addition of diltiazem or atenolol is warranted. Overly aggressive dosing of atenolol or atenolol coadministered with diltiazem can produce bradycardia, heart block, and hypotension. Intravenous administration of digoxin is not recommended because of the high likelihood of toxicity. In patients that require immediate rate control because of extremely rapid ventricular rates, oral loading of digoxin (0.006 mg/kg for the first 1 to 2 doses) or intravenous diltiazem (0.1 to 0.2 mg/kg bolus then 2 to 6 µg/kg/min CRI) can be attempted.

- The ideal heart rate for dogs with DCM and atrial fibrillation is not known; however, most clinicians use a value of 150 beats/min as their threshold between an acceptable rate and need for more aggressive treatment.
- A 24-hour ambulatory ECG (Holter) monitoring is the preferred method to determine mean heart rate and efficacy of long-term oral treatment.

ADDITIONAL ORAL MEDICATIONS

In addition to combinations of diuretics, ACE inhibitors, and digoxin, other medications are likely beneficial in DCM. The use of these medications is based on beneficial effects demonstrated in human or animal model studies. As clinical data become increasingly available in dogs, the use of these medications will continue to grow. The following recommendations are based on a limited number of reports in dogs and the author's own experience.

- In addition to their antiarrhythmic use, beta-adrenergic blockers such as metoprolol and carvedilol are used to slow progression of heart enlargement and systolic dysfunction. Initiation of these drugs is done in patients with clinically stable heart disease; beta-blocking agents should not be used in patients with active signs of congestion (the exception would be emergency beta blocker use to control rapid atrial fibrillation). Initiation of beta blockade can acutely worsen contractility, and therefore patients are gradually titrated onto the medications over 4 to 8 weeks. Adverse side effects include bradycardia, hypotension, and exacerbation of CHF. Clinicians who prescribe beta blockers must be prepared to manage acute heart failure secondary to drug initiation. In humans, beta blockers slow progression of disease and improve survival, but they do not dramatically improve quality of life. Beneficial effects require several months of continuous treatment, and in dogs with end-stage disease, treatment may not be practical. Accordingly, both the maximum benefit and the minimum risk of beta blocker use are probably early in the disease course.

- Metoprolol (initial dose of 0.1 to 0.2 mg/kg q12h followed by gradual titration to 0.4 to 0.8 mg/kg q12h over 4 to 8 weeks).
- Carvedilol (initial dose of 0.1 mg/kg q12h followed by gradual titration to 0.5 mg/kg q12h over 4 to 8 weeks).

KEY POINTS

Beta blockade is one of the cornerstones of treatment in humans with DCM. In these patients, beta blockers slow progression of disease, improve systolic function, and prolong survival. These benefits are dose-dependent, and aggressive therapy yields the greatest results. In canine patients, little is known about the ideal timing, dose, and drug that should be used. In healthy dogs, oral carvedilol doses ranging from 0.5 to 1.5 mg/kg q12h blunt response to sympathetic stimulation with isoproterenol. The appropriate dose for dogs with heart disease is unknown, but it is likely to be lower than that used in healthy dogs. In dogs with experimental mitral valve disease, oral carvedilol at 0.4 mg/kg q24h reduced heart rate, whereas in a small study of dogs with advanced naturally occurring DCM, oral carvedilol at 0.3 mg/kg q12h did not result in any measurable improvement in echocardiographic heart size or systolic function. Thus the effective dose of carvedilol in affected dogs is likely to be >0.3 mg/kg q12h.

- Aldosterone antagonists, such as spironolactone, act as mild diuretics but, even more important, reduce the proliferative effects of aldosterone within the myocardium and vasculature. Other beneficial properties include blunting of sympathetic nervous activity and normalization of baroreceptor function. In the presence of severe heart disease, ACE inhibition alone may not be sufficient in suppressing aldosterone production, and in humans with heart failure, spironolactone improves survival.
  - Spironolactone (1 to 2 mg/kg q12h) is commonly prescribed in combination with hydrochlorothiazide in dogs with severe DCM. Because of its antiproliferative effects, spironolactone may also be beneficial in the occult and early symptomatic stages of disease.
- Amino acid deficiency is present in some breeds with DCM (e.g., American Cocker Spaniels).

- Taurine supplementation (500 mg q12h for Cocker Spaniels) is recommended in dogs with a low plasma taurine concentration.
- Concurrent L-carnitine supplementation (1 g q12h for Cocker Spaniels) is recommended in dogs with taurine deficiency. Alternatively, because of the relative expense of L-carnitine compared with taurine, L-carnitine is withheld during the initial 3 months of taurine treatment and administered only to those dogs that have not responded to taurine alone.
- L-Carnitine deficiency was detected in a family of Boxers with LV dilation and systolic dysfunction. Supplementation (50 mg/kg q8 to 12h) should be considered in dogs with this presentation. The value of supplementation in Boxers with arrhythmias and no LV dilation (which is the most common presentation) is doubtful.
- Dogs that respond to amino acid supplementation can often reduce or discontinue conventional heart failure medications (e.g., furosemide, ACE inhibitors, digoxin); however, taurine or carnitine supplementation should continue indefinitely.
- Heart disease is accompanied by elevations of circulating cytokines and alterations of energy production, both of which may contribute to the heart failure syndrome of weight loss, muscle wasting, and poor appetite.
  - Fish oil supplements can reduce interleukin concentrations and help improve cardiac cachexia.
  - Coenzyme Q_{10} is part of the mitochondrial respiratory transport chain and supplementation may improve quality of life.
  - The benefit of supplementary antioxidant vitamins E, A, or C is unknown.

PROGNOSIS

The time course from occult to symptomatic DCM is highly variable and can be years. During this phase, serial echocardiograms and ECGs are recommended. Sudden death can occur during the occult phase, especially in Boxers and Doberman Pinschers. Once clinical signs such as CHF develop, long-term prognosis is poor. Survival times derived from clinical studies are difficult to assess because of nonstandardized treatment, lack of ACE inhibitor use, and statistical issues surrounding euthanasia. Median survival time is likely 3 to 4 months in Doberman Pinschers and 5 to 6 months in other breeds. Dogs that survive more than 7 months may do well for an extended period of time. One-year survival is approximately 10% to 15%. Atrial fibrillation, biventricular CHF, and young age at time of presentation (<5 years) are associated with worse prognosis. Although the overall survival rate is disheartening, it is difficult to assess how any individual dog may fare. I suggest aggressive intravenous management of dogs with fulminant heart failure and reevaluation after 24 to 72 hours of therapy.

HYPERTROPHIC CARDIOMYOPATHY

HCM is an uncommon myocardial disease of dogs. HCM is characterized by idiopathic concentric LV hypertrophy and can lead to heart failure or sudden death. HCM, if accompanied by systolic anterior motion of the mitral valve and LV outflow tract obstruction, is specifically referred to as hypertrophic obstructive cardiomyopathy. Most dogs reported to have HCM are male and young (typically <3 years), suggesting a heritable etiology. The LV hypertrophy associated with HCM can be symmetric (i.e., affecting both the interventricular septum and LV posterior wall equally) or asymmetric (in humans, the septum is typically more affected than the posterior wall). In my experience, most cases of canine HCM involve symmetric LV hypertrophy. Significant LV hypertrophy causes diastolic dysfunction, left atrial enlargement, heart failure, and arrhythmias. Most dogs with HCM are asymptomatic, and the diagnosis is made during evaluation of a heart murmur or arrhythmia. Echocardiography is the diagnostic method of choice. Treatment is aimed at abolishing the obstructive component of disease with beta-blocking agents (atenolol 0.5 to 1.0 mg/kg orally q12 to 24h), alleviating heart failure with diuretics, and suppressing arrhythmias. Sudden death appears to be more common than CHF. Many dogs with HCM remain asymptomatic for years.

FREQUENTLY ASKED QUESTIONS

What causes DCM?

The etiology of primary DCM is unknown. DCM is a description of the heart's response to injury (i.e., dilation and systolic dysfunction) and as such may be the end result of multiple causes. In fact, given the forms of DCM that are unique to different breeds, it is likely that more than one cause exists. Possible causes include genetic/familial, immune-mediated, infectious, toxic, or nutritional. DCM in Doberman Pinschers may involve specific components of the cytoskeleton or extracellular matrix. Cellular energy production is markedly reduced in affected Doberman Pinschers, but whether these changes are primary abnormalities or secondary changes has yet to be determined. Boxers with ARVC are thought to possess abnormal calcium

cycling, which is detected in certain forms of ARVC in humans.

When should I use pimobendan in dogs with DCM?

Pimobendan is indicated in two clinical circumstances in dogs with DCM. The first is for the treatment of CHF secondary to DCM in commonly affected dog breeds, such as Doberman Pinschers, Irish Wolfhounds, Great Danes, and other giant-breed dogs. The second is for the treatment of select cases of preclinical DCM in Doberman Pinschers. Clinicians must remember that the natural history of DCM in the Doberman Pinscher and the subsequent diagnosis of preclinical disease can involve presence of ventricular arrhythmias without evidence of decreased LV contractility. Note that the PROTECT study, which showed that pimobendan delayed onset of sudden death or CHF, was performed in a very select group of Doberman Pinschers. Dobermans whose only indication of preclinical DCM was ventricular arrhythmias (e.g., they had arrhythmias but had normal echocardiographic LV contractility), with a history of syncope, and with severe ventricular arrhythmias, such as ventricular tachycardia regardless of their echocardiographic findings, were excluded. Thus the results of the PROTECT study only apply to Doberman Pinschers with decreased echocardiographic LV contractility and without significant amounts of ventricular arrhythmia. This represents just a proportion of Doberman Pinschers that are diagnosed with preclinical disease. Thus, in many instances, clinicians must still use their best judgment as to whether pimobendan is indicated. In the absence of decreased contractility, one of the main purported benefits of pimobendan, that of positive inotropy, is likely diminished, and clinicians might chose to monitor progression using serial echocardiography. In cases with severe arrhythmias, concurrent therapy with pimobendan and the anti-arrhythmic agent sotalol could be considered. Close monitoring for clinical signs, such as activity intolerance, syncope, inappetence, and respiratory effort, is advisable. In Boxers with ARVC, there are no studies to date examining the safety and efficacy of pimobendan, and routine use of pimobendan in them is discouraged.

Is combination therapy possible with beta blockers and pimobendan?

There is a wealth of data supporting use of beta blockers in humans with DCM. Although these agents are effective at slowing pathologic ventricular remodeling and improving survival, they do relatively little to improve quality of life or exercise tolerance. In contrast, pimobendan, though not proven to improve survival in humans, has a marked benefit on quality of life in dogs. Some cardiologists combine pimobendan and a beta blocker in dogs with symptomatic DCM. The positive inotropic effect of pimobendan may increase the likelihood of successful titration of and tolerance to beta blockers and thereby achieve both increased quality and quantity of life.

SUGGESTED READINGS

Borgarelli M, Tarducci A, Tidholm A, Haggstrom J: Canine idiopathic dilated cardiomyopathy. Part II: Pathophysiology and therapy, Vet J 162:182–195, 2001.

Hairu CD, Carpenter DH Jr: Arrhythmogenic right ventricular cardiomyopathy in Boxers, Compend Contin Educ Vet 32:E3, 2010.

Meurs KM, Lahmers S, Keene BW, et al.: A splice site mutation in a gene encoding for PDK4, a mitochondrial protein, is associated with the development of dilated cardiomyopathy in the Doberman Pinscher, Hum Genet 131:1319–1325, 2012.

Meurs KM, Stern JA, Sisson DD, et al: Association of dilated cardiomyopathy with the striatin mutation genotype in Boxer dogs, J Vet Intern Med 27:1437–1440, 2013.

O'Grady MR, O'Sullivan ML: Dilated cardiomyopathy: an update, Vet Clin North Am Small Anim Pract 34:1187–1207, 2004.

Stephenson HM, Fonfara S, Lopez-Alverez J, et al: Screening for dilated cardiomyopathy in great Danes in the United Kingdom, J Vet Intern Med 26:1140–1147, 2012.

Summerfield NJ, Boswood A, O'Grady MR, et al: Efficacy of pimobendan in the prevention of congestive heart failure or sudden death in Doberman Pinschers with preclinical dilated cardiomyopathy (the PROTECT study), J Vet Intern Med 26:1337–1349, 2012.

Tidholm A, Haggstrom J, Borgarelli M, Tarducci A: Canine idiopathic dilated cardiomyopathy. Part I: Aetiology, clinical characteristics, epidemiology and pathology, Vet J 162:92–107, 2001.

Wess G, Maurer J, Simrak J, Hartmann K: Use of Simpson's method of disc to detect early echocardiographic changes in Doberman Pinschers with dilated cardiomyopathy, J Vet Intern Med 24:1069–1076, 2010.

Feline Cardiomyopathy

9

Kristin MacDonald

The term *cardiomyopathy* literally means heart muscle disease and designates a disorder of the heart that primarily affects the cardiac muscle (myocardium). *Primary* indicates that the myocardial disease is not secondary to valvular disease, pericardial disease, coronary vascular disease, systemic or pulmonary hypertension, congenital abnormalities, or systemic disease. Most primary cardiomyopathies are of unknown etiology (idiopathic). However, in human medicine, recent advances in genetic testing have identified causative mutations in many cardiomyopathies previously categorized as idiopathic. A secondary cardiomyopathy is a disease that affects the myocardium secondary to infectious, toxic, metabolic, or other disease processes that affect multiple body systems. In 1995, the World Health Organization categorized the types of cardiomyopathies according to the dominant pathophysiologic features produced by the myocardial disease, which has since then been revised by the American Heart Association in 2006. Veterinary medicine has adopted much of the human categorization of cardiomyopathies because they seem to clinically fit the diseases we see in feline cardiology.

FELINE CARDIOMYOPATHIES

GENERAL COMMENTS

- Cardiomyopathies are classified into functional pathophysiologic categories on the basis of echocardiographic evaluation, including hypertrophic cardiomyopathy (HCM; i.e., left ventricular concentric hypertrophy), dilated cardiomyopathy (DCM; i.e., systolic myocardial failure), restrictive cardiomyopathy (RCM; i.e., marked diastolic dysfunction in the face of a relatively normal left ventricle [LV]), arrhythmogenic right ventricular cardiomyopathy (ARVC), and unclassified cardiomyopathy (UCM; i.e., atrial dilation without other functional myocardial abnormalities).
- Most cardiomyopathies diagnosed in cats are idiopathic (primary). HCM often has a heritable basis and may be caused in some cats within the Maine Coon and Ragdoll breeds

by sarcomeric mutations of the individual contractile unit of the heart muscle. The only nutritional cause of a cardiomyopathy in cats is taurine deficiency causing DCM. Although ARVC, DCM, and RCM are currently defined as idiopathic in veterinary medicine, there may be genetic causes that have yet to be identified in cats, just as there have been in people.

- UCM and RCM are poorly defined clinical entities in cats. These "diagnoses" have been assigned to many feline patients with presumed primary myocardial disease that do not meet the criteria for making a diagnosis of HCM or DCM.
- Echocardiography is the essential diagnostic test to diagnose the specific cardiomyopathies in cats and is essential for early and accurate morphologic classification of the cardiomyopathy.

KEY POINT

Cardiomyopathies represent the overwhelming majority of heart diseases in cats. Other diseases such as valvular disease or pericardial disease are very uncommon. In one study, 62% of 408 cats presenting for cardiology workup were diagnosed with a primary cardiomyopathy. The most common feline cardiomyopathy is HCM, which accounts for approximately 58% to 68% of feline cardiomyopathy cases. The other cardiomyopathies are less common, including RCM (5% to 21%), UCM (10%), DCM (10%), and ARVC (<1% of cases).

CLASSIFICATION

- Cardiomyopathies are classified according to their morphologic appearance, typically based on echocardiography (Table 9.1). Within each classification, a wide range of morphologic and clinical presentations may be seen. Primary cardiomyopathies (genetic, nongenetic, and acquired) are confined to the heart muscle. Conversely, secondary cardiomyopathies show myocardial involvement as part of more widespread multiorgan systemic disorders, and were previously referred to as "specific" cardiomyopathies.

Table 9.1 Echocardiographic Abnormalities in Feline Cardiomyopathy

Cardiomyopathy	Echocardiographic Abnormalities	Heart Failure
HCM	LV wall or septal wall thickness >6 mm, papillary muscle hypertrophy, normal systolic function. Left atrial dilation may or may not be present.	Diastolic heart failure Left heart failure Pulmonary edema or pleural effusion
HOCM	HCM with SAM of the mitral valve present, creating mild to severe LVOT obstruction and MR.	
DCM	Systolic myocardial failure (FS <26%, ESD >11 mm, EPSS >4), compensatory LV eccentric hypertrophy (EDD >20 mm), LA +/− RA dilation, +/− RV eccentric hypertrophy and myocardial failure.	Systolic heart failure Left-sided + right-sided heart failure Pulmonary edema, pleural effusion, +/− ascites
RCM Myocardial form	Normal LV wall thickness, normal systolic function. LA or biatrial dilation. Restrictive filling pattern of mitral inflow (E/A >2, short deceleration time).	Diastolic heart failure Left-sided +/− right-sided heart failure; pulmonary edema or pleural effusion
EMF form	Large fibrotic bridging band or scar of the LV, severe LA +/− RA dilation.	
UCM	Normal to equivocal LV wall thickness (<6mm), normal to mild systolic myocardial failure. LA +/− RA dilation; +/− diastolic dysfunction.	Probable diastolic heart failure Left-sided +/− right-sided heart failure Pulmonary edema or pleural effusion
ARVC	Severe RV eccentric hypertrophy and myocardial failure, severe RA dilation, normal to mild LA dilation.	Systolic heart failure Right-sided heart failure; pleural effusion and ascites

ARVC, Arrhythmogenic right ventricular cardiomyopathy; *DCM,* dilated cardiomyopathy; *E/A,* peak E to E wave velocity ratio; *EDD,* end diastolic diameter; *EMF,* endomyocardial fibrosis; *ESD,* end systolic diameter; *EPSS,* E point to septal separation; *FS,* fractional shortening; *HCM,* hypertrophic cardiomyopathy; *HOCM,* hypertrophic obstructive cardiomyopathy; *LA,* left atrium; *LV,* left ventricle; *LVOT,* left ventricular outflow tract; *MR,* mitral regurgitation; *RA,* right atrium; *RCM,* restrictive cardiomyopathy; *RV,* right ventricle; *SAM,* systolic anterior motion of the mitral valve; *UCM,* unclassified cardiomyopathy.

PRIMARY CARDIOMYOPATHIES

- Hypertrophic cardiomyopathy (HCM)
- Idiopathic dilated cardiomyopathy (DCM)
- Restrictive cardiomyopathy (RCM)
- Unclassified cardiomyopathies (UCM)
- Arrhythmogenic right ventricular cardiomyopathy (ARVC)

A limitation in the functional classification of cardiomyopathies based on diastolic function, systolic function, and left ventricular hypertrophy is that there may be considerable overlap encountered between categories and the potential to shift between categories based on their subsequent echocardiographic appearance. Therefore, although the cardiomyopathies are presented as distinct categories in this text, there may be overlap and changes in functional abnormalities over time. Although there are specific criteria used to diagnose restrictive diastolic-filling physiologic processes seen in some cardiomyopathies, there is not a clear clinical categorization or differentiation of RCM from UCM in cats, and the two categories are often merged together.

SECONDARY CARDIOMYOPATHIES

- Nutritional (taurine deficiency–induced DCM)
- Metabolic (hyperthyroidism, acromegaly)
- Infiltrative (neoplasia, amyloidosis)
- Inflammatory (toxins, immune reactions, infectious agents)
- Toxic (doxorubicin, heavy metals)

CLINICAL CLASSIFICATION AND PATHOPHYSIOLOGY

- Most feline cardiomyopathies (HCM, RCM, and UCM) are caused by abnormalities of diastolic function or the ability of the heart to actively relax and passively fill with blood. The cause of the diastolic function in these cardiomyopathies may differ, but the clinical effect of severe diastolic dysfunction is the same: elevated left ventricular pressure, variable elevation of right ventricular filling pressures (UCM and +/− RCM), and development of congestive heart failure (CHF) (see Table 9.1).
- Systolic myocardial failure (DCM, +/−ARVC, and +/− RCM) is caused by a primary contractile abnormality of the ventricle whereby it cannot contract and eject blood out of the heart, leading to decreased stroke volume and cardiac output. This is seen on an echocardiogram as

an increased left ventricular systolic dimension and decreased fractional shortening (FS) (see Table 9.1). Systolic myocardial failure also increases diastolic filling pressure because excess blood remains in the ventricle after systole and because of expansion of the blood volume by renin-angiotensin-aldosterone system (RAAS) activation.

- Left-sided CHF (i.e., backward failure) is manifested by elevated left-sided heart filling pressure and increased pulmonary capillary wedge pressure >20 to 25 mm Hg, leading to the development of pulmonary edema and pleural effusion in cats. Right-sided CHF is caused by elevated right-sided heart filling pressures (>10 to 15 mm Hg), leads to systemic venous hypertension, and is manifested by pleural effusion, jugular venous distension, and often ascites in cats. Peripheral edema is not a typical characteristic of right-sided heart failure in cats. A combination of left-sided and right-sided heart failure is common in cats with biatrial dilation caused by various cardiomyopathies (DCM, UCM, and RCM).
- Low output heart failure (i.e., forward failure) is caused by marked decrease in cardiac output and systemic arterial hypotension and is manifested by cold peripheral extremities, weak pulses, tachycardia, pale mucous membranes, weakness, or collapse. Low output heart failure is typically seen in end-stage heart disease.
- High output heart failure in cats is most commonly associated with thyrotoxicosis causing excessive blood flow through the capillary beds and is associated with tachycardia, a gallop heart sound, bounding pulses, and CHF (pulmonary edema or pleural effusion).
- Arterial thromboembolism (ATE) may occur in cats with cardiomyopathy and left atrial dilation of various severities. Left atrial and left auricular blood flow stasis can cause platelet aggregation and formation of a thrombus. Other potential contributing causes of ATE in cats with cardiomyopathy include left atrial/auricular endothelial cell damage, and/or a hypercoagulable state caused by increased platelet activation or increased blood coagulation proteins. The ATE that most cats have has a cardiogenic origin.
- Heart disease is not synonymous with heart failure (congestive or low-output). Many cats with heart disease, especially HCM, never have heart failure. Heart failure is the end result of severe heart disease with many causes. Often, cats with DCM, RCM, or UCM miss early detection because a murmur may be absent on auscultation and are often only diagnosed at an end stage once severe symptoms of heart failure are present.

SIGNALMENT AND PRESENTING COMPLAINTS

KEY POINT

The clinical presentation, physical examination findings, radiographic findings, and electrocardiographic (ECG) findings are similar for all forms of myocardial disease and generally cannot be used to differentiate among them. Echocardiography is necessary to determine the specific disorder that is present.

- Presenting complaints in cats with cardiomyopathies are often referable to the presence of CHF or other sequelae such as ATE or, rarely, severe arrhythmias that causes syncope or collapse. Cardiomyopathies may be mild to severe, with a wide spectrum of potential clinical presentations ranging from asymptomatic to severely affected cats. The typical clinical presentation, physical examination findings, radiographic findings, and ECG findings are discussed in this section, but echocardiographic findings are discussed within the specific cardiomyopathy category.
- Common presenting complaints in cats with severe cardiomyopathy may include the following:
  - Dyspnea/tachypnea
  - Weight loss, weakness, lethargy
  - Anorexia
  - Acute paresis or paralysis of pelvic limbs or a thoracic limb consistent with ATE
- Uncommon complaints may include syncope, collapse, coughing, or abdominal distension.
- A precipitating event is common in cats that have heart failure. Recent fluid administration, anesthesia or surgery, or repositol corticosteroid administrations are among the most common antecedent events.
- Cats may be symptom free for cardiomyopathy and have no presenting complaint referable to heart disease but may be examined for other systemic disease or for a wellness examination.

PHYSICAL EXAMINATION

- Early detection of disease should be a primary goal, before signs of fulminant heart failure or ATE occur. A thorough physical examination, with careful attention to auscultation, should be performed.

Cardiac auscultation abnormalities in cats with cardiomyopathy commonly include the following:

- Systolic murmur (commonly heard along the left sternal border). Murmur intensity does not relate to severity of underlying disease. This murmur is often caused by mitral regurgitation or left ventricular outflow tract obstruction. Presence of a murmur does not definitively diagnose the cat with cardiomyopathy, but raises suspicion of underlying cardiomyopathy.

- Gallop sound: an additional heart sound heard in diastole either during early diastolic filling (S_3) or during atrial systole (S_4). Given the rapid heart rates (HRs) in cats, differentiation of S_3 and S_4 heart sounds is impossible and unnecessary. Presence of a gallop is abnormal and may occur when there is diastolic or systolic dysfunction or volume overload to the ventricle. It is more commonly auscultated in cats with heart failure than in symptom-free cats. Aside from cardiomyopathy, other important causes of gallop heart sounds include: anemia and hyperthyroidism.
- Arrhythmia: premature beats, runs of tachycardia, or irregularly irregular tachycardia (i.e., atrial fibrillation) may be present. Bradycardia (HR <150 beats/min) may be present if there is hyperkalemia associated with reperfusion syndrome in cats with ATE or in cats with third degree atrioventricular (AV) block that have underlying cardiomyopathy.

Clinical signs often seen in cats with heart failure include the following:

- Respiratory abnormalities
  - Tachypnea, dyspnea, orthopnea
  - Muffled or harsh lung sounds
- Hypothermia
- Jugular pulses/distention: uncommon but present in cats with right-sided heart failure

Clinical signs associated with ATE

- Acute paresis of pelvic limbs or thoracic limb associated with pain
- Cold peripheral extremity
- Absent femoral arterial pulse of the affected pelvic limb
- Cyanotic toe pads
- Firm painful muscles of affected limb
- Neuropathy, typically with absent CPs

ANCILLARY TESTS

- Thoracic radiography and electrocardiography may direct or reinforce suspicion that a cardiac disorder is present. They may also further characterize the disorder and alert the clinician to secondary ramifications that may require attention; however, neither electrocardiography nor thoracic radiography provides adequate evidence for ruling out, confirming, or classifying feline cardiac disease. Echocardiography is required to confirm or rule out and categorize myocardial disease.
- Electrocardiography is indicated for evaluation of an arrhythmia identified on auscultation, or for evaluation of cats with episodic weakness, syncope, or collapse. However, an electrocardiogram should not be used as a method to screen for underlying cardiomyopathy.
- ECG abnormalities seen in cats with cardiomyopathy
  - Ventricular arrhythmias: ventricular premature complexes (VPCs) are common but typically mild and often do not warrant antiarrhythmic therapy. Ventricular tachycardia or complex ventricular arrhythmias may be seen in cats with cardiomyopathy and warrant antiarrhythmic therapy.
  - Atrial tachyarrhythmias: atrial premature complexes are less common than VPCs and do not warrant treatment. Supraventricular tachycardia with high sustained rates >300 beats/min may be seen in cats with cardiomyopathy and warrants treatment. Atrial fibrillation may be present in cats with severe cardiomegaly and left atrial dilation and warrants negative chronotropic therapy.
  - Left axis deviation or left anterior fascicular block pattern may be present in some cats with HCM, although either may also be present in some normal cats or hyperthyroid cats.
- Increased amplitude of R waves may be present in cats with left ventricular enlargement or concentric hypertrophy and is insensitive for diagnosis of cardiomyopathy.
- Thoracic radiography is most useful for detecting gross cardiac enlargement and CHF (e.g., pulmonary venous distension, pulmonary edema, pleural effusion, or dilated caudal vena cava) (Figures 9.1 and 9.2). Restraint for radiographic procedures can be life threatening to dyspneic cats. Extreme caution should be taken before proceeding with radiography. Severely dyspneic cats may require emergency stabilization before radiographs are obtained.
- While the cat is in sternal recumbency, a brief "triage" thoracic ultrasound is a less stressful initial diagnostic tool than radiography for detection of severe pleural effusion and also directs the optimal location for thoracocentesis.
- Systemic blood pressure measurement is also a necessary test to evaluate for systemic hypertension or hypotension and helps direct acute and long-term medical therapy. Systemic hypertension can create mild left ventricular concentric hypertrophy, which may mimic HCM on echocardiography.

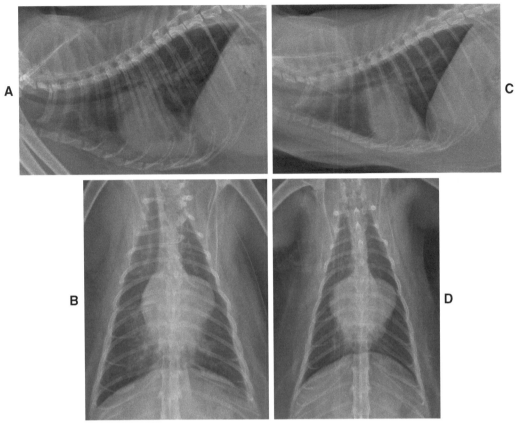

Figure 9.1 Thoracic radiographs of a cat with severe hypertrophic cardiomyopathy (HCM) and left heart failure. There is severe cardiomegaly and left atrial dilation seen on lateral (**A**) and ventrodorsal (VD) (**B**) views. The lateral view (**A**) depicts patchy interstitial infiltrates, especially of the caudal lung lobes and pulmonary venous distension, which are consistent with left-sided heart failure. Recheck radiographs (**C** and **D**) postfurosemide therapy show resolution of the pulmonary edema and pulmonary venous distension but persistent cardiomegaly.

KEY POINTS

- A thoracic radiograph with normal findings does not preclude the diagnosis of a cardiomyopathy. Many symptom-free cats with mild changes and normal LA size will have a thoracic radiograph with normal findings.
- Echocardiography, including Doppler echocardiography, is essential for noninvasive determination of a functional and anatomic diagnosis. Before a diagnosis of cardiomyopathy is assigned solely on the basis of morphologic/functional appearance, a concerted effort should be made to rule out cardiac and extracardiac diseases that might mimic the echocardiographic appearance of primary myocardial diseases.
- Other diagnostic tests do not usually contribute to the diagnosis of myocardial disease but are important for determining the overall status of the patient, identifying concomitant disorders, and assessing the efficacy or untoward effects of therapy. When possible, routine biochemistries, urinalysis, thyroxine level, and a complete blood count should be performed before pharmacologic intervention to establish baseline values for the patient and to rule

out concurrent, secondary metabolic, or hematologic disturbances.
- Pleural effusion fluid analysis, including chemical and cytologic evaluation, can help determine whether heart failure may be causing pleural effusion accumulation. Cardiogenic pleural effusion may be characterized as a transudate, modified transudate, pseudochylous effusion, or true chylous effusion but is not a hemorrhagic effusion or an exudate.
- Plasma and whole blood taurine concentrations should be measured in all cats with echocardiographically documented myocardial failure (see the section on taurine deficiency–induced myocardial failure).
- N-terminal pro–B-type natriuretic peptide (NT-ProBNP) is a sensitive and accurate blood screening test for detection of heart failure in cats with cardiomyopathy and may be used to help distinguish whether the dyspnea is caused by heart failure or primary respiratory disease. Currently, a quantitative ELISA (enzyme-linked immunosorbent assay) and point-of-care assay are commercially available (see Chapter 6). In a large scale study of 425 cats diagnosed with mild to end-stage

cardiomyopathy, NT-ProBNP correlated with a stage of cardiac disease severity and survival time, with levels >270 pmol/L, which were suggestive of clinically significant disease. There are variable results in studies in which symptom-free cats were evaluated. The NT-ProBNP test does not replace the need for further diagnostic testing with an echocardiogram or radiographs but helps assess the likelihood of underlying cardiac disease.

THERAPY

- Therapy should be based on the clinical and functional classification of the disease process in the individual patient and not by following a standard approach based solely on the diagnosis.
- With only two exceptions, the indications for, and benefits of, therapeutic intervention in symptom-free cats with myocardial disease are controversial. These exceptions are the following:
  - Myocardial failure secondary to taurine deficiency
  - Thyrotoxic heart disease
- Dyspneic cats are easily stressed and may acutely deteriorate and die if stressful diagnostic or therapeutic interventions are initiated too early. A triage level thoracic ultrasound should be done if available in the severely dyspneic cat to evaluate for severe pleural effusion. If an ultrasound is unavailable and the cat is too unstable to safely obtain radiographs, thoracocentesis may be attempted at the right caudal thorax. The severely dyspneic cat can then receive oxygen and be given a parenteral dose of furosemide to stabilize before radiographs. If physical abnormalities and history are suggestive of lower airway disease (asthma), the cat may be given steroids and bronchodilators parenterally and receive oxygen.
- All patients with evidence of significant and life-threatening CHF (pulmonary edema, pleural effusion) require immediate therapy (i.e., appropriate combinations of thoracocentesis, parenteral furosemide, and oxygen). Cats with significant pleural effusion will benefit most from immediate thoracocentesis.
  - **Furosemide** is the diuretic of choice in cats. Furosemide should be administered intravenously (2 to 4 mg/kg q12-4h then rapidly tapered to 1 to 2 mg/kg q6-8h on the basis of resting respiratory rate and effort) or intramuscularly (2 to 4 mg/kg q2h until an intravenous catheter can be placed) depending on the stress level of the cat. Dosing must be dramatically reduced once the respiratory rate begins to decrease. In general, aggressive diuretic therapy is continued until the respiratory rate is below 40 breaths per minute.
  - Enriched fraction of inspired oxygen (FiO$_2$ 50%) can be administered with an oxygen cage, which controls temperature and humidity and removes excess carbon dioxide.
  - Transdermal nitroglycerin (⅛ to ¼ inch QID ≤2 days) is a venodilator whose efficacy is unknown in cats. It may lessen pulmonary venous hypertension, thereby decreasing the formation of pulmonary edema.
  - Sedation with a low dose opioid such as butorphanol or buprenorphine may be administered to calm distressed patients.
- Chronic heart failure therapy
- Maintenance therapy is generally aimed at minimizing clinical signs (e.g., dyspnea, tachypnea) and preventing an acute respiratory crisis. Oral furosemide may be uptitrated according to the severity of heart failure. The oral doses range

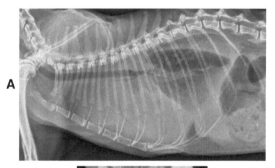

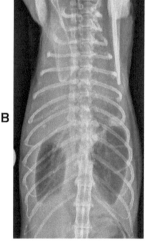

Figure 9.2   A and **B,** Thoracic radiographs of a cat with severe dilated cardiomyopathy (DCM) and biventricular heart failure. Severe pleural effusion is present in this cat with severe DCM and biventricular heart failure, which obscures visualization of the heart, pulmonary vasculature, and pulmonary parenchyma. Repeat thoracic radiographs after palliative thoracocentesis may allow visualization of the intrathoracic structures. An echocardiogram is needed to definitively diagnose the heart failure causing the pleural effusion and to determine the origin of the cardiac disease.

from 1 to 3 mg/kg q24h BID, and may uptitrate from TID in refractory heart failure to a maximum in cats that can tolerate high furosemide doses, of 4 mg/kg TID for severe refractory heart failure. Often a typical oral dose of furosemide is 6.25 mg BID. Recheck radiographs are helpful to assess the presence and severity of pulmonary edema or pleural effusion after heart failure treatment and aids in furosemide dose titration (see Figure 9.1, C and D).

- Angiotensin-converting enzyme (ACE) inhibitors (enalapril 0.5 mg/kg PO q24h BID, ramipril 0.5 mg/kg PO q24h, and benazepril 0.5 mg/kg PO q24h) may provide adjunctive benefit for treatment of chronic heart failure.
- Antiarrhythmic drugs may be indicated to control significant arrhythmias such as atrial fibrillation, ventricular tachycardia, or supraventricular tachycardia.
- Positive inotropic agents such as pimobendan (0.25 mg/kg PO BID or 1.25 mg per cat PO BID) may be indicated in patients with myocardial failure identified by echocardiography or low-output heart failure (i.e., hypotension and signs of poor perfusion).
- All cats with myocardial failure identified by echocardiography should be supplemented with **taurine** (250 mg PO BID; see the section on taurine deficiency–induced myocardial failure) until proved to have a normal taurine blood concentration or a lack of response after several months of supplementation on the basis of a recheck echocardiogram.

ARTERIAL THROMBOEMBOLISM THERAPY

- Prophylactic therapy may be instituted in cats with a high risk for having ATE, including those cats that have recovered from an ATE event, cats that have spontaneous echocardiographic contrast or thrombus in the atrium on echocardiography, or cats that have moderate or severe atrial dilation.
  - Clopidogrel (18.75 mg PO q24h) is a potent platelet receptor antagonist that is currently favored for prophylaxis of ATE and was superior to aspirin in the FATCAT (Feline Arterial Thromboembolism: Clopidogrel vs. Aspirin Trial) clinical study for time to development of recurrent ATE in cats recovering from ATE.
  - **Aspirin** (5 to 81 mg PO every 3 days) may be used for ATE prophylaxis, although it appears inferior to clopidogrel in cats that had ATE in the FATCAT clinical study. Recurrence of thromboembolic events in aspirin-treated cats were as high as 75% in another study. Aspirin may be added to clopidogrel in cats with

refractory spontaneous contrast or thrombus seen on an echocardiogram.
  - **Enoxaparin** (1.5 mg/kg SC BID-TID), a low molecular weight heparin, has shown promise in anecdotal clinical settings. No large clinical trials have been completed.

ACUTE THERAPY FOR ARTERIAL THROMBOEMBOLISM

- Left untreated, the outcome of arterial occlusion will depend on the extent of occlusion and time to spontaneous reperfusion, either through the primary vessel or the collateral circulation. Cats may lose the affected leg(s) because of ischemic necrosis, die of reperfusion syndrome or toxemia, remain paralyzed from peripheral nerve damage, or regain full or partial function of the leg. Overall response to presently available conservative or aggressive clinical intervention has been poor. Survival of cats receiving treatment ranges from 45% to 73%. Positive predictors for better survival include a single limb affected and presence of motor function at presentation. Negative predictors for survival include refractory heart failure, malignant arrhythmias, multiorgan embolization, presence of an intracardiac thrombus, progressive azotemia, disseminated intravascular coagulation, and unresponsive hypothermia. In cats recovering from ATE, the most common cause of death is CHF, followed by recurrent ATE.
- Invasive therapeutic options such as surgical removal of emboli, rheolytic embolectomy, or catheter embolectomy are not currently recommended because of similar survival in medical therapy.
- Medical therapies—most are untested and unproven
  - Anticoagulation with **heparin** (220 U/kg IV followed 3 hours later by a maintenance dose of 66-200 U/kg SQ four times a day) is used to prevent further thrombosis. Adjust the dose to maintain the activated partial thromboplastin time at or slightly above the upper limit of the normal reference range. **Enoxaparin** (1.5 mg/kg SC TID q6h) is another option that does not require coagulation panel monitoring because it affects factor X activity.
  - Thrombolytic therapy (e.g., tissue plasminogen activator, streptokinase, or urokinase) is rarely recommended because of expense of the drug, life-threatening complications, and lack of effective prevention of recurrent ATE.
  - Pain management: Analgesia is crucial for cats with ATE, particularly in the first 2 days

after the ATE. Various opioids may be chosen, including fentanyl (2 to 5 µg/kg/h constant rate infusion [CRI] for 12 to 18 hours until fentanyl patch takes effect) or buprenorphine (0.005- to 0.015 mg/kg IV q6h).

- Vasodilators such as acepromazine and hydralazine may not increase arterial blood flow to the affected limb but may lead to systemic hypotension and have therefore fallen out of clinical favor.
- Reperfusion syndrome: Cats may have acute reperfusion syndrome characterized by life-threatening hyperkalemia and acidosis caused by spontaneous autogenous or exogenous thrombus lysis. This may occur any time over the first several days to 1 week after ATE and must be treated aggressively and immediately. Continuous ECG monitoring may be useful to detect acute onset of bradycardia that occurs with life-threatening hyperkalemia. Electrolytes and pH should be measured at least daily to twice daily in hospitalized cats.
- Acute treatment
  - 10% calcium gluconate: 0.5 to 1.5 mL/kg IV slowly over 5 to 10 minutes
  - Sodium bicarbonate: 1 to 2 mEq/kg IV slowly over 15 minutes
  - 25% dextrose: 0.7 to 1 g/kg IV over 3 to 5 minutes
  - 25% dextrose with insulin: regular insulin 0.5 U/kg IV with dextrose 2 g/U of insulin administered
  - Atropine: 0.02 to 0.04 mg/kg IV if bradycardia present

PROGNOSIS

- Within the broad category of feline cardiomyopathy there is a wide range of diseases and severity, which makes it impossible to predict accurate prognosis. Although subclinical cats may live many years with cardiomyopathy, once heart failure occurs, prognosis is typically limited to months. Cats with ATE have the gravest prognosis, with a median survival time (MST) ranging from 77 to 254 days, which is dependent on the presence of heart failure (former MST).
- Prognosis for each form of cardiomyopathy is discussed in that respective section.

PATHOLOGY

- Gross examination of the heart provides useful anatomic information and should be performed when possible to confirm antemortem findings.
- Cats with severe cardiomyopathy often have gross evidence of left atrial enlargement and

CHF. Edematous lungs are heavy and red and sink when placed in water or formalin. Pulmonary edema may be identified as frothy fluid exuding from the cut surface of the lung or filling the trachea or smaller airways. Pleural effusion may be readily identified on opening the thorax.

- Increased heart weight or heart weight indexed to body weight (29 to 37 g [HCM] compared with <20 g [normal]; ≥6.4 +/− 0.1 g heart weight per kilogram of body weight [HCM] compared with ≤4.8 +/− 0.1 g/kg [normal]) is often seen in cats that die from HCM and may also be present in cats with enlarged hearts from other cardiomyopathies.
- In most cases, histopathologic evaluation adds little useful information, and unless readily available at low cost, it is not recommended unless specific indications are present (see the section on specific diseases). Hallmark histopathologic abnormalities of HCM include cardiomyocyte hypertrophy, myofiber disarray (in 30% of cases in one study, involving at least 5% of the septum), interstitial and replacement fibrosis, and small coronary arteriosclerosis.

PRIMARY CARDIOMYOPATHIES

HYPERTROPHIC CARDIOMYOPATHY

HCM is a disease of the ventricular (primarily left ventricular) myocardium characterized by mild to severe thickening (concentric hypertrophy) of the papillary muscles, interventricular septum, and LV free wall. The word *primary* in this context means that the hypertrophy results from an inherent problem in the myocardium and is not secondary to a pressure overload (systemic hypertension or aortic stenosis) or to hormonal stimulation (T4).

GENERAL COMMENTS

- When any other disease process that may lead to concentric hypertrophy is present, the diagnosis of HCM is excluded. Secondary disorders typically produce symmetric concentric hypertrophy, usually only with a maximum increase in wall thickness of <50%, even with severe disease. If severe or asymmetric concentric hypertrophy is present in a patient with one of these disorders, then concomitant HCM should be considered. Likewise if heart failure is present, HCM should be suspected because secondary causes of left ventricular concentric hypertrophy do not usually independently cause heart failure. If left ventricular concentric hypertrophy does not regress after several months of effectively treating the underlying problem such as hypertension or hyperthyroidism, HCM should also be suspected as being a concurrent disease.

- HCM is the most commonly diagnosed cardiac disease in cats, and its prevalence appears to be increasing (ranging from 15% to 30% of healthy cats); however, echocardiographic screening for the disease has also become more common during this time.
- The cause of HCM is idiopathic, yet heritable familial HCM is identified in several predilected breeds, including Maine Coon, Ragdoll, Persian, British Shorthair, American Shorthair, Norwegian Forest, Turkish Van, Sphynx, Bengal, and Scottish Fold cats.
- Two different missense mutations in cardiac myosin-binding protein C gene *(MYBPC3)* have been identified to cause HCM in some families of Maine Coon and Ragdoll cats, and a commercial assay is available for genetic screening (through the Cardiac Genetics Laboratory at the North Carolina State College of Veterinary Medicine). Heterozygous affected cats may not have phenotypic evidence of disease (i.e., no concentric ventricular hypertrophy on echocardiography) but may transmit the defect to progeny or develop HCM later in life. Homozygous affected cats often develop severe disease earlier in life.

CLINICAL CLASSIFICATION AND PATHOPHYSIOLOGY

- HCM is characterized by increased left ventricular myocardial wall thickness in the absence of other secondary causes. Papillary muscle hypertrophy is subjectively assessed on echocardiogram and may range from mild to severe. Concentric hypertrophy may include the interventricular septum and the left ventricular free wall and may be either global (symmetric) or segmental (asymmetric). Hypertrophy may range from mild (6 to 6.5 mm) to severe (>7.5 mm). The concentric hypertrophy may also result in a decrease in afterload because of the increase in wall thickness, which may result in a decreased end-systolic volume, often to zero (end-systolic cavity obliteration).
- Impaired diastolic filling during early active relaxation or during passive ventricular filling caused by increased ventricular stiffness leads to diastolic dysfunction. Diastolic dysfunction in cats with HCM is caused by increased wall stiffness because of hypertrophy, myocyte disarray, myocardial fibrosis, and possible impaired calcium handling causing impaired active diastolic relaxation. Reduced myocardial perfusion may lead to myocardial ischemia and myocardial necrosis, with subsequent replacement fibrosis of the myocardium. Small vessel coronary artery disease

and activated neurohormonal systems such as RAAS may lead to interstitial myocardial fibrosis. Myocardial fibrosis may also cause ventricular arrhythmias and potentially sudden death.

- Systolic anterior motion (SAM) of the mitral valve is often (67% of cats with HCM in one study) but not always present in cats with HCM and may range from mild to severe. Cats with HCM and SAM are commonly said to have the obstructive type of HCM or to have hypertrophic obstructive cardiomyopathy (HOCM). It is typically the cause of the left parasternal systolic murmur in HCM. SAM of the mitral valve develops secondary to anterior ventrally displaced, hypertrophied papillary muscles that pull the mitral valve into the left ventricular outflow tract during systole. Other factors that may exacerbate or worsen SAM of the mitral valve include severe basilar septal concentric hypertrophy, increased contractility, and tachycardia.
- SAM of the mitral valve produces a dynamic subaortic stenosis that increases systolic intraventricular pressure in mid to late systole and is worsened with increased contractility. The dynamic subaortic stenosis increases the velocity of blood flow through the subaortic region and produces turbulence in the left ventricular outflow tract and aorta. Simultaneously, when the septal leaflet is pulled toward the interventricular septum, a gap is left in the mitral valve creating mitral regurgitation, which is typically only mild to moderate in severity. Moderate or severe SAM of the mitral valve greatly increases left ventricular systolic pressure, which increases the severity of concentric left ventricular hypertrophy and potentiates the vicious cycle of hypertrophy and the potential for worsened diastolic function.
- Diastolic heart failure is caused by severe diastolic dysfunction in cats with severe HCM. Severe diastolic dysfunction leads to elevated left ventricular filling pressure and left atrial dilation, ultimately leading to left-sided CHF when the pulmonary venous pressure exceeds 20 to 25 mm Hg. Approximately half of cats with CHF have concurrent pulmonary edema and pleural effusion. Pleural effusion is common in cats with heart failure. It can be classified as a modified transudate, pseudochylous, or true chylous effusion. The exact pathophysiologic processes of pleural effusion secondary to left heart failure is unknown in cats. The most likely possibility is that feline visceral pleural veins drain into the pulmonary veins such that elevated pulmonary venous pressure causes the formation of pleural effusion.
- Sudden death may occur in any cat and may be unrelated to disease severity. The incidence

of sudden death in cats with HCM is unknown. Sudden death may be caused by severe ventricular arrhythmia that causes fibrillation or from massive ATE that occludes the proximal aorta.

- Left atrial or auricular thrombi may form in cats with HCM, typically when the left atrium (LA) is dilated. Left atrial thrombi commonly break loose (become emboli) and are carried by blood flow most commonly to the terminal aorta where they lodge. These arterial thromboemboli occlude aortic blood flow and elaborate vasoactive substances that constrict collateral vessels. The net result is cessation of blood flow to the caudal legs resulting in acute paresis/paralysis and pain. The incidence of ATE in cats with HCM is approximately 12% to 17% and is associated with varying degrees of left atrial enlargement. Thrombus formation may occur when there is an abnormality in one or more of the components of a Virchow triangle, which include hypercoagulability, endothelial disruption, and blood stasis. When the LA becomes moderately to severely dilated, the blood flow velocity is reduced, resulting in red cell aggregation, platelet activation, and subsequent thrombus formation. Blood flow stasis may be the most important factor for development of left atrial thrombi in cats with cardiac disease. Hypercoagulability has been reported in cats with cardiomyopathy or ATE.

SIGNALMENT AND PRESENTING COMPLAINTS

- There is a wide range of patient characteristics in feline HCM, with any age being possible for HCM to develop. Although the average age of cats diagnosed with HCM is reportedly 5.5 to 6.5 years, cats may range from several months of age to geriatric. With increased awareness of the disease and more frequent echocardiographic screening of predisposed breeds, cats are being diagnosed earlier in the disease course, often as young juveniles.
- Familial autosomal dominant heritable HCM occurs in Maine Coon and Ragdoll cats as a result of mutations in (MYBPC3) (see Chapter 6). In a family of Maine Coon cats with familial HCM caused by MYBPC3 mutation, homozygous affected cats had phenotypic echocardiographic evidence of left ventricular hypertrophy between 4 and 6 months of age and severe left ventricular hypertrophy by 7 to 12 months of age. Heart failure usually developed by 20 months of age, and most of these cats died by 4 years of age. Male Maine Coon cats that are homozygous affected typically have more severe disease at an earlier age. Heterozygously

affected Maine Coon cats may live many years with moderate left ventricular hypertrophy and atrial dilation without development of CHF or sudden death. Ragdoll cats can have a severe, early onset form of familial HCM, with a mean age of diagnosis of 15 months in one study (ages range from 6 months to 2 years). In a genetic study, Ragdoll cats that were homozygously affected with the MYBPC3 mutation had HCM 18 months earlier than heterozygously affected cats.

- Other predisposed breeds include Persian, Himalayan, Birman, American Shorthair, British Shorthair, Sphinx, Bengal, Siberian, Norwegian Forest, and Scottish Fold cats. Despite certain breed predispositions, the domestic Shorthair cat is the most commonly affected breed. The average age of onset and rate of progression in mixed breed cats is unknown.
- Although there is no sex-linked heritability pattern, approximately three fourths of cats diagnosed with HCM are neutered males.
- Presenting complaints are variable, depending on the severity of HCM. Because cats are often symptom free, they may be seen by the veterinarian for other problems or for a routine health examination or preanesthetic evaluation. Other cats with severe HCM may have a complaint referable to heart failure, including difficulty breathing, anorexia, lethargy, or weight loss. A precipitating event was identified in approximately half of cats diagnosed with CHF in one study. The most common precipitating event was fluid administration (28%), followed by anesthesia/surgery (25%), and recent corticosteroid administration (21%) with methylprednisolone (70% of cats) or an injectable form of triamcinolone (30% of cats) given 1 to 2 weeks before diagnosis of heart failure.
- Sometimes the first presenting complaint is sudden death or acute paralysis caused by ATE.

PHYSICAL EXAMINATION

- Auscultation abnormalities: A systolic murmur is the most common physical examination abnormality in cats with HCM and has been reported in 31% to 72% of cats. Murmur grades range from soft (1) to loud (4), often depending on the presence and severity of SAM of the mitral valve. A gallop is less frequently auscultated (33%), and an arrhythmia is uncommon (7%). A small percentage (5%) of cats have no clinical abnormalities. Please refer to the previous general section of cardiomyopathies for a complete discussion of physical examination abnormalities.

ECHOCARDIOGRAPHY

- The defining abnormality seen on echocardiography in cats with HCM is an increased end-diastolic left ventricular wall thickness of 6 mm or greater, which may include the interventricular septum or the left ventricular free wall in the absence of other secondary causes of concentric hypertrophy. Papillary muscle hypertrophy is commonly present and is subjectively assessed (Figure 9.3, *A*). Sometimes papillary muscle hypertrophy is the only abnormality present. Cats may have generalized (global) concentric hypertrophy or asymmetric

(segmental) concentric hypertrophy of the septum or free wall (Figure 9.3, *A* and *C*). Because of these various patterns of hypertrophy, HCM is a diagnosis that should be made by examining several two-dimensional echocardiographic views and measuring wall thicknesses in diastole from the thickest region or regions on the two-dimensional images. M-mode echocardiography may miss regional thickening unless it is guided by the two-dimensional view. Often the basilar interventricular septal hypertrophy is best assessed with the right parasternal long axis view (Figure 9.3, *C*). The left ventricular end-diastolic or end-systolic dimension may be normal or decreased, and end-systolic cavity obliteration may occur. End-systolic cavity obliteration is seen as an obliterated end-systolic chamber lumen as a result of the marked increase in left ventricular hypertrophy and reduction in afterload (Figure 9.3, *B*).

- Left atrial dilation may be identified as a left atrial to aortic diameter ratio (measured at the first frame of aortic valve closure) with two-dimensional echo of >1.5. An enlarged LA indicates increased left ventricular end-diastolic pressure and risk of CHF. Typically left atrial dilation is moderate or severe (left atrial/aortic ratio >1.8) in cats with CHF. Occasionally a thrombus is identified in the LA or its appendage. Spontaneous red cell aggregation (i.e., smoke) should be carefully assessed within the LA and auricle in both right parasternal views and the left parasternal cranial view where the auricle is positioned close to the body wall.

- SAM of the mitral valve may be identified by two-dimensional echocardiography in the right parasternal long axis left ventricular outflow tract view. Often the abnormality may be detected most easily by color flow Doppler interrogation of the left ventricular outflow tract and mitral valve. The characteristic color flow Doppler abnormality is a double jet of turbulence arising from a single point in the left ventricular outflow tract in mid to late systole, causing both mitral regurgitation and turbulent blood flow in the left ventricular outflow tract out to the aorta (Figure 9.4). With the left apical five-chamber view, continuous wave Doppler is used to measure the velocity of aortic blood flow and quantifies the severity of obstruction. The modified Bernoulli equation (pressure gradient = $4 \times velocity^2$) is used to calculate the LV to aortic pressure gradient and determine the severity of obstruction (mild <50 mm Hg, moderate 50 to 80 mm Hg, severe >80 mm Hg). The obstruction is dynamic, worsens through systole, and creates a characteristic shape of a "dagger" on continuous wave

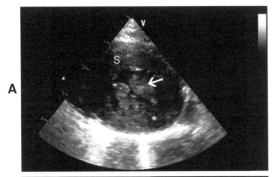
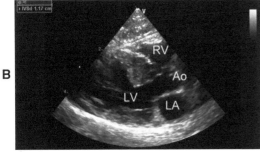
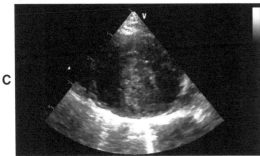

Figure 9.3 Echocardiogram of the left ventricle (*LV*) of a cat with severe hypertrophic cardiomyopathy (HCM). HCM consists of concentric left ventricular hypertrophy (>6 mm) that may be global or asymmetric. Asymmetric hypertrophy may mainly include the papillary muscles and left ventricular free wall (**A**) or the basilar interventricular septum (**B**). There is often end-systolic cavity obliteration (**C**) where there is no chamber lumen remaining at end diastole because of marked concentric hypertrophy and reduced afterload. *Ao,* Aorta; *LA,* left atrium; *RV,* right ventricle.

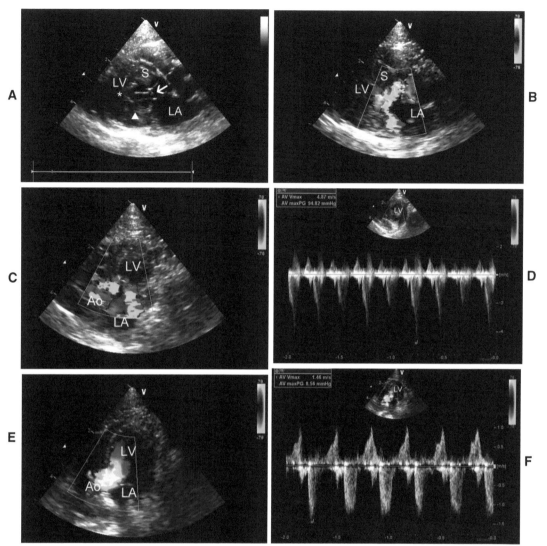

Figure 9.4 Echocardiographic assessment of systolic anterior motion (SAM) of the mitral valve in a cat with severe hypertrophic obstructive cardiomyopathy (HOCM). The right parasternal long axis left ventricular outflow tract view allows visualization of the anterior mitral valve and shows SAM of the mitral valve (**A**). Papillary muscles (*) are severely hypertrophied and anteriorly displaced, which pull the chordae tendineae and the anterior leaflet (*arrow*) toward the severely hypertrophied basilar interventricular septum (*S*). The left ventricle (*LV*) free wall (*triangle*) also has concentric hypertrophy. Color flow Doppler imaging of the left ventricular outflow tract shows a double turbulent jet where the anterior mitral leaflet obstructs the left ventricular outflow tract and also creates mitral regurgitation seen on right parasternal long-axis left ventricular outflow tract view (**B**) and left apical five-chamber view (**C**). From the left apical five-chamber view, continuous wave Doppler imaging is used to measure the aortic blood flow velocity, which is 4.87 m/sec, corresponding to a severely increased LV/aortic pressure gradient of 95 mm Hg with the modified Bernoulli equation (**D**). After 2 weeks of atenolol administration, a recheck echocardiogram shows minimal SAM on color flow Doppler imaging (**E**), and continuous wave Doppler imaging shows normal left ventricular outflow tract velocity of 1.5 m/sec corresponding to a normal LV/aortic pressure gradient of 8.5 mm Hg (**F**). *Ao,* Aorta; *LA,* left atrium.

Doppler interrogation, with a peak velocity at end-systole (see Figure 9.4). The pressure gradient roughly correlates with the severity of the SAM, although it can be quite labile, changing with the cat's level of excitement.

- Diastolic dysfunction in cats with severe HCM has been documented with tissue Doppler imaging and measures of transmitral flow and relaxation time. Cats with severe HCM routinely have a decrease in early diastolic wall motion of the LV free wall and mitral valve annulus using tissue Doppler imaging. Pulsed wave (PW) Doppler measurement of mitral inflow velocity from the left apical four-chamber view often

shows a delayed relaxation pattern (early diastolic filling wave [E] to atrial systole [A] wave
ratio of <1, prolonged isovolumic relaxation
time, and prolonged deceleration time) in cats
with HCM. Delayed relaxation is the first level
of diastolic dysfunction when there is impaired
early diastolic filling but normal left atrial pressures. As diastolic dysfunction worsens, left
atrial pressure increases, leading to a pseudonormal filling pattern on mitral inflow velocity
measurement. A restrictive filling pattern may
be seen in cats with severe diastolic dysfunction
and severely elevated left atrial pressure and is
evidenced by E/A ratio >2, decreased deceleration time, and shortened isovolumic relaxation
time. Assessment of mitral inflow patterns of
diastolic function is fraught with challenges
such as summation of E and A waves in cats with
HRs >150 beats/min and is affected by changes
in preload and afterload.

ADDITIONAL TESTING

- Assessment of secondary (reversible) causes of
concentric ventricular hypertrophy such as systemic hypertension or hyperthyroidism is necessary in cats with echocardiographic evidence
of left ventricular concentric hypertrophy. Systemic blood pressure should be measured in all
cats with left ventricular concentric hypertrophy, and the serum thyroxine level measured in
cats >5 years of age with left ventricular concentric hypertrophy.
- Genetic testing for a *MYBPC3* mutation may be
considered in Maine Coon cats or Ragdoll cats
to assess the risk of developing HCM and is recommended for Maine Coon and Ragdoll cats
intended for breeding. There is a high prevalence, 34%, of genetically affected symptom-
free Maine Coon cats in the general breeding
population. A test with negative results does not
rule out HCM because cats may have HCM from
other causes or unidentified genetic mutations.
Cats with positive test results should be evaluated by echocardiography to assess whether
there is phenotypic evidence of disease, and
echocardiography should be repeated annually
in genotypically affected cats.

THERAPY

- There is a lack of studies in which the impact
of treatment on the clinical course of disease in
symptom-free cats with HCM is evaluated. The
clinician is forced to form an opinion, often
based on personal experience, on the anecdotal
experience of an expert, or on small studies in
which specific echocardiographic variables that
may not actually pertain to the overall course
of the disease are examined. Therefore there

is great controversy about whether symptom-
free cats should be treated and with what specific medical therapy. Ideally the fundamental
goals in treatment of symptom-free cats would
include reduction in left ventricular hypertrophy, improvement in diastolic function, reduction in risk of ATE, and prolongation to time
of heart failure. However, there are little data
that confirm or deny that any particular treatment has a considerable effect on these goals.
It is likely that many cats with mild to moderate HCM may live long lives without any clinical
consequences of the disease, and committing
to lifelong daily to twice daily medications may
be unnecessary. However, many veterinarians
feel compelled to treat a patient with a disease,
and some owners demand treatment for their
pets, even if there is only a theoretic case for
using a drug. Consequently, whenever HCM
is diagnosed in a cat, the veterinarian must
explain the pros and cons of treatment options
to each owner and try to let the owners make
an informed decision based on their wishes and
lifestyle.
- The decision of whether to treat a symptom-
free cat with HCM may include severity of
SAM of the mitral valve, severity of left ventricular hypertrophy, size of the LA, presence
of tachyarrhythmias, client factors associated
with medicating daily to twice daily indefinitely, and patient temperament. Often the
choice lies between beta blockers (atenolol)
and calcium channel blockers (diltiazem).
Whatever the initial choice, response to therapy should dictate whether dose adjustment,
changing drug class, or discontinuation of
therapy is warranted.
- In a prospective, blinded, placebo-controlled
study, the effects of atenolol compared with
diltiazem in symptom-free cats with HCM were
evaluated. Results were relatively underwhelm-
ing. Atenolol had modest effects to improve
one variable of diastolic function and slightly
reduced septal thickness, and there were no
significant effects of diltiazem on diastolic
function, left atrial size, or left ventricular
hypertrophy. Atenolol also reduced the severity of SAM of the mitral valve, and diltiazem
did not. An earlier uncontrolled pilot study
reported a reduction in left ventricular hypertrophy, which has not been demonstrated in
subsequent controlled studies. The AQUA
study reported that atenolol improved the
owner's subjective overall assessment of their
cat's quality of life compared with placebo but
had no effect in mobility quantified by an accel-
erometer, or in a detailed questionnaire about
quality of life.

- Prophylactic antiplatelet agents such as clopidogrel are indicated in cats with any of the following: moderate to severe left atrial dilation, spontaneous echocardiographic contrast or a thrombus on an echocardiogram, or a previous episode of ATE.
- ACE inhibitors are unlikely to impact the severity of left ventricular hypertrophy or diastolic function on the basis of a placebo-controlled, prospective, blinded clinical study. However they may be considered in cats with severe HCM and severe left atrial dilation with impending heart failure.
- Once heart failure develops, use of furosemide and an ACE inhibitor are standard therapies. Unfortunately, heart failure typically represents the end stage of the disease, and survival time is often limited to several months to a year despite medical therapy. Beta blockers are not started in acute heart failure because these patients may have a poorer outcome when receiving beta blockers. Cats already receiving a beta blocker may continue to receive it, but the dose or frequency may need to be reduced.
- Controversy exists regarding the use of pimobendan for cats with HCM and heart failure. Potential pharmacodynamic benefits of pimobendan could include preload reduction and positive lusitropy (increases diastolic relaxation) and positive inotropy (in cats with myocardial failure from end-stage HCM). A retrospective study documented survival benefit in cats with heart failure secondary to HCM with no myocardial failure that were treated with pimobendan and other standard cardiac medications (MST, 626 days) compared with cats not given pimobendan (MST, 103 days). However, the group of cats not receiving pimobendan had a shorter survival time than is often clinically expected, yet literature reports highly variable survival times in retrospective studies (92 to 654 days) in cats with heart failure caused by HCM.

BETA BLOCKERS

Atenolol is currently the preferred beta blocker and is a selective B1 blocker administered BID usually but sometimes q24h depending on HR.

- **Atenolol:** 6.25 to 12.5 mg per cat q12h. Atenolol is supplied as 25-mg tablets.

CALCIUM CHANNEL BLOCKERS

- **Diltiazem** is currently the preferred calcium channel blocker and is available in three forms:
  - **Cardizem:** 7.5 mg PO q8h. This product is supplied as 30-mg tablets. One-quarter tablet is given q8h.
  - **Dilacor XR:** 30 mg PO q12h. This product is supplied as 120-, 180-, and 240-mg capsules. Each large capsule can be opened to yield two, three, or four 60-mg tablets, which are then halved to achieve a 30-mg dose.
  - **Cardizem CD:** 45 mg PO q24h. Cardizem CD is supplied as 180-mg capsules that contain many smaller capsules. The larger capsule can be opened and the smaller capsules divided into a number that produces an appropriate dose; this should be done by a compounding pharmacy.

KEY POINT

I prefer to use atenolol for treatment of symptom-free cats with moderate to severe left ventricular hypertrophy, moderate to severe SAM, or concurrent tachyarrhythmias and HCM.

PROGNOSIS

- Left atrial size, CHF, intracardiac thrombus, or ATE is a negative prognostic indicator in cats with HCM. The MST of cats with HCM surviving more than 24 hours from time of diagnosis was 709 days in one study but varies tremendously depending on the stage of disease. The MST was 1129 days in symptom-free cats, 654 days in cats with heart failure, and only 184 days in cats with ATE. The REVEAL study evaluated 1362 cats with HCM over 5 years and reported the incidence rates of CHF as 3.4% per year (17% at 5 years), ATE as 1.7% per year (8.5% at 5 years), and all-cause cardiac death as 4.4% per year (22% at 5 years). MST was 4.97 years (2.6 to 6.2 years) for HCM compared with 5.45 years for normal cats, likely because of sampling from an aged feline population. Risk factors for development of CHF were septal hypertrophy (HR, 1.36 beats/min) and left atrial dilation (HR, 1.05 beats/min), and risk factors for ATE were septal and free wall hypertrophy (HR, 1.36 and 1.28 beats/min, respectively) and left atrial dilation (HR, 1.07 beats/min).
- Symptom-free cats with mild to moderate hypertrophy and no LA enlargement are thought to have a good long-term prognosis. Reported average survival times are generally in the range of 4 to 6 years. Symptom-free cats with obvious wall thickening and LA enlargement are likely at higher risk for developing heart failure. These cats are also thought to be at risk for developing thromboembolic disease.
- In general, cats that have heart failure have a poor prognosis. Typical survival times are several months but vary depending on the patient's response to therapy.

- In general, cats with aortic thromboembolism have a poor to grave prognosis. Typical survival times in cats that are not euthanized at the time of the diagnosis may be several months. Prolonged survival times have been recently reported by the FATCAT clinical study of cats with ATE (from various cardiomyopathies) treated with clopidogrel (442 days) compared with those treated with aspirin (192 days). Cats that survive the thromboembolic episode may do well for an extended period of time; however these cats are at high risk for recurrence of thromboembolism.
- Owners should always be warned of the potential for sudden death in cats with HCM, even symptom-free cats with mild HCM. The exact incidence of sudden death in cats with HCM is unknown, but postulated causes are ventricular arrhythmia or large intracardiac thrombus.

FELINE (IDIOPATHIC) DILATED CARDIOMYOPATHY

DCM is a disease of the ventricular myocardium (predominantly left) characterized by *primary* systolic myocardial failure.

GENERAL COMMENTS

- Before 1987, DCM was one of the most commonly diagnosed heart diseases in cats. Most cases at that time were likely a secondary cardiomyopathy associated with nutritional taurine deficiency. In current times, DCM is uncommon in cats and is most often caused by primary idiopathic DCM.
- Idiopathic DCM is a diagnosis of exclusion, ruling out secondary causes of myocardial failure such as taurine deficiency, tachycardiomyopathy, severe volume overload leading to secondary myocardial failure (i.e., severe mitral insufficiency or large left to right shunting congenital heart diseases), or toxicity such as doxorubicin cardiotoxicity.
- The underlying etiology of idiopathic DCM remains unknown and may represent a common endpoint to many processes. A heritable cause has not been identified in cats but is an important cause of DCM in humans where 30% to 50% of cases are caused by mutations in more than 30 genes.
- Another secondary and reversible cause of myocardial failure that mimics idiopathic DCM is severe hypocalcemia and was reported in a cat with primary hypoparathyroidism.

TAURINE DEFICIENCY–INDUCED MYOCARDIAL FAILURE

- Taurine deficiency–induced myocardial failure is associated with low plasma, whole blood,

and tissue taurine concentrations that may be reversible after taurine supplementation.
- Taurine is an essential sulfur-containing amino acid in cats and has an obligatory role in bile salt conjugation. Taurine is synthesized by the liver and brain from dietary sulfur amino acids (cysteine), and the rate of synthesis in the cat is much lower than its loss though conjugation of cholic acid. Taurine homeostasis in cats depends on dietary intake, endogenous synthesis, enterohepatic turnover, microbial degradation in the large intestine, and urinary and fecal losses.
- Typical diet history may include feeding home cooked diets low in taurine (such as chicken breast) or feeding solely one canned food for many years.
- Not all taurine-deficient cats have myocardial failure (20% to 65% of cats). The other factors required for taurine deficiency causing myocardial failure are unknown.
- The role that taurine, an essential amino acid in the cat, plays in the maintenance of myocardial function remains unknown. Taurine has diverse functions, with the most important including modulation of contractility (possibly through myocardial calcium homeostasis), metabolic and osmotic regulation of the myocardium, membrane stabilization of photoreceptor cells of the retina, and neuroinhibitor actions in the central nervous system.

KEY POINT

Although myocardial failure secondary to taurine deficiency is now quite rare in cats, all cats with myocardial failure should be assumed to be taurine deficient until shown not to be taurine responsive.

PATHOPHYSIOLOGY

- The underlying abnormality leading to clinical manifestations in cats with idiopathic DCM is primary systolic myocardial failure. End-systolic left ventricular volume increases, owing to a reduction in myocardial pump function. As a result, stroke volume and cardiac output decrease. Neurohumoral compensatory mechanisms promote an increase in intravascular volume and end-diastolic pressures, stimulating eccentric hypertrophy (dilation). At these larger left ventricular end-diastolic volumes, the geometry of the ventricle is such that small changes in chamber dimension during systole provide adequate stroke volume and cardiac output; however, working at these larger volumes is energetically inefficient for the ventricle. At any point in this degenerative process that end-diastolic pressures rise too high or cardiac output drops too low, the patient may have signs of CHF or low-output heart failure respectively. Biventricular failure, including pulmonary edema and pleural effusion, is common in cats because both the left and right ventricles are affected.

- Often cats are not diagnosed until they have symptoms for heart failure at an end stage of the disease.

SIGNALMENT AND PRESENTING COMPLAINTS

- Strong breed predispositions are not observed in DCM but it has been reported in the following breeds: Persian, Domestic Shorthair, Domestic Longhair, Birman, Siamese, and Burmese.
- It is an adult onset disease, with mean age reported to range from 7 to 9 years but with a wide range of 5 months to 14 years.
- No sex predilection is evident.
- Cats with DCM may have a variable period of lethargy, anorexia, and malaise before overt signs of CHF, including dyspnea and tachypnea.
- Cats may have no prior signs of an acute onset of CHF or systemic thromboembolism.

PHYSICAL EXAMINATION

- A gallop heart sound is the most common auscultation finding (79% of cats), and a soft left parasternal systolic murmur is less commonly present (17% of cats). Most cats with DCM have heart failure, with pleural effusion more common than pulmonary edema (91% compared with 36%). Cats usually exhibit tachypnea, dyspnea, and orthopnea, and lung sounds are often muffled. Femoral arterial pulses are usually weak. Right-sided heart failure may also be present, including signs of jugular distension and a pendulous abdomen. A retinal examination is necessary to evaluate for taurine deficiency–associated central retinal lesions because taurine deficiency is the main differential for idiopathic DCM. Please refer to the previous general section of cardiomyopathies for a complete discussion of physical examination abnormalities.

ANCILLARY TESTS

- Measurement of whole blood and plasma taurine blood concentration is an essential test for cats with echocardiographic evidence of myocardial failure.
- Ideally, both whole blood and plasma levels are measured, but if only one can be measured because of financial constraint, whole blood is

recommended. Plasma taurine concentration is subject to significant fluctuations depending on the fasted state of the cat. In cats fed diets adequate in taurine, plasma taurine concentration was critically low (<30 nmol/mL) in 9 (26%) of 35 normal cats that were fasted for 71 hours and in 2 normal cats that were fasted for only 23 hours.

- Taurine deficiency is defined as plasma taurine concentration <50 nmol/mL or whole blood taurine concentration of ≤250 nmol/mL. There are strict guidelines for obtaining and handling blood samples for taurine analysis; please refer to laboratory specifications.

ECHOCARDIOGRAM

DCM is defined as primary myocardial failure, which is diagnosed by a decreased FS of <26% and an increased end-systolic diameter >11 mm (Figure 9.5; see Table 9.1). There is a secondary compensatory eccentric hypertrophy that is identified as an increased end-diastolic left ventricular diameter (>18 mm). E-point to septal separation is another index of systolic function and is increased (>4 mm). Left atrial dilation occurs secondary to elevated left ventricular filling pressure and is identified as a left atrial/aortic ratio >1.5. Other subjective findings often include right atrial dilation and right ventricular eccentric hypertrophy, mild pericardial effusion, and pleural effusion. Mild centrally arising AV valvular insufficiency secondary to decreased AV valve coaptation is also commonly present. Spontaneous echocardiographic contrast or an atrial thrombus may be present.

THERAPY

- For acute CHF, see the earlier section on treatment of CHF in the discussion of therapy in the general information section. In addition, I am adding pimobendan (1.25 mg PO BID or 0.25 mg/kg PO BID) to the acute heart failure treatment in cats with DCM or other secondary causes of myocardial failure. In cats with low-output heart failure (cardiogenic shock), dobutamine CRI and pimobendan are indicated.
- Chronic therapy for cats with DCM and heart failure is similar to other cardiomyopathies except for the addition of pimobendan and possibly digoxin (0.007 mg/kg PO q48h or ¼ of a 0.125-mg tablet orally once a day for cats weighing >4 kg, or q48h for cats weighing <4 kg). Avoidance of negative inotropes such as beta blockers is necessary to avoid life threatening decompensation. Clopidogrel is also likely necessary for prevention of possible ATE, which is common in cats with DCM (18% of

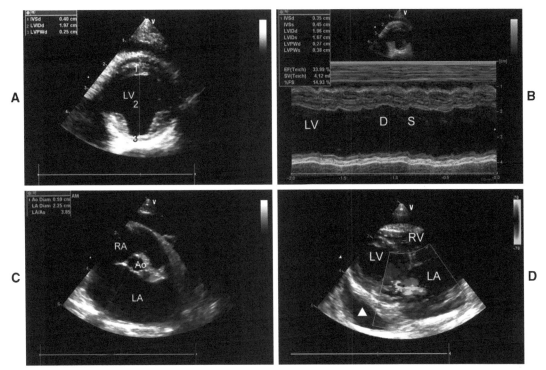

Figure 9.5 Echocardiogram of a cat with severe dilated cardiomyopathy (DCM). This two-dimensional echocardiogram from the right parasternal cross-sectional view at the level of the papillary muscles shows severe eccentric hypertrophy of the left ventricle (*LV*), which is a compensatory mechanism to normalize stroke volume in the face of severe biventricular systolic myocardial failure (**A**) and a thin left ventricular free wall (*LVPWd*). **B,** Placing the cursor through the septum and free wall in this view, an M-mode tracing is obtained, which allows measurement of the left ventricular chamber diameter in end-diastole (*D*) and end-systole (*S*) and calculation of fractional shortening (*FS*). This M-mode shows severe myocardial failure evidenced by increased end-systolic diameter, marked reduction in FS (15%), and compensatory increase in left ventricular end-diastolic diameter (eccentric hypertrophy). **C,** There is severe left atrial dilation, which is assessed by measurement of the aortic and left atrial diameters on the first frame of aortic valve closure with two-dimensional echocardiography, and with calculation of the left atrial to aortic ratio, which in this cat is severely increased at 3.85 (<1.5 normal). Color flow Doppler interrogation of the mitral valve often shows mild centrally arising functional mitral regurgitation secondary to severe ventricular volume overload and pleural effusion (*triangle*) (**D**). *Ao,* Aorta; *RA,* right atrium; *RV,* right ventricle.

cats had echocardiographic evidence of intracardiac thrombi in one study).

- Treatment of taurine deficiency–induced myocardial failure
  - Taurine 250 mg PO BID is empirically administered until results of the blood taurine levels are obtained, and if deficiency is documented, taurine supplementation may be continued long term. Clinical signs typically improve within 2 weeks, and by 3 to 6 weeks there is echocardiographic evidence of decreased end-systolic left ventricular diameter, increased FS, and decreased end-diastolic left ventricular diameter. Myocardial failure should improve but may persist for up to a year after supplementation.
  - Most taurine-responsive cats have complete reversal of echocardiographic and clinical evidence of myocardial failure after supplementation with taurine after several months.

Occasionally cats may have residual mild myocardial failure (left ventricular shortening fraction, 25% to 30%); however, these cats are generally symptom free and rarely require any form of therapy other than maintaining normal plasma taurine concentrations.

- Diuretics and ACE inhibitors can be discontinued when clinical signs resolve and cardiac size is smaller on radiographs or echocardiogram, usually after several months of therapy. The ACE inhibitor should be removed first and then the diuretic tapered over a period of 2 weeks. The owner should be taught to monitor the respiratory rate while withdrawing heart failure medications, and clinical and radiographic evaluation should be repeated 1 week after withdrawing medications to detect any decline in the cat's condition. Likewise, positive inotropes (pimobendan +/– digoxin) may be weaned off after several months, once the heart size reduces and the myocardial failure improves.

- The diet should be altered to maintain normal plasma taurine concentrations (>60 nmol/mL). Taurine supplementation can be discontinued once echocardiographic values return to within normal limits and the cat is eating a diet with adequate amounts of taurine, although some patients continue lifelong taurine administration.
- Taurine concentration in plasma and whole blood should be monitored periodically to be certain that the diet fed is maintaining concentrations within acceptable limits. If taurine concentrations are depleted again, then many cats will again have myocardial failure.

PROGNOSIS

- Prognosis for idiopathic DCM is grave, but there are minimal data documenting clinical characteristics and outcome. MST in one study was 11 days, and my overall experience is that cats with heart failure caused by DCM may survive for weeks or up to 3 months. Preclinical cats with myocardial failure are rarely identified, but these cats may live months to years before succumbing to heart failure or ATE. Cats with signs of low-output heart failure or fulminant heart failure have a grave prognosis. These cats usually either die soon after admission from cardiogenic shock or succumb quickly to refractory CHF or ATE.
- Taurine deficiency–induced myocardial failure confers a good prognosis if the cat can survive the first several weeks of therapy. In one large study, 30% of cats with myocardial failure died within the first week after diagnosis. Hypothermia and thromboembolic disease were associated with a poor prognosis. Early cardiovascular death within the first month occurs in approximately 38% of treated cats. However, if a cat survives after the first 2 weeks of therapy, there is a 96% chance of long-term survival with complete recovery if there is documented taurine deficiency.

FELINE RESTRICTIVE CARDIOMYOPATHY

RCM is a diverse group of conditions characterized by restriction of diastolic filling caused by an increased ventricular stiffness. The clinical picture is of a normal ventricle with normal wall thickness, normal ventricular size and systolic function, but presence of left atrial or biatrial dilation with normal AV valves. Specific clinical and morphologic criteria for this diagnosis in the cat have not been as clearly defined as they have in humans.

GENERAL COMMENTS

- In human medicine, RCM is divided into two main categories: endomyocardial fibrosis and interstitial myocardial fibrosis. Without the use of invasive diagnostic procedures such as endomyocardial biopsy or necropsy examination, it is impossible to differentiate the myocardial fibrosis form of RCM from UCM; therefore the two diseases in cats are often combined in the literature as RCM/UCM.
- Etiology in cats remains idiopathic, and no familial basis has been reported in cats.

PATHOPHYSIOLOGY

- The characteristic functional abnormality of RCM is increased left ventricular stiffness causing impaired diastolic filling and elevated diastolic filling pressure. Fibrosis occurs within the myocardium, subendocardium, or endocardium, with an end result of marked diastolic dysfunction. Once left ventricular filling pressure increases to >25 mm Hg, pulmonary edema or pleural effusion develops (i.e., left CHF). Tachyarrhythmias may accentuate the diastolic dysfunction and contribute to further increase in diastolic filling pressure.
- LV disease predominates. In most cases, systolic function is preserved. In the endomyocardial fibrosis form of RCM, a fibrotic band may bridge the LV and distort the mitral valve to create both mitral regurgitation and systolic obstruction of blood flow in the LV.

SIGNALMENT AND PRESENTING COMPLAINTS

- Signalment is difficult to report accurately because there is little agreement among cardiologists as to which cases fall within this classification compared with patients with UCM. Recently, the myocardial fibrosis form has been described as an animal model of human RCM in 35 cats at the Animal Medical Center. RCM represented 4.5% of all feline cardiac cases seen at the Animal Medical Center in that report. Seventy-one percent of cats were male, with a mean age of 10 +/−4 years (range, 1.5 to 17.1 years). In contrast, a previous case series reported a female predisposition (71% of cats) and a mean age of 7.1 years +/−3 years. A majority of cats (32/35 in one report) have clinical signs of heart failure.

PHYSICAL EXAMINATION

- Auscultation abnormalities are invariably present and less common than those in cats with HCM; 36% of cats with RCM had a murmur, 23% of cats had a gallop, and 14% of cats had an arrhythmia in one report. Please refer to the previous general section of cardiomyopathies for a complete discussion of physical examination abnormalities.

ECHOCARDIOGRAM

- Left atrial or biatrial dilation in the face of normal left ventricular size, normal systolic function, and minimal left ventricular hypertrophy are hallmark echocardiographic findings. Intracardiac thrombi or spontaneous echocardiographic contrast are common (reported in 23% of cases). In cats with endomyocardial fibrosis, the endocardium is hyperechoic, thickened, and there is often a fibrotic band bridging from the papillary muscles/free wall to the interventricular septum. This fibrotic band often distorts the papillary muscle shape and involves the mitral valve apparatus to create both mitral regurgitation and intraventricular systolic obstruction of blood flow out the LV (Figure 9.6).

- A restrictive filling pattern is the characteristic functional abnormality seen in patients with RCM and occurs when there is severe diastolic impairment leading to markedly elevated left atrial pressure and a high left atrial to left ventricular diastolic pressure gradient. It is characterized by an increased early diastolic filling velocity (>1 m/sec), a decreased atrial filling velocity (<0.4 m/sec), an increased E/A ratio (>2), a shortened deceleration time (normal is 59 +/− 14 m/sec), and decreased isovolumic relaxation time (normal is 55 +/− 13 m/sec).

ANCILLARY TESTS

- As with other forms of myocardial disease, ancillary tests rarely help discriminate the diagnosis from other cardiomyopathies.

- Arrhythmias appear to be common in cats with RCM and may include supraventricular tachycardia (reported in 8/35 cats), VPCs or ventricular tachycardia (10/35 cats), or atrial fibrillation (1/35 cats).

- There is often dramatic atrial dilation seen on thoracic radiographs. Radiographic evidence of heart failure is common (32/35 cats) and may include cardiogenic pulmonary edema and pulmonary venous distension (13/35 cats), signs of right heart failure (pleural effusion, dilated caudal vena cava, hepatomegaly, +/- ascites in 6/35 cats), or biventricular failure (13/35 cats).

THERAPY

- For acute CHF see the earlier section on treatment of CHF in the discussion of therapy in the general information section.

- No specific therapy for controlling the fibrous tissue reaction is available.

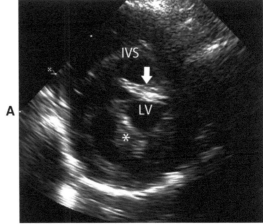

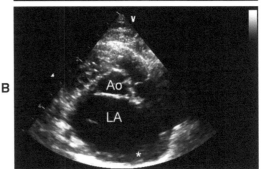

Figure 9.6 Echocardiogram of a cat with severe endomyocardial fibrosis and restrictive cardiomyopathy (RCM). **A,** This two-dimensional echocardiogram of the left ventricle (*LV*) at the level of the papillary muscles shows a large fibrotic bridging band (*arrow*) tethering the anterior left ventricular free wall and papillary (*) to the interventricular septum (*IVS*). **B,** There is severe left atrial dilation, which is assessed by measurement of the aortic and left atrial diameters on the first frame of aortic valve closure in the right parasternal cross-sectional view with two-dimensional echocardiography and with calculation of the left atrial to aortic ratio, which in this cat is severely increased at 2.74 (≤1.5 normal). Spontaneous echocardiographic contrast (*) is also seen within the left atrium. *Ao,* Aorta; *LA,* left atrium.

- Beta blockers or calcium channel blockers are not effective for improving diastolic function caused by fibrosis but may be of benefit to control persistent significant tachycardia if present Likewise, antiarrhythmic medications are indicated for treatment of ventricular or supraventricular tachyarrhythmias.

- Anticoagulant therapy is recommended in cats with moderate to severe atrial dilation, intracardiac thrombus, or spontaneous echocardiographic contrast. Cats with RCM have a high risk of ATE (45% incidence in one study), likely because they are often diagnosed at an end stage where there is severe atrial dilation.

- Pimobendan may be considered in cats with RCM and CHF because it may decrease preload and has positive lusitropic effects (improves relaxation). However, overall diastolic function is unlikely to be improved because the main problem is increased ventricular stiffness from fibrosis.

PROGNOSIS

- Prognosis is typically poor because most cats are diagnosed at an end stage when there are signs of heart failure or ATE. In a report of 35 cats, MST was 3.4 months (0.1 to 52 months). Heart failure (18/35 cats), +/– ATE (5/18 cats), and sudden cardiac death (3/35 cats) are the most common causes of death.

PATHOLOGY

- Endocardial, subendocardial, and/or myocardial fibrosis are hallmark lesions of RCM (Figure 9.7). Diffuse interstitial fibrosis is commonly present within the myocardium, and some cats have larger patchy regions of replacement fibrosis. In addition, many cats have evidence of myocyte disarray, which is also seen in cats with HCM. Endocardial fibrosis may cause fibrous adhesions between papillary muscles and the myocardium, with distortion and fusion of the chordae tendineae and mitral valve leaflets. Extreme LA and left auricular enlargements are common, and right atrial dilation may also be present.

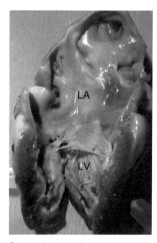

Figure 9.7 Gross disease of a cat with severe endomyocardial fibrosis and restrictive cardiomyopathy (RCM). Gross pathologic examination of a heart with severe endomyocardial fibrosis of the left ventricle (*LV*). There is diffuse, thick endocardial and subendocardial fibrosis of the LV, causing severely increased left ventricular diastolic filling pressures and leading to severe left atrial dilation and heart failure. *LA*, Left atrium.

UNCLASSIFIED FELINE CARDIOMYOPATHIES

UCM is a nebulous category including cats with significant left atrial or biatrial dilation despite normal to near-normal systolic function and normal to near-normal LV wall thickness in the absence of severe AV valvular dilation. This description is very similar to RCM, and many consider combining categories to UCM/RCM unless there is obvious endomyocardial fibrosis or a restrictive filling pattern on mitral inflow measured by PW Doppler interrogation. A restrictive filling pattern may be impossible to detect in cats with tachycardia and fusion of the early and late diastolic filling waves on PW Doppler interrogation of mitral inflow. Therefore many clinicians use the term *UCM* to include cats with atrial or biatrial enlargement with normal LV size and function. There is a lack of specific criteria for diagnosis of UCM.

GENERAL COMMENTS

- In recent years, increasing numbers of cats have been recognized with obviously abnormal hearts, many having heart failure, but not fitting into any recognized disease classification such as HCM or DCM. There is a lack of specific criteria for diagnosis of UCM. It is likely the abnormalities are acquired, but the etiology remains unknown.
- Although no controlled studies have been performed, taurine deficiency or metabolic abnormalities (e.g., hyperthyroidism) have not been consistent findings in affected cats.

PATHOPHYSIOLOGY

- The pathophysiologic condition is unknown; however, clinical observations suggest diastolic dysfunction similar to that described for RCM is the predominant functional abnormality in these cats. Atrial myopathy is another hypothesis for the atrial dilation, but this has not been confirmed.

SIGNALMENT AND PRESENTING COMPLAINTS

- There is no sex or breed predisposition for UCM, and mean age in a case series of 11 cats was 8.8 +/– 4.8 years.
- Similar to RCM, many cats have clinical signs of dyspnea (64%), tachypnea, and nonspecific signs of lethargy (27%), anorexia, or weight loss.

PHYSICAL EXAMINATION

- A murmur is variably present in cats (50% in one case series). An arrhythmia is less common (18% in one case series), and a gallop heart sound may also be present. Physical examination is similar to that of other forms of myocardial disease.

ECHOCARDIOGRAM

By nature of the definition, the echocardiographic findings are extremely variable. Left atrial or biatrial dilation is the hallmark abnormality seen on echocardiogram in the face of a relatively normal LV (i.e., normal chamber size, no significant left ventricular concentric hypertrophy, and normal to nearly normal systolic function) (Figures 9.8 and 9.9). There may be mild systolic dysfunction with mildly increased end-systolic left ventricular internal diameter and mildly decreased FS. Various patterns of mild regional myocardial hypertrophy may be observed in the septum or LV free wall of some cats. Enlargement of the right heart is variable but may be marked in some cases. Mild AV valvular insufficiency is often present on color flow Doppler imaging. Diastolic dysfunction may be evident on tissue Doppler imaging or PW Doppler interrogation of mitral inflow. Atrial thrombus or spontaneous contrast may be seen in cats with atrial dilation.

ANCILLARY TESTS

- Thoracic radiographs often reveal severe cardiomegaly and atrial dilation. Pleural effusion is also common (50% of cats in a case series of 22 cases), and pulmonary edema was reported less frequently (9% of cases).
- An electrocardiogram may show arrhythmias such as VPCs (50% of cases), supraventricular tachycardia, atrial premature complexes, or atrial standstill (18% of cases). Atrial standstill is rare in cats and may be the cause of the atrial dilation and atrial myopathy in some cats with UCM.

THERAPY

- For acute CHF, see the earlier section on treatment of CHF in the discussion of therapy in the general information section. For cats with chronic CHF, furosemide and ACE inhibitors are recommended (see previous section).
- Treatment is essentially the same as outlined in the previous RCM section.
- Anticoagulant therapy is often recommended because atrial dilation is present in cats with UCM.

PROGNOSIS

- The prognosis is generally based on clinical presentation, echocardiographic and radiographic evidence of elevated diastolic pressures, and response to therapy.
- Symptom-free cats with mild LA enlargement are thought to have a good long-term prognosis. Symptom-free cats with marked LA enlargement are likely to be at higher risk for developing heart failure.
- In general, cats that have heart failure have a poor prognosis. However, cats that have heart failure and respond favorably to therapy may do well for prolonged periods of time.

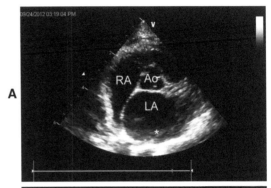

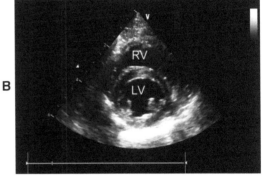

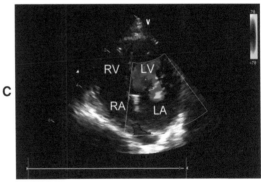

Figure 9.8 Echocardiogram of a cat with severe unclassified cardiomyopathy (UCM) and severe left atrial dilation. **A,** This cat with severe UCM has severe left atrial dilation, evidenced by a marked increase in left atrial diameter to aortic diameter ratio of 2.47 (≤1.5 normal) measured in the right parasternal cross-sectional view with two-dimensional echocardiography. There is also spontaneous echocardiographic contrast (*) in the left atrium. **B,** The left and right ventricles appear normal, with normal left ventricular wall thickness and normal systolic function. **C,** Color flow Doppler imaging of the mitral valve from the left apical four-chamber view depicts mild centrally arising mitral regurgitation and severe left atrial dilation. *Ao,* Aorta; *LA,* left atrium; *LV,* left ventricle; *RA,* right atrium; *RV,* right ventricle.

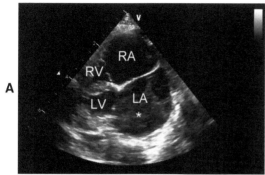
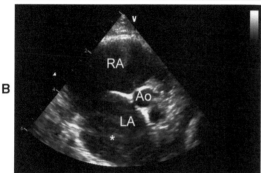

Figure 9.9 Echocardiogram of a cat with severe unclassified cardiomyopathy (UCM) and biatrial dilation. UCM may cause biatrial dilation, which is seen in this right parasternal four-chamber view (**A**) and in the right parasternal cross-sectional view (**B**). There is spontaneous echocardiographic contrast (*) within the left atrium. With the right parasternal cross-sectional view, the left atrial diameter to aortic diameter ratio is severely increased at 3.42 (≤1.5 normal), indicating severe left atrial dilation, and the right atrium (*RA*) is subjectively assessed and is severely dilated. *Ao,* Aorta; *LA,* left atrium; *LV,* Left ventricle; *RV,* right ventricle.

- Cats with ATE have a poor prognosis. Cats that survive the thromboembolic episode may do well for extended periods; however, these cats are generally at high risk for recurrence of ATE.

ARRHYTHMOGENIC RIGHT VENTRICULAR CARDIOMYOPATHY

ARVC is a rare myocardial disease in cats (diagnosed in 2 of 287 cats with cardiomyopathy) and is more commonly seen in humans and Boxer dogs. ARVC is characterized by fatty or fibrofatty replacement of cardiomyocytes in the right ventricle and right atrium, sometimes extending in a milder degree to the left ventricular myocardium. No familial pattern has been reported in cats, and etiology remains unknown in cats.

GENERAL COMMENTS

Little is known about ARVC in cats, and there is only one case series of 12 cats diagnosed with

ARVC in the medical literature. Unlike other cardiomyopathies, the predominant feature of ARVC is right heart enlargement, with left atrial dilation also possible in some cats. ARVC causes signs of right heart failure, including pleural effusion, jugular venous distension, ascites, and hepatomegaly.

PATHOPHYSIOLOGY

Fatty or fibrofatty replacement of cardiomyocytes in the right atrial and ventricular myocardium causes systolic myocardial failure, chamber dilation, and elevated right heart filling pressures. Once right ventricular diastolic pressure exceeds approximately 15 mm Hg, right-sided heart failure develops, including pleural effusion and ascites. The fatty replacement of the cardiomyocytes also leads to malignant ventricular and sometimes supraventricular tachyarrhythmias, which may cause sudden cardiac death. The same disease may also occur in the left atrial myocardium and cause left atrial dilation.

SIGNALMENT AND PRESENTING COMPLAINTS

- There is no breed or sex predilection for ARVC in cats, and a mean age of diagnosis was 7.3 +/– 5.2 years in one case series of 11 cats with ARVC.
- Presenting complaints are often referable to heart failure and include dyspnea, tachypnea, abdominal distension, lethargy, anorexia, or weight loss.

PHYSICAL EXAMINATION

- A majority of cats have clinical evidence of right-sided heart failure (67% of cats in a case series). A right parasternal holosystolic murmur is commonly present (67% of cats) and is caused by functional tricuspid regurgitation.

ECHOCARDIOGRAM

- Severe right atrial dilation and right ventricular eccentric hypertrophy (increased end-diastolic diameter of the right ventricle) are the classic echocardiographic abnormalities (Figure 9.10). Sometimes ventricular aneurysms may be identified. Mild to moderate centrally arising tricuspid regurgitation is often present, secondary to right ventricular and atrial dilation and functional tricuspid regurgitation. Varying degrees of left atrial dilation may be present. Pleural effusion, hepatic venous distension, and possibly ascites are common in cats with severe ARVC and right-sided heart failure. Mild pericardial effusion also may be present secondary to right-sided heart failure. Intraatrial thrombus or spontaneous echocardiographic contrast is also commonly seen.

- The main differential diagnosis for ARVC is tricuspid valve (TV) dysplasia. Therefore careful evaluation of the TV for malformations seen in TV dysplasia is needed because TV dysplasia confers a better prognosis than ARVC.

ANCILLARY TESTS

- Thoracic radiographs typically show severe right-sided heart enlargement and evidence of right-sided heart failure, including pleural effusion (67% of cats), ascites (33% of cats), and +/– dilated caudal vena cava (17% of cats).
- Arrhythmias are very common in cats with ARVC, which may include VPCs (75% of cats in a case series), ventricular tachycardia (38% of cats), or atrial fibrillation (50% of cats).

THERAPY

Therapy is identical to cats with DCM; please refer to that section.

PROGNOSIS

Prognosis for cats with ARVC is grave. In a case series of 12 cats with ARVC, 75% of cats died or were euthanized because of profound right-sided heart failure or ATE, with an MST of 1 month.

SECONDARY CARDIOMYOPATHIES

THYROTOXIC HEART DISEASE

Thyrotoxic heart disease is a secondary cardiomyopathy caused by direct and indirect effects of high-circulating thyroid hormone on the cardiovascular system. In the current era of earlier detection of hyperthyroidism, most cardiac changes seen on echocardiography (i.e., thick left ventricular and septal walls) are mild and are reported in 37% of hyperthyroid cats.

GENERAL COMMENTS

- Thyrotoxic heart disease is a frequently recognized secondary cardiomyopathy that may be confused with HCM, a primary myocardial disease.
- Thyrotoxic heart disease or hyperthyroidism does not cause HCM.
- The prevalence and severity of thyrotoxic heart disease has been decreasing in recent years, likely as a result of increased awareness and, as a consequence, early diagnosis and treatment of hyperthyroidism.
- Isolated hyperthyroidism rarely causes CHF in current times, but cats may also be affected with a concurrent (additional) cardiomyopathy that has been exacerbated by hyperthyroidism.

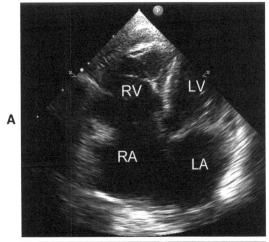
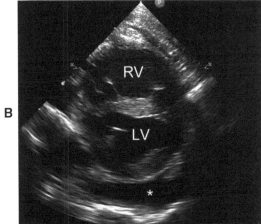
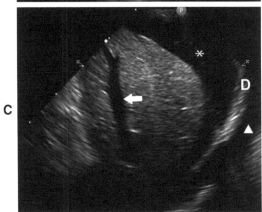

Figure 9.10 Echocardiogram of a cat with severe arrhythmogenic right ventricular cardiomyopathy (ARVC) and right-sided heart failure. Two-dimensional echocardiograms from the left apical four-chamber view (**A**) and right parasternal cross-sectional view at the level of the papillary muscles (**B**) show severe right ventricular eccentric hypertrophy secondary to the severe right ventricular myocardial failure, severe right atrial dilation, and pleural effusion (*). **C,** Right-sided heart failure is present, including hepatomegaly, hepatic venous distension (*arrow*), ascites (*), and pleural effusion (*triangle*). *D,* Diaphragm; *LA,* left atrium; *LV,* left ventricle; *RA,* right atrium; *RV,* right ventricle.

PATHOPHYSIOLOGY

- The effects of thyroid hormone on the heart are thought to be both direct and indirect.
- The sum effect of excess thyroid hormone (hyperthyroidism) is a heart that operates at a faster rate (tachycardia), is hypertrophied, can contract faster and more powerfully (enhanced contractility), and has a propensity to abnormal electrical depolarizations (arrhythmias).
- Although these might at first glance sound like beneficial changes (bigger, faster, stronger, more excitable), the thyrotoxic state greatly strains the energy economy of the heart and increases the overall work of the heart. In addition, the thyrotoxic heart, although hyperkinetic when the patient is at rest, has less "reserve capacity" available for when increased cardiac work is necessary (e.g., exercise). This situation placed on top of preexisting cardiac disease (e.g., HCM, RCM, DCM, valvular disease) can lead to decompensation of a previously well-compensated cardiac disease.
- Reduced systemic vascular resistance in the presence of an increased intravascular volume (not documented in cats) associated with significant increases in cardiac output are what define the high-output state of the cardiovascular system in hyperthyroid cats. This high-output state can (especially in the presence of underlying primary cardiac disease) progress, resulting in clinically apparent signs of CHF in hyperthyroid cats.

SIGNALMENT AND PRESENT COMPLAINTS

- There is no sex or breed predisposition. Affected cats are typically adult to geriatric, with a mean age reported as 13 years (range: 4 to 22 years).
- Most cats are seen for routine examination or because of signs referable to increased metabolic activity, such as polyphagia, polyuria/polydipsia, or weight loss.
- On rare occasions, cats may have CHF or low-output heart failure.
- Cats with acute exacerbation of thyrotoxicosis, (thyroid storm) may have collapse, weakness, dyspnea, or sudden death.

PHYSICAL EXAMINATION

- Classic signs of hyperthyroidism include evidence of weight loss and unkempt hair coat.
- Systolic heart murmur (53% to 54%) or gallop heart sound may be present.
- Sinus tachycardia is often present.
- A thyroid nodule is usually palpable (83% to 90% of cases), typically bilateral (2/3 of cases).
- Normal to increased femoral pulse strength and increased strength of apical cardiac beat (precordial impulse) are also commonly identified.

ANCILLARY TESTS

- Electrocardiography
  - Sinus tachycardia is commonly present.
  - There are tall R waves, which are suggestive of left ventricular hypertrophy or dilation.
  - Variable arrhythmias, including atrial premature complexes and VPCs, are present.
  - Uncommonly, intraventricular conduction disturbances are seen.
- Thoracic radiography: common findings include the following:
  - Generalized cardiomegaly may be present, with or without LA enlargement.
  - When CHF is present, pulmonary edema and pleural effusion are equally likely to be present.
- Echocardiography
  - Reported echocardiographic changes in cats with hyperthyroidism include increased aortic root dimension, LA enlargement, increased end-diastolic or end-systolic left ventricular dimensions, mild to moderate concentric hypertrophy of the LV free wall or septum, and an increased (or, rarely, decreased) left ventricular shortening fraction. Typical echocardiographic changes in current times include mild left ventricular concentric hypertrophy. SAM of the mitral valve, if seen, may suggest that there is also unrelated primary HCM because it is rarely due to thyrotoxic heart disease alone.
  - There are reports of cats with myocardial failure demonstrating marked increases in left ventricular end-diastolic and end-systolic dimensions, moderate to severe LA enlargement, and a reduction in shortening fraction. The relationship of this presentation to a deficiency of the amino acid taurine is unknown, but it may also represent late irreversible changes associated with hyperthyroidism.

THERAPY

- For acute CHF, see the section on treatment of CHF in the discussion of therapy in the general information section.
- Signs of CHF may be difficult to control before beginning to control the hyperthyroid state. Begin with pharmacologic manipulations, including methimazole, furosemide, and an ACE inhibitor in cats with CHF. Untreated cats should not be anesthetized or isolated for iodine-131 until their acute hyperthyroid state has been attenuated with medical therapy.
- In cats with asymptomatic thyrotoxicosis, therapy is aimed at controlling the hyperthyroid

state (i.e., methimazole or radioactive iodine therapy). Typically ^{131}I therapy is delayed until the renal function is assessed during euthyroid state achieved by methimazole.

- Beta-adrenergic blockade is a common recommendation in the literature. There is no contraindication to its use, but benefits have not been documented in most cases. In fact, in hypertensive hyperthyroid cats, beta blockers effectively controlled tachycardia but were ineffective at controlling hypertension in 70% of cats.
- Beta-adrenergic blockade may be considered in the following situations:
  - For the management of significant supraventricular or ventricular tachyarrhythmias.
  - In hyperthyroid cats undergoing anesthetic procedures.
  - In the treatment of suspected concurrent severe HCM. However, the addition of atenolol is often postponed until a recheck echocardiogram is done several months after the euthyroid state to assess for potential improvement in the echocardiographic abnormalities, before adding atenolol.
- Antihypertensive treatment with amlodipine (0.625 to 1.25 mg per cat q24h to BID, uptitrating based on follow-up BP measurements) is needed in cats showing target organ damage resulting from hypertension, in cats with persistent systolic arterial blood pressure >180 mm Hg posthyperthyroid treatment, or in cats with new onset of hypertension after a euthyroid state is achieved.

PROGNOSIS

- Symptom-free cats can be managed very well without the use of specific cardiovascular therapy before appropriate therapy for the hyperthyroid state, and most evidence indicates that the cardiovascular changes are reversible.
- Many cats with CHF can be managed successfully if the hyperthyroid state is controlled, unless there is concurrent severe and unrelated primary cardiac disease.
- Most cats with severe systolic myocardial failure have a poor prognosis because the changes appear to be irreversible, unless influenced by taurine deficiency.

ACROMEGALIC HEART DISEASE

Acromegalic heart disease is a secondary cardiomyopathy caused by direct and indirect effects of increased circulating growth hormone (hypersomatotropism).

GENERAL COMMENTS

- Acromegaly is a rare disorder in cats, with between 100 to 200 cases reported worldwide to date.

- It is caused by a growth hormone–secreting tumor of the pituitary gland.
- Clinical suspicion of acromegaly is increased in cats with severe insulin-resistant diabetes mellitus.
- In a case series of 14 cats, all had insulin-resistant diabetes mellitus and enlargement of the liver, heart, kidneys, or tongue. Various cardiovascular abnormalities were seen in most of the affected cats.

PATHOPHYSIOLOGY

- The pathogenesis of heart disease in cats with acromegaly is unclear. Growth hormone causes anabolic effects of increased myocardial hypertrophy, abdominal organomegaly (liver, kidneys), excess growth of pharyngeal tissues that results in stertor, enlarged tongue, and broadening and flattening of the forehead. Growth hormone also antagonizes the effects of insulin and causes insulin-resistant diabetes mellitus.

SIGNALMENT AND PRESENTING COMPLAINTS

- Presenting complaints commonly include polyuria/polydipsia, polyphagia, and weight loss referable to uncontrolled diabetes.
- Although no breed predilections have been identified, almost all of the reported cases have occurred in older neutered male cats.

PHYSICAL EXAMINATION

- Systolic murmurs were noted in 9 (64%) of the 14 cats described.
- Physical features of acromegaly include prognathia inferior, cranial and abdominal enlargement, organomegaly (especially kidneys and liver), increased body size, and weight gain.
- Signs of CHF may develop late in the course of the disease and have been reported in 6 (43%) of 14 cats with acromegaly, including pulmonary edema (5/6), ascites (2/6), and pleural effusion (1/6).
- Central nervous system signs (i.e., circling and seizures) caused by enlargement of the pituitary tumor may be seen (2/14 cats in one report).

ANCILLARY TESTS

- Electrocardiography: abnormalities were not detected in any of the 14 cats reported.
- Thoracic radiography: mild to moderate cardiomegaly was identified in 12 of 14 (86%) cats.
- Echocardiography: septal and left ventricular wall concentric hypertrophy, resembling HCM, was identified in seven of eight cats examined.

- Diagnosis of acromegaly
  - A tentative diagnosis is made based on the presence of severe insulin-resistant diabetes mellitus or renal failure in a cat with clinical features of acromegaly.
  - Documentation of a pituitary mass on computed tomographic scan or magnetic resonance imaging provides further support.
  - The diagnosis of acromegaly is confirmed by demonstration of extremely high basal serum growth hormone concentrations (22 to 131 μg/L reported in all 14 cats in one study).

THERAPY

- In general, therapy is aimed at controlling the diabetic state and renal failure. If CHF is present, supportive care (diuretics and ACE inhibitors) may also be beneficial.
- Successful therapy for feline acromegaly has not been reported. Potential therapeutic modalities include radiation therapy, medical therapy with somatostatin analog octreotide, or hypophysectomy.
- Supportive therapy for CHF should be used in those cats with consistent clinical findings. (See the section on treatment of CHF in the discussion about therapy in the general information section.) Of the six reported cases of CHF, four of these cats died, three of which had concurrent renal failure.

PROGNOSIS

- The short-term prognosis is good. Pituitary tumors grow slowly, and neurologic signs are uncommon. Diabetes can be relatively well controlled with high doses of insulin.
- Mild to moderate CHF responds fairly well to symptomatic therapy.
- Most cats eventually died or were euthanized owing to refractory CHF or renal failure. Reported survival ranged from 4 to 24 months after diagnosis.

NEOPLASTIC INFILTRATION OF THE HEART

GENERAL COMMENTS AND HISTORICAL PERSPECTIVE

- Neoplastic infiltration of the heart is rare in cats.
- Echocardiography is generally required for nonsurgical detection.
- Cardiac tumors reported in cats include the following:
  - Lymphoma
  - Chemodectoma
  - Hemangiosarcoma
  - Metastatic pulmonary carcinoma
  - Metastatic mammary gland carcinoma

- Lymphoma is the most common tumor of the feline myocardium. Reported cardiac abnormalities in cats with lymphoma include complete heart block, pericardial effusion, and CHF.
- Echocardiographic findings in cats with diffuse neoplastic infiltration of the myocardium can mimic those of HCM, although often the myocardium is irregular and has abnormal echogenicity compared with normal adjacent regions of the myocardium.
- Regression of neoplastic infiltration was reported in one cat with lymphoma after treatment with combination chemotherapy.

DRUGS, TOXINS, AND PHYSICAL INJURY

- A large number of drugs and toxins are reported to cause myocardial injury in domestic animals, but very few are likely to be encountered in a clinical small animal practice. Of these, doxorubicin has received the most attention in cats.
- Decreased FS and increased left ventricular end-systolic dimensions were reported in four of six experimental cats given cumulative doses of doxorubicin of 170 to 240 mg/m². However, clinical signs of heart failure were not observed even after a cumulative dose of 300 mg/m², and no cat showed ECG abnormalities during the study. As in other species, pathologic studies revealed extensive areas of myocyte vacuolization and myocytolysis. Similar clinical observations have been reported in cats with malignancies treated with doxorubicin. None had overt heart failure, and arrhythmias were only rarely observed.

INFECTIOUS MYOCARDITIS

- Infectious myocarditis is a rare myocardial disease in cats and is characterized by the presence of myocardial necrosis +/− degeneration and inflammation. Liu and associates described a syndrome of acute nonsuppurative myocarditis in 25 young cats (mean age, 2.6 years). Most cats died unexpectedly, and necropsy revealed focal or diffuse infiltration of the endocardium and myocardium with mononuclear cells and a few neutrophils. A viral cause was suspected but never identified.
- One report describes a transmissible myocarditis/diaphragmitis in cats. No organism has been isolated, but transmission between cats by injecting blood from infected cats into other cats does reliably reproduce the disease. All cats had high fever (103.8° to 105.7° F), were lethargic, and were partially anorexic. Complete blood counts and chemistries were normal in all cats for 6 weeks, except for an elevation of creatine phosphokinase in three of seven cats.

The disease resolved on its own in these cats. Necropsy revealed pale 1- to 3-mm discrete foci surrounded by hemorrhage on ventricular myocardium and on the diaphragm. No clinical signs referable to the cardiovascular system were noticed.

- The relationship of endomyocarditis to the other cardiomyopathies of cats is unknown. Other reported causes of myocarditis in cats include toxoplasmosis, *Streptococcus canis* myocarditis, lymphoplasmacytic myocarditis secondary to *Bartonella* infection, and metastatic infection from sepsis or bacterial endocarditis.
- Echocardiographic abnormalities seen in infectious myocarditis may include hyperechoic, hypertrophied regions of the ventricular myocardium, a nodular or granular appearance of the myocardium, ventricular and atrial dilation, myocardial failure, or pericardial effusion.

SUMMARY

- HCM is very common in cats and represents the largest percentage of cardiac diseases currently diagnosed in the cat.
- Unclassified and RCMs are the next most common feline myocardial diseases and are often combined into one group because of difficulty in differentiation of the two cardiomyopathies in many cats. Treatment is likely the same for UCM and RCM.
- DCM is infrequently diagnosed, and most cases are idiopathic. Taurine deficiency–induced myocardial failure mimics DCM and must be tested for by measurement of blood taurine concentration because it is a curative disorder.
- Treatment of CHF is essentially the same for all forms of cardiomyopathy and includes furosemide, an ACE inhibitor, and often an anticoagulant for prophylaxis of ATE. Additional disease-specific therapies are prescribed on the basis of the underlying cardiac disease or contributing factors.
- Of the secondary cardiomyopathies discussed, only nutritional (taurine responsive) myocardial failure and thyrotoxic heart disease are encountered with any frequency. Both of these disorders have been well classified, and both respond dramatically to appropriate specific therapy. The other secondary cardiomyopathies occur infrequently and are generally poorly understood. The general approach, diagnosis, and therapy for these disorders are similar to those for other feline cardiomyopathies.
- One must recognize that the associated clinical and diagnostic findings frequently overlap, often making a definitive diagnosis difficult. Echocardiography is the one diagnostic aid that reliably allows differentiation among the different cardiomyopathies encountered in cats; however, even with a thorough ultrasound examination, distinctions may often still be unclear.

FREQUENTLY ASKED QUESTIONS

A murmur has been recently incidentally auscultated in an overtly healthy cat. What are appropriate recommendations to the owner?

Murmurs are commonly auscultated in cats and may be caused by either pathologic abnormalities, such as underlying cardiomyopathy, or may be benign. It is impossible to distinguish the cause of the murmur by auscultation alone. Presence of a gallop heart sound or an arrhythmia further increases suspicion of underlying cardiac disease and strengthens the need for an echocardiogram. HCM is a common cause of murmurs in symptom-free cats, with prevalence rates of 18% to 62% (depending on criteria used for diagnosis of HCM) in overtly healthy cats with murmurs. An echocardiogram is recommended to evaluate the cause of a murmur in cats because some symptom-free cats have severe underlying cardiac disease warranting treatment. If an echocardiogram is not possible, the NT-ProBNP biomarker blood test is a test to assess the likelihood of underlying cardiomyopathy.

Do cats with suspected heart failure require an echocardiogram before medical therapy is started?

Furosemide and usually an ACE inhibitor are standard medical therapy for cats with CHF. If CHF is likely according to clinical signs, auscultation abnormalities, and thoracic radiographs, furosemide and an ACE inhibitor may be started without having a confirmatory echocardiogram. Ideally, an echocardiogram would be performed in the near future to refine the diagnosis and help aid in treatment decisions for additional diagnostic therapy.

Should I empirically treat a cat with a newly diagnosed murmur with cardiac medications if the owner declines further diagnostic testing?

No, because the cause of the murmur is not known, empiric treatment with cardiac medications is not justified in cats with murmurs incidentally diagnosed. Murmurs may be benign or caused by underlying heart disease of many causes. Not all cats with heart disease require medications; therefore empiric treatment of a cat with a murmur is not recommended. However, if the cat shows signs of CHF such as dyspnea, tachypnea, lethargy, anorexia, and weight loss, thoracic radiographs would be necessary to evaluate for presence of pulmonary edema or pleural effusion and, if present, should be treated with furosemide and likely an ACE inhibitor.

What type of anesthetic protocol modifications are needed in cats with heart disease?

Cats with cardiomyopathy may be at risk for fluid overload, so the fluid rate is often decreased to a lower rate of 5 to 6 mL/kg/hr. Anticholinergic medications should not be empirically given but may be administered if there is bradycardia. ACE inhibitors should not be given for 12 to 24 hours before anesthesia is administered because they may contribute to refractory hypotension while the patient is under anesthesia. Atenolol may be continued the morning of the procedure in patients chronically medicated with it. Typical acceptable protocols include premedication with an opioid and induction with propofol and benzodiazepine or midazolam. There are various risk categories for anesthesia depending on the underlying cardiac disease, severity of disease, and the presence of heart failure or significant arrhythmias. Protocol adjustments are often based on the underlying cardiomyopathy and severity.

SUGGESTED READINGS

Atkins CE, Gallo AM, Kurzman ID, Cowen P: Risk factors, clinical signs, and survival in cats with a clinical diagnosis of idiopathic hypertrophic cardiomyopathy: 74 cases (1985-1989), J Am Vet Med Assoc 201:613–618, 1992.
Cote E, MacDonald KA, Meurs KM, Sleeper MM: Feline cardiology, Iowa, Ames, 2011, Wiley Blackwell.
Ferasin L, Sturgess CP, Cannon MJ, Caney SM: Feline idiopathic cardiomyopathy: a retrospective study of 106 cats (1994-2001), J Feline Med Surg 5:151–159, 2003.
Fox PR, Basso C, Thiene G, Maron BJ: Spontaneously occurring restrictive nonhypertrophied cardiomyopathy in domestic cats: a new animal model of human disease, Cardiovasc Pathol 23:28–34, 2014.
Liu SK, Tilley LP: Animal models of primary myocardial disease, Yale J Biol Med 53:191, 1980.
MacDonald KA: Feline myocardial diseases, In Ettinger SJ, Feldman ED, eds: Textbook of veterinary internal medicine, ed 7, Philadelphia, 2010, WB Saunders, pp 1328–1341.
Maron BJ, Towbin JA, Thiene G, et al: Contemporary definitions and classification of the cardiomyopathies: an American Heart Association Scientific Statement from the Council on Clinical Cardiology, Heart Failure and Transplantation Committee; Quality of Care and Outcomes Research and Functional Genomics and Translational Biology Interdisciplinary Working Groups; and Council on Epidemiology and Prevention, Circulation 113:1807–1816, 2006.
Paige CF, Abbott JA, Elvinger F, Pyle RL: Prevalence of cardiomyopathy in apparently healthy cats, J Am Vet Med Assoc 234:1398–1403, 2009.
Pion PD, Kittleson MD, Rogers QR, Morris JG: Myocardial failure in cats associated with low plasma taurine: a reversible cardiomyopathy, Science 237:764–768, 1987.
Riesen SC, Kovacevic A, Lombard CW, Amberger C: Prevalence of heart disease in symptomatic cats: an overview from 1998 to 2005, Schweiz Arch Tierheilkd 149:65–71, 2007.
Rush JE, Freeman LM, Fenollosa NK, Brown DJ: Population and survival characteristics of cats with hypertrophic cardiomyopathy: 260 cases (1990-1999), J Am Vet Med Assoc 220:202–207, 2002.

Cor Pulmonale and Pulmonary Thromboembolism

10

Lynelle R. Johnson

Cor pulmonale is defined as right-sided heart failure caused by pulmonary or thoracic disease. It is characterized by clinical signs related to fluid accumulation, or by radiographic or echocardiographic evidence of right ventricular overload. By definition, pulmonary hypertension (PH) must be present in cor pulmonale in order for the right heart to fail. Heartworm disease with pulmonary vascular obstruction is the most common cause of cor pulmonale in dogs, although any cause of PH, including pulmonary arterial obstruction, pulmonary venous hypertension from cardiac disease, or pulmonary arterial hypertension associated with vascular remodeling from global hypoxic vasoconstriction, can result in cor pulmonale.

Pulmonary embolism can lead to acute or chronic PH. Pulmonary arterial obstruction can result from lodging of clot material (pulmonary thromboembolism [PTE]) or from embolization of fat, septic material, neoplastic cells, or heartworms in the pulmonary arteries or capillary bed. PTE is a complication of many commonly encountered diseases and is associated with a grave prognosis.

COR PULMONALE AND PULMONARY THROMBOEMBOLISM

PHYSIOLOGY

- Pulmonary circulatory pressures are maintained at a level much lower than systemic pressures to reduce the workload on the thin-walled right ventricle. Normal pressures in dogs and cats are reported as a systolic pulmonary artery pressure of 15 to 25 mm Hg, end-diastolic pulmonary artery pressure of 5 to 10 mm Hg, and a mean pulmonary artery pressure of 10 to 15 mm Hg. The pulmonary circulation maintains a low right ventricular pressure in the face of increases in cardiac output through recruitment of closed capillaries and distension of existing capillaries.

- Distribution of pulmonary blood flow is controlled by hypoxic pulmonary vasoconstriction and is also modulated by endothelial release of vasoconstrictors and vasodilators. Hypoxic pulmonary vasoconstriction is a protective mechanism that prevents deoxygenated blood from entering the circulation by preferentially constricting vascular supply to poorly ventilated lung regions. Thus, regional alveolar hypoxia results in local vascular constriction that preserves gas exchange. However, global hypoxia or diseases that disrupt the normal vascular response to hypoxia can result in a deleterious rise in pulmonary artery pressure. Alterations in endothelium-derived mediators can also impact pulmonary artery pressures. The most potent vasoconstrictor is endothelin-1; thromboxane A2 and superoxide also mediate vasoconstriction. Vasodilators produced by the endothelium include nitric oxide and prostacyclin. Altered release and activity of these vasoreactive mediators in disease or imbalance in concentrations of the various mediators can result in a rise in pulmonary artery pressure.

- PTE results in abnormal gas exchange, altered vascular reactivity, changes in pulmonary mechanics, and loss of ventilatory control. Physical obstruction of large pulmonary arteries leads to increased vascular pressure and reactive pulmonary vasoconstriction caused by release of clot-associated factors such as thromboxane that increase vascular resistance. Secondary alterations in pulmonary physiology worsen and perpetuate derangements in gas exchange. Release of humoral mediators such as serotonin from platelets results in bronchoconstriction and increased airway resistance. Surfactant function is altered by embolization, resulting in loss of elastic recoil and atelectasis, decreased pulmonary compliance, and a progressive increase in right-to-left shunting. These factors, along with an expansion of alveolar dead space from an increase in nonperfused lung regions, lead to an increase in the work of breathing. Altered central control of ventilation contributes to relentless tachypnea.

ETIOLOGY

- Cor pulmonale can result from disorders that affect the pulmonary vasculature, such as obstructive or obliterative diseases of the pulmonary circulation, or from sustained hypoxic vasoconstriction associated with chronic parenchymal or tracheobronchial disease. Rarely, an increase in pulmonary blood flow will result in PH. Not all animals with pulmonary vascular, airway, or parenchymal disorders will develop PH and cor pulmonale, and it is likely that genetic or other influences contribute to the pathophysiology. PH and cor pulmonale appear to be encountered more commonly in dogs than in cats. Primary PH is relatively uncommon; however, various pulmonary conditions can lead to secondary PH in the dog or cat, including chronic tracheobronchial disorders, pneumonia, or interstitial lung disease (Box 10.1). Often, definitive characterization of the respiratory disease resulting in PH cannot be achieved. A minority of these animals will have overt clinical signs of right-sided heart failure (cor pulmonale).
- PTE is a secondary condition seen in association with diseases that cause stasis of blood flow, alter endothelial integrity, or increase coagulability. PTE has been linked most commonly with immune-mediated hemolytic anemia, neoplasia, sepsis, protein-losing nephropathy, cardiac disease, and hyperadrenocorticism (Box 10.2). Clinically silent pulmonary embolism occurs in a majority (82%) of dogs undergoing total hip replacement surgery. It might also occur in other diseases but could go unrecognized until signs associated with chronic thromboembolic disease or massive embolization occur. Small pulmonary thromboemboli are rapidly lysed and removed by the local fibrinolytic system; however, occlusion of larger pulmonary arteries or massive showering of emboli to a large circulatory volume can lead to acute right ventricular overload.

CLINICAL PRESENTATION

HISTORY AND CLINICAL SIGNS

- Dogs or cats with PH and cor pulmonale can be of any age, depending on the underlying cause of elevated pulmonary artery pressures. In general, there is a history of signs referable to the pulmonary system or to congestive heart failure. Animals can display any combination of signs, including lethargy, weakness, cough,

---

> **Box 10.1   Causes of Pulmonary Hypertension**
>
> Pulmonary vascular disease
> Heartworm disease
> Chronic pulmonary thromboembolism
> Chronic pulmonary disease
> Tracheobronchial disease or collapse
> Pulmonary fibrosis/interstitial pneumonia
> Pneumonia
> Primary pulmonary hypertension

> **Box 10.2   Predisposing Conditions for Pulmonary Thromboembolism**
>
> Immune-mediated hemolytic anemia
> Neoplasia
> Sepsis
> Protein-losing nephropathy/enteropathy
> Cardiac disease
> Hyperadrenocorticism
> Central catheter use
> Hemodialysis
> Total parenteral nutrition
> Hip replacement surgery

respiratory distress, tachypnea, abdominal distention, and syncope. Historical features and clinical signs are not specific for PH or cor pulmonale but might suggest the underlying cardiopulmonary disease.

- PTE is generally a disorder of older animals, and history and clinical signs reflect the underlying disease process. Clinical recognition of this disorder is difficult because of nonspecific systemic and cardiorespiratory signs. Animals with PTE can demonstrate weight loss, lethargy, and anorexia caused by the primary disease process with acute or gradual development of tachypnea and breathlessness. Certainly, secondary PTE should be suspected in an animal with a predisposing condition (see Box 10.2) that has acute-onset tachypnea, cyanosis, or hypoxemia that is refractory to oxygen therapy.

KEY POINT

PTE occurs secondary to a variety of underlying conditions. Affected animals have signs reflecting the primary systemic disease or refractory respiratory distress.

PHYSICAL EXAMINATION

- Animals with cor pulmonale will generally display tachypnea or respiratory distress caused by fluid accumulation (ascites or pleural effusion) or caused by an underlying cardiopulmonary disease. A systolic heart murmur due to mitral or tricuspid regurgitation is found in most dogs with PH and cor pulmonale. Animals that have clinical signs of overt right-sided heart failure can display jugular venous distention, hepatomegaly, ascites, or, less commonly, subcutaneous edema.
- Dogs and cats with PTE have tachypnea and hyperpnea that is not alleviated by oxygen administration. Cough is relatively uncommon. Harsh lung sounds or loud bronchovesicular sounds can be detected; crackles or wheezes are less frequent. Physical examination abnormalities, such as pale mucous membranes in the case of immune-mediated hemolytic anemia or a pot-bellied appearance caused by hyperadrenocorticism, reflect the underlying disease.

DIAGNOSTIC TESTING
LABORATORY TESTING

- Basic laboratory tests generally reflect the underlying disease and do not add to the diagnosis of PH, cor pulmonale, or PTE. The diagnosis of PTE is particularly problematic. Testing for plasma D-dimer, a breakdown product resulting from the action of plasmin on cross-linked fibrin, has been shown in human medicine to have high sensitivity but low specificity in the diagnosis of PTE. In veterinary medicine, several diseases can result in a positive D-dimer test, although the magnitude of the elevation might enhance the suspicion of pulmonary embolization. However, a negative test result does not entirely exclude the possibility of PTE.
- Hypercoagulability can be assessed with performance of thromboelastography, a test that assesses the kinetics of clot formation, clot stability, and clot strength. Although this test appears useful in establishing a hypercoagulable state, there is no information available on its correlation with embolization.
- Pulse oximetry and arterial blood gas analysis are useful for detecting abnormal gas exchange. Hemoglobin saturation with oxygen (S_pO_2) is related to arterial oxygen partial pressure by a sigmoidal relationship, with values above 95% indicating normoxemia. Below 95%, values for S_pO_2 lie on the exponential part of the curve, and small changes in S_pO_2 reflect very large changes in arterial oxygen. Thus, pulse oximetry provides only a crude estimate of lung function.

Arterial blood gas analysis provides a more precise assessment of oxygenation and can be used to follow response to therapy. Arterial blood gas analysis in the animal with PTE often reveals hypoxemia, hypocapnia, and increased alveolar-to-arterial gradient; however, normal arterial oxygenation does not exclude the diagnosis of PTE. Some animals with PTE will respond to supplemental oxygen administration with normalization of arterial oxygen, although many have continued tachypnea because of altered control of ventilation. Animals with additional cardiac or pulmonary pathology that increases shunt fraction will not necessarily have a complete response to exogenous oxygen supplementation.

RADIOGRAPHS

- Radiographic evidence of right ventricular enlargement in an animal with lung or pulmonary vascular disease is supportive of cor pulmonale (Figure 10.1). Retrospective review of radiographs in animals with PTE might reveal regional oligemia, lack of normal vascular tapering, or enlarged central pulmonary arteries; however, in the clinical setting, radiographic changes appear less obvious because PTE is not suspected in a large proportion of animals that die from embolization.
- Thoracic radiographic abnormalities are common in PTE but are rarely specific. Pulmonary infiltrates can be interstitial, alveolar, or lobar in dogs and cats. Alveolar infiltrates can represent hemorrhage, edema, or infarction. Cardiomegaly and mild to moderate pleural effusion are common in dogs and cats. Importantly, normal chest radiographs are reported in 7% to 27% of dogs and cats with necropsy-confirmed PTE, and PTE should be a top differential diagnosis in an animal with marked respiratory distress and normal thoracic radiographs.

KEY POINT

Normal thoracic radiographic findings in a tachypneic animal that fails to respond to oxygen administration should raise suspicion of pulmonary embolism.

ELECTROCARDIOGRAPHY

- Reported abnormalities with right ventricular enlargement caused by PH or PTE include deep S waves in leads II and aVF and a right axis deviation. Right atrial enlargement is supported by tall or peaked P waves; however, electrocardiographic evaluation of right ventricular enlargement is insensitive, and abnormalities

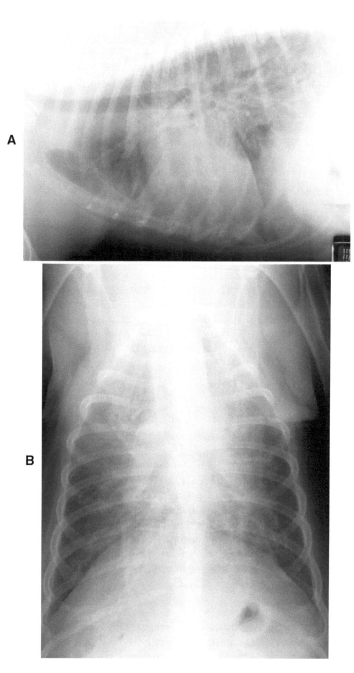

Figure 10.1   There is generalized enlargement of cardiac silhouette on the right lateral (**A**) and dorsoventral (**B**) views. Pulmonary arteries are enlarged and appear to taper slowly. Numerous pleural fissure lines are identified, and there is a diffuse heavy interstitial and peribronchial pattern identified within the lung.

have been reported in <15% of dogs with PH. The electrocardiogram should be closely examined for rhythm disturbances that can be found in dogs with PH.

ECHOCARDIOGRAPHY

- Two-dimensional echocardiography can provide subjective evidence of PH leading to cor pulmonale (when pulmonic stenosis has been ruled out). Supportive evidence of right ventricular overload includes right ventricular concentric hypertrophy and dilation, dilation of the main pulmonary artery, systolic flattening of the interventricular septum, and paradoxical septal motion. Doppler echocardiography can be used to estimate pulmonary artery pressure when tricuspid regurgitation or pulmonic insufficiency is present (Figure 10.2). With use of the modified Bernoulli equation (pressure gradient = $4 \times velocity^2$), spectral Doppler allows reasonably accurate estimation of right ventricular systolic pressure through measurement of tricuspid regurgitation velocity and estimation of pulmonary artery diastolic pressure through measurement of pulmonic

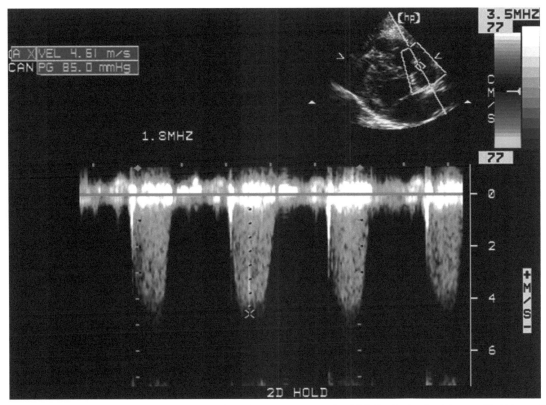

Figure 10.2   Tricuspid regurgitant jet in a dog with pulmonary hypertension (PH). On the basis of the modified Bernoulli equation, the right-ventricular-to-right-atrial-pressure gradient is 85 mm Hg. (Courtesy Dr. Fiona Campbell, University of Queensland.)

insufficiency velocity. PH is documented by a tricuspid regurgitant jet >2.8 m/sec or a pulmonic insufficiency jet >2.2 m/sec.

- Echocardiographic features consistent with pulmonary embolization overlap with those found in PH. In some cases, a thrombus can be visualized within the heart or great vessels. Therefore echocardiography should be considered in animals with predisposing conditions for PTE that have an acute onset of respiratory distress because right ventricular dilation, pulmonary artery enlargement, or septal flattening could suggest pulmonary embolization.

Echocardiography should be considered in dogs suspected of having PTE.

CATHETERIZATION AND ADVANCED IMAGING

- Direct measurement of pulmonary artery pressure through right-heart catheterization is the gold standard for diagnosing PH. Unfortunately, it requires sedation or general anesthesia, and animals with PH are at increased risk for anesthetic complications. Therefore catheterization is rarely performed in this clinical situation.

- Pulmonary angiography has been considered the gold standard for diagnosis of PTE in humans; however, use of contrast helical computed tomography to confirm PTE is increasing. Definitive angiographic diagnosis of PTE depends on visualization of an intraluminal filling defect in a pulmonary artery or loss of visualization of an artery. However, neither modality is commonly used in veterinary medicine because each requires anesthesia.

- Ventilation/perfusion scanning uses technetium-99m–labeled macroaggregated albumin as a vascular marker and technetium-99m–labeled diethylenetriamine pentaacetic acid as a ventilatory marker to define segmental or lobar perfusion defects in areas of normal ventilation. Ventilation scans are rarely performed in nonanesthetized animals; however, perfusion scanning alone can be completed without anesthesia and can assist in documentation of perfusion deficits. This is a safe, noninvasive technique for evaluation of PTE, although it is somewhat nonspecific because perfusion deficits could reflect thrombosis or simply a lung region experiencing hypoxic pulmonary vasoconstriction.

THERAPY

- Currently, little is known about the optimal therapy for either PH or PTE. In animals with cor pulmonale, cautious diuretic therapy is warranted to reduce fluid accumulation, and judicious use of thoracocentesis or abdominocentesis can improve respiration. Excessive removal of fluid should be avoided because animals could have volume contraction or systemic hypotension. Pimobendan, a phosphodiesterase 3 inhibitor, acts as an inodilator and lowers pulmonary pressure in dogs with PH secondary to chronic mitral valve disease. Although not evaluated in clinical trials, the positive inotropic effects of pimobendan may be beneficial in cor pulmonale by improving right ventricular systolic function.
- Definitive treatment of PTE is challenging, and the decision to pursue aggressive therapy is complicated by the fact that the diagnosis of embolization is difficult to confirm. Agents that cause clot lysis locally (tissue plasminogen activator) or systemically (streptokinase, urokinase) are expensive, require intensive monitoring, and can be associated with complications. In addition, efficacy is questionable. Ancillary therapies, including control of the primary disease process and oxygen supplementation, are essential in management. In practice, effort is directed toward preventing the occurrence of PTE through prophylactic therapy with drugs such as aspirin, clopidogrel, and low molecular weight heparin (see Frequently Asked Questions).
- Therapy for PH has not been well defined in veterinary medicine. Standard treatment of the underlying cardiopulmonary condition should be used and can lessen signs related to cardiopulmonary dysfunction and PH. Anticoagulant therapy is sometimes recommended to treat PH associated with chronic thromboembolic disease in humans or to limit in situ thrombosis that can result in progressive vascular obstruction. Little information is available on efficacy and use of anticoagulants or antiplatelet drugs in veterinary medicine, and their use remains controversial.
- Insight into various therapies for PH in animals has been gained by reviewing treatment of primary PH in humans, which is partially mediated by alterations in endothelium-derived vasodilators and constrictors and by vascular proliferation. Intravenous or inhaled prostacyclin (a breakdown product of arachidonic acid metabolism) and inhaled nitric oxide are among the drugs used. These vasodilators are selective for the pulmonary circulation and have more pronounced impact on pulmonary pressures than systemic pressures. However, they require sophisticated or complicated delivery and result in only minimal reductions in pulmonary artery pressures. Although these reductions are statistically significant and provide some clinical benefit in human patients, it is unclear whether these small changes in pulmonary arterial pressures would be beneficial in veterinary patients.
- Use of sildenafil in dogs with PH has been associated with clinical improvements in exercise tolerance and quality of life, although pulmonary artery pressures are not always changed. Sildenafil is a phosphodiesterase 5 inhibitor, acting by accumulation of cyclic guanosine monophosphate in vascular smooth muscle, resulting in vasodilation.

FREQUENTLY ASKED QUESTIONS

What clinical findings would support the diagnosis of cor pulmonale, and how could this be confirmed?

Animals with clinical signs relative to cor pulmonale generally display respiratory abnormalities (tachypnea, hyperpnea, and/or cough) and also exhibit signs of right-sided heart failure (ascites, jugular venous distention, and/or subcutaneous edema). A history of syncope should raise suspicion for PH. Radiographically, cor pulmonale is evident as right-sided heart enlargement. Right atrial enlargement and dilation of the caudal vena cava support the diagnosis. Two-dimensional echocardiography reveals eccentric dilation of the right ventricle most commonly. With chronic PH or PH in a young animal, right ventricular hypertrophy can be noted. Doppler echocardiography can confirm PH by detection of a velocity jet >2.8 or 2.2 m/sec in the presence of tricuspid regurgitation or pulmonic insufficiency, respectively.

What tests confirm the diagnosis of PTE and provide support for institution of anticoagulant therapy?

Unfortunately, antemortem diagnosis of PTE remains challenging, and definitive diagnosis is often not achieved in the clinical setting. Suspicion for PTE should be present when an animal with a recognized predisposing condition (see Box 10.2) develops acute-onset respiratory distress. Normal thoracic radiographic findings do not preclude the diagnosis. Supportive evidence of PTE would include a positive D-dimer test, echocardiographic evidence of right ventricular overload, and perfusion deficits on pulmonary scintigraphy in an animal with refractory respiratory distress. Anticoagulant therapy with low molecular weight heparin is often instituted in a patient with these findings to limit further deposition of clot material and to enhance clot breakdown. Thrombolytic therapy is rarely used because of the risk of generating a systemic fibrinolytic state or creating ischemia-reperfusion injury. Because of the difficulty in establishing a diagnosis of PTE and the morbidity and mortality associated with this secondary complication, prophylactic antithrombotic therapy should be considered in animals with recognized predisposing conditions.

What drugs can be used as prophylaxis for PTE?

The drug historically used to inhibit platelet aggregation is aspirin, although the dose that achieves this effect has not been clearly identified and not all animals exhibit reduced platelet function. A low dose of 1.0 mg/kg/day (dog) or every third day (cat) has been suggested, although this dose only inhibits platelet function in one third of healthy dogs. Aspirin doses of 5 to 10 mg/kg q24-48h (dogs) and 25 mg/kg every 3 days (cats) have also been used. Newer drugs such as clopidogrel have some effect on platelet aggregation, although the precise dosing in dogs is unclear and efficacy in PTE has not been established. Although not evaluated in the setting of PTE, clopidogrel at a dose of 18.75 mg per cat appears to decrease the risk of aortic thromboembolism in animals with cardiomyopathy. Low molecular weight heparin (enoxaparin, dalteparin) acts through inhibition of coagulation, with enhanced factor X versus factor II inhibition compared with unfractionated heparin. This class of drug can be used concurrently with antiplatelet drugs; however, the pharmacokinetics are not fully understood, and pharmacodynamic studies in PTE are lacking.

What type of treatment can be considered for PH?

Aggressive management of underlying cardiopulmonary conditions should be instituted. Animals with chronic bronchitis or small airway collapse often require steroids (oral or inhaled) and extended-release theophylline (10 mg/kg PO q12h [dog] or 15 to 19 mg/kg PO in the evening [cat]). Interstitial lung diseases are less likely to respond to medical therapy. In either group of animals with respiratory dysfunction, supplemental oxygen therapy either at home or in the hospital can improve clinical presentation. Use of sildenafil (1 to 3 mg/kg PO q8-12h) can be considered for animals with signs related to PH. Clinical signs and quality of life are improved with therapy, although echocardiographic estimates of pulmonary artery pressure can remain unchanged.

SUGGESTED READINGS

Bach JF, Rozanski EA, MacGregor J, et al: Retrospective evaluation of sildenafil citrate as a therapy for pulmonary hypertension in dogs, J Vet Intern Med 20:1132, 2006.

Boyle KL, Leech E: A review of the pharmacology and clinical uses of pimobendan, J Vet Emerg Crit Care 22:398–408, 2012.

Dudley A, Thomason J, Fritz S, et al: Cyclooxygenase expression and platelet function in healthy dogs receiving low-dose aspirin, J Vet Intern Med 27:141, 2013.

Epstein SE, Hopper K, Mellema MS, Johnson LR: Diagnostic utility of D-dimers in dogs with pulmonary embolism, J Vet Intern Med 27:1646, 2013.

Glaus TM, Soldati G, Maurer R, Ehrensperger F: Clinical and pathological characterisation of primary pulmonary hypertension in a dog, Vet Rec 154:786, 2004.

Googs R, Wiinberg B, Kjelgaard-Hansen M, Chan DL: Serial assessment of the coagulation status of dogs with immune-mediated haemolytic anaemia using thromboelastography, Vet J 191:347, 2012.

Johnson L, Boon J, Orton EC: Clinical characteristics of 53 dogs with Doppler derived evidence of pulmonary hypertension: 1992-1996, J Vet Intern Med 13:440, 1999.

Johnson LR, Lappin MR, Baker DC: Pulmonary thromboembolism in 29 dogs: 1985-1995, J Vet Intern Med 13:338, 1999.

Kellum HB, Stepien RL: Sildenafil citrate therapy in 22 dogs with pulmonary hypertension, J Vet Intern Med 12:1258, 2007.

Koblik PD, Hornoff W, Harnagel SH, et al: A comparison of pulmonary angiography, digital subtraction angiography, and 99mTc-DTPA/MAA ventilation-perfusion scintigraphy for detection of experimental pulmonary emboli in the dog, Vet Radiol Ultrasound 30:159, 1989.

La Rue MG, Murtaugh RJ: Pulmonary thromboembolism in dogs: 47 cases (1986-1987), J Am Vet Med Assoc 197:1369, 1990.

Liska WD, Poteet BA: Pulmonary embolism associated with canine total hip replacement, Vet Surg 32:178, 2003.

Nelson OL, Andreason C: The utility of plasma D-dimer to identify thromboembolic disease in the dog, J Vet Intern Med 17:830, 2003.

Norris CR, Griffey SM, Samii VF: Pulmonary thromboembolism in cats: 29 cases (1987-1997), J Am Vet Med Assoc 215:1650, 1999.

Pyle RL, Abbott J, MacLean H: Pulmonary hypertension and cardiovascular sequelae in 54 dogs, Int J Appl Res Vet Med 2:99, 2004.

Schermerhorn T, Pembleton-Corbett JR, Kornreich B: Pulmonary thromboembolism in cats, J Vet Intern Med 18:533, 2004.

Schober K, Baade H, Ludewig E, et al: Cor pulmonale in terrier breed dogs with chronic-progressive, idiopathic pulmonary fibrosis: 19 cases (1996-2001), Tierarztliche Praxis Ausgabe K, Kleintiere/Heimtiere 30:180, 2002.

Uehara Y: An attempt to estimate the pulmonary artery pressure in dogs by means of pulsed Doppler echocardiography, J Vet Med Sci 55:307, 1993.

Weinkle TK, Center SA, Randolph JF, et al: Evaluation of prognostic factors, survival rates, and treatment protocols for immune-mediated hemolytic anemia in dogs: 151 cases (1993-2002), J Am Vet Med Assoc 226:1860, 2005.

11

Heartworm Disease

Justin D. Thomason | Clay A. Calvert

Heartworm infection, primarily in the dog and cat, has been reported in many countries and occurs throughout the United States. Infections are most common in tropical and semitropical regions, and the risk is greater in dogs that live outside. Most infected dogs are medium to large breeds and 3 to 8 years of age at the time of diagnosis.

Numerous mosquito species serve as vectors after acquiring microfilariae (larval stage 1, L_1) while feeding on a canine host. Cats living either indoors or outdoors are infected by mosquitoes that have acquired microfilariae from infected dogs. The infection rates in cats are lower than the rates in dogs, although in some regions the infection rates in cats are higher than expected.

Development of microfilariae (L_1) to infective larvae (L_3) within the mosquito occurs in 1 to 4 weeks, requiring less time as the ambient temperature increases. Infective larvae are deposited on the host's skin as the mosquito feeds and the larvae enter the bite wound in small numbers, usually less than 10 larvae per mosquito.

In dogs, infective larvae (L_3) migrate through host tissue while molting (to L_4 and L_5), and L_5 (1 to 2 cm in length) arrive in the pulmonary arteries in approximately 100 days. Adult worms develop largely in the caudal lobar arteries by 150 to 200 days after L_3 inoculation. Adult *Dirofilaria immitis* are long (approximately 15 cm, males; 25 cm, females) nematodes that reside primarily in the pulmonary arteries but can move into the right ventricle when the worm burden is high. Microfilariae (L_1) are produced by gravid females 6 to 7 months after infection.

Microfilariae (L_1) are usually detectable in infected dogs not receiving monthly or injectable prophylaxis. However, in highly endemic regions, from 25% to 50% of infected dogs do not have circulating microfilariae because they are entrapped in the pulmonary capillaries by host immune mechanisms. The number of circulating microfilariae does not correlate to adult heart worm burden. Adult heartworms can live 3 to 5 years, while microfilariae (L_1) live for 1 to 3 years.

Most dogs are highly susceptible to heartworm infection, and most infective larvae (L_3) develop

into adults. A lower percentage of cats inoculated with L_3 have adult infections, and the burden is often only one to three worms, but it can be higher in highly endemic regions. Further evidence of resistance in cats is the short survival time of many L_5 in the pulmonary arteries, and adult worms probably survive no longer than 2 years. Another difference between heartworm disease in dogs and cats is that in the cat, larvae are more likely to migrate to ectopic sites such as the brain, systemic arteries, and subcutaneous (SC) sites.

KEY POINT

Adult heartworms are present in the pulmonary arteries approximately 6 months after transmission from the mosquito.

PATHOPHYSIOLOGY

- Heartworms damage the pulmonary arterial endothelial lining within 3 days of experimental heartworm transplantation. Pulmonary arteries containing heartworms have endothelial swelling, widened intercellular junctions, sloughing of longitudinal strips of endothelium, and adhesion of many activated leukocytes and platelets to the damaged areas. Endothelial damage decreases nitric oxide production and increases endothelin production (endothelial dysfunction). Endothelial dysfunction also increases permeability to serum proteins and water, permitting leakage of small arterioles into the perivascular interstitium. Trophic factors are released by damaged endothelium and activated platelets and leukocytes. These factors (such as platelet-derived growth factor) stimulate migration and multiplication of smooth muscle cells within the tunica media. Endothelin causes vasoconstriction and vascular fibrosis. Pathognomonic villi of heartworm disease consist of the rapidly dividing smooth muscle cells and the collagen produced by them.
- Arteriographic abnormalities are seen within weeks of heartworm transplantation into dogs.

Lobar arteries, especially those to the caudal and accessory lung lobes, dilate, become tortuous, and develop aneurysms. Smaller distal arteries lose their normal tapering and may be occluded. Arteries with a diameter smaller than the adult heartworms frequently appear to be abruptly pruned. Blood flow is frequently obstructed and diverted to nonaffected lung lobes.

- Increased permeability of the vascular surfaces of smaller vessels produces perivascular fluid infiltration, which can be seen as an alveolar pattern on radiographs. An interstitial pattern is also frequently seen and is probably a combination of vascular disease, perivascular fluid leakage, and inflammation.
- The severity of cardiopulmonary disease is determined by worm numbers, host immune response, duration of infection, and host activity level. Active dogs have more disease than inactive dogs for any given worm burden. Sedentary dogs can harbor more than the typical 10 to 20 worms associated with infections in endemic regions without developing clinical signs. However, frequent exertion/activity increases pulmonary arterial disease and can precipitate clinical signs and even right-sided congestive heart failure (CHF). Pulmonary disease is also exacerbated by natural or drug-induced worm death. High worm burdens are most often the result of inoculation from many mosquitoes over one season. Very large exposure over a short time span can result in vena cava syndrome the following year, typically in young dogs. Decreased flow and inadequate recruitment of collateral arterioles result in inadequate pulmonary flow in response to exertion. Pulmonary hypertension results and then right ventricular afterload increases, resulting in right heart dilation and hypertrophy and, in active dogs, right-sided CHF. Right-sided CHF is characterized by high central venous pressure, hepatic congestion, and ascites. In general, small dogs tolerate infections and treatment less well than large dogs.
- Heartworm-associated inflammatory mediators induce immune responses in the lungs and kidneys (immune complex glomerulonephritis). Leakage of plasma and inflammatory mediators from small vessels and capillaries causes parenchymal lung inflammation and edema. Pulmonary arterial constriction causes increased flow velocity, especially with exertion, and resultant shear stresses further damage the endothelium. The process of endothelial damage, vasoconstriction, increased flow velocity, and local ischemia is a vicious cycle. Inflammation with ischemia can result in irreversible interstitial fibrosis.

PATHOPHYSIOLOGY IN CATS

- Pulmonary arterial disease in the cat is similar to that in the dog, although small arteries develop more severe muscular hypertrophy. Arterial thrombosis is caused by both blood clots and worms lodged in narrow lumen arterioles.
- Immature heartworms can reach the lungs of cats within 100 days, at which time pneumonitis develops. Clinical signs are coughing and wheezing, which resemble asthma and usually improve spontaneously. The feline heartworm antibody test usually becomes positive at this time. Subsequently, when L_5 mature to adult heartworms 6 to 7 months after infection, cats usually begin to experience episodic coughing and dyspnea. As worms die, an intense pneumonitis develops, and even one dead worm can produce severe pneumonitis, thromboembolism, and death.
- The worst pulmonary disease is seen after adult heartworms have died and their fragments are swept distally into the small pulmonary arteries. The response at the pulmonary arterial surface is an exacerbation of that seen with live heartworms. Villous proliferation is exuberant, and there are thrombi and a granulomatous inflammatory reaction around the dead heartworms. Blood flow is severely reduced, sometimes with no pulmonary arterial flow going to the caudal lung lobes. The caudal lung lobes frequently consolidate and fail to function as blood gas exchangers.

CLINICAL SYMPTOMS

- Clinical signs are a reflection of the number of infecting heartworms, the duration of infection, and the response of the canine host. Most dogs are symptom free. Coughing and dyspnea are the most common signs and are usually associated with parenchymal disease in the caudal lung lobes. This disease is focused around the pulmonary arteries, with inflammatory fluids accumulating, owing to increased vascular permeability to serum proteins and fluids.
- Decreased ability to exercise and the sequence of right ventricular dilation, hypertrophy, and failure are the responses to fixed vascular resistance and PH. This fixed resistance impedes arterial flow and increases the work of the right ventricle. Severe disease restricts the ability to recruit arteries to transport the high blood flow needed for exercise and decreases the ability to exercise. This resistance to flow is complicated by the exaggerated hypertensive response to alveolar hypoxia (arteriolar constriction) that accompanies heartworm infection. Patients with heart failure frequently

have had increased exercise before presentation with overt signs and demonstrate ascites and hepatomegaly. Cardiac cachexia develops within a few weeks.

- Hemoptysis may occur, especially after the heartworms have been killed by adulticide, and is the result of vascular and airway wall rupture. This blood loss normally starts in an area of severe vascular and parenchymal disease in the caudal lung lobes, probably when coughing ruptures vascular and airway walls.

DIAGNOSIS

- Monthly oral prophylaxis induces embryo stasis, and serologic antigen testing is required for diagnosis. Antigen detection tests are all very sensitive and specific. Infections acquired during the previous mosquito season are first detected by antigen testing 7 to 8 months later. The level of antigenemia is directly related to the number of mature female worms that are present. At least 90% of dogs harboring three or more adult females will test positive. For low-worm-burden suspects, a commercial laboratory-based microwell titer test (Diro-CHEK by Synbiotics, Kansas City, Mo.) is most sensitive. In general, strong, quick, positive reactions correlate with relatively high worm burdens. However, strong reactions also occur following worm death.

ANCILLARY TESTS
ECHOCARDIOGRAPHY

- In dogs, echocardiography is relatively unimportant as a diagnostic tool. Worms seen in the right heart and vena cava are associated with high-burden infection and with or without caval syndrome. With severe disease, changes associated with PH are often present. The following are a number of abnormalities on the echocardiogram that support a diagnosis of PH:
  - Underloaded left ventricle
  - Underloaded pulmonary veins
  - Underloaded left atrium
  - Right ventricular dilation with hypertrophy
  - Right atrial dilation
  - Flattening of the interventricular septum
  - Paradoxic septal motion
  - High-velocity tricuspid regurgitation
  - High-velocity pulmonic regurgitation
  - Upward diastolic billowing of the pulmonic valve leaflets
  - Prolonged duration from initial to maximum right ventricular outflow tract systolic flow velocity

ELECTROCARDIOGRAPHY

- Usually the electrocardiogram of a heartworm-infected dog is normal. Right ventricular hypertrophic patterns are seen when there is severe, chronic PH and are associated with overt or impending right-sided CHF. Heart rhythm disturbances are usually absent or mild, but atrial fibrillation is an occasional complication of severe PH.

DIAGNOSIS OF FELINE HEARTWORM INFECTION

- The diagnosis is based on historical and physical findings, index of suspicion, echocardiography, and serologic findings. Cats may have a positive antigen test result 8 months after L_3 inoculation. However, less than 50% of infected cats will test positive if they have less than 3 adult female worms or immature infections. Antiheartworm antibodies are produced by 90% of infected cats and may first appear 2 to 3 months post-L_3 infection and are usually present by 5 months. This test is most useful when the result is negative. Antibodies can persist for at least 6 months after worm death. Also, antibodies induced by larvae can persist after macrolide prophylaxis has been instituted and has killed the pre-adults. Thus a positive antibody test result is consistent with L_4 and L_5 larvae, adult infection, or persisting antibody following death of larvae or adults. A negative heartworm antibody test result indicates a 90% probability of absence of infection. Microfilaremia is unusual and typically transient in cats.

KEY POINT

The combination of vomiting, eosinophilia, and hyperglobulinemia warrant a high index of suspicion of heartworm infection in cats.

ECHOCARDIOGRAPHY

- In cats, echocardiography is useful because worms can usually be imaged. Parallel white echogenic lines may be seen in the right heart and pulmonary arteries. The best view is obtained in the right parasternal short-axis angulated to image the right and left main pulmonary arteries. High worm burdens may be associated with worms in the right heart.

MICROFILARIAL TESTS IN DOGS

- The problems with microfilarial detection tests are related to their sensitivity and the incidence of occult or nonmicrofilaremic infections.

DIRECT SMEAR

- This is a simple test wherein a drop of anticoagulated blood is placed on a slide and examined under the microscope. The test is quick and simple and, if microfilariae of *D. immitis* are detected, the diagnosis of heartworm disease is made. A positive test result eliminates the need for a microfilarial concentration test. However, the following are shortcomings of the direct smear:
  - It is 20% to 25% less sensitive in detecting microfilariae than the concentration tests (i.e., false-negative result).
  - It will be negative in the 25% to 50% of heartworm infections wherein circulating microfilariae are absent (so-called occult or amicrofilaremic infections).

CONCENTRATION TESTS

- Although a drop of blood is usually held back for the direct smear (which, if positive, means that the more time-consuming and more expensive concentration test does not have to be performed), the direct smear test result is usually negative because most dogs are not infected and a negative direct smear test result does not rule out heartworm infection.
- The two types of concentration tests are the modified Knott test and the filter test. Both are of similar sensitivity, specificity, cost, and labor. The choice between the two is largely one of tradition, habit, or practice. Both tests require that the examiner be able to distinguish the microfilariae of *D. immitis* from *Acanthocheilonema reconditum*. This challenge may be more difficult with the filter tests. Between 25% and 50% of infected dogs lack circulating microfilariae and thus concentration tests often fail to identify infection.

FALSE-NEGATIVE ANTIGEN TESTS IN DOGS

- Although false-negative antigen test results occur, the incidence is less than that of microfilaria tests and occult infections. False-negative results may be caused by the following:
  - Infections <7 months after L_3 inoculation
  - Few worms (< 3)
  - No female worms
  - Examiner interpretation
- In most cases, false-negative test results are associated with early or mild infections; microfilarial test results will also be negative, and radiographic changes will be absent or minimal.
- Heartworm-infected dogs living in highly endemic regions have a higher worm burden than infected dogs in regions where infections are less common. Heartworm-infected

dogs that have never received prophylaxis have higher worm burdens than those that have been receiving prophylaxis. The heartworm burden can be estimated by the degree of antigenemia, and this burden is often directly proportional to the severity of disease. The potential utility of worm-burden estimate is that the risk of post-adulticide thromboembolic complications is greater in high heartworm burden infections. Nonetheless, thoracic radiographs are probably more predictive of this complication risk, and antigen level alone is not to be used to assess the risk of pulmonary thromboembolism.

MINIMUM DATABASE

- Thoracic radiographs are the single test that provides the most information as to the severity of disease. All dogs with symptomatic infections have visible abnormalities. Dogs with severe disease have a worse prognosis and require an alternative treatment protocol.
- Complete blood count.
- Serum chemistry profile.
- Urinalysis.

THORACIC RADIOGRAPHS

In dogs, the thoracic radiograph is the single test that provides the most information as to disease severity. Attention should be given mostly to the main pulmonary artery segment (the 1 o'clock position on the ventrodorsal [VD] or dorsoventral [DV] projection) and the caudal lobar pulmonary arteries. The latter are best evaluated on the DV projection. Severe disease is characterized by a large main pulmonary artery segment and dilated, tortuous caudal lobar pulmonary arteries. If the latter are twice the diameter of the ninth rib at their point of superimposition, then the infection has produced severe disease. Normally these arteries are not larger than the ninth rib.

Fluffy, ill-defined parenchymal infiltrates of variable extent often surround the caudal lobar arteries and are usually worst in the right caudal lobe. The infiltrate may improve with cage confinement with or without antiinflammatory dosages of a corticosteroid.

In cats, the caudal lobar arteries normally appear relatively large but are larger still with heartworm infection. Patchy parenchymal infiltrates may also be present in cats with respiratory signs. The main pulmonary artery segment usually is not visible because of its relatively midline location.

COMPLETE BLOOD COUNT

- Eosinophilia and basophilia are common during heartworm infection and other more common parasitic infections. *A. reconditum* infection produces an eosinophilia of even greater magnitude than *D. immitis* infection. Anemia is a marker of severe heartworm disease.

SERUM CHEMISTRIES

- Serum chemistries are often unremarkable with uncomplicated heartworm infection. However, hyperglobulinemia can be present with chronic heartworm infections, and hemoglobinemia is often evident with caval syndrome and less often with thromboembolism. Increased BUN and serum creatinine may be the result of dehydration. However, both renal amyloidosis and immune complex glomerulopathy eventually cause azotemia.

URINALYSIS

- Proteinuria is common in animals with severe and chronic infections and is caused by immune-complex glomerulonephritis or amyloidosis. Hemoglobinuria is evident with caval syndrome or severe lysis associated with pulmonary thromboembolism or microangiopathy (severe, class 3, disease).

KEY POINT

Thoracic radiography is the most important diagnostic test for determining the severity of heartworm disease.

CLASSIFICATION OF HEARTWORM DISEASE

- Class 1
  - No or minimal signs
  - Normal or equivocal radiographic abnormalities
  - Absence of anemia
  - Absence of thrombocytopenia
  - Absence of hemoglobinuria
- Class 2
  - Mild to moderate symptoms
  - Symptoms usually are intermittent
- Class 3
  - Cough often severe and at rest
  - Weight loss-unthrifty
  - Syncope
  - Exercise intolerance
  - Ascites (right-sided CHF)
  - Anemia
  - Thrombocytopenia
  - Hemoglobinuria

THERAPY

- Before adulticide administration, it is recommended to initiate doxycycline (10 to 20 mg/kg q12h) for approximately 4 weeks in combination with a monthly macrocyclic lactone. The aim of doxycycline treatment is to eliminate *Wolbachia,* a gram-negative, intracellular, intrafilarial bacterium that is believed to incite pulmonary vasculature and possibly renal inflammation. This inflammation is believed to contribute to heartworm death–associated clinical signs. *Wolbachia* organisms are largely eliminated by this treatment and are unlikely to reappear in less than 3 months. The concentration of microfilaria, if present, will also be reduced. If doxycycline is not available then minocycline (5 to 10 mg/kg q12h) may be used.

- It is also recommended to initiate a monthly macrocyclic lactone, such as ivermectin, at the time that doxycycline treatment is started. Not only will the macrocyclic lactone gradually eliminate microfilariae (L_1), but also, the combination of doxycycline and a macrocyclic lactone is believed to kill some of the adult heartworms. Many microfilariae are removed from the circulation, and those that are ingested by mosquitos and subsequently molt produce L_3 that are noninfectious. The monthly macrocyclic lactone will close a window of opportunity for reinfection. In addition, during the one month of doxycycline and macrocyclic lactone treatment, more melarsomine-resistant immature worms will mature to melarsomine-sensitive age (at least 4 months after L_3 infection).

- Melarsomine should be administered to most infected dogs. The first injection is recommended after 4 weeks of doxycycline and macrocyclic lactone treatment. For all class 1 and 2 patients, one injection of melarsomine is administered intramuscularly at 2.5 mg/kg, deep in the epaxial musculature with a 22-gauge needle (1-inch for large dogs). After drawing up the dose of melarsomine, place a new needle on the syringe. Pressure is applied during and for 1 minute after the needle is withdrawn to prevent the drug from seeping into SC tissues. Approximately one month later, two injections of melarsomine (by the previous method) separated by 24 hours are administered. These two injections are administered on alternate sides. This protocol is sometimes referred to as graded kill.

- After each melarsomine injection, patients must be kept strictly confined and inactive for 4 to 6 weeks to minimize the risk of pulmonary thromboembolism. The adverse effects of melarsomine are otherwise limited to local inflammation, brief low-grade fever, and ptyalism. Hepatotoxicity is a rare complication.

- We have encountered a high proportion of toy and miniature breed dogs that experience severe pulmonary thromboembolic complications after the double melarsomine injections (third and fourth injections). It is our practice to administer melarsomine as single injections 4 to 6 weeks apart to a total of 3 injections to toy and miniature dogs. Postadulticide thromboembolic complications have been less with this protocol.

- Class 3 patients should be stabilized before melarsomine administration. However, doxycycline and a macrocyclic lactone treatment should be initiated if possible. Stabilizing treatment variably includes cage confinement, oxygen, corticosteroid (prednisone, 1mg/kg once daily) and heparin (100 to 300 U/kg SC q6h for 1 to 3 weeks before the graded-kill melarsomine protocol). Consider sildenafil (1.5 to 2.0 mg/kg q8h) to reduce pulmonary hypertension and improve pulmonary perfusion. Sildenafil (20-mg tablets) is commercially available at reasonable cost.
- Some class 3 patients have overt right-sided CHF (hepatic congestion and ascites). These patients require additional drugs to reduce pulmonary hypertension, increase right ventricular contractility, suppress renin-angiotensin-aldosterone activity, and reduce sodium and fluid overload. The labor intensiveness and numbers of drugs administered to these patients is daunting. Clinical judgment is required.

KEY POINT

Use the graded-kill melarsomine protocol.

PATIENTS WITH RIGHT-SIDED CONGESTIVE HEART FAILURE

- Dogs with ascites may need to be treated with furosemide (1 to 2 mg/kg BID), low-dose angiotensin-converting enzyme (ACE) inhibitor such as enalapril (0.25 mg/kg BID and possibly increased to 0.5 mg/kg BID after 1 week), sildenafil and pimobendan (0.2 to 0.3 mg/kg BID). Spironolactone (1 to 2 mg/kg BID) may be used in combination with furosemide. Digoxin, digitoxin, and arteriolar dilators, such as hydralazine and amlodipine, should not be administered. Digoxin is not effective for cor pulmonale, and arteriolar dilators (occasionally even ACE inhibitors) are likely to cause systemic hypotension. In our experience, treatment of the PH and cage confinement will often result in resolution of the right-sided CHF.

POSTADULTICIDE THROMBOEMBOLIC COMPLICATIONS

- Pulmonary thromboembolism can occur from 2 to 30 days after treatment, and signs are most likely from 10 to 21 days after treatment. Clinical signs are coughing, hemoptysis, dyspnea-tachypnea, lethargy, and anorexia. Physical findings variably include pale or gray mucous membranes, pulmonary crackles, and fever. Abnormal laboratory data may include an inflammatory leukogram, thrombocytopenia, and prolonged activated clotting time or prothrombin time. Local or disseminated intravascular coagulation may be occurring. Treatments to consider include oxygen, cage confinement, prednisone at an antiinflammatory dosage (1.0 mg/kg once daily), heparin (100 to 300 U/kg SC TID), and/or antiplatelet therapy (aspirin or clopidogrel) for several days to 1 week. Aspirin (5 to 7 mg/kg once daily) or clopidogrel (0.5 to 1.0 mg/kg once daily) is less labor intensive than heparin treatment but is probably less effective.

CONFIRMING ADULTICIDE EFFICACY

- The graded-kill melarsomine protocol kills all or most worms in approximately 75% of dogs. Antigen testing is performed 4 to 6 months after the third dose of the graded-kill protocol. Many test results will be negative at 4 months, but some will become negative only after 6 months. A strongly positive test result after 6 months should be followed by retreatment (two injections 24 hours apart).

EFFECT OF IVERMECTIN ON ADULT HEARTWORMS IN DOGS

- Ivermectin administered monthly for 2 to 3 years to dogs beginning at 5 to 7 months after L_3 inoculation eradicates most adult worms. Further, during this time period, some older worms are also killed. However, the use of ivermectin is not a substitute for melarsomine treatment because the "slow-kill" may allow pulmonary disease to progress in the interim. We have encountered some disastrous outcomes in dogs treated in this fashion. In addition, this treatment may contribute to macrocyclic lactone resistance (see the following on lack of efficacy).

TREATMENT OF FELINE HEARTWORM INFECTION

- There is no current satisfactory approach to heartworm infections in cats. Although infection often is lethal, a safe and effective melarsomine protocol has not been developed. Thus, all cats in heartworm-endemic regions should receive drug prophylaxis. The adult heartworm lifespan in cats is probably no longer than 2 years. Cats may remain symptom free, experience episodic vomiting or episodic dyspnea (resembling asthma), may die suddenly from pulmonary thromboembolism, or, rarely, have CHF. With each heartworm death, pulmonary complications occur.

- Cats are managed conservatively with restricted activity and corticosteroid therapy, such as prednisone or prednisolone (1.0 to 2.0 mg/kg once daily). Steroids reduce the severity of vomiting and respiratory signs. The hope is that episodes of pulmonary complications will not prove fatal as the worms die. Barring superinfection, it is thought that 25% to 50% of cats can survive with this approach. Serial antibody testing can be used to monitor heartworm status.

- Surgical retrieval of worms from the right atrium, right ventricle, and vena cavae can be attempted in patients with high worm burden detected by echocardiography. An endoscopic basket or horsehair catheter can be advanced through the right jugular vein under fluoroscopy.

MICROFILARICIDE TREATMENT IN DOGS

- Treatment aimed at killing microfilariae acutely is not recommended; rather, it is sufficient to eliminate microfilariae, when present, during the process of treatment with doxycycline and a macrocyclic lactone. Arguments in favor of not attempting to kill microfilariae acutely include the following:
  - Lack of proven disease associated with microfilaremia.
  - Potential for adverse reactions.
  - Monthly prophylactic drugs, in combination with doxycycline, result in gradual disappearance of microfilariae from the blood, even if gravid female worms persist.

- High-dose ivermectin (50 µg/kg) and standard dose milbemycin oxime (0.5 mg/kg, one dose) are acutely microfilaricidal. In the face of high microfilarial counts (>40,000/mL), adverse reactions are common. Usually the microfilarial concentration is <10,000/mL, and mild adverse reactions occur in only approximately 10% of dogs. Most adverse reactions are limited to brief ptyalism and defecation occurring within hours and lasting up to several hours.

- However, some dogs, especially small dogs, with high microfilariae counts may develop tachycardia, tachypnea, pale mucous membranes, diarrhea, and even shock. Treatment includes intravenous fluids and a soluble corticosteroid. Recovery is rapid when treatment is administered quickly. Microfilariae counts are not

routinely performed, and thus severe reactions are seldom expected. If microfilaricide treatment is chosen, it should be administered in the morning, and the patient observed for the day and discharged in the late afternoon or evening.

- Most veterinarians have chosen not to administer a microfilaricidal drug but rather to use doxycycline and a macrocyclic lactone, realizing that the microfilariae will gradually disappear. Milbemycin oxime should not be used under this logic because the prophylactic dose is microfilaricidal. The primary argument for adhering to the traditional approach (i.e., treating microfilariae) is that microfilaremic dogs serve as a reservoir for mosquitoes to acquire the microfilariae and possibly transmit them to another dog or cat. However, we are of the opinion that this risk is small.

KEY POINT

Rapid kill of microfilaria is unnecessary.

VENA CAVA SYNDROME IN DOGS

- Vena cava syndrome is uncommon except in very highly endemic regions such as Florida and the Gulf Coast. This syndrome typically occurs in young adult dogs that have received a massive exposure to L_3 over a short time. Thus, large numbers (>100) of worms mature in the heart and pulmonary arteries at the same time. The right-sided heart chambers become engorged with worms, and many extend into the venae cavae. Tricuspid regurgitation occurs, and pulmonary outflow tract and right-sided heart inflow become abnormal. Cardiovascular collapse results. Secondary complications include hemolysis, hemoglobinuria, acute hepatic failure, and renal failure.

- Unless appropriate treatment is provided, death usually occurs within 24 hours. Treatment is removal of the worms (with minimum sedation) through the right jugular vein with a long (preferably flexible) alligator forceps or horsehair catheter. Subsequent to worm removal, supportive fluid therapy is provided. Adulticide treatment of some remaining worms may be required after recovery (i.e., in 1 to 3 weeks). The success rate of this treatment is excellent, but experience is essential.

ANCILARY TREATMENTS FOR CANINE HEARTWORM DISEASE

Several ancillary drugs or treatments are sometimes used in the treatment of heartworm disease. They are usually limited to the treatment of severe

Table 11.1   Indications and Actions of Ancillary Treatments for Canine Heartworm Disease

Treatment	Effect	Indication
Doxycycline or minocycline	*Wolbachia* therapy; impairs microfilaria development	Often recommended in all cases of heartworm infection
Aspirin	Platelet inhibition	Severe pulmonary arterial disease
Heparin	Anticoagulant	Thrombosis Hemoglobinuria
Steroids	Antiinflammatory	Parenchymal lung disease secondary to pulmonary thromboembolism Allergic pneumonitis

(class 3) heartworm disease. The indications and actions of these treatments are summarized in Table 11.1.

HEPARIN

- Heparin should be considered for dogs with class 3 disease with the following conditions:
  - Symptomatic pulmonary thromboembolism
  - Hemoglobinuria
  - Severe thrombocytopenia
- Heparin (100 to 300 U/kg SC TID for 3 to 7 days) helps reduce the severity of pulmonary thrombosis; thus it helps improve blood flow, and by inhibiting fibrin production, it reduces platelet consumption, red blood cell damage, hemolysis, anemia, and hemoglobinuria. Heparin is combined with cage confinement.

CAGE CONFINEMENT

- For class 3 disease, it is important to minimize the need for cardiac output and pulmonary blood flow. Exertion increases the strain on the right ventricle and increases the risk of pulmonary thrombosis. Cage confinement or another form of severe confinement should be continued for 4 to 6 weeks.

OXYGEN

- Oxygen promotes pulmonary arterial dilation and is a useful component for dogs that are severely debilitated caused by class 3 disease and whenever symptomatic pulmonary thromboembolism occurs, either before or following adulticide treatment. Some class 3 disease patients have been kept in oxygen-cage confinement for as long as 3 weeks. Such patients usually also receive heparin.

CORTICOSTEROIDS

- These drugs reduce the inflammation associated with pulmonary thromboembolism but do not improve pulmonary arterial disease itself. With extended use, they actually reduce pulmonary blood flow by promoting coagulation.

When pulmonary thrombosis occurs, plasma and inflammatory cells leak out of the smaller arterioles, leading to granulomatous inflammation. Corticosteroids help reduce the severity of inflammation. The question arises as to whether corticosteroids should be given prophylactically because all dogs with heartworm disease will experience at least mild granulomatous inflammation and pulmonary thrombosis, which occurs from 3 to 21 days after administration of adulticide (most severe from 10 to 17 days). Some clinicians prescribe prednisone (1.0 mg/kg once daily) beginning a few days after adulticide treatment and continuing for 1 to 2 weeks. Reduced fever and improved appetite are potential benefits.

- Corticosteroids are indicated whenever there is clinical, laboratory, and radiographic evidence of moderate to severe pulmonary thromboembolism (whether before or after adulticide treatment). Clinical signs include dyspnea, pale or gray mucous membranes, coughing, and hemoptysis. An inflammatory leukogram and thrombocytopenia are usually present. The duration of use is generally 5 to 10 days, until there is clinical and radiographic evidence of significant improvement. Potential adverse actions of corticosteroids are GI ulceration and decreased pulmonary blood flow resulting from enhanced thrombosis. These effects are both time and dose related.

COMPLICATIONS OF HEARTWORM DISEASE

- Most complications of heartworm disease are the result of severe pulmonary myointimal proliferation and are thus associated with or indicative of class 3 infections.

PULMONARY THROMBOEMBOLISM

- Preadulticide and postadulticide thrombosis is common. Clinical signs are the following:
  - Coughing
  - Dyspnea

- Pyrexia
- Hemoptysis
- Leukocytosis
- Thrombocytopenia
- Pulmonary thromboembolism, although possible at any time, is most likely to occur and is most severe during the first month after adulticide treatment. Diagnosis can be assisted with thoracic radiographs and D-dimer assay. Treatment is cage confinement, corticosteroids, and heparin.

THROMBOCYTOPENIA

- Variable reductions of platelet counts are commonly seen, especially with class 3 disease. Thrombocytopenia may occur before but is most common and severe after adulticide treatment. Thrombocytopenia is consumptive as the result of thromboembolism and disseminated intravascular coagulopathy (DIC). Treatment is heparin.

HEMOGLOBINURIA

- Red blood cell lysis caused by severe pulmonary thromboembolism and fibrin deposition is an occasional complication of class 3 disease and the caval syndrome. Treatment is heparin for class 3 disease and worm retrieval for the caval syndrome.

CARDIAC CIRRHOSIS

- Severe PH leading to chronic right-sided CHF can cause gradually progressive hepatic congestion, leading to fibrosis and failure. There is no effective treatment.

EOSINOPHILIC PNEUMONITIS

- Approximately 10% to 20% of dogs with occult heartworm infection experience allergic or eosinophilic pneumonitis. The syndrome produces severe respiratory signs (coughing-dyspnea). However, this is an early syndrome and is usually not associated with severe PH. The pathophysiologic process involves immune entrapment of microfilariae in the pulmonary capillaries (occult infection results) with an unusually severe eosinophilic infiltrate. Pulmonary crackles may be ausculted and radiograph interpretation may be confused for cardiogenic pulmonary edema (left-sided CHF), *Pneumocystis carinii* infection, or pulmonary blastomycosis. The treatment is corticosteroids, and the response is rapid and complete. Adulticide treatment should be administered as soon as the symptoms have resolved.

EOSINOPHILIC GRANULOMATOSIS

- A small percentage of dogs with immune mediated occult disease have eosinophilic inflammation and infiltration of numerous organs, with the most severe manifestation being multiple,

variable sized pulmonary eosinophilic granulomas. Granulomas may develop in bronchi and the trachea. Eosinophilic pleural effusion may develop. This syndrome responds initially to corticosteroids, but relapse with progressive pulmonary disease is usual. The addition of azathioprine, cyclophosphamide, or mycophenolate has been beneficial. However, death is the end result in most cases, even after the heartworms have been killed.

KEY POINT

Exercise restriction and controlled leash walks are recommended for 4 to 6 weeks after melarsomine therapy.

HEARTWORM PROPHYLAXIS

- Heartworm prophylaxis is recommended for all dogs and cats at risk of infection. Heartworm testing is an integral component of prophylactic therapy. All dogs given heartworm prophylaxis for the first time should be both microfilaria free and antigen free. Annual antigen testing is recommended in all dogs regardless of the type of heartworm prophylaxis used. Although some have questioned the need for annual testing, poor compliance is an ongoing problem. In addition, some strains of larvae are resistant to treatment, and this resistance will result in adult infection. Failure to properly increase the drug dosage in large, rapidly growing puppies may also cause prophylactic failure.

MONTHLY PROPHYLAXIS

- A number of drugs are available for heartworm prophylaxis in dogs and cats, with some providing extended parasite control. They are very effective when administered monthly because larvae up to 4 months of age post-L_3 inoculation are readily killed by these agents. Adult infection is unlikely if a monthly dose is occasionally missed. The monthly use of these drugs causes gradual disappearance, over 5 to 9 months, of circulating microfilariae in dogs with adult heartworms. Thus antigen-detecting serologic tests should be used for annual screening. It is best to test 7 to 8 months either after the mosquito season begins or after the previous mosquito season ends.
- Invermectin, milbemycin oxime, moxidectin, and selamectin are recommended. All are safe as prescribed for all breeds. Milbemycin oxime, however, kills microfilariae (L_1) quickly, and shock can occur in the face of high L_1 concentrations.

Thus milbemycin oxime is not administered as a preventative to dogs with microfilariae.

REPORTS OF LACK OF EFFICACY

- Lack of efficacy (LOE) of a heartworm preventive product is defined as an animal testing heartworm positive regardless of appropriateness of dosage or administration consistency. There are many possible reasons for LOE, including resistance to macrocyclic lactones, inadequate compliance, variation in pharmocodynamics, variation in pharmacokinetics, or combinations of these.
- In vitro studies have identified microfilariae that are less susceptible to high doses of all the macrocyclic lactones. These microfilariae exhibit an allele on the P-glycoprotein gene that differs from the general population.
- In addition, studies have demonstrated decreased susceptibility of the MP3 strain (originally collected in northeast Georgia) to single monthly doses of commercial heartworm products. It is possible that the adulticide treatment of dogs with macrocyclic lactones, rather than melarsomine, may be selecting for populations of resistant microfilariae through prolonged drug exposure. Therefore it is recommended to treat dogs with adult heartworms with melarsomine and avoid the "slow-kill" protocol when possible.

KEY POINT

Because of reported lack of efficacy of heartworm preventative product, avoid the "slow-kill" protocol when possible.

SUGGESTED READING

American Heartworm Society: Current canine guidelines. Available at: www.heartwormsociety.org.

Bowman D: Heartworms, macrocyclic lactones, and the specter of resistance to prevention in the United States, Parasit Vectors 5:138, 2012.

Bowman DD, Atkins CE: Heartworm biology, treatment, and control, Vet Clin North Am Small Animal Pract 39:1127–1158, 2009.

Carreton E, Morcho R, Gonzalez-Miguel J, et al: D-dimer deposits in lungs and kidneys suggest its use as a marker in the clinical workup of dogs with heartworm (Dirofilaria immitis) disease, Vet Parasitol 191:182–186, 2013.

Carreton E, Morcho R, Gonzalez-Miguel J, et al: Variation of D-dimer values as assessment of pulmonary thromboembolism during adulticide treatment of heartworm disease in dogs, Vet Parasitol 195:106–111, 2013.

12

Pericardial Disorders and Cardiac Tumors*

Amanda E. Coleman | Gregg S. Rapoport

- Most clinically significant pericardial disorders in small animals are associated with pericardial effusion, defined as fluid accumulation within the pericardial space that is in excess of normal. Excessive intrapericardial fluid may result in cardiac tamponade, a life-threatening phenomenon characterized by compromised cardiac filling and output.
- The most common causes of pericardial effusion in dogs are neoplastic, accounting for 38% to 71% of cases.
- Hemodynamically significant pericardial effusion seldom occurs in cats. In this species, pericardial effusions most commonly occur in association with congestive heart failure, are of small volume, and do not produce cardiac tamponade. Consequently, these effusions are most often an incidental manifestation of underlying disease rather than the primary cause for presenting signs.

PERICARDIAL EFFUSION AND CARDIAC TAMPONADE

INCIDENCE AND PATIENT SIGNALMENT

- In a university referral veterinary hospital (University of Minnesota Veterinary Medical Center), pericardial effusions were confirmed as the primary cause for clinical signs in 1 of every 233 new canine admissions from January 1999 to December 2001, accounting for approximately 7% of dogs with clinical signs of heart disease and representing an incidence of 0.43%.
- Symptomatic pericardial effusions most commonly occur in older and larger dogs, with median age and body weight at the time of presentation ranging from 9.1 to 9.7 years and 31.2 to 34.8 kg, respectively.
- Golden Retriever, Labrador Retriever, German Shepherd, Saint Bernard, Newfoundland, and Great Dane dog breeds appear to be predisposed to the development of pericardial

effusion. In one report, the Saint Bernard breed with symptomatic pericardial effusion was diagnosed at a younger age than other commonly represented breeds.

PATHOPHYSIOLOGY

- In health, the pericardial space contains a small amount of fluid, an ultrafiltrate of plasma that serves to lubricate the heart during the cardiac cycle. Normal intrapericardial pressure is subatmospheric and mirrors that of the pleural space.
- Small increases in the volume of intrapericardial fluid may be tolerated without hemodynamic consequence. However, once the reserve volume of the pericardium is exceeded, further increases are associated with a potentially dangerous rise in intrapericardial pressure.
- *Cardiac tamponade,* a phenomenon that occurs during the decompensated phase of pericardial effusion development, results from intrapericardial pressure elevations that are sufficient to compress the right-sided cardiac chambers during diastole, interfering with normal systemic venous return. The result is a reduction in cardiac stroke volume and impaired cardiac output.
- The volume of pericardial effusion that can be tolerated without development of cardiac tamponade is closely related to rate of fluid accumulation. In experimental canine models involving the rapid infusion of fluid or air into the pericardial space, volumes of 60 to 80 mL of fluid and 8.7 ± 1.9 cm^3 of air per kilogram of body weight are sufficient to produce cardiac tamponade. In contrast, dogs with slowly developing pericardial effusions may have fluid volumes exceeding 1 to 1.5 L, which reflect the ability of the pericardium to adapt over a longer time course, stretching to allow greater increases in fluid volume with less incremental pressure rise.

CLINICAL PRESENTATION

Historical and physical examination findings in patients with hemodynamically significant pericardial effusion are attributable to the consequences of increased systemic venous pressure

---

*The authors wish to acknowledge Drs. Anthony Tobias and Elizabeth McNeil for their contributions to the previous edition of this chapter.

and decreased forward cardiac output (systemic hypotension).

HISTORY AND PRESENTING COMPLAINTS

- In most cases, clinical signs in dogs with pericardial effusions are nonspecific and have an apparently acute onset.
- The clinical presentation of patients with symptomatic pericardial effusion is influenced by the rate of pericardial fluid accumulation. For those in which fluid development is gradual, time allows for pericardial stretch and compensatory neurohormonal mechanisms, which struggle to maintain cardiac output at the expense of elevated systemic venous pressures. In these patients, signs of right-sided congestive heart failure predominate. Owners may report weakness or lethargy, decreased exercise tolerance, exertion-related syncope, reduced appetite, or abdominal distension caused by ascites.
- In contrast, dogs affected by acute cardiac tamponade have a clinical picture that is characterized by a sudden decline in cardiac output, with signs of weakness, collapse, increased respiratory effort, or shock.
- Less common presenting complaints include cough, vomiting, diarrhea, polyuria, and polydipsia.

PHYSICAL EXAMINATION FINDINGS

- Dogs with pericardial effusion may have clinical signs ranging from subtle to those associated with hemodynamic collapse caused by severe cardiac tamponade. Because the clinical picture of these patients can be nonspecific in nature, a thorough physical examination is critical to detect signs that appropriately raise the clinician's index of suspicion for pericardial effusion.
- Common physical examination findings include muffled heart sounds, generalized weakness, poor pulse quality, tachycardia, and tachypnea. Abdominal distention with a palpable fluid wave caused by ascites is also noted in 49% to 63% of cases.
- In dogs with cardiac tamponade, careful physical examination usually discloses jugular venous distension, a consequence of elevated right-sided cardiac filling pressures. In dogs with long or thick hair coats, clipping of the jugular furrow may help to make this more obvious.
- *Pulsus paradoxus*, defined as a phasic variation in pulse quality associated with respiration and characterized by a decline in pulse quality during inhalation, may be identified.

The finding of a combination of muffled heart sounds, jugular venous distension, and weak pulse quality or pulsus paradoxus should heighten concern for the presence of pericardial effusion.

DIAGNOSTIC FINDINGS
THORACIC RADIOGRAPHY

- Thoracic radiography is a valuable tool for the diagnostic evaluation of suspected pericardial effusion. In addition to facilitating a diagnosis of pericardial effusion in a number of cases, radiographs may demonstrate the presence of pulmonary metastases, radiopaque intrapericardial foreign bodies, or lymphadenomegaly.
- In patients with small to moderate volumes of pericardial effusion, as occur in cases of acute cardiac tamponade, the cardiac silhouette may be normal or variably enlarged; in fact, cardiomegaly may be absent in up to 48% of such cases. Pericardial effusion may remain undetected without additional diagnostic testing, such as echocardiography, in these cases.
- Radiographic signs that support a diagnosis of pericardial effusion include the following: (Figure 12.1):
  - An enlarged and rounded ("globoid") cardiac silhouette without evidence of specific chamber enlargement pattern(s)
  - Sharply delineated margins of the cardiac silhouette, attributable to the absence of significant motion during the cardiac cycle
  - Bilateral contact between the cardiac silhouette and thoracic wall on the dorsoventral or ventrodorsal projection
  - Signs consistent with right-sided congestive heart failure, including widening of the caudal vena cava, hepatomegaly, ascites, and small-volume pleural effusion
  - Reduced size of the pulmonary vasculature caused by pulmonary undercirculation

ELECTROCARDIOGRAPHY

- Electrocardiography has poor sensitivity for the detection of pericardial effusion. Most dogs with pericardial effusion have a normal sinus rhythm, often with sinus tachycardia.
- QRS complexes may be of low voltage (R wave amplitude <1 mV in all limb leads), a finding that is present in 50% to 57% of cases (Figure 12.2, *A, B*).
- Ventricular ectopy and, far less commonly, supraventricular tachycardia and atrial fibrillation may also be noted.

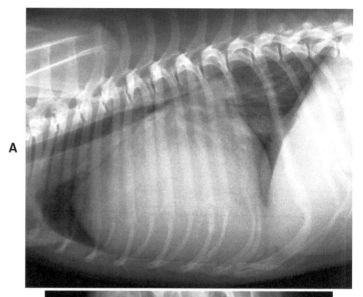

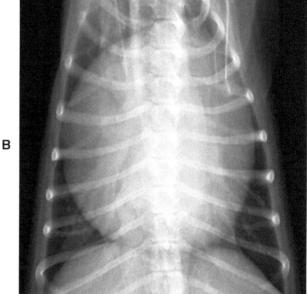

Figure 12.1 Thoracic radiographs from a dog with pericardial effusion. **A,** The lateral projection shows a markedly enlarged cardiac silhouette, tracheal elevation, and overlap of the cardiac silhouette and diaphragm. **B,** The ventrodorsal projection shows bilateral contact between the pericardial sac and the costal margins. The edge of the cardiac silhouette is sharply delineated, and the lung fields are clear of any infiltrate that would indicate the presence of left-sided congestive heart failure.

- *Electrical alternans,* defined by a beat-to-beat variation in the contour and amplitude of the QRS complex (Figure 12.2, *C*), is strongly suggestive of the presence of pericardial effusion. This phenomenon results from the to-and-fro swinging of the heart within the fluid-filled pericardial sac relative to stationary limb leads. Electrical alternans is present in only 20% to 64% of dogs with pericardial effusion.
- ST segment elevation is a well-described finding in the earliest stages of acute human pericarditis. Although mentioned in one study of canine pericardial effusion, ST segment change has not been well characterized in this species.

ECHOCARDIOGRAPHY

- Echocardiography is the most sensitive and specific noninvasive diagnostic tool for confirmation and semiquantitative estimation of pericardial effusion, in addition to allowing for characterization of its hemodynamic significance.
- With two-dimensional echocardiography, pericardial effusion is typically seen as a circumferential anechoic or hypoechoic space surrounding the heart, the size of which is proportional to the volume of effusion. In large volume pericardial effusions, the heart may "swing" freely within the pericardial space: this beat-to-beat change in cardiac position is responsible for the

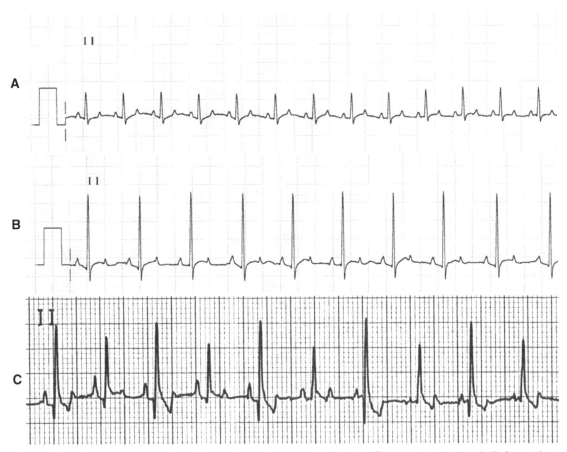

Figure 12.2 Electrocardiograms (lead II) from dogs with pericardial effusion. Calibration box, 1 mV. **A,** Before pericardiocentesis, the QRS complexes are of low voltage (R wave <1 mV) and heart rate is 140 beats/min. **B,** After pericardiocentesis, R wave amplitude is almost 2 mV and heart rate is 100 beats/min. **C,** Beat-to-beat variations in amplitude and contour of the QRS complexes characteristic of electrical alternans. (**A** and **B,** Modified from Tobias AH: Pericardial disorders. In Ettinger SJ, Feldman EC, eds: Textbook of veterinary internal medicine, ed 6, St Louis, 2005, Saunders. **C,** Courtesy Dr. Teresa DeFrancesco, Raleigh, N.C.)

surface electrocardiographic finding of electrical alternans.

- It is occasionally difficult to differentiate pericardial and pleural effusions; the former are characterized by a smooth, round outer contour, whereas the latter are more irregularly marginated. In cases with both pericardial and pleural effusion, the pericardium is easily perceived with fluid on either side.
- Echocardiographic evidence of cardiac tamponade is seen as collapse of the free wall of the right atrium or right ventricle during diastole. The right atrial free wall should be outwardly curved throughout the cardiac cycle, reflecting the normal positive transmural distending pressure. Although the right atrium normally contracts in volume with atrial systole, pronounced inversion or collapse of the right atrial free wall that persists throughout atrial diastole provides evidence of elevated intrapericardial pressure and transient reversal of transmural pressure

(Figure 12.3). In severe cases, the right ventricle may be affected as well, with echocardiographic signs ranging from transient and localized concavity of the right ventricular free wall to near-complete right ventricular chamber obliteration throughout diastole (see Figure 12.3).

- The left ventricular cavity may be reduced in size and its walls may be thickened during diastole, a consequence of decreased venous return to the left-sided cardiac chambers and the phenomenon of "pseudohypertrophy."
- In addition to confirming the presence and estimating the quantity of pericardial effusion, echocardiography is valuable for the detection of associated intrapericardial masses. Whereas histopathologic examination is necessary to confirm and definitively establish tumor type, the echocardiographic location and characteristics of an intrapericardial mass provide information about its most probable classification. This is particularly important given that

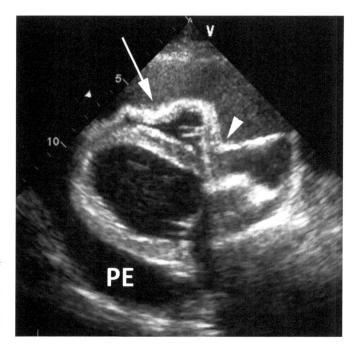

Figure 12.3   Echocardiographic evidence of tamponade in a dog with pericardial effusion (*PE*). This image was recorded from the right parasternal location and shows diastolic inversion of the right atrial (*arrowhead*) and right ventricular (*arrow*) walls.

prognoses associated with the various causes of pericardial effusion differ tremendously with tumor origin. Echocardiographic findings specific to the two most common tumor types identified in dogs are discussed in detail later.

- In a recent study, the reported sensitivity and specificity of echocardiography for detection of a cardiac mass of any type, when performed by a board-certified veterinary cardiologist or cardiologist in training, was 82% and 100%, respectively. With repeat examinations, sensitivity of this test increased to 88%. Older studies report sensitivity values ranging from 17% to 63%, and in a recent report on surgical outcomes in dogs with right atrial hemangiosarcoma (HSA) undergoing surgical resection, only 48% had a mass evident on echocardiography.

The presence of pericardial fluid facilitates the detection of intrapericardial masses, which is particularly relevant to the delineation of HSA and heart base tumors. Pericardial fluid forms an echolucent zone around the right atrium and auricle and the ascending aorta, the locations from which these tumors most commonly arise. In the absence of pericardial fluid, these locations are obscured by lung interference. *Consequently, whenever the clinical condition of the patient permits, pericardiocentesis should be deferred until a thorough echocardiographic examination has been completed.*

- Echocardiography may also demonstrate findings consistent with other less common underlying causes of pericardial effusion, including intrapericardial cysts, thrombi associated with left atrial perforation, and the presence of abdominal viscera within the pericardial sac in cases of peritoneopericardial diaphragmatic hernia.

ECHOCARDIOGRAPHIC FEATURES OF SPECIFIC TUMOR TYPES

CARDIAC HEMANGIOSARCOMA

- The positive and negative predictive values of echocardiography for detection of right atrial HSA vary from 92% to 100% and 64% to 87%, respectively; false-negative studies are therefore considered common.
- The following features are characteristic for cardiac HSA (Figure 12.4):
  - These tumors most commonly arise from the wall of the right atrium or right atrial appendage, protrude into the pericardial space, and move with the heart. They may also protrude into the right atrial lumen, spread to involve other areas of the heart base and pericardium, and involve the right atrioventricular groove.
  - Right atrial masses are usually visible from right parasternal echocardiographic windows. However, these tumors may be small and elusive. Imaging from left parasternal locations to provide alternate imaging planes, especially of the right auricle, is necessary to

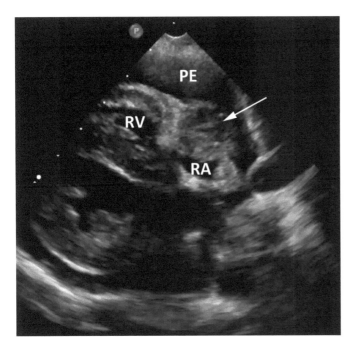

Figure 12.4 Echocardiographic image from a dog with cardiac hemangiosarcoma (HSA) recorded in the short-axis view from the right parasternal location. A cavitary and cystic mass *(arrow)* is associated with the right atrial *(RA)* wall. *PE*, Pericardial effusion; *RV*, right ventricle.

demonstrate the presence of HSA in some cases.

- HSA typically contains small hypoechoic spaces, giving the tumor a mottled or cavitary appearance, and these tumors are occasionally cystic.

HEART BASE TUMORS

- The reported positive and negative predictive values of echocardiography for detection of heart base tumors are 89% and 93%, respectively.
- The following features are characteristic for heart base tumors (Figure 12.5):
  - Heart base tumors are usually associated with the ascending aorta.
  - They vary from small ovoid structures attached to the ascending aorta to very extensive masses that surround the aorta and main pulmonary artery. Compression or invasion of the atria and major blood vessels may be seen.

ADVANCED IMAGING TECHNIQUES

- Advanced cross-sectional imaging modalities, including computed tomography (CT) and cardiac magnetic resonance (CMR), are used in cases of human pericardial effusion as superior means for characterization of cardiac tumors. CMR is considered a gold standard for evaluating pericardial disease and cardiac masses in human patients. Currently, these tools are not widely used, nor have they been extensively evaluated, in veterinary patients with pericardial effusion.

- Recently, the diagnostic utility of multidetector CT was evaluated in 11 dogs with naturally occurring pericardial effusion. Although CT did not improve the investigators' ability to detect cardiac tumors over echocardiography, it did expose noncardiac metastatic and concurrent neoplastic disease, offering a potential advantage over traditional techniques by allowing more complete disease staging. Because histopathologic analysis was not performed on all dogs, sensitivity and specificity of the technique could not be determined from this study.

- The utility of CMR for enhancing the detection of cardiac masses has also been evaluated in a small number of dogs with pericardial effusion. In these cases, CMR was not able to substantially improve the diagnosis of cardiac tumors over echocardiography. However, the authors did describe a significant learning curve and suggested that with substantial training, the accuracy of this modality may improve.

- Future studies may elucidate a benefit of these modalities in cases of pericardial effusion in which a cardiac mass is not detected or findings are equivocal with transthoracic echocardiography alone.

PERICARDIAL FLUID ANALYSIS

- Pericardial effusions in dogs are nearly always hemorrhagic or serosanguineous, sterile, inflammatory exudate, irrespective of cause.

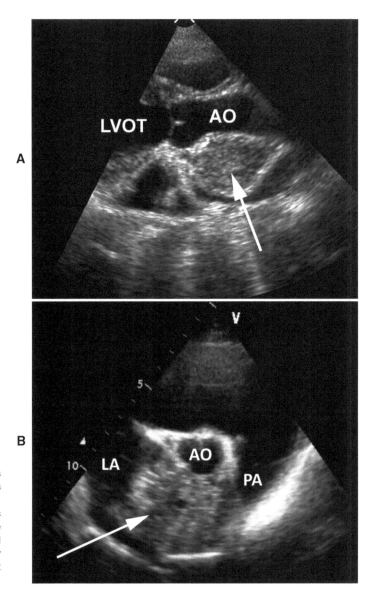

Figure 12.5 Echocardiographic images from two dogs with heart base tumors recorded from the left parasternal location. **A**, A large homogeneous mass *(arrow)* is seen adjacent to the caudal aspect of the aorta *(AO)*. **B**, A similar well-circumscribed mass is noted between the AO, pulmonary artery *(PA)*, and left atrium *(LA)*. *LVOT*, Left ventricular outflow tract.

- Total nucleated cell count, red cell count, protein concentration, pH, and lactate of pericardial fluid overlap extensively between the various neoplastic and non-neoplastic causes of pericardial effusion. Therefore these characteristics are rarely useful in establishing etiology.
- Cytologic examination is also typically unrewarding for distinguishing between potential causes of pericardial effusion. In fact, fluid analysis is able to establish an etiologic diagnosis in only 7.7% to 12.8% of cases. In a recent study, the diagnostic utility of cytologic examination was found to increase to 20.3% in cases with an effusate hematocrit <10%, reflecting a threefold increased chance of obtaining a diagnosis in these cases.
- The most common tumor types associated with pericardial effusions in dogs, HSA and aortic body tumors (ABTs), are poorly exfoliating and therefore associated with a high incidence of false-negative cytologic diagnoses. Further, pericardial diseases that lead to effusion often result in dramatic mesothelial proliferation, with exfoliated reactive mesothelial cells often bearing characteristics that mimic malignancy. For these reasons, a fluid cytologic evaluation must be interpreted very cautiously.
- Nonetheless, some of the less common causes of pericardial effusion, such as infectious pericarditis and lymphosarcoma, are diagnosed primarily on the basis of pericardial fluid cytologic evaluation. Consequently, we submit pericardial fluid for analysis in all cases, despite the generally low diagnostic yield of this test.

- Pericardial effusion should be cultured in cases in which an infectious cause is suspected on the basis of a cytologic examination.

INITIAL PATIENT STABILIZATION: PERICARDIOCENTESIS

- Pericardiocentesis is life-saving in cases of pericardial effusion that are associated with significant hemodynamic compromise caused by cardiac tamponade. This procedure is performed in an effort to remove as much fluid from the pericardial space as possible and to obtain fluid samples for diagnostic purposes.
- Medical interventions are rarely successful in resolving signs of symptomatic pericardial effusion and should be used alone only while preparations for pericardiocentesis are made. Fluid resuscitation may provide transient benefit by supporting systemic venous return, particularly in acute tamponade associated with hemorrhage, and is usually administered rapidly through the intravenous route. The exception to this is in animals with hemopericardium caused by rupture of the left atrium.
- The most serious potential complications of pericardiocentesis include laceration or perforation of the myocardium or coronary vasculature. Additional risks include the development of life-threatening ventricular arrhythmias or pneumothorax.
- We prefer to hospitalize cases for 12 to 24 hours following pericardiocentesis to monitor for signs of potential complications or rapid re-effusion.

APPROACH TO PERICARDIOCENTESIS

- Our preferred approach is to restrain the animal in left lateral or sternal recumbency and to approach the pericardium from the right side. This technique avoids the major coronary arteries, reducing the risk of laceration, and provides a lung-free window through the cardiac notch.
- Dogs usually tolerate pericardiocentesis without sedation; however, it may be necessary in

some cases. We prefer to administer butorphanol (0.1 to 0.2 mg/kg intravenously [IV]) when mild sedation is required.

- Continuous electrocardiographic monitoring should be performed during pericardiocentesis because ventricular arrhythmias commonly occur because of contact between the catheter and epicardium and may require treatment. For this reason, we prefer to have 1 to 2 preprepared doses (2 mg/kg of body weight) of 2% lidocaine available for administration, if needed.
- We prefer a 14-gauge or 16-gauge over-the-needle catheter system to perform pericardiocentesis in dogs, although through-the-needle catheters are also effective. With the former system, two small side holes may be made near the tip of the catheter to minimize the chance of obstruction or aspiration of the myocardium against a single end hole. The catheter system is coupled to a large volume syringe via an extension tube and a three-way stopcock.
- The right thorax is shaved, and with ultrasound guidance, a location that provides the shortest distance between the pericardium and chest wall without intervening lung tissue is chosen as the ideal site for entry. If ultrasound is not available, thoracic radiographs can be used to identify the ideal intercostal space. This usually corresponds to the fifth or sixth intercostal space, just ventral to the costochondral junction.
- The skin, intercostal muscles, and parietal pleura are infiltrated with 2% lidocaine, and the area is surgically prepared.
- A small stab incision is made in the skin (Figure 12.6, A), and the catheter system is advanced towards the pericardium, maintaining an orientation perpendicular to the body wall (Figure 12.6, B). During advancement, slight negative pressure is applied and maintained with the syringe and extension tube; this allows the operator to detect access to the pericardial space by observing fluid movement into the extension tubing and syringe.
- The catheter is then advanced over the needle into the pericardial space, with care taken to immobilize the stylet to avoid inadvertent laceration of the heart (Figure 12.6, C). The stylet is removed, the extension tube is connected to the catheter (Figure 12.6, D), and a small amount of fluid is aspirated (Figure 12.6, E).
- Pericardial fluid is typically hemorrhagic in appearance. For confirmation that the tip of the catheter is in the pericardial space and not within a cardiac chamber, an aliquot of fluid is placed in an activated clotting time tube. Blood will normally clot in an activated clotting time

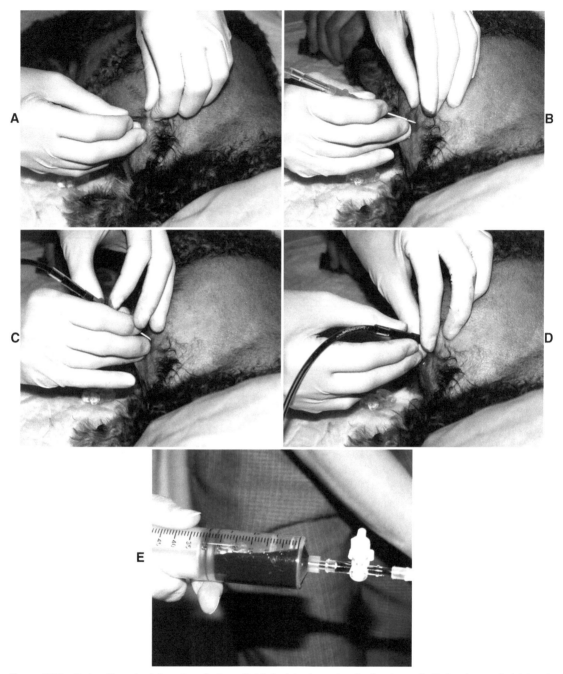

Figure 12.6   Pericardiocentesis in a dog. **A,** A small skin incision is made after local anesthetic has been administered. **B,** An over-the-needle catheter system with two side holes is advanced toward the pericardium. Slight negative pressure is applied with a syringe coupled to the needle by extension tubing. **C,** Pericardial fluid flows into the extension tubing, and the catheter is advanced over the needle into the pericardial space. **D,** The extension tubing is removed from the needle and coupled to the catheter. **E,** Pericardial effusion is aspirated.

tube within 60 to 90 seconds. In contrast, hemorrhagic effusions in body cavities are rapidly depleted of clotting factors and thrombocytes so that pericardial fluid should not clot. If no clots form within the activated clotting tube, samples are collected for fluid analysis and

culture, and all of the pericardial fluid is aspirated. The catheter is then removed.

• In virtually all cases with pericardial effusion, pericardiocentesis results in rapid and marked hemodynamic improvement; this is manifested as improvement in clinical signs, pulse quality, and mucous membrane perfusion, and a decline in heart rate.

CHRONIC MANAGEMENT OF RECURRENT PERICARDIAL EFFUSION

The approach to the chronic management of pericardial effusion varies with the underlying cause; the value of identifying its likely cause by use of echocardiography, if possible, is emphasized.

CONSERVATIVE MANAGEMENT

- In 21% to 50% of dogs with idiopathic pericardial effusion (IPE), long-term resolution is achieved after a single pericardiocentesis.
- Intermittent pericardiocentesis may be used to palliate clinical signs in dogs with recurrent effusion. The reported median survival time of 6 dogs with IPE treated conservatively with repeated pericardiocentesis was 1834 days; in this group, a median of 2.5 (range, 2 to 11) treatments was required. Despite these results, there is concern for the eventual development of constrictive or effusive-constrictive pericarditis with this approach. Some authors, therefore, recommend pericardiectomy (surgical removal of the pericardial sac) in all dogs with recurrent pericardial effusion to avoid this potential complication.

PERICARDIECTOMY

- Pericardiectomy is indicated in cases of recurrent pericardial effusion that are *not* associated with disorders of active bleeding (i.e., not associated with HSA, left atrial rupture, or hypocoagulable states). Significant survival benefit of pericardiectomy has been demonstrated in patients with IPE and pericardial effusion associated with ABTs; however, survival time is not significantly improved in those with cardiac HSA treated with this approach alone.
- Removal of all or a portion of the pericardium decreases its surface area, thereby reducing fluid production in disease states in which it directly participates. Furthermore, this procedure creates a connection between the pericardial and pleural spaces. Because of the larger resorptive surface area of the latter, fluid reaccumulation is generally avoided.
- Direct examination during pericardiectomy allows the surgeon to identify any previously undetected masses in equivocal or presumed idiopathic cases. In addition, diagnostic samples of the pericardium and any identified masses may be obtained.
- The most common technique for pericardiectomy is the subphrenic (subtotal) technique, whereby the pericardium is transected just ventral to the phrenic nerves bilaterally. This is performed directly through a median sternotomy or lateral thoracotomy; alternatively, thoracoscopic techniques, although technically challenging, may be used. Perioperative mortality rate for surgical subtotal pericardiectomy is approximately 13%.
- Less invasive approaches for pericardial resection or fenestration, including thoracoscopic techniques and balloon pericardiotomy, have been described in dogs with neoplastic and nonneoplastic pericardial effusion.
  - Thoracoscopic techniques provide theoretical advantages over open-chest approaches, including less tissue trauma and superior visualization (afforded by magnification and illumination), and they are associated with less postoperative pain. Pericardial window techniques, by which a small (at least 3 cm × 3 cm) portion of the pericardium is excised, have been described; however, it appears that the creation of a window is likely inferior to subphrenic techniques for cases of IPE, as discussed later.
- Percutaneous balloon pericardiotomy may be a reasonable alternative to more invasive techniques in dogs with recurrent effusion, although this procedure has been associated with stoma closure and recurrence of pericardial effusion in some cases.

SPECIFIC CAUSES OF PERICARDIAL EFFUSIONS: EPIDEMIOLOGY, MANAGEMENT, AND PROGNOSIS

NEOPLASTIC CAUSES

Neoplastic diseases are the most common causes of clinically significant pericardial effusion. Of these, cardiac HSA, chemodectoma (ABT), mesothelioma, and ectopic thyroid carcinoma are reported with the greatest frequency. In general, dogs with neoplastic effusions tend to have a worse prognosis than those dogs with effusions due to nonneoplastic causes. Cardiac tumors are not always associated with the presence of pericardial effusion; they may cause clinical signs by obstructing blood flow within the heart or great vessels or by impairing myocardial contractile function. Neoplastic diseases most commonly associated with pericardial effusion are discussed later.

CARDIAC HEMANGIOSARCOMA
DESCRIPTION AND DIAGNOSTIC FEATURES

- HSA, a highly aggressive and malignant neoplasm of vascular endothelium or hematopoietic precursor cells, is the most commonly diagnosed canine cardiac tumor. In this species, it occurs with a nearly tenfold greater incidence than does the ABT, the second most common cardiac neoplasm. Cardiac HSA also represents the most common cause of symptomatic canine pericardial effusion.

- Cardiac HSA is most often associated with the right atrial free wall/right atrial appendage, comprising the majority (88%) of masses affecting the right atrium. However, this tumor may also occur at other cardiac locations, including the heart base.
- These tumors produce pericardial effusion and cardiac tamponade when they rupture, rapidly bleeding into the pericardial space. Often the effusion is of small or moderate volume when clinical signs associated with cardiac tamponade manifest.
- HSA is a highly metastatic disease and by the time of diagnosis should be considered systemic. Among dogs with cardiac HSA presenting to a referral center for signs attributable to cardiac tamponade, the prevalence of detectable, concurrent, noncardiac HSA is approximately 55%. Two necropsy-based studies of dogs dying or euthanized because of HSA-related pericardial effusion found similar metastatic rates of 68% to 75%.

EPIDEMIOLOGY

- Pericardial effusion associated with cardiac HSA tends to affect older, large-breed dogs, with a mean and median age at the time of diagnosis of approximately 9 years (range, 3 to 13) and a mean body weight of 32 kg.
- Reported breed predispositions for HSA include Golden Retriever and German Shepard dogs.
- No clear gender predilection for cardiac HSA has been reported, although within gender, intact dogs, particularly females, appear to be at greater risk for development of these tumors.

TREATMENT AND PROGNOSIS

- The presence of cardiac HSA confers a grave long-term prognosis.
- Many owners of dogs with cardiac HSA choose palliation with pericardiocentesis alone. Pericardiocentesis is predictably associated with marked clinical improvement; however, clinical signs of tamponade typically recur within a few days or weeks, often resulting in death or prompting euthanasia. Median survival time for dogs with pericardial effusion due to

HSA, treated with either pericardiocentesis or pericardiectomy alone, is approximately 16 days.

- Pericardiectomy alone is not associated with survival benefit in dogs with cardiac HSA and pericardial effusion. This may be due to the fact that removal of the pericardium increases the risk of exsanguination.
- More aggressive approaches to the treatment of cardiac HSA include various combinations of tumor resection, pericardiectomy, and chemotherapy.
  - Various authors have noted median survival times of 42 days to 4 months in dogs treated by mass resection alone.
  - Adjuvant chemotherapy after tumor resection may prolong survival in dogs with cardiac HSA. A retrospective study of 23 dogs with right atrial HSA in which tumor resection and pericardiectomy was performed reported a median survival time of 56 days in all dogs. However, eight dogs receiving adjuvant chemotherapy lived significantly longer than those who did not, with median survival times of 175 days and 42 days, respectively. In this study, no dog lived >7.6 months.
  - A recent report retrospectively examined the use of doxorubicin-based chemotherapy protocols alone for the treatment of right atrial masses presumed to be HSA on the basis of echocardiography. These patients did not undergo pericardiectomy or mass resection, and only one had histopathologic confirmation of tumor type. Median survival time in this population was 139 days (range, 2 to 302).
- Management of cardiac HSA should always include consultation with a veterinary oncologist to take advantage of continually evolving and emerging modalities for the treatment of this highly malignant tumor.

HEART BASE TUMORS
DESCRIPTION AND DIAGNOSTIC FEATURES

- The term *heart base tumor* is used to designate any mass located at the base of the heart in association with the great vessels.
- Most heart base tumors in dogs are ABTs (also known as aortic body chemodectoma and nonchromaffin paraganglioma), although other tumor types are reported in this location. These include HSA, tumors arising from ectopic thyroid tissue, and mesothelioma, which may account for up to 35%, 26%, and 17% of heart base tumors, respectively.
- ABTs are neuroepithelial in origin, arising from the chemoreceptor cells of the aortic bodies,

small clusters of cells situated within the adventitia of the aortic root. These cells respond to alterations in blood oxygen and carbon dioxide tensions and pH by modifying respiration and blood pressure.

- ABTs tend to be slowly growing and locally expansive, although local invasion and metastasis do occur. In one study, metastasis was noted in 50% of cases at the time of necropsy, with the lungs, spleen, and liver being the sites most commonly affected.
- Clinical signs associated with ABT are typically related to the development of pericardial effusion or to compression of adjacent structures. ABT may be noted as incidental findings in patients undergoing echocardiography or thoracic radiography for other indications. These tumors are nonfunctional and so are not associated with cardiovascular disruption through mechanisms other than those described above.

EPIDEMIOLOGY

- Despite being the second most common cardiac tumor in dogs, the incidence of ABT is approximately tenfold lower than that of cardiac HSA, accounting for approximately 8% of all cardiac tumors.
- Brachycephalic breeds, the English Bulldog, Boxer, and Boston Terrier, in particular, are predisposed to ABTs, although dogs of nonbrachycephalic breeds may be affected as well. In various studies, brachycephalic breeds have accounted for 39% to 85% of dogs with ABTs. It has been postulated that the chronic hypoxia experienced by dogs of these breeds may explain this predisposition; in both dogs and humans, chronic hypoxia is known to induce hyperplasia of the chemoreceptor organs.
- Among the predisposed breeds, males may be at increased risk of having ABTs, but differences in sex predisposition are not statistically significant in all studies.
- Median age at time of diagnosis of ABTs is 9 years (range, 7 to 12).

TREATMENT AND PROGNOSIS

- Complete surgical resection of heart base tumors is seldom possible because the tumors are highly vascular, invariably located close to major blood vessels, and usually extensive by the time of diagnosis.
- Palliation with pericardiectomy alone often results in prolonged survival with an excellent quality of life in dogs with ABT.

- In one study, median survival times among dogs with biopsy-confirmed ABT was 730 days in those undergoing subtotal pericardiectomy at the time of surgical biopsy and only 42 days in those not treated with pericardiectomy.
- Curiously, the survival benefit conferred by this procedure was enjoyed regardless of whether pericardial effusion was present at the time of diagnosis. The authors suggested that pericardiectomy might act to prolong the time to onset of clinical signs, avoiding early euthanasia at the time of cardiac tamponade development. Indeed, 8 of the 10 dogs not undergoing pericardiectomy were euthanized because of persistent or progressive pericardial effusion.
- External-beam radiation therapy may provide an additional treatment option for dogs with ABTs, especially those with compressive effects of these tumors. There is a paucity of available data regarding the safety and efficacy of this treatment option in veterinary patients. The authors of a single case report describe the use of radiation therapy for a dog with progressive cough related to a large ABT; improvement in the cough and a 50% reduction in tumor volume were noted at 25 months after treatment, and the dog was alive 3.5 years after diagnosis despite the need for pericardiectomy and additional radiation therapy.

MESOTHELIOMA

DESCRIPTION AND DIAGNOSTIC FEATURES

- Mesothelioma, a malignant neoplasm that affects the epithelial cells lining the serosal surfaces of body cavities (including the pericardial space) is emerging as an increasingly important cause of pericardial effusion. In recent studies, mesothelioma has been responsible for up to 21% of neoplastic pericardial effusions identified.
- Mesothelioma represents a significant diagnostic challenge because differentiation from IPE (see later) is often very difficult, even when histopathologic analysis of the pericardium is possible.
  - Three (43%) of seven dogs with an ultimate diagnosis of mesothelioma were misclassified as having IPE on initial biopsy in one study.
  - Typically a diffuse neoplasm, mesothelioma is only infrequently associated with the presence of a discrete mass, which further complicates its differentiation from IPE on the basis of echocardiographic findings. When a discrete mass is noted, it most often manifests as a heart base tumor.
- The clinical course of a patient with mesothelioma can be very helpful in determining the

origin of the effusion. The accumulation of significant amounts of unrelenting pleural effusion within 4 to 6 months of pericardiectomy should increase the index of suspicion for mesothelioma in a dog that previously received a diagnosis of IPE.

EPIDEMIOLOGY

- Mesothelioma is most common among older dogs of all sizes. Mean age among affected cases at the time of presentation was 8.6 years (range, 4 to 14) in one study, with both genders equally represented.
- Breed predispositions have not been widely suggested, although one report has described the eventual development of pericardial mesothelioma in five Golden Retrievers that received long-term treatment with intermittent pericardiocentesis for presumed IPE.

TREATMENT AND PROGNOSIS

- The long-term prognosis for dogs with pericardial effusion caused by mesothelioma is grave.
- Pericardiectomy, with or without adjuvant chemotherapy, may be used to palliate signs of cardiac tamponade in dogs with mesothelioma. Ultimately, in the vast majority of cases, dogs undergoing pericardiectomy die or are euthanized because of the development of severe, recurrent pleural effusion that requires frequent thoracocentesis to alleviate clinical signs.
- Adjuvant chemotherapy may prolong survival in these cases, although additional studies are needed to confirm this.
  - In one study of 8 dogs with mesothelioma, for which a median survival time of 60 days (range, 15 to 300) was reported, only dogs receiving chemotherapy lived >120 days; the dog who survived the longest (300 days) was treated with pericardiectomy, doxorubicin, and intracavitary cisplatin.
  - In another study of five dogs with mesothelioma that underwent pericardiectomy, of which three also were treated with adjuvant chemotherapy, median survival time was 13.6 months.
  - Long-term survival has been reported in a dog in which a histopathologic diagnosis of pericardial mesothelioma was made after pericardiectomy for recurrent pericardial effusion. Treatment was initiated 48 hours after surgery with intracavitary cisplatin and intravenous doxorubicin, and the dog was disease free 27 months later.

Pericardial mesothelioma represents both a diagnostic and therapeutic challenge. Unlike other cardiac tumors, mesothelioma does not typically form discrete tumor masses that are readily detectable with echocardiography. Even with pericardial biopsy and histopathologic analysis, the diagnosis may be elusive, and only after recurrent pleural or pericardial effusions result in mortality and postmortem examination is the diagnosis confirmed in many cases.

OTHER CARDIAC TUMORS

- Cardiac lymphoma, rhabdomyosarcoma, and fibrosarcoma with pericardial effusion have been reported in both dogs and cats.
- Cardiac lymphoma is diagnosed in approximately 1% of dogs with pericardial effusion. Among the various cardiac tumors, cardiac lymphoma is unique because cytologic evaluation of the pericardial fluid establishes the diagnosis in many cases. Treatment with adjuvant chemotherapy, with or without pericardiectomy, appears to increase survival time; in one study of 12 dogs with pericardial effusion due to cardiac lymphoma, the median survival times of dogs receiving (n = 5) or not receiving (n = 7) adjuvant chemotherapy were 157 days and 22 days, respectively.
- An 18-month-old dog with an intrapericardial lipoma, pericardial effusion, and cardiac tamponade has also been reported.

IDIOPATHIC PERICARDIAL EFFUSION

DESCRIPTION AND DIAGNOSTIC FEATURES

- IPE, also referred to as idiopathic hemorrhagic pericardial effusion, idiopathic pericardial hemorrhage, and idiopathic pericarditis, is a diagnosis of exclusion, made in cases in which no intrapericardial masses are identified after thorough echocardiographic evaluation or exploratory surgery, and the results of ancillary tests such as pericardial fluid analysis fail to disclose etiology.
- As with any idiopathic disease, the diagnosis should be made with caution.
  - Small intrapericardial tumors may elude detection, especially in cases where echocardiography is performed following pericardiocentesis.
  - As discussed previously, mesothelioma should always be considered an important differential diagnosis for IPE.
- Pericardial histopathologic examination from dogs with IPE demonstrates changes consistent

with pericarditis of undetermined etiology. Pericardial tissue from dogs with IPE may exhibit a spectrum of changes that include extensive fibrosis, mixed inflammatory cell infiltrate, and perivascular lymphoplasmacytic aggregates, nonspecific findings that are often indistinguishable from those seen in dogs with neoplastic pericardial effusion.

- An immune-mediated autoreactive process has been identified in certain cases of human idiopathic pericarditis; however, immunohisto-chemistry-based investigations in dogs have not clearly identified a similar process.

EPIDEMIOLOGY

- IPE is the second most common cause of hemo-dynamically significant pericardial effusion, accounting for 19% to 45% of cases and second only to cardiac HSA in most reports.
- Middle-aged large or middle-aged giant dogs (mean body weight, 29 to 35 kg) appear to be predisposed to the development of IPE, with some, but not all, authors noting a male gender predilection.
- In general, dogs with IPE tend to be younger at the time of presentation than dogs with neo-plastic pericardial effusion, with a median age of approximately 6 to 7.9 years (range, 2 to 14 years) described over various studies, although there was no age difference between dogs with IPE and mesothelioma in one report.
- Breeds that appear to be predisposed to IPE include the Golden Retriever, Saint Bernard and Great Dane. Saint Bernards with symp-tomatic pericardial effusion are reportedly diagnosed at a younger age than the other commonly represented breeds (mean age, 2.6 years).

TREATMENT AND PROGNOSIS

- In 21% to 50% of dogs with IPE, long-term res-olution is achieved following a single pericardi-ocentesis. In the remainder, time to recurrence is variable but typically occurs within one year (median, 16 weeks; range, 1 to 250 weeks).
- In dogs with recurrent large-volume pericardial effusion due to IPE, intermittent pericardio-centesis has been used to palliate clinical signs. In one study that described the use of intermit-tent pericardiocentesis in six dogs managed conservatively for recurrent PE, a median sur-vival time of 5 years was noted, with a median of 2.5 (range, 2 to 11) treatments required. Other authors have observed median survival times of 3 to 4.5 years in dogs treated with pericardio-centesis alone.

- Despite these encouraging results, many clini-cians, including us, recommend treating first episodes of IPE with pericardiocentesis, fol-lowed by pericardiectomy in cases that develop recurrent effusion.
  - This recommendation is based on a desire to reduce the risk for recurrent life-threatening tamponade and the potential for development of constrictive or effusive-constrictive pericar-ditis, a serious complication that has been noted in association with long-standing IPE.
  - Furthermore, surgical pericardiectomy per-mits examination of thoracic and intraperi-cardial structures to rule out other causes of pericardial effusion, such as previously unde-tected tumors or foreign bodies.
- Pericardiectomy significantly improves survival times in dogs with IPE. In most studies in which the use of this treatment was examined, median survival time could not be accurately ascer-tained because most dogs were still living at the time of writing; however, among eight dogs with IPE undergoing subtotal pericardiectomy in one report, there was a 100% chance of survival at 2 years after the procedure.
  - Subtotal (subphrenic) techniques appear to be superior to pericardial window tech-niques for the treatment of dogs with IPE, with significantly longer median survival time and disease-free intervals noted with the former. This may be due to the higher risk of inaccurate diagnosis or "healing" of the pericardium to the epicardium (reseal-ing the pericardial space and allowing recurrence of pericardial effusion) with the window technique.

KEY POINT

Prognosis is very good in dogs with recurrent IPE that undergo pericardiectomy and survive the perioperative period.

- Nonsteroidal antiinflammatories, with or with-out colchicine, are routinely prescribed to humans with idiopathic pericarditis. Colchi-cine, when used as an adjunctive therapy, has proven effective in reducing the number of recurrences in these patients, although use of this drug may be limited in some by the development of gastrointestinal side effects. In severe cases or in patients who fail to respond to these measures, systemic corticosteroids may also be prescribed; however, in general, corti-costeroids are avoided in the absence of known autoimmune disease because there is evidence that they may increase the incidence of relapse.

The safety and efficacy of colchicine, nonsteroidal antiinflammatories, corticosteroids, and any other medical therapies in the management of IPE in small animals have yet to be established.

LEFT ATRIAL RUPTURE

DESCRIPTION AND DIAGNOSTIC FEATURES

- Left atrial rupture (also known as left atrial perforation, left atrial tear, and left atrial splitting) is an uncommon cause of pericardial effusion that occurs as a complication of severe, chronic degenerative valve disease. Affected animals have advanced mitral valve disease that includes significant left atrial dilatation.
- Pericardial effusion results from linear splits of the left atrial endocardial and myocardial layers, with dissecting hemorrhage and perforation of the epicardium.
- Affected patients have a history consistent with acute pericardial effusion, with most owners reporting an acute onset of generalized weakness or collapse. Sudden death may occur as well; 4 (30%) of 11 dogs with left atrial rupture in one study had cardiopulmonary (3) or pulmonary (1) arrest.
- A loud left apical systolic murmur is usually apparent, even if muffling of the heart sounds is noted.
- Typical echocardiographic findings include small- to moderate-volume pericardial fluid with a hyperechoic, mobile thrombus within the pericardial space, severe mitral insufficiency, and enlargement of the left atrium.
- The findings of necropsy-based studies suggest that ruptured mitral valve chordae tendineae are frequently noted in dogs with left atrial rupture; therefore it has been postulated that chordal rupture may be an important acute event that precipitates left atrial rupture through creation of a sudden rise in left atrial pressure. This observation may also help to explain the frequent concurrence of acute cardiogenic pulmonary edema in these patients at the time of diagnosis (57% in one retrospective report), which is unexpected in the setting of cardiac tamponade and in clear contrast to other causes of pericardial effusion.
- Left atrial rupture should be suspected in small dog breeds with a history of advanced mitral valve disease or a heart murmur on physical examination that experience an episode of weakness or collapse and in which pericardial effusion, especially with evidence of blood clot formation, is present on echocardiography. In some cases, the dog may be recovering or even clinically normal at the time of evaluation, and relatively little pericardial fluid may be present.

EPIDEMIOLOGY

- Dogs affected by left atrial rupture are typically older, small dog breeds with chronic degenerative mitral valve disease.
- In two recent retrospective studies, median age was 11.6 to 12 years (range, 5.8 to 19 years) and median body weight was 5.8 to 11 kg (range, 4 to 30 kg).

TREATMENT AND PROGNOSIS

- Reported survival times for dogs affected by left atrial rupture vary considerably, although the long-term prognosis for this condition is considered poor, in general.
- In a retrospective study of 14 dogs with left atrial rupture that were seen at a referral emergency service, only 5 dogs (36%) survived to discharge, with the majority of the nonsurvivors being either dead at the time of arrival or euthanized during hospitalization. However, as the investigators note, there was likely selection bias in this study because five of the dogs included were identified through a necropsy database.
- In contrast, the authors of a recent retrospective study of 11 dogs with left atrial rupture noted a median survival time of 203 days (range, 0 to 760 days). Four of the 10 dogs did not require hospitalization, and each of the 10 dogs that survived the first 24 hours after diagnosis lived at least 30 days. The authors note the possibility of selection bias in their survival results, as well because only dogs stable enough to undergo echocardiography were included. However, these findings illustrate the fact that a number of dogs affected by left atrial rupture can survive the hemodynamic insult of left atrial rupture.
- For cases in which the patient is recovering or clinically normal after an episode of collapse, no specific therapy is necessary, other than congestive heart failure medications, if appropriate (i.e., for those dogs with concurrent left-sided congestive heart failure). In these cases, complete resolution of both the pericardial effusion and the intrapericardial thrombus is often noted at recheck in 7 to 14 days.
- Pericardiocentesis is required for cases with hemodynamic compromise as a result of tamponade. As the possibility of continued hemorrhage exists, blood transfusion and repeated pericardiocentesis may be necessary, with thoracotomy to remove larger clots from the pericardial space and to repair the left atrium in the most severe of cases; the prognosis in such instances is grave.

HYPOCOAGULABLE CONDITIONS

- Pericardial effusions secondary to coagulation disorders are rare causes of clinically significant tamponade.
- Two cases of pericardial effusion and cardiac tamponade secondary to anticoagulant rodenticide toxicity have been reported in the dog; both were successfully treated with pericardiocentesis, vitamin K_1 therapy, and supportive care.
- We routinely measure coagulation parameters in patients in which an intrapericardial mass is not identified with echocardiography.

INFECTIOUS CAUSES

- Bacterial and fungal infections are occasionally associated with pericardial effusions in dogs, accounting for up to 8.5% of cases of pericardial effusion in some parts of the United States.
- Many cases of septic pericardial effusion associated with bacterial pathogens arise or are thought to arise from intrapericardial foreign body penetration, usually by migrating foxtails (*Hordeum* species). A perforating esophageal foreign body was responsible in one reported case. In contrast to most other causes of pericardial effusion, pericardial fluid cytologic and culture results are crucial for the diagnosis of infectious cases.
- In the largest series of bacterial pericarditis reported in dogs (5 cases), treatment involved pericardiectomy and removal of foreign bodies, chest drainage, and antibiotic therapy for up to 6 months. All dogs recovered without complications, suggesting that dogs with bacterial pericarditis have a good prognosis when treated aggressively with a combination of surgical and medical therapy.
- Systemic coccidioidomycosis in dogs has been associated with the development of effusive-constrictive pericarditis. Coccidioidomycosis should be considered in young large dog breeds with pericardial thickening and effusion that reside in or have a travel history that includes areas where the soil fungus *Coccidioides immitis* is endemic, such as the southwestern United States.
  - Treatment involves pericardiectomy (with or without epicardial excision), chest drainage, and antifungal therapy.
  - On the basis of limited published information, the prognosis for cases of coccidioidomycosis with pericardial involvement is guarded. In one case series that examined outcomes in 17 dogs treated with pericardiectomy and epicardial excision, perioperative mortality was 23.5%. However, in dogs that survived to discharge and for which follow-up was available, 82% survived at least 2 years after surgery.
  - A single case of effusive-constrictive pericarditis caused by *Aspergillus niger* has been reported in a dog.

MISCELLANEOUS CAUSES OF PERICARDIAL EFFUSION

- Right-sided congestive heart failure and uremia are known to cause small-volume pericardial effusion in dogs; however, the effusion is typically not of sufficient volume to cause hemodynamic compromise.
- A case of cholesterol-based pericardial effusion has been reported in a dog with hypothyroidism and cardiac tamponade.
- Intrapericardial granulation tissue, mimicking a tumor and likely representing a resolving hematoma or abscess, was diagnosed in an 8-month-old dog with a 2-week history of lethargy and increased respiratory effort.

FELINE PERICARDIAL EFFUSION

- Hemodynamically significant pericardial effusion rarely occurs in cats. Instead, pericardial effusion in this species occurs most commonly in association with congestive heart failure, is of small volume, and does not produce cardiac tamponade. Consequently, these effusions are rarely the primary cause for presenting signs; in a study examining 146 cats with pericardial effusion, only 3 (2%) had effusions that where characterized as greater than mild.
- In addition to congestive heart failure, diseases associated with pericardial effusion in cats include the following:
  - Neoplastic diseases, including lymphoma and metastatic carcinoma. Thymoma, mesothelioma, primary and metastatic cardiac HSA, and ABTs are rare but reported causes of pericardial effusion in cats.
  - Uremia.
  - Feline infectious peritonitis.
  - Disseminated intravascular coagulation.
  - Warfarin toxicity.
- IPE has not been reported in cats.

CONSTRICTIVE PERICARDIAL DISEASE

DESCRIPTION AND DIAGNOSTIC FEATURES

- Constrictive pericardial disease (also known as constrictive pericarditis) is a rare condition in small animals, thought in most cases to be a complication of chronic pericardial inflammation. The term *effusive-constrictive pericardial disease* has been used to distinguish those cases in which pericardial effusion is also present.

- Pericardial constriction occurs when a thickened, fibrotic pericardium impairs cardiac filling and limits total diastolic volume by creating a noncompliant "shell" in which the heart is encased. The hallmark of constrictive pericarditis is rapid early ventricular diastolic filling that abruptly halts when the limit of ventricular distensibility is reached, a point that is set by the constraining pericardium.
- Signs of right-sided congestive heart failure dominate the clinical picture of patients affected by constrictive pericardial disease, and these patients may also have tachypnea, weakness, syncope, weight loss, and diminished exercise tolerance.
- Constrictive pericardial disease is most often idiopathic, but it has also been associated with the following:
  - Infectious agents, including *C. immitis*, *Actinomyces* organisms, *Mycobacterium* organisms, and *A. niger*
  - Chronic, recurrent IPE
  - Metallic foreign bodies
  - Osseous metaplasia
- Constrictive pericardial disease represents a significant diagnostic challenge. The disease is suspected in patients with signs of right-sided congestive heart failure in which other causes have been ruled out. Although echocardiographic findings may support the diagnosis, the most reliable proof of pericardial constriction is obtained by documenting characteristic abnormalities on invasive catheter-based hemodynamic studies.

EPIDEMIOLOGY

Medium- to large-breed dogs of various ages seem to be predisposed to the development of constrictive pericardial disease. Mean age in one study was 6.6 years (range, 2.5 to 9.5 years).

TREATMENT AND PROGNOSIS

- Treatment of constrictive pericardial disease consists of surgical pericardiectomy. In many cases, the visceral pericardium (epicardium) is spared or only minimally affected, and removal of the pericardium is essentially curative. However, for those in which the visceral pericardium is also involved, as seems to be the case particularly in dogs with infectious forms of the disease, epicardial excision may also be required.
- In a study of 10 dogs treated for constrictive pericardial disease with pericardiectomy, 6 had complete resolution of clinical signs and long-term survival. In the remaining 4, the most common cause of death in the postoperative period was pulmonary thromboembolism.

- In a case series that examined outcomes in 17 dogs with *C. immitis* treated with pericardiectomy and epicardial excision, perioperative mortality was 23.5%. However, in dogs that survived to discharge and for which follow-up was available, 82% survived at least 2 years after surgery.

MISCELLANEOUS PERICARDIAL DISEASES

PERITONEOPERICARDIAL DIAPHRAGMATIC HERNIA

DESCRIPTION AND DIAGNOSTIC FEATURES

- Peritoneopericardial diaphragmatic hernia (PPDH) is an uncommon condition defined by an abnormal communication between the peritoneal cavity and pericardial sac, which allows the movement of abdominal structures into the pericardial space. In affected animals, clinical signs are a manifestation of the compressive effects of the displaced abdominal organs on cardiopulmonary structures or of their entrapment, strangulation, or obstruction.
- In dogs and cats, PPDH is almost exclusively a congenital anomaly, likely caused by abnormal formation or incomplete fusion of the septum transversum during embryogenesis.
- Commonly herniated structures include the liver, gallbladder, omentum, and small intestine.
- Clinical signs in affected animals may be nonspecific in nature or may relate to the respiratory (more common in cats) or gastrointestinal (more common in dogs) systems. Tachypnea, dyspnea, exercise intolerance, vomiting, or anorexia are common clinical signs noted by owners. In up to 50% of cases, PPDH may be an incidental radiographic finding in symptom-free animals or those with apparently unrelated clinical signs.
- Radiographic signs suggestive of PPDH include enlargement of the cardiac silhouette, indistinct diaphragmatic borders (diaphragmatic "discontinuity"), the presence of soft tissue or fat opacity between the heart and diaphragm, or gas-filled structures within the pericardial space.

EPIDEMIOLOGY

- Prevalence rates of up to 0.59% have been reported in cats and dogs. The prevalence of PPDH in a large referral population was significantly greater for cats than for dogs (0.062% and 0.015%, respectively).
- Affected animals are usually mature at the time of diagnosis, with median ages of 1 to 4 years and 1.2 to 2.5 years noted for cats and dogs, respectively.

- In retrospective studies of PPDH, cats of long-haired breeds and dogs of the Weimaraner breed appear to be overrepresented. Domestic short-hair cats were underrepresented in two reports.
- Although no sex predilection has been reported in cats, some authors have noted a possible predisposition in male dogs.

TREATMENT AND PROGNOSIS

- Dogs and cats with PPDH that have symptoms may undergo surgical herniorrhaphy, which is associated with resolution of clinical signs in 85% of cases. Perioperative mortality rates of 5.5% to 14% have been reported for this procedure.
- In a recent retrospective study of dogs and cats with PPDH treated with surgery (n = 34) or with medical management alone (n = 24), long-term survival was similar between treatment approaches. The authors of this study suggest that nonsurgical management of PPDH may therefore be appropriate for animals without clinical signs.

CONGENITAL INTRAPERICARDIAL CYSTS

- Congenital intrapericardial cysts have been reported sporadically in veterinary patients. In two of these cases, the histologic appearance was similar to that of human coelomic pericardial cysts, thought to be formed by abnormal fetal development of the pericardial mesoderm. However, in most veterinary cases, these structures appear to be cystic hematomas, either associated with PPDH or with a stalk of tissue that attaches them to the parietal pericardium. For this reason, it has been postulated that these cysts may be a result of omental or falciform fat entrapment during fetal development.
- Clinical signs in affected patients are similar to those noted in other pericardial diseases and are caused by cardiac tamponade caused by compression from the cyst itself and/or any associated pericardial effusion.
- Echocardiography can be used to identify a mass in the pericardial space that is often loculated in appearance. Pericardial effusion may be present as well.
- Surgical removal of these structures with pericardiectomy is typically associated with resolution of clinical signs and an excellent long-term prognosis in affected animals. Percutaneous centesis of cystic fluid may be required to stabilize the patient before surgery.

SUMMARY AND CONCLUSIONS

- Chief complaints, histories, and physical examination findings in dogs with pericardial effusions are diverse and often vague.

- Thoracic radiography and electrocardiography may be helpful to diagnose the presence of pericardial effusion; however, these techniques are relatively insensitive. Echocardiography is considered the most sensitive and specific diagnostic tool for the diagnosis and semiquantification of pericardial effusion.
- Most symptomatic pericardial effusions in dogs are neoplastic in origin, with cardiac HSA representing the most common cause.
- Echocardiography is the diagnostic test of choice for the detection of cardiac tumors. This test should be performed before pericardiocentesis if the patient's clinical condition permits.
- In most patients with hemodynamically significant pericardial effusion, pericardiocentesis is necessary for initial stabilization.
- Fluid analysis and cytologic evaluation are rarely helpful in determining the underlying etiology of pericardial effusion; nonetheless, these tests are warranted because they may provide a diagnosis in patients with cardiac lymphoma or infectious pericarditis.
- Depending on the underlying cause, the prognosis for dogs with pericardial effusion varies from grave to excellent. Pericardiectomy is the cornerstone of therapy in most cases that have prolonged survival.

FREQUENTLY ASKED QUESTIONS

Is there a role for the use of diuretics in the treatment of pericardial effusion?

Because many dogs with pericardial effusion show signs of right-sided congestive heart failure, it might seem that diuretic agents would be indicated to mobilize accumulated fluid. However, their use is contraindicated in patients with hemodynamically significant pericardial effusion because these agents significantly reduce preload, a determinant of cardiac output on which these animals heavily rely. In this setting, diuretics may significantly worsen systemic hypotension and increase the risk of cardiogenic shock and azotemia. The exception to this rule is in dogs with left atrial rupture associated with advanced degenerative mitral valve disease; these dogs frequently have respiratory difficulty associated with concurrent left-sided congestive heart failure and can benefit from cautious diuretic therapy. After pericardiocentesis, fluid accumulation in the abdominal and thoracic cavities due to right-sided congestive heart failure will typically spontaneously resolve without the need for diuretic therapy.

Why do dogs with pericardial effusion have pulsus paradoxus?

Pulsus paradoxus refers to the phasic change in peripheral arterial pulse quality that corresponds to the patient's phase of respiration. Specifically, it is defined as a decline in systemic arterial pressure of >10 mm Hg during inhalation; therefore dogs demonstrating pulsus paradoxus have stronger pulse quality during exhalation and weaker or absent palpable pulses during inhalation. Pulsus paradoxus is due to the limitation to cardiac filling imposed by the presence of significant pericardial effusion. When the patient inhales, intrathoracic pressure falls, and venous return to the thorax and right side of the heart is augmented. As the right-sided heart is constrained by the presence of the pericardial effusion, right-sided heart filling occurs at the expense of left-sided heart volume. This phenomenon causes left-sided heart volume and systemic cardiac output to fall during inhalation, resulting in poor systemic arterial pulse quality. The opposite effect occurs in exhalation, during which the quality of the systemic arterial pulse increases.

What are the primary clinical signs in a dog with clinically significant pericardial effusion?

Commonly, dogs with significant pericardial effusion have three cardinal signs, historically referred to as the Beck triad. These include muffled heart sounds, weak femoral pulses, and jugular venous distension. Careful examination of dogs suspected to have pericardial effusion usually reveals the presence of all three components. Inspection of the jugular veins sometimes necessitates shaving the hair from the patient's jugular groove to properly visualize the vein. Inspection of the jugular vein should be done with the patient standing. Jugular venous distension is often overlooked, but it is a quick and reliable way to help distinguish cardiac from noncardiac causes of abdominal effusion.

SUGGESTED READINGS

Adler Y, Finkelstein Y, Guindo J, et al: Colchicine treatment for recurrent pericarditis: a decade of experience, Circulation 97:2183, 1998.

Alleman AR: Abdominal, thoracic, and pericardial effusions, Vet Clin Small Anim Pract 33:89, 2003.

Aronsohn MG, Carpenter JL: Surgical treatment of idiopathic pericardial effusion in the dog: 25 cases (1978-1993), J Am Anim Hosp Assoc 35:521, 1999.

Aronsohn AR, Gregory CR: Infectious pericardial effusion in five dogs, Vet Surg 24:402, 1995.

Banz AC, Gottfried SD: Peritoneopericardial diaphragmatic hernia: a retrospective study of 31 cats and eight dogs 46:398–404, 2010.

Berg RJ, Wingfield W: Pericardial effusion in the dog: a review of 42 cases, J Am Anim Hosp Assoc 20:721, 1983.

Boddy KN, Sleeper MM, Sammarco CD: Cardiac magnetic resonance in the differentiation of neoplastic and nonneoplastic pericardial effusion, J Vet Intern Med 25:1003–1009, 2011.

Bonagura JD: Electrical alternans associated with pericardial effusion in the dog, J Am Vet Med Assoc 178:574, 1981.

Boston SE, Higginson G, Monteith G: Concurrent splenic and right atrial mass at presentation in dogs with HSA: a retrospective study, J Am Anim Hosp Assoc 47:336–341, 2011.

Buchanan JW: Spontaneous left atrial rupture in dogs, Adv Exp Med Biol 22:315–334, 1972.

Burns CG, Bergh MS, McLoughlin MA: Surgical and non-surgical treatment of peritoneopericardial diaphragmatic hernia in dogs and cat: 58 cases (1999-2008), J Am Vet Med Assoc 242:643–650, 2013.

Cagle LA, Epstein SE, Owens SD, et al: Diagnostic yield of cytologic analysis of pericardial effusion in dogs, J Vet Intern Med 28:66–71, 2014.

Case JB, Maxwell M, Aman A, et al: Outcome evaluation of a thoracoscopic pericardial window procedure or subtotal pericardiectomy via thoracotomy for the treatment of pericardial effusion in dog, J Am Vet Med Assoc 242:493–498, 2013.

Churg A, Colby TV, Cagle P, et al: The separation of benign and malignant mesothelial proliferations, Am J Surg Pathol 24:1183, 2000.

Closa JM, Font A, Mascort J: Pericardial mesothelioma in a dog: long-term survival after pericardiectomy in combination with chemotherapy, J Small Anim Pract 40:383, 1999.

Constantino-Casas P, Rodriguez-Martinez HA: Guterrez Diaz-Ceballos ME: A case report and review: the gross, histological, and immunohistochemical characteristics of a carcinoma of ectopic thyroid in a dog, Br Vet J 152:669, 1996.

Davidson BJ, Paling AC, Lahmers SL, et al: Disease association and clinical assessment of feline pericardial effusion, J Am Anim Hosp Assoc 44:5–9, 2008.

Day MJ, Martin MWS: Immunohistochemical characterization of the lesions of canine idiopathic pericarditis, J Small Anim Pract 43:383, 2002.

Dunning D, Monnet E, Orton EC, et al: Analysis of prognostic indicators for dogs with pericardial effusion: 46 cases (1985-1996), J Am Vet Med Assoc 212:1276, 1998.

Ehrhart N, Ehrhart EJ, Willis J, et al: Analysis of factors affecting survival in dogs with aortic body tumors, Vet Surg 31:44, 2002.

Ghafferi S, Pelio DC, Lange AJ, et al: A retrospective evaluation of doxorubicin-based chemotherapy for dogs with right atrial masses and pericardial effusion, J Small Anim Pract 55:254–257, 2014.

Fine DM, Tobias AH, Jacob KA: Use of pericardial fluid pH to distinguish between idiopathic and neoplastic effusions, J Vet Intern Med 17:525, 2003.

Hall DJ, Shofer F, Meier CK, et al: Pericardial effusion in cats: a retrospective study of clinical findings and outcome in 146 cats, J Vet Intern Med 21:1002–1007, 2007.

Hayes HM, Sass B: Chemoreceptor neoplasia: a study of the epidemiological features of 357 canine cases, J Vet Med 35:401, 1988.

Heinritz CK, Gilson SD, Soderstrom MJ, et al: Subtotal pericardiectomy and epicardial excision for treatment of coccidioidomycosis-induced effusive-constrictive pericarditis in dogs: 17 cases (1999-2003), J Am Vet Med Assoc 227:435, 2005.

Holt D, Van Winkle T, Schelling C, et al: Correlation between thoracic radiographs and findings in dogs with hemangiosarcoma: 77 cases (1984-1989), J Am Vet Med Assoc 200:1535, 1992.

Jackson J, Richter KP, Launer DP: Thoracoscopic partial pericardiectomy in 13 dogs, J Vet Intern Med 13:529, 1999.

Johnson KH: Aortic body tumors in the dog, J Am Vet Med Assoc 152:154, 1968.

MacDonald KA, Cagney O, Magne ML: Echocardiographic and clinicopathologic characterization of pericardial effusion in dogs: 107 cases (1985-2006), J Am Vet Med Assoc 235:1456–1461, 2009.

MacGregor JM, Faria MLE, Moore AS, et al: Cardiac lymphoma causing pericardial effusion in 12 dogs: 12 cases (1994-2004), J Am Vet Med Assoc 227:1449, 2005.

MacGregor JM, Rozanski EA, McCarthy RJ, et al: Cholesterol-based pericardial effusion and aortic thromboembolism in a 9-year-old mixed-breed dog with hypothyroidism, J Vet Intern Med 18:354, 2004.

Maisch B, Seferovic PM, Ristić AD, et al: Guidelines on the diagnosis and management of pericardial disease: executive summary, Eur Heart J 25:587–610, 2004.

McDonough SP, MacLauglin NJ, Tobias AH: Canine pericardial mesothelioma, Vet Pathol 29:256, 1992.

Mellanby RJ, Herrtage ME: Long-term survival of 23 dogs with pericardial effusions, Vet Record 156:568–571, 2005.

Nakamura RK, Tompkins E, Russell NJ, et al.: Left atrial rupture secondary to myxomatous mitral valve disease in 11 dogs, J Am Anim Hosp Assoc 50(50):405–408, 2014.

Owen TJ, Bruyette DS, Layton CE: Chemodectoma in dogs, Compend Cont Ed Pract Vet 18:253, 1996.

Petrus DJ, Henik RA: Pericardial effusion and cardiac tamponade secondary to brodifacoum toxicosis in a dog, J Am Vet Med Assoc 215:647, 1999.

Ployart S, Libermann S, Doran I, et al: Thoracoscopic resection of right auricular masses in dogs: 9 cases (2003-2011), J Am Vet Med Assoc 242(2):237–241, 2013.

Rajagopalan V, Jesty SA, Craig LE, et al: Comparison of presumptive echocardiographic and definitive diagnosis of cardiac tumors in dogs, J Vet Intern Med 27:1092–1096, 2013.

Rancilio NJ, Higuchi T, Gagnon J, et al: Use of three-dimensional conformal radiation therapy for treatment of a heart base chemodectoma in a dog, J Am Vet Med Assoc 241:472–476, 2012.

Reineke EL, Burkett DE, Drobatz KJ: Left atrial rupture in dogs: 14 cases (19990-2005), J Vet Emerg Crit Care 18:158–164, 2008.

Rush JE, Keene BW, Fox PR: Pericardial disease in the cat: a retrospective evaluation of 66 cases, J Am Anim Hosp Assoc 26:39, 1990.

Scollan KF, Bottorff B, Stieger-Vanegas S, et al: Use of multidetector computed tomography in the assessment of dogs with pericardial effusion, J Vet Intern Med 29:79–87, 2015.

Shubitz LF, Matz ME, Noon TH, et al: Constrictive pericarditis secondary to Coccidioides immitis infection in a dog, J Am Vet Med Assoc 218:537, 2001.

Sidley JA, Atkins CE, Keene BW, et al: Percutaneous balloon pericardiotomy as a treatment for recurrent pericardial effusion in 6 dogs, J Vet Intern Med 16:541–546, 2002.

Sisson D, Thomas WP, Reed J, et al: Intrapericardial cysts in the dog, J Vet Intern Med 7:364, 1993.

Sisson D, Thomas WP, Ruehl WW, et al: Diagnostic value of pericardial fluid analysis in the dog, J Am Vet Med Assoc 184:51, 1984.

Stafford Johnson M, Martin M, Binns S, et al: A retrospective study of clinical findings, treatment and outcome in 143 dogs with pericardial effusion, J Small Anim Pract 45:546–552, 2004.

Stepien RL, Whitley NT, Dubielzig RR: Idiopathic or mesothelioma-related pericardial effusion: clinical findings and survival in 17 dogs studied retrospectively, J Small Anim Pract 41:342, 2000.

Thake DC, Cheville NF, Sharp RK: Ectopic thyroid adenomas at the base of the heart of the dog, Vet Pathol 8:421, 1971.

Thomas WP, Reed JR, Bauer TG, et al: Constrictive pericardial disease in the dog, J Am Vet Med Assoc 184:546–553, 1984.

Walsh PJ, Remedios AM, Ferguson JF, et al: Thoracoscopic versus open partial pericardiectomy in dogs: comparison of postoperative pain and morbidity, Vet Surg 28:472, 1999.

Ware WA, Hopper DL: Cardiac tumors in dogs: 1982-1995, J Vet Intern Med 13:95, 1999.

Weisse C, Soares N, Beal MW, et al: Survival time in dogs with right atrial hemangiosarcoma treated by means of surgical resection with or without adjuvant chemotherapy: 23 cases (1986-2000), J Am Vet Med Assoc 226:575, 2005.

Yamamoto S, Hoshi K, Hirakawa A, et al: Epidemiological, clinical and pathological features of primary cardiac hemangiosarcoma in dogs: a review of 51 cases, J Vet Med Sci 75:1433–1441, 2013.

Yates WD, Lester SJ, Mills JH: Chemoreceptor tumors diagnosed at the Western College of Veterinary Medicine: 1967-1979, Can Vet J 21:124, 1980.

13 Congenital Heart Disease

Keith N. Strickland | Mark A. Oyama

INCIDENCE

- The incidence of congenital heart disease in dogs has been reported to be 6.8 to 8.0 per 1000 hospital admissions. On average, this equates to 1 case per 15 litters. The actual incidence is likely higher as some defects result in neonatal death and are unreported.
- The most common congenital heart defects in dogs include patent ductus arteriosus (PDA), pulmonic stenosis (PS), aortic stenosis, ventricular septal defect (VSD), and tetralogy of Fallot (Table 13.1). Several breed predispositions have been identified (see Appendix 1).
- Less common defects in dogs include mitral valve dysplasia, atrial septal defects, tricuspid valve dysplasia, cor triatriatum dexter, double chambered right ventricle, and mitral stenosis. Rare defects include persistent truncus arteriosus, tricuspid stenosis, double outlet right ventricle, and transposition of the great vessels.
- Congenital heart disease is less common in cats than in dogs. The reported incidence is 0.2 to 1.0 per 1000 hospital admissions. No consistent breed or gender predilections have been adequately demonstrated.
- The most common congenital heart defects in cats include mitral valve dysplasia, tricuspid valve dysplasia, PDA, VSD, aortic stenosis, tetralogy of Fallot, persistent common atrioventricular canal, and endocardial fibroelastosis.
- Less common defects in cats include persistent truncus arteriosus, PS, atrial septal defect, tricuspid stenosis, and double chambered right ventricle.

HEREDITARY ASPECTS

- Congenital heart diseases are the most common type of heart disease in young dogs and cats but are occasionally diagnosed in adult animals.
- Congenital heart defects are generally recognized in the young animal and usually represent a heritable trait or a defect that originated during gestation. A primary genetic mutation

or environmental influences may exist, resulting in significant variation of disease severity.
- The following are four common forms of congenital heart disease that have been shown to be inherited in dogs:
  - PDA in the Poodle
  - Subaortic stenosis (SAS) in the Newfoundland
  - Tetralogy of Fallot in the Keeshond
  - PS in the Beagle

DIAGNOSIS

- In general, a congenital heart defect is suspected when a heart murmur is detected in a young dog or cat (Table 13.2).
- Other supporting clinical features may include the following:
  - Failure to thrive
  - Cyanosis
  - Collapse or seizure
  - Intolerance to activity or exercise
  - Jugular venous distention
  - Electrocardiographic (ECG) abnormalities
  - Radiographic evidence of cardiac enlargement
- A tentative diagnosis can often be made on the basis of results of a complete cardiovascular physical examination, routine ECG, and radiography (see Table 13.2).
- The specific diagnosis is confirmed in most cases by echocardiography and rarely by cardiac catheterization, angiography, or oximetry. Information obtained from the echocardiogram is also helpful in determining the severity of the defect, especially if Doppler techniques are used (measurement of blood velocities within the heart).

THERAPY

- Advances since the early 1990s allow for the treatment of certain stenotic lesions by balloon valvuloplasty, which is a technique in which a small balloon located at the end of a cardiac catheter is used, and transcatheter occlusion of PDA with an occluding device. Surgical correction or palliation is possible for certain defects.

Table 13.1 Classification of Congenital Defects According to Pathophysiology

Canine	Feline
Defects Primarily Causing Volume Overload	**Defects Primarily Causing Volume Overload**

Systemic to pulmonary (left-to-right) shunting
  Common
    Patent ductus arteriosus
    Ventricular septal defect
  Uncommon
    Atrial septal defect
    Endocardial cushion defect
    (Pseudo) truncus arteriosus
Valvular regurgitation
  Common
    Mitral dysplasia
    Tricuspid dysplasia
  Uncommon
    Pulmonic insufficiency
    Aortic insufficiency
	Common
	  Ventricular septal defect
	  Patent ductus arteriosus
	  Atrial septal defect
	  Endocardial cushion defect
	Uncommon
	  Truncus arteriosus
	  Valvular regurgitation
	Common
	  Mitral dysplasia
	  Tricuspid dysplasia

Defects Primarily Causing Pressure Overload	**Defects Primarily Causing Pressure Overload**

Common
  Pulmonic stenosis
  Subaortic stenosis
Uncommon
  Valvular aortic stenosis
  Coarctation and interruption of the aorta
  Cor triatriatum dexter
	Common
	  Dynamic subaortic stenosis
	Uncommon
	  Pulmonic stenosis
	  Pulmonary artery branch stenosis
	  Fixed subaortic stenosis
	  Valvular aortic stenosis
	  Cor triatriatum dexter
	  Cor triatriatum sinister

Defects Primarily Causing Cyanosis	**Defects Primarily Causing Cyanosis**

Common
  Tetralogy of Fallot
Uncommon
  Pulmonary to systemic shunting (ventricular septal defect [VSD])
  Pulmonary to systemic shunting (patent ductus arteriosus [PDA])
  Tricuspid atresia/right ventricular hypoplasia
  Double outlet right ventricle
  Transposition of the great vessels
  Truncus arteriosus
  Aorticopulmonary window
	Common
	  Tetralogy of Fallot
	  Endocardial cushion defect
	Uncommon
	  Pulmonary to systemic shunting (VSD)
	  Pulmonary to systemic shunting (PDA)
	  Double outlet right ventricle
	  Truncus arteriosus

Miscellaneous Cardiac and Vascular Defects	**Miscellaneous Cardiac and Vascular Defects**

Common
  Peritoneopericardial diapharagmatic hernia
  Persistent right aortic arch
  Persistent left cranial vena cava
Uncommon
  Endocardial fibroelastosis
  Pericardial defects
  Anomalous pulmonary venous return
  Double aortic arch
  Retroesophageal left subclavian artery
  Situs inversus
	Common
	  Peritoneopericardial diapharagmatic hernia
	  Endocardial fibroelastosis
	Uncommon
	  Persistent right aortic arch

Table 13.2   Auscultatory Findings in Congenital Heart Disease

Lesion	Timing	Features	Point of Maximum Intensity	Comments
Atrial septal defect	Systolic (diastolic)	Ejection (diastolic rumble)	Left base	Systolic murmur ends before S_2, which is usually split; murmur (or murmurs) caused by relative pulmonic (tricuspid) stenosis
(Sub) aortic stenosis	Systolic*	Ejection (crescendo-decrescendo)	Left base	Often nearly as loud at the right base; diastolic murmur of aortic regurgitation may also occur
Mitral valve dysplasia[†]	Systolic	Regurgitant (holosystolic)	Left apex	May radiate widely
Patent ductus arteriosus	Continuous	Machinery	Left base	Murmur peaks at S_2, often radiates to right base and thoracic inlet
Pulmonary hypertension (Eisenmenger syndrome)	None (systolic)	Split S_2 (ejection)	Left base	Accentuated and split S_2; systolic murmur of tricuspid regurgitation or blowing, decrescendo diastolic murmur of pulmonic regurgitation may also occur
Pulmonic stenosis	Systolic	Ejection (crescendo-decrescendo)	Left base	Occasional systolic ejection sound; blowing, decrescendo diastolic murmur of pulmonic regurgitation may occur
Tetralogy of Fallot	Systolic	Ejection (crescendo-decrescendo)	Left base	Murmur due to pulmonic stenosis; may be soft or absent with pulmonary artery hypoplasia
Tricuspid valve dysplasia[†]	Systolic	Regurgitant (holosystolic)	Right midprecordium	Often low pitched and rumbling
Ventricular septal defect	Systolic*	Regurgitant (holosystolic)	Right base	Often higher pitched and more cranially located than tricuspid regurgitation; may also be loud at left base

From Ettinger SE, Feldman EF: Textbook of veterinary internal medicine, ed 7, St Louis, 2010, Saunders.
*At times a diastolic murmur of aortic regurgitation may also be present.
[†]Mitral stenosis and tricuspid stenosis are rare but may cause diastolic murmurs over the affected valve and ventricle.

- Medical treatment is primarily for the control or prevention of complications, such as congestive heart failure (CHF), arrhythmias, and endocarditis, rather than for correction of the defect. Medical therapy is discussed briefly in this chapter.

INNOCENT (FUNCTIONAL) MURMUR

Not all young dogs and cats with heart murmurs have congenital heart disease. Innocent or functional murmurs are created by mild turbulence within the heart and great vessels, and usually diminish in intensity or resolve by 4 to 5 months of age.

The following characteristics of innocent murmurs help differentiate them from pathologic murmurs.

- Innocent murmurs are systolic in timing, usually occurring early in systole and of short duration (ejection-type). They are "soft" (i.e., grade 2I/6 or less in intensity) and often have a low-pitched, vibrating, or musical quality.
- Innocent murmurs are usually loudest along the left sternal border and are poorly transmitted. Their intensity may vary with changes in position, with the phase of respiration, with exercise, and from examination to examination.

- The most important characteristic of the innocent murmur is that it is heard in the absence of any other demonstrable evidence of cardiovascular disease (e.g., lack of clinical signs or radiographic abnormalities).
- More intense systolic murmurs (grade 3I/6 or greater) and diastolic murmurs are indicative of cardiac disease and should prompt further diagnostics.

SPECIFIC DEFECTS

PATENT DUCTUS ARTERIOSUS

- In fetal circulation, the ductus arteriosus serves to shunt maternally oxygenated blood into the aorta, thereby bypassing the nonfunctional lungs. Shortly after birth, several factors contribute to cause closure of the ductus. Pulmonary vascular resistance drops, vasodilatory prostaglandin levels decrease, and oxygen tension increases, resulting in a marked increase in pulmonary blood flow and vasoconstriction of the ductus. After closure by vasoconstriction, the ductus is permanently closed by fibrous contracture, which produces the ligamentum arteriosum. Failure of the ductus to close is termed *patent ductus arteriosus (PDA)* or *persistent ductus arteriosus.*

PATHOPHYSIOLOGY

- The consequences of a PDA depend primarily on the diameter of the ductus and the pulmonary vascular resistance, with the large majority of PDA cases resulting in left-to-right shunting.
- Failure of ductal closure is due to an abnormal amount of elastic fibers compared with contractile smooth muscle fibers (so-called extension of the noncontractile wall structure of the aorta into the ductus arteriosus). Varying amounts of normal smooth muscle causes varying degrees of ductal closure; this creates a structure that ranges from a funnel-shaped ductus that narrows on the pulmonary artery side of the ductus (Figure 13.1) to a tubelike structure without narrowing.
- Blood flow through the ductus is dependent on the relative resistances of the systemic and pulmonary circulation. When pulmonary vascular resistance is normal, blood continually shunts from the aorta (high resistance) into the pulmonary circulation (low resistance). Shunting in this fashion (systemic to pulmonary) is referred to as left-to-right and represents the most common pattern in PDA (Figure 13.2). When pulmonary vascular resistance increases and exceeds systemic vascular resistance, blood will shunt from the pulmonary artery into the aorta (so-called right-to-left or reversed PDA). With a very small diameter ductus, the volume of blood shunted is small, and there may be no hemodynamic effects.

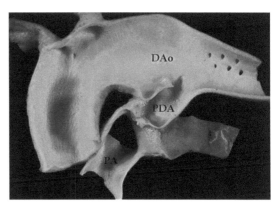

Figure 13.1 Postmortem specimen, from a young German Shepherd, of the transverse and proximal descending aorta (*DAo*) on top, the pulmonary artery (*PA*) branches ventrally, and a left-to-right shunting patent ductus arteriosus (*PDA*) between them. The aortic end of the PDA is wide open. The PA end is partially constricted. This results in a funnel shape to the PDA. (From Kittleson MD, Kienle RD: Small animal cardiovascular medicine, St. Louis, 1998, Mosby. With permission from Dr. Mark D. Kittleson).

In most cases there is significant shunting and one of two major consequences occurs. In cases of persistent left-to-right shunting, volume overloading of the left atrium and left ventricle results in eventual left-sided failure. In the rare case of a very large diameter ductus (sometime referred to as nonresistive), excessive pulmonary blood flow induces dramatic increases in pulmonary vascular resistance, pulmonary hypertension, and shunt reversal (Eisenmenger syndrome), resulting in right-to-left shunting, systemic hypoxemia to the caudal half of the body, and differential cyanosis. If it is going to occur, shunt reversal takes place within the first 6 months of life. Long-term effects of reversed PDA include polycythemia, activity intolerance, and organ failure, as opposed to CHF, which is rare.

DIAGNOSIS

ETIOLOGY AND BREED DISPOSITION

- PDA occurs in both the dog and cat, with higher frequency in the dog. There is also a higher frequency in the female.
- Breeds predisposed or at increased risk include Bichon Frisé, Chihuahua, Cocker Spaniel, Collie, English Springer Spaniel, Keeshond, Labrador Retriever, Maltese, Newfoundland, Poodle, Pomeranian, Shetland Sheepdog, and Yorkshire Terrier.
- The defect has been shown to be inherited in the Miniature Poodle, transmitted as a polygenic trait.
- The German Shepherd often exhibits a large tubular ductus that is prone to shunt reversal and is difficult to close with catheter-based occlusion devices.

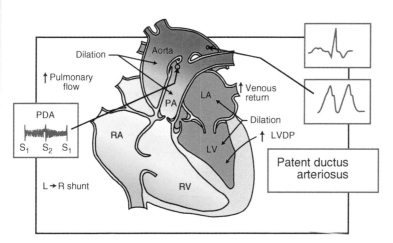

Figure 13.2 Pathophysiology and genesis of clinical findings in patent ductus arteriosus (*PDA*). *LA,* Left atrium; *LV,* left ventricle; *LVDP,* left ventricular developed pressure; *PA,* pulmonary artery, *RA,* right atrium; *RV,* right ventricle. (Modified from Fox PR, Sisson D, Moise N, eds: Textbook of canine and feline cardiology: principles and clinical practice, ed 2, Philadelphia, 1999, WB Saunders.)

HISTORY AND CLINICAL SIGNS

- Clinical signs are related to the degree and direction of shunting and may range from none to severe CHF in left-to-right PDA, or signs of hypoxia and polycythemia in right-to-left PDA.
- Cats seldom display signs of cardiac failure until decompensation is advanced and life threatening.

PHYSICAL EXAMINATION
PALPATION

- "Water-hammer" or bounding arterial pulses are usually present in animals with left-to-right shunting PDA. This type of pulse represents a widened pulse pressure secondary to the loss of diastolic pressure through the ductus and elevation of systolic blood pressure from the volume-overloaded left ventricle. Usually the larger the ductus (and therefore the shunt), the more prominent the arterial pulse.
- In most left-to-right PDA cases, a precordial thrill can be palpated over the cranial left-heart base, and the left apical impulse is prominent. In cases with right-to-left shunting, there is no precordial thrill and the right apical impulse is more prominent.

GENERAL

- Caudal or differential cyanosis is an important physical finding in animals with right-to-left shunting PDA. Owing to the location of the ductus (distal to the arteries supplying the head and forelimbs), cyanosis is limited to the caudal half of the body. Differential cyanosis is best appreciated by examining caudal mucous membranes of the prepuce or vulva as compared with mucous membranes of the mouth.
- Polycythemia (packed cell volume greater than 60) is usually present in cases with right-to-left

shunts but can be absent in animals younger than a year of age.

AUSCULTATION

- A continuous-type machinery murmur is a hallmark of left-to-right shunting PDA. The murmur is loudest in mid-to-late systole and gradually decreases in intensity through diastole. In cases with a very small diameter ductus, this characteristic murmur is restricted to the cranial left-heart base and may be missed if auscultation is limited to the apex. The systolic component of the murmur is usually quite prominent at the cardiac apex; however, a systolic murmur secondary to mitral regurgitation because of annular dilation as the heart enlarges is also possible.
- In cases with a right-to-left shunting PDA, there is no murmur associated with the shunt; however, a split second heart sound or diastolic murmur of pulmonic insufficiency as a result of pulmonary hypertension can be present. A murmur of tricuspid regurgitation may be present in some cases. Because right-to-left PDAs start as large left-to-right PDAs that gradually reverse, there is initially a typical continuous murmur early in life, followed by loss of the diastolic component of the continuous murmur and then loss of the systolic component.

DIAGNOSTIC TESTING
ELECTROCARDIOGRAM

ECG abnormalities are present in most cases of PDA and include evidence of left ventricular and left atrial enlargement such as the following:

- Tall R waves are present in leads II (>3.0 mV), III, and aV$_F$.
- P mitrale (widened P wave) is often present.

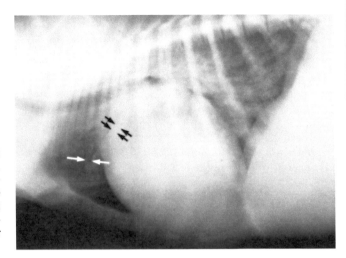

Figure 13.3 Patent ductus arteriosus (PDA) (lateral projection) in a 3-month-old Poodle. There is generalized heart enlargement, engorgement of the right cranial lobar artery (*white arrows*), and engorgement of the right cranial lobar vein (*black arrows*). Vascular engorgement, perivascular congestion, and alveolar edema are seen in the caudal lung lobes.

- Atrial fibrillation and ventricular arrhythmias may occur in association with CHF.
- Animals with pulmonary hypertension may show evidence of right ventricular hypertrophy such as deep S waves in leads I, II, III, and aV_F and a right shift of the mean electrical axis.

THORACIC RADIOGRAPHS

- The radiographic signs of PDA (Figures 13.3 and 13.4) vary considerably with the volume of blood being shunted, the age of the animal, and the degree of cardiac decompensation.
- Dorsoventral radiographs often reveal three prominences along the left cardiac silhouette
  - The aneurysmal bulge of the aortic arch
  - The enlarged pulmonary outflow tract
  - The enlarged left atrial appendage
- Mild to moderate left ventricular and left atrial enlargement are usually present.
- Overcirculation of the lung field can often be visualized.
- Severe cardiomegaly, pulmonary congestion, and pulmonary edema will be present when there is CHF.
- Right ventricular enlargement and prominent tortuous pulmonary arteries are seen in animals with severe pulmonary hypertension and right-to-left PDA.

ECHOCARDIOGRAPHY

- Echocardiographic changes reflect the volume-overloaded state of the left side of the heart and include left atrial dilation, left ventricular dilation, and normal to excessive wall motion (fractional shortening). In most cases, the ductus can be visualized. Transthoracic or transesophageal echocardiography of the ductal shape is an essential diagnostic tool

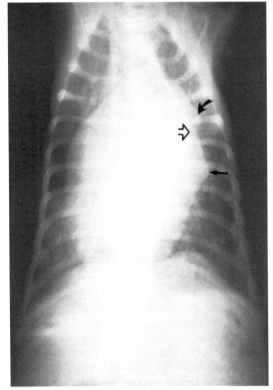

Figure 13.4 Patent ductus arteriosus (PDA) (dorsoventral projection) in a 3-month-old Poodle. There is generalized heart enlargement, an aneurysm-like bulge of the descending aorta (*open arrow*), a bulge of the main pulmonary artery (*curved arrow*), and enlargement of the left auricle (*straight arrow*). Alveolar infiltrate due to pulmonary edema is present in the caudal lung lobes.

when contemplating catheter-based occlusion of the PDA.
- Shunting of left-to-right blood flow through the ductus can be detected by Doppler echocardiography and can be visualized with color-flow Doppler echocardiography.

- In cases with pulmonary hypertension and reversed-shunting, right ventricular hypertrophy is evident along with enlargement of the main pulmonary artery; Doppler echocardiography may reveal pulmonic insufficiency.
- Contrast echocardiography can be used to confirm the presence of a right-to-left shunting PDA. In this technique, agitated saline is injected into a peripheral vein during echocardiographic examination of the abdominal aorta to detect right-to-left shunting of blood. The absence of intracardiac shunting with the presence of microbubbles within the abdominal aorta is diagnostic of reversed PDA.

CARDIAC CATHETERIZATION AND ANGIOCARDIOGRAPHY

- Cardiac catheterization and angiocardiography are rarely needed for diagnosis but are routinely performed to characterize and measure the ductus before catheter-based occlusion.
- The diagnosis of a left-to-right PDA can be made by injecting contrast media into the aortic arch. The simultaneous filling of the main pulmonary artery and the aorta is diagnostic for PDA. Likewise, a main pulmonary artery contrast injection can be used to confirm the diagnosis of a right-to-left shunt (simultaneous filling of the main pulmonary artery and aorta).
- Nonselective angiocardiography is performed by injecting contrast material through a large-diameter venous catheter and may be used to support the diagnosis of a right-to-left shunting PDA; however, this technique is of limited value in the diagnosis of left-to-right shunts.

DIFFERENTIAL DIAGNOSIS

- Echocardiography or angiocardiographic studies may be used to differentiate PDA from other congenital cardiac defects. Two cardiac defects that can resemble PDA are as follows:
  - Aorticopulmonary window
    - A round or oval communication between the aorta and the main pulmonary artery close to their origin from the heart base. This rare defect usually results in severe pulmonary hypertension and might require angiography or transesophageal echocardiography for differentiation from PDA.
  - Concurrent aortic stenosis and insufficiency
    - The systolic murmur of aortic stenosis and the diastolic murmur of aortic insufficiency combine to mimic the machinery murmur of PDA. Echocardiography easily differentiates this condition from PDA.

NATURAL HISTORY

- Mortality is high in affected, untreated dogs; approximately 64% die before 1 year of age if left untreated.
- Constant volume overload of the left atrium and left ventricle results in chamber dilation, myocardial dysfunction, and arrhythmias.
  - Left-sided cardiac strain and pulmonary congestion lead to CHF.
  - Sudden death following exertion has been observed in young affected dogs.
- When there is right-to-left shunting, progressive polycythemia and hypoxemia occur. Survival to 3 to 5 years of age is not uncommon. Phlebotomy is indicated if the packed cell volume is elevated to greater than 65% and symptoms are present.

THERAPY AND PROGNOSIS

SURGERY

- Because of the high risk of CHF, the vast majority of left-to-right shunting PDA cases should be either surgically ligated or occluded.
- In symptom-free animals with left-to-right shunting PDA, surgical correction of the ductus should be performed as soon as possible. Current surgical ligation success rates are >95%.
- In cases with mild to moderate left-sided heart failure, resolution of pulmonary edema must precede anesthesia and surgery.
- In cases with severe heart failure, patient stabilization should be attempted; however, these patients are poor anesthetic risks. Presence of myocardial failure and atrial fibrillation are negative prognostic indicators.

Advantages

- Best approach for patients with a large PDA with tubular shape (e.g., German Shepherds)
- May be the best approach for very small dogs that are too small for catheter-based occlusion

Disadvantages

- Requires thoracotomy and hospitalization for 48 to 72 hours with postoperative analgesia.
- Success depends on the experience of the surgeon.
- Correction of PDA is contraindicated when right-to-left shunting is present. Acute right ventricular failure and death will occur because the patent ductus functions as a relief valve for the right ventricle.

CATHETER-BASED OCCLUSION

- Shunting through the ductus may be obviated by a minimally invasive, catheter-based occlusion device. This procedure uses delivery of a coil or ductal occluding device into the lumen of the ductus resulting in embolization of the ductus.

- Coils or occlusion devices are selected on the basis of the approximate size of the ductus (as determined by angiography or echocardiography). The device is typically delivered from a catheter passed up the femoral artery and into the ductus (Figure 13.5), or less commonly through a transvenous approach that accesses the ductus from the pulmonary artery side. Multiple coils may be needed for full occlusion of the ductus, whereas only a single ductal occlusion device (e.g., Amplatz Canine Ductal Occluder) is used.

Advantages

- A less invasive procedure with a shorter hospitalization period and reduced postoperative morbidity as compared with surgical ligation

- Success rate very similar to ligation by an experienced surgeon

Disadvantages

- Might be difficult to catheterize the femoral artery of very small dogs
- Ineffective in patients with a large, tubular PDA (e.g., PDA in German Shepherds)
- Requires fluoroscopy or transesophageal echocardiography
- Includes possible complications of embolization of coils or occlusion device, or incomplete closure

MEDICAL MANAGEMENT

- In cases with CHF before correction, or in cases deemed unacceptable anesthetic-surgical candidates, medical management of CHF is indicated

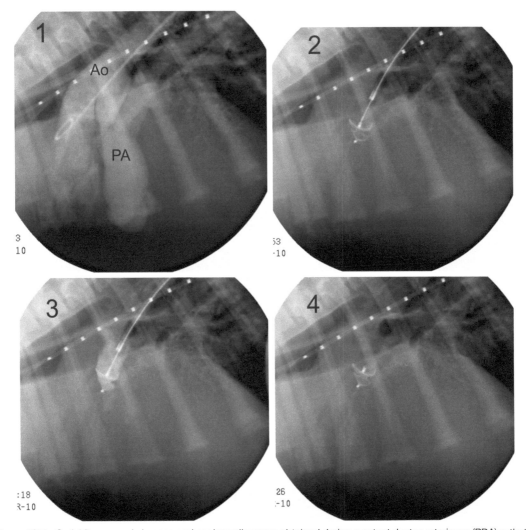

Figure 13.5 Serial fluoroscopic images and angiocardiograms obtained during a patent ductus arteriosus (PDA) catheter-based device occlusion procedure. *1)* Angiogram reveals funnel-shaped PDA and left-to-right shunting from the aorta (*Ao*) to the pulmonary artery (*PA*). *2)* Catheter-based device is positioned across the PDA. *3)* Angiogram reveals occlusion of the PDA by the device. *4)* Device is disconnected from the catheter and remains properly positioned across the PDA.

(see Chapter 15). In cases with advanced CHF, medical therapy might be continued beyond closure, especially if severe mitral regurgitation or myocardial failure is present.

- There are no drugs currently effective for closing the patent ductus in dogs and cats.

SUBAORTIC STENOSIS

ANATOMY

- Aortic stenosis is a narrowing or reduction of the left ventricular outflow tract (LVOT) at the subvalvular (fibrous ring or muscular) level, fusion of the aortic valve leaflets as the valvular level, or stenosis of the aorta at the supravalvular level. The subvalvular form (SAS) is the most common form in the dog. With this defect, a fibrous band or ring located just below the aortic semilunar valves impedes left ventricular systolic ejection and causes left ventricular concentric hypertrophy.
- Valvular and supravalvular stenosis are relatively rare in the cat and dog. Valvular aortic stenosis is most commonly reported in the Bull Terrier.
- Some patients demonstrate a dynamic SAS associated with systolic anterior motion of the anterior mitral valve leaflet. This condition has been described in patients with fixed aortic stenosis/ SAS, hypertrophic cardiomyopathy, mitral valve dysplasia, and other conditions that cause hypertrophy of the interventricular septum.
- Some breeds (Boxers, Bull Terriers, Golden Retrievers) have mildly decreased LVOT areas that result in mild elevations of transvalvular blood velocity without other structural abnormalities.

PATHOPHYSIOLOGY

- Stenosis of the LVOT results in pressure overload and concentric hypertrophy of the left ventricle (Figure 13.6). As blood is forced through

the stenotic area, velocity increases, resulting in turbulence, a systolic ejection murmur, and a poststenotic dilation of the aorta. The velocity of blood through the lesion is directly proportional to the severity (i.e., cross-sectional area of the LVOT) of disease. Left ventricular hypertrophy results in increased myocardial oxygen demand and ischemia, as well as diastolic dysfunction.

- Myocardial hypertrophy, decreased capillary density, and increased wall tension all contribute to produce myocardial hypoxia/ischemia. Focal areas of myocardial infarction and fibrosis, particularly involving the papillary muscles, small coronary vessels, and subendocardium, are common in patients with severe stenosis. These cases are prone to sudden death, presumably from fatal ventricular arrhythmias induced by hypoxia.
- Left-sided CHF is uncommon.
- The presence of aortic stenosis or SAS increases the risk of the development of infective endocarditis.

DIAGNOSIS

ETIOLOGY AND BREED PREDISPOSITION

- An autosomal dominant inheritance pattern has been identified in the Newfoundland and is associated with mutation of the *PICALM* gene.
- Other commonly affected breeds include Bouvier de Flandres, Boxer, English Bulldog, German Shepherd, German Shorthair Pointer, Golden Retriever, Great Dane, Rottweiler, and Samoyed.
- Bull Terriers are predisposed to valvular aortic stenosis characterized by thickened and calcific aortic valve leaflets and a hypoplastic aortic valve annulus.

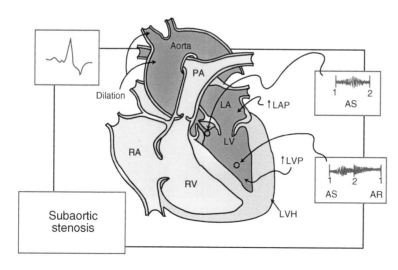

Figure 13.6 Pathophysiology and genesis of clinical signs in congenital subaortic stenosis (SAS). *LA,* Left atrium; *LAP,* left arterial pressure; *LV,* left ventricle; *LVH,* left ventricular hypertrophy; *LVP,* left ventricular pressure; *PA,* pulmonary artery; *RA,* right atrium; *RV,* right ventricle. (From Fox PR, Sisson D, Moise NS, eds: Textbook of canine and feline cardiology: principles and clinical practice, ed 2, Philadelphia, 1999, WB Saunders.)

HISTORY AND CLINICAL SIGNS

- In mildly to moderately affected cases, there are often no clinical signs, and the suspicion of aortic stenosis occurs when a murmur is detected during routine examination.
- In severe cases, owners may report failure to thrive, exercise intolerance, collapse, and labored breathing. In some cases, the first clinical sign is sudden death.

PHYSICAL EXAMINATION

PALPATION

- Animals with aortic stenosis can have increased left ventricular precordial impulses, and those with severe stenosis usually have a palpable precordial thrill over the aortic valve area. Femoral pulses are often weak and late rising (pulsus parvus et tardus).

AUSCULTATION

- SAS causes a systolic ejection-type murmur heard best over the left fourth intercostal space at the level of the costochondral junction (aortic valve area). Frequently, the murmur radiates up the carotid artery and can be auscultated in the midcervical area. Occasionally, the murmur may be loudest in the right third or fourth intercostal space midway up the thorax. Rarely, a concurrent diastolic murmur of aortic insufficiency is present.

DIAGNOSTIC TESTING

ELECTROCARDIOGRAM

- The ECG may be normal. Alternatively, there may be evidence of left ventricular hypertrophy (tall R waves in leads II [>3.0 mV], III, and aV$_F$).
- Ventricular or supraventricular arrhythmias are occasionally detected.
- ST segment depression or elevation at rest or after exercise is occasionally detected in severe cases and indicative of myocardial ischemia.

THORACIC RADIOGRAPHS

- Radiographic changes tend to parallel severity of the stenosis. Characteristic features include enlargement of the aortic arch (poststenotic dilation) and prominent left ventricle (Figures 13.7 and 13.8).
- Left atrial enlargement is rare but can be present in advanced cases with concurrent mitral insufficiency.

ECHOCARDIOGRAPHY

- Echocardiography is the most sensitive noninvasive method to visualize the narrowed LVOT and secondary cardiac changes. In most cases, there is significant left ventricular hypertrophy. In severe cases, the papillary muscles and myocardium become hyperechoic secondary to ischemia and fibrosis.
- Doppler echocardiography allows measurement of blood flow velocity through the stenosis and provides data regarding severity. The velocity of blood through the stenosis, measured by Doppler echocardiography, provides a noninvasive measure of the pressure gradient across the stenosis. The pressure gradient (in mm Hg) can be readily derived with the modified Bernoulli equation: pressure gradient between LV and aorta (mm Hg) =4× velocity of LVOT flow (m/s)^2.
- Pressure gradients <50 mm Hg are considered mild, 50 to 80 mm Hg are considered moderate, and >80 mm Hg are considered severe.

KEY POINT

The differentiation between patients with trivial to mild stenosis and normal patients with physiologic-induced accelerated transaortic velocities can be difficult, if not impossible. A diagnosis of trivial to mild subaortic/aortic stenosis based solely on elevations of transaortic velocity can be problematic; the diagnosis should include a combination of the following: accelerated transvalvular velocities, turbulent blood flow, visualization of an anatomical lesion, concurrent aortic insufficiency, or a distinct "step up" in velocity across a discreet region of the outflow tract. Most examiners consider LVOT velocity >2.25 m/s as indicative of SAS.

CARDIAC CATHETERIZATION

- Cardiac catheterization and angiography are occasionally used when multiple cardiac defects are suspected.
- Angiography illustrates the stenosis and poststenotic dilation. Pressure measurements obtained during selective catheterization are used to determine the location and pressure gradient across the stenosis.

NATURAL HISTORY

- The clinical manifestations of SAS are variable. Up to 70% of dogs with severe stenosis may die suddenly during the first 3 years of life. Cardiac arrhythmias are common in affected dogs. In others, CHF may develop later in life. Dogs with

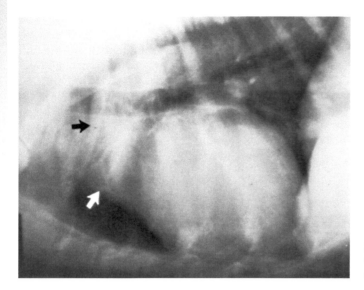

Figure 13.7 Aortic stenosis (lateral projection). There is marked enlargement of the aortic arch cranial to the heart base (*arrows*).

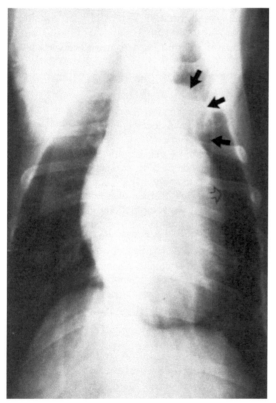

Figure 13.8 Aortic stenosis (dorsoventral projection). The enlarged aortic arch extends to the heart base (*arrows*). The left auricle (*open arrow*) extends beyond the cardiac border, and there is slight left ventricular enlargement.

SAS are predisposed to infective endocarditis or the aortic valve, which is often a life-threatening complication. Other affected individuals may demonstrate symptoms such as syncope or lack of exercise capacity.

THERAPY AND PROGNOSIS

SURGERY

- Surgical resection of the SAS lesion requires cardiopulmonary bypass and is not indicated for patients with mild stenosis. Surgery in cases of severe SAS has not been associated with improved long-term survival and is rarely performed because of the expense and morbidity associated with the procedure.

BALLOON DILATION

- Balloon valvuloplasty is infrequently performed and most often contemplated in cases with discrete and membranelike stenosis. Special cutting and high-pressure balloons can be used. Significant reductions in the pressure gradient across the stenosis can be achieved immediately after balloon dilation; however, restenosis is likely, and balloon dilation has not been consistently associated with improved long-term outcome.

MEDICAL MANAGEMENT

- Because of the lack of effective interventional techniques, medical management forms the basis of therapy in most cases of SAS. Beta blockers (propranolol or atenolol) are used to reduce myocardial oxygen demand. They might also be of some benefit in reducing the frequency of arrhythmias. Renin-angiotensin-aldosterone antagonists or inhibitors such as spironolactone or angiotensin-converting enzyme (ACE) inhibitors are occasionally prescribed in an attempt to reduce myocardial remodeling or fibrosis. The benefits of medical therapy are largely theoretic in nature and have

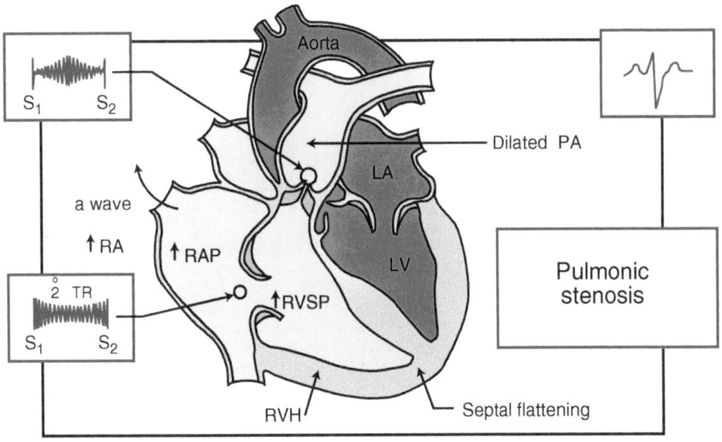

Figure 13.9 Pathophysiology and genesis of clinical signs in pulmonic stenosis (PS). *LA,* Left atrium; *LV,* left ventricle; *PA,* pulmonary artery; *RAP,* right atrial I pressure; *RVH,* right ventricular hypertrophy; *RVSP,* right ventricular systolic pressure. (Modified from Fox PR, Sisson D, Moise NS, eds: Textbook of canine and feline cardiology: principles and clinical practice, ed 2, Philadelphia, 1999, WB Saunders.)

not been consistently shown to improve long-term outcome.

- Antibiotics should be administered when bacteremia is suspected or likely (e.g., dental procedures) to reduce the chance of infective endocarditis.
- Diuretic therapy is indicated in cases of CHF.
- Positive inotropes such as digoxin and pimobendan are contraindicated in SAS and in other forms of outflow obstruction and should not be used.

PULMONIC STENOSIS

PS is the third most commonly reported congenital defect in the dog. PS is most often caused by fusion of the aortic valve leaflets at the valvular level. In Bulldogs and Boxers, stenosis of the pulmonary artery can occur at the subvalvular level because of an anomalous origin of the left coronary artery. Supravalvular PS is uncommon.

PATHOPHYSIOLOGY

- The consequences of this defect are in direct proportion to the severity of the obstruction. The major clinical manifestations are secondary to pressure overload of the right ventricle.
- Hemodynamically, valvular PS results in a pressure gradient across the stenotic valve because of resistance to right ventricular outflow (Figure 13.9). The severity of the lesion is directly related to this pressure gradient. Right ventricular hypertrophy is almost always present; the degree varies with the severity of stenosis.
- Turbulence associated with the increase in velocity of blood across the stenotic valve is the cause of the poststenotic dilation in the main pulmonary artery segment.
- The valvular lesion may be characterized by fusion of the valve leaflets, dysplasia of the valvular apparatus, or both.

- Depending on the severity of the right ventricular hypertrophy, some patients will have a dynamic, infundibular stenosis in addition to the fixed valvular stenosis.

DIAGNOSIS

ETIOLOGY AND BREED DISPOSITION

- PS occurs more often in the dog than in the cat.
- The defect is more common in the following breeds: Airedale Terrier, Beagle, Boykin Spaniel, Boxer, Chihuahua, Cocker Spaniel, English Bulldog, Bull Mastiff, Samoyed, Schnauzer, and West Highland White Terrier.
- A polygenic inheritance pattern has been identified in the Beagle.

HISTORY AND CLINICAL SIGNS

- Animals with mild or moderate PS are usually symptom free, and many live apparently normal lives with mild disease.
- Animals with PS that have symptoms also have clinical signs of fatigue secondary to low cardiac output. Exercise-induced syncope may occur because of the limitation in cardiac output imposed by the stenotic valve. Decompensation and signs of right-sided heart failure may occur. Approximately 35% of dogs with severe stenosis have clinical signs.
- Severe right ventricular hypertrophy can result in myocardial hypoxia and ventricular arrhythmias.

PHYSICAL EXAMINATION

PALPATION

- Animals with moderate to severe PS have easily palpable right ventricular impulses. A precordial thrill is usually present at the left lower third or fourth intercostal space.

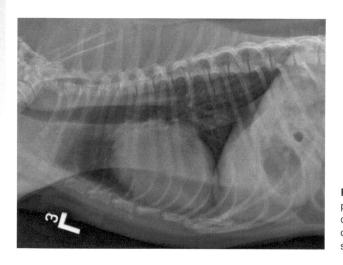

Figure 13.10 Pulmonic stenosis (PS) (left lateral projection) in a dog. There is increased sternal contact of the right side of the heart because of right-sided heart enlargement and normal to slightly diminished pulmonary vasculature.

- Jugular venous distention and pulsations may be present if tricuspid regurgitation or CHF is present.

AUSCULTATION

- A systolic, ejection murmur is heard best at the left lower third or fourth intercostal space. If the murmur is severe, it may radiate over the cranial thorax and be audible at the thoracic inlet.
- A split second heart sound due to delayed closure of the pulmonic valve may also be present.
- It can be difficult to differentiate between the murmurs of subaortic/aortic stenosis and PS.

DIAGNOSTIC TESTING

ELECTROCARDIOGRAM

- Signs of right ventricular hypertrophy are present in the majority of cases. There are deep S waves present in leads I, II, and III, and a right shift of the mean electrical axis in the frontal plane.
- Ventricular arrhythmias may be present.

THORACIC RADIOGRAPHS

- The primary radiographic features (Figures 13.10 and 13.11) include right atrial and ventricular enlargement and enlargement of the main pulmonary segment. Decreased pulmonary vascularity with pulmonary arteries smaller than normal is detected in severe cases.

ECHOCARDIOGRAPHY

- Echocardiography is highly sensitive in the diagnosis and determination of severity of PS.
- Characteristic findings include the following:
  - Right ventricular dilation and hypertrophy of the right ventricular wall and interventricular

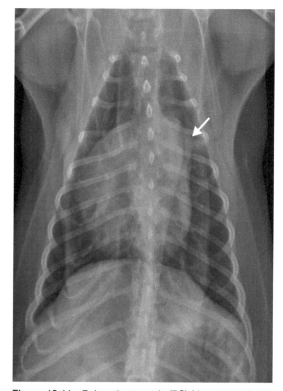

Figure 13.11 Pulmonic stenosis (PS) (dorsoventral projection) in a dog. There is marked right-heart enlargement and prominence of the main pulmonary artery (*arrow*).

septum. Because of increased pressures within the right ventricle, the septum is typically flattened (Figure 13.12).
- The right ventricular outflow tract is often dilated, and in cases of valvular stenosis, the pulmonic valve cusps are thickened and immobile. A poststenotic dilation of the main pulmonary artery is usually evident.
- Doppler echocardiography provides a sensitive and noninvasive method to determine the

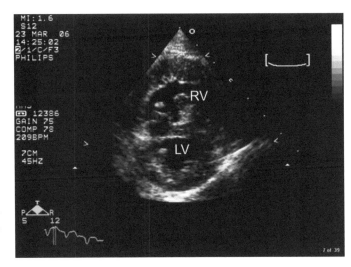

Figure 13.12 Right parasternal short-axis, two-dimensional (2D) echocardiogram obtained from a West Highland White Terrier with severe pulmonic stenosis (PS). Note the severely thickened right ventricle *(RV)*. *LV,* Left ventricle.

severity of stenosis by estimating the pressure gradient across the obstruction in a similar manner as with aortic stenosis: mild (<50 mm Hg), moderate (50 to 80 mm Hg), and severe (>80 mm Hg).

OTHER DIAGNOSTIC TECHNIQUES

- Cardiac catheterization and angiography are performed routinely before an interventional procedure such as balloon valvuloplasty. Selective coronary angiography is required to rule out the presence of an anomalous left main coronary artery in English Bulldogs and Boxers, if surgery or balloon valvuloplasty is considered.

DIFFERENTIAL DIAGNOSIS

- Atrial septal defect: The right ventricular volume overload associated with a left-to-right shunting atrial septal defect may result in a systolic ejection murmur over the pulmonic valve. Such murmurs are usually softer than those associated with PS.
- Innocent or physiologic murmurs: These murmurs are usually much softer than typical PS murmurs and do not typically persist beyond 6 months of age.

NATURAL HISTORY

- Uncomplicated survival to adulthood is common in dogs with mild to moderate PS. In general, the natural history correlates with disease severity (pressure gradient) and the degree of right ventricular hypertrophy. Dogs with moderate to severe PS may have signs of right-sided CHF, cardiac arrhythmias, syncope with exertion, or sudden death (rare). Concurrent tricuspid valve dysplasia increases the risk of the development of CHF.

THERAPY AND PROGNOSIS

- The need for treatment and the prognosis are dependent on the severity of the defect as determined by Doppler echocardiography or cardiac catheterization. Cases with mild stenosis do not require treatment and have a favorable prognosis. Those with severe stenosis are candidates for balloon valvuloplasty, and may have a poor prognosis if uncorrected. Intermediate cases should be followed to monitor for progression of the stenosis.

SURGERY

- The method of surgical correction depends on the type of stenosis present and its severity.
- Some forms of PS may be palliated by circumventing the stenosis with a conduit or by placing a patch graft in young animals with valvular PS. In general, surgical correction is not commonly performed.

BALLOON VALVULOPLASTY

- A special cardiac catheter is guided from a jugular or femoral vein approach and through the stenotic valve. A balloon situated at the end of the catheter is inflated to break open the stenosis. Balloon valvuloplasty is most effective for valvular stenosis when valves are thin and fused and hypoplasia of the annulus is not present. Balloon valvuloplasty is generally contraindicated in cases of subvalvular PS due to a main left coronary artery anomaly because avulsion of the coronary artery from the aortic root can occur during balloon inflation.
- In general, balloon valvuloplasty results in a significant (40% to 60%) decrease in the pressure

gradient and is maintained in 60% to 70% of patients; however, the long-term effects on survival improvement have not been definitely determined.

- This procedure is generally recommended for patients with moderate to severe stenosis, particularly those patients with symptoms such as syncope or decreased exercise capacity.

English Bulldogs and some Boxers may have an anomalous left main coronary artery arising from a single right coronary artery associated with the stenosis that precludes surgical or catheter-based intervention because of the risk of avulsion of the left coronary artery and subsequent death.

MEDICAL MANAGEMENT

- Signs of right-sided CHF should be treated as described in Chapter 15.
- Beta blocker therapy (atenolol 0.25 to 1.5 mg/kg PO q12h) is routinely administered to patients with moderate to severe right ventricular hypertrophy in an effort to decrease myocardial oxygen consumption and to suppress ventricular arrhythmias.

VENTRICULAR SEPTAL DEFECT

ANATOMY

- The interventricular septum separates the left ventricle and the right ventricle. It is muscular at the apex and tapers to a membranous portion at the heart base near the origin of the aorta. VSDs may occur in any area of the septum but are most commonly located in the membranous portion.
- VSDs may occur as isolated defects, may coexist with concurrent defects (e.g., PDA and atrial septal defect), or may be a component of more complex cardiac anomalies.

PATHOPHYSIOLOGY

- The two major factors that determine the consequences of a VSD are the cross-sectional area of the VSD and the relative pressures (or resistances) of the right or left ventricles and pulmonary and systemic circulations, respectively. When left and right ventricular pressures and vascular resistances are normal, blood will shunt left to right, as the left ventricular systolic pressure is roughly five times greater than right ventricular systolic pressure (Figure 13.13). In the typical VSD (left-to-right shunting membranous

defect), most of the blood is shunted into the right ventricular outflow tract, or the main pulmonary artery. This shunt creates a large volume overload to the pulmonary circulation, the left atrium, and the left ventricle. Thus when pulmonary resistance remains relatively normal, despite the left-to-right shunting, the right ventricle is spared most of the effects of the shunting.

- Small left-to-right shunting VSDs may be of no hemodynamic significance, although they may predispose the animal to the development of endocarditis. In rare cases, some small defects close spontaneously.
- Moderately sized defects may allow significant shunting and produce clinical signs of left-sided CHF.
- Very large defects may create a functional single ventricle with equilibration of left and right ventricular pressures and net right-to-left shunting. Similarly, if right ventricular resistance increases (e.g., PS, pulmonary hypertension), right ventricular pressure will increase proportionately, thereby decreasing the shunt volume. If right ventricular pressure increases to a point where it exceeds left ventricular pressure, blood will shunt right to left, and signs of generalized cyanosis and polycythemia may develop.

DIAGNOSIS

ETIOLOGY AND BREED PREDISPOSITION

- Breed studies in the Keeshond have shown the defect to be polygenic.
- The English Bulldog appears to have a higher incidence than other breeds, but the defect is seen in many purebred and mixed-breed dogs.

HISTORY AND CLINICAL SIGNS

- The clinical course of animals with VSD is variable and to a large extent dependent on the size of the defect and the ventricular pressures. Small defects may cause little or no functional disturbances and may cause no clinical signs. Moderate to large defects usually produce signs of left-sided failure subsequent to the chronic left-sided volume overload. In cases that develop pulmonary hypertension, signs of right-sided failure and cyanosis will predominate.

PHYSICAL EXAMINATION

PALPATION

- In many cases, a precordial thrill is present at the right-sided heart base (third to fourth

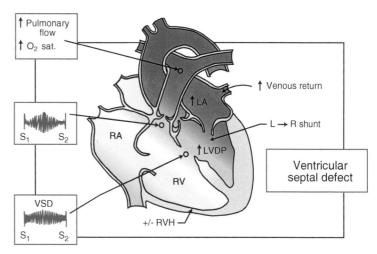

Figure 13.13 Pathophysiology and genesis of clinical findings in VSD. *LA,* Left atrium; *LVDP,* left ventricular developed pressure; *RA,* right atrium; *RV,* right ventricle; *RVH,* right ventricular hypertrophy. (Modified from Fox P.R., Sisson D., Moise N.S., eds: Textbook of canine and feline cardiology: principles and clinical practice, ed 2, Philadelphia, 1999, WB Saunders.)

intercostal spaces, just above the costochondral junctions). Volume overloading of the left ventricle often accentuates the left-sided impulse. In cases with significant pulmonary hypertension, precordial thrills are unusual, and the right apical impulse is accentuated.

AUSCULTATION

- Typically the murmur is harsh, holosystolic, and heard best at the right sternal border, at the second through fourth intercostal spaces.
- A murmur of functional PS may be heard over the pulmonic valve area. This is a result of the extra volume of blood passing through the pulmonic valve and not related to a structural valve problem.
- A split-second heart sound occasionally is present because of a slightly prolonged right ventricular ejection time.
- When the defect causes destabilization of an aortic valve cusp, a diastolic murmur of aortic insufficiency may be present in addition to the systolic murmur. This combination is referred to as a to-and-fro murmur rather than a continuous murmur.
- In cases with progressive pulmonary hypertension, elevations in right ventricular resistance result in diminished shunting. With very large defects, severe pulmonary hypertension, or both, a murmur may be absent because of the lack of a pressure differential across the septum.

DIAGNOSTIC TESTING

ELECTROCARDIOGRAM

- ECG abnormalities usually parallel the degree of hemodynamic compromise.
- The ECG may be normal when a small defect is present.

- The ECG may show evidence of left, right, or biventricular enlargement, depending on hemodynamic consequences of the shunt.
- Right bundle branch block or a splintered QRS complex indicative of a ventricular conduction abnormality may also be observed.

THORACIC RADIOGRAPHS

- Small defects usually do not cause radiographic changes.
- Left ventricular enlargement, left atrial enlargement, and increased pulmonary artery prominence are seen with larger defects resulting in significant left-to-right shunting.
- Right ventricular enlargement accompanied by prominent tortuous pulmonary arteries may be present in cases of pulmonary hypertension and right-to-left shunting.

ECHOCARDIOGRAPHY

- The diagnosis of VSD can usually be confirmed by routine echocardiography. Typical findings for a moderate to large shunt include left ventricular and left atrial dilation and a defect in the interventricular septum with two-dimensional (2D) echocardiography. Distinguish the septal dropout normally present in the membranous septum from a VSD. In most VSD cases, the interventricular septum is slightly blunted just apical to the defect, whereas the septum tapers gradually in normal animals.
- Contrast echocardiography will confirm the presence of a right-to-left shunting VSD. Agitated saline is rapidly injected into a peripheral vein, resulting in the appearance of microbubbles (contrast) within the heart. In the absence of a right-to-left shunt, all contrast

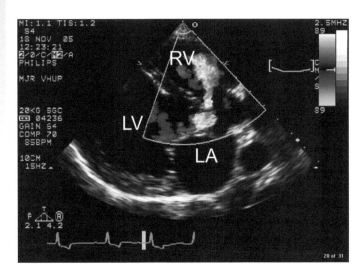

Figure 13.14 Right parasternal long-axis, two-dimensional echocardiogram obtained from a 9-week-old Golden Retriever puppy with a right-sided systolic murmur. Note the aliased color flow pattern crossing the interventricular septum. This finding is consistent with a left-to-right shunting ventricular septal defect (VSD). *LA,* Left atrium; *LV,* left ventricle; *RV,* right ventricle.

remains right-sided. In right-to-left shunting VSD, microbubbles will be seen traversing the defect.

- Doppler echocardiography will confirm the shunting of blood through the defect (Figure 13.14).

KEY POINT

- High-velocity flow across the VSD and normal transpulmonic valvular velocities typically indicate that the defect is associated with a small shunting volume. These "restrictive" shunts are often hemodynamically insignificant and are unlikely to be associated with clinical signs.
- Low-velocity flow across the VSD and increased transpulmonic valvular velocities typically indicate that the defect is associated with a large shunting volume. These "unrestrictive" shunts are often hemodynamically significant and are likely to be associated with clinical signs.

OTHER DIAGNOSTIC PROCEDURES

- Cardiac catheterization and determination of oxygen saturation of blood from individual cardiac chambers may be used to confirm shunting. Left-to-right shunts produce a step-up in oxygen saturation in the right ventricle compared with the right atrium.

THERAPY AND PROGNOSIS

- The prognosis and need for therapy are dependent on the severity of the defect. Small defects are usually well tolerated with little to no effect on longevity. Larger septal defect with significant shunting might require surgical or catheter-based device closure or eventual medical therapy for CHF. The proximity of the VSD to the aortic valve increases risk of infectious

endocarditis, and antibiotic prophylaxis before procedures likely to produce bacteremia (e.g., dental cleaning) is recommended.

SURGERY OR CATHETER-BASED DEVICE CLOSURE

- Open heart techniques to surgically close or patch the VSD are curative; however, these techniques are available at a very limited number of locations and are often prohibitively expensive. Palliative reduction of the shunt can be accomplished by pulmonary artery banding, a technique resulting in elevation of the right ventricular systolic pressure. As right ventricular pressure increases, the shunt volume decreases, and the pulmonary circulation is spared the deleterious effects of chronic volume overload. Catheter-based closure of the VSD with an occlusion device is reported but technically difficult because of the proximity of the VSD to the aortic valve.

MEDICAL MANAGEMENT

- In patients with significant shunting, medical management of CHF may be required. Treatment should be tailored to the type and degree of failure (see Chapter 15). In cases of right-to-left VSD, the long-term consequences of hypoxemia and polycythemia are managed with activity restriction and periodic phlebotomy.

PROGNOSIS

- Prognosis is excellent for animals with small defects or for those with surgically corrected defects. Cases with moderate to large defects have a variable clinical course and prognosis depending on shunt volume.

TETRALOGY OF FALLOT

Tetralogy of Fallot is a cyanosis-producing defect and results from a combination of PS, VSD, right ventricular hypertrophy, and varying degrees of dextroposition and overriding of the aorta. The right ventricular hypertrophy is secondary to the obstruction in right ventricular outflow. The PS may be valvular, infundibular, or both.

PATHOPHYSIOLOGY

The hemodynamic consequences of tetralogy of Fallot depend primarily on the severity of the PS and the size of the VSD.

- The direction and magnitude of the shunt through the septal defect are dependent on the degree of right ventricular obstruction. If the PS is mild and right ventricular pressures are only modestly elevated, then blood will shunt primarily from left to right. Pathophysiologically, these cases are similar to VSD cases with pulmonary artery banding (i.e., the mild right ventricular obstruction protects the pulmonary vasculature from excessive shunting).
- When PS is severe, the elevated right ventricular pressures will result in right-to-left shunting. Consequences include reduced pulmonary blood flow (resulting in fatigue and shortness of breath) and generalized cyanosis (resulting in weakness).
- Because of the shunting of venous blood into the aorta and consequent hypoxemia, the kidneys are stimulated to release erythropoietin. Chronic elevations in erythropoietin result in polycythemia. The increased blood viscosity associated with polycythemia can have significant hemodynamic effects, resulting in sludging of blood and poor capillary perfusion. Animals with severe polycythemia may seizure.

DIAGNOSIS
ETIOLOGY AND BREED PREDISPOSITION

- Breeds predisposed to tetralogy of Fallot include the English Bulldog, Keeshond, Miniature Poodle, Miniature Schnauzer, and Wire-Haired Fox Terrier. This defect has also been recognized in other canine breeds and in cats.

HISTORY AND CLINICAL SIGNS

- Typical historical features include stunted growth, exercise intolerance, cyanosis, collapse, and seizure activity.

PHYSICAL EXAMINATION
PALPATION

- A precordial thrill may be felt in the third left intercostal space near the costochondral junction.

AUSCULTATION

- In most cases, a murmur of PS is present. The intensity of the murmur is attenuated when severe polycythemia is present.

DIAGNOSTIC TESTING
ELECTROCARDIOGRAM

- A right ventricular enlargement pattern is usually present.
- Arrhythmias may be present.

THORACIC RADIOGRAPHS

- Variable right-sided heart enlargement is present.
- Pulmonary vessels are undersized, and the main pulmonary artery is often diminished.

ECHOCARDIOGRAPHY

- Echocardiography will confirm the diagnosis. Contrast echocardiography will demonstrate right-to-left shunting at the level of the VSD. Flow through the defect can also be determined by Doppler echocardiography.

CARDIAC CATHETERIZATION

- Selective angiocardiography of the right ventricle demonstrates simultaneous filling of the aorta and pulmonary artery in cases with right-to-left shunts. Oximetry can be performed to help quantify the degree of right-to-left shunting.

THERAPY AND PROGNOSIS
SURGERY

- Surgical correction of tetralogy of Fallot is not commonly performed because of the attendant mortality and expense. Palliative surgical options include the modified Blalock-Taussig anastomosis, wherein a vascular graft is placed between the left subclavian artery and pulmonary artery to increase pulmonary blood flow. This procedure is generally effective in reducing signs of pulmonary hypoperfusion and systemic hypoxia. In some cases, palliation can be provided by reducing the severity of the PS with balloon valvuloplasty.

MEDICAL MANAGEMENT

- Nonselective beta-adrenergic blockade (e.g., propranolol) has been used to reduce the dynamic component of right ventricular outflow obstruction and to attenuate beta-adrenergic–mediated decreases in systemic vascular resistance, which increase the magnitude of right-to-left shunting during activity.
- Polycythemia should be controlled by periodic phlebotomy. When the packed cell volume exceeds 68, intervention is indicated. Up to 20 mL/kg of blood can be removed and replaced with a crystalloid solution such as lactated Ringer solution or saline.
- If the required frequency of phlebotomy is poorly tolerated by the patient hydroxyurea, an oral myelosuppressive agent can be used. However, administration of this drug requires close patient monitoring with periodic complete blood and platelet counts.

ATRIOVENTRICULAR VALVE DYSPLASIA

Congenital malformation of the mitral and tricuspid valves has been reported in dogs and cats. Malformation of the valve may result in a range of hemodynamic consequences, including valvular regurgitation, mitral or tricuspid stenosis, and dynamic left ventricular outflow obstruction. Congenital malformation of the mitral valve complex (mitral valve dysplasia) is a common congenital cardiac defect in the cat. In addition, several canine breeds are predisposed, including Bull Terriers, German Shepherds, and Great Danes. Tricuspid valve dysplasia has been shown to have a genetic basis in Labrador Retrievers.

ANATOMY

- Mitral valve dysplasia most commonly results in valvular insufficiency and systolic regurgitation of blood into the left atrium.
- Any component of the atrioventricular valve complex (valve leaflet, chordae tendineae, papillary muscles) may be malformed. Often more than one component is defective. A wide spectrum of valvular malformations has been described: thickening of the valve leaflets; incomplete separation of the valvular structures from the ventricular wall; shortening or elongation, thickening, and fusion of the chordae tendineae; and malpositioning or malformation of the papillary muscles.

PATHOPHYSIOLOGY

- Malformation of the atrioventricular valve complex can result in significant valvular

insufficiency. In the case involving the mitral valve, chronic mitral regurgitation leads to volume overload to the left heart, which results in dilation of the left ventricle and atrium in the same manner that occurs in chronic degenerative valvular disease (see Chapter 7).
- When mitral regurgitation is severe, cardiac output decreases, resulting in signs of cardiac failure.
- Dilation of the left-sided chambers predisposes affected animals to arrhythmias. Severe atrial enlargement increases the risk of tachyarrhythmias such as atrial fibrillation.
- In some cases, malformation of the mitral valve complex causes a degree of valvular stenosis and insufficiency.
- If the tricuspid valve is involved, then atrial and ventricular enlargement secondary to volume overload with subsequent systemic venous hypertension and right-sided CHF is a likely outcome, if regurgitation is severe.

DIAGNOSIS

HISTORY AND CLINICAL SIGNS

- Clinical signs correlate with the severity of the defect. Affected animals usually display signs of left-sided heart failure, including weakness, cough, and exercise intolerance if the mitral valve is affected. Alternatively, signs of right heart failure (abdominal distention associated with ascites) may be present if the tricuspid valve is affected.

PHYSICAL EXAMINATION
PALPATION

- Affected animals may have a precordial thrill over the left cardiac apex (mitral valve) or right cardiac apex (tricuspid valve).

AUSCULTATION

- A holosystolic murmur of mitral regurgitation is most prominent at the left cardiac apex. A diastolic heart sound (gallop) is present in some cases. The murmur of tricuspid regurgitation is heard most clearly at the right cardiac apex. Some patients with clinically significant tricuspid regurgitation may have "silent" regurgitation.

DIAGNOSTIC TESTING
ELECTROCARDIOGRAM

- Atrial arrhythmias (atrial premature contractions, atrial fibrillation) are common.
- Evidence of left atrial enlargement (widened P waves) and left ventricular enlargement may be present.

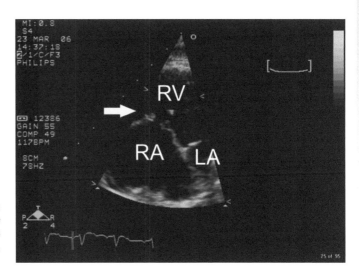

Figure 13.15 Echocardiogram from a dog with tricuspid valve dysplasia. Note the severely thickened tricuspid valve leaflets (*arrow*). *LA,* Left atrium; *LV,* left ventricle; *RV,* right ventricle.

- Splintered QRS complexes are common ECG findings in cats and dogs with tricuspid valve dysplasia. Right-sided heart enlargement patterns may also be present.

THORACIC RADIOGRAPHS

- The most prominent abnormality with mitral valve dysplasia is severe left atrial enlargement. Left ventricular enlargement is also present. Pulmonary veins may be distended, and evidence of left-sided CHF may be present.
- Right atrial and ventricular enlargement may be evident if severe tricuspid valve regurgitation is present. Distention of the caudal vena cava may be noted if right-sided CHF is present.

ECHOCARDIOGRAPHY

- Echocardiography demonstrates malformation of the mitral valve complex (fused chordae tendineae and thickened, immobile valve leaflets) and left atrial and ventricular dilation.
- Doppler echocardiography demonstrates severe mitral regurgitation. If present, mitral stenosis can be identified.
- The echocardiographic findings with tricuspid valve dysplasia mirror those changes seen with mitral valve dysplasia and only involve the right heart instead (Figure 13.15).

THERAPY AND PROGNOSIS

- Prognosis for severely affected animals with clinical signs is poor. Mildly affected animals may remain free of clinical signs for several years. Therapy for progressive CHF is detailed in Chapter 15.

FREQUENTLY ASKED QUESTIONS

Which is the best approach for treatment of PDA: surgical ligation or catheter-based device occlusion?

Both approaches have been demonstrated to be effective and safe when performed by experienced individuals; therefore the best approach is the approach that is most readily available (there are geographical limitations for device occlusion because there are a limited number of individuals trained to perform catheter-based interventional procedures).

Does the intensity of a cardiac murmur associated with congenital heart disease correlate with the severity of the disease?

In general, the intensity of the murmur roughly approximates the severity of the defect; however, there are some exceptions. Patients with small, restrictive VSDs often have very loud systolic murmurs but are unlikely to be clinically affected. With regard to defects that cause obstruction to ventricular outflow, presence of myocardial failure can decrease the intensity of the murmur. Some patients with tricuspid valve dysplasia have "silent" regurgitation that can only be detected by echocardiography or angiocardiography. Patients with reversed PDA have severe cardiovascular derangement but often have no audible cardiac murmurs.

What is the most important diagnostic test for a patient suspected of having a congenital heart defect?

Echocardiography is the most important part of the evaluation of a patient suspected of having a congenital heart defect. Two-dimensional echocardiography provides an anatomic image of the cardiac structures that can be observed in real time for assessment of structural and functional abnormalities.

M-mode echocardiography can be used to quantify cardiac dimensions and function. Doppler echocardiography is a critical part of the echocardiographic evaluation of a patient with a cardiac murmur. Color flow Doppler allows for rapid detection of abnormal flow patterns, and spectral Doppler can be used for quantification of blood flow characteristics such as velocity.

SUGGESTED READINGS

Bonagura JD, Lehmkuhl L: Congenital heart disease. In Fox PR, Sisson D, Moise NS, eds: Textbook of canine and feline cardiology, Philadelphia, 1999, WB Saunders.

Eason BS, Fine DM, Leeder D, et al: Influence of beta-blockers on survival in dogs with severe subaortic stenosis, J Vet Intern Med 28:857–862, 2014.

Kittleson MD, Kienle RD, eds: Small animal cardiovascular medicine, St Louis, 1998, Mosby.

Oliveira P, Domenech O, Silva J, et al: Retrospective review of congenital heart disease in 976 dogs, J Vet Intern Med 25:477–483, 2011.

Oyama MA, Sisson DD, Thomas WP, Bonagura JD: Congenital heart disease. In Ettinger SJ, ed: Textbook of veterinary internal medicine, ed 7, Philadelphia, 2010, Elsevier.

Stern JA, White SN, Lehmkuhl LB, et al: A single codon insertion in PICALM is associated with development of familial subvalvular aortic stenosis in Newfoundland dogs, Hum Genet 133:1139, 2014.

Cardiovascular Effects of Systemic Diseases

14

Francis W. K. Smith, Jr. | Donald P. Schrope | Carl D. Sammarco

Many systemic diseases are capable of profoundly affecting cardiovascular structure and function (Box 14.1). The veterinarian may detect cardiovascular abnormalities as the predominant clinical sign, or systemic disease manifestations may overshadow cardiac abnormalities. Although cardiovascular manifestations may sometimes be of no clinical significance, at other times they may constitute the major medical concern. Detection of cardiovascular involvement may be based on clinical signs, radiographic changes, electrocardiographic (ECG) or echocardiographic abnormalities, or laboratory findings. Emphasis in this chapter is given to diseases having the greatest cardiovascular effects or incidence in veterinary practice. The focus of discussion is the cardiovascular effects and their treatment.

ENDOCRINE DISEASES

HYPERTHYROIDISM

- Hyperthyroidism is the most common systemic disturbance to affect cardiac function in cats and is rare in dogs. Hyperthyroid heart disease can be a severe problem, leading to heart failure in some animals.
- Hyperthyroidism is a disease of middle-aged to geriatric cats (range, 4 to 22 years; mean, 13 years) that is generally caused by a thyroid adenoma. Clinical evidence of thyrotoxic heart disease is unusual before the age of 6 years.
- There is a declining reported incidence of cardiovascular complications from hyperthyroidism. This change is probably related to earlier diagnosis, as measurement of T_4 concentrations are now a common component of geriatric screening profiles.
- Thyroid tumors in dogs are generally rare and nonfunctional adenocarcinomas that do not cause hyperthyroidism. Iatrogenic hyperthyroidism can result from over supplementation of thyroxin in hypothyroid dogs.

CARDIAC PATHOPHYSIOLOGY

DIRECT EFFECTS

- Positive inotropic effects (i.e., increased contractility) result from an increased sodium-potassium exchanging adenosine triphosphatase (Na^+, K^+-ATPase) activity, increased mitochondrial protein synthesis, and increased synthesis and enhanced contractile properties of myosin. Thyroid hormone favors the production of the alpha heavy chain myosin isoenzyme, which has the fastest ATPase activity but is less efficient at converting ATP to mechanical energy. Thyroid hormones increase the number of L-type calcium channels and expression of sodium calcium ATPase, which improves the recycling of calcium by the sarcoplasmic reticulum. Both systolic and diastolic functions are altered.
- Positive chronotropic effects (i.e., increased heart rate) result from an increased rate of sinoatrial firing, decreased threshold of atrial activation, and shortened refractory period of the conduction tissue. The effect on atrial activation may increase the risk for atrial arrhythmias.

INDIRECT EFFECTS

- The effect of thyroid hormones on the adrenergic system is controversial. The number of myocardial beta-adrenergic receptors and their affinity are increased in hyperthyroid animals. However, this does not always explain or result in an increased responsiveness to catecholamines. Postreceptor effects of thyroid hormone are probably mediated by changes in intracellular G protein populations that result in an enhanced response to adrenergic agonists. Circulating catecholamine levels are normal.
- Hyperthyroidism results in an increased metabolic rate and, consequently, an increased tissue oxygen demand. The need for increased tissue perfusion and oxygen delivery requires greater

Box 14.1   Classification of Important Systemic Disorders That Affect the Heart

Endocrine

Thyroid gland
  Hyperthyroidism
  Hypothyroidism
Adrenal gland
  Hyperadrenocorticism
  Hypoadrenocorticism
  Pheochromocytoma
Pituitary
  Acromegaly (hypersomatotropism)
Pancreas
  Diabetes mellitus (hyperglycemia)

Metabolic

Hypercalcemia
Hypocalcemia
Hyperkalemia
Hypokalemia
Hypoglycemia
Uremia
Anemia

Neoplastic and Infiltrative Heart Diseases

Physical and Chemical Agents

Hyperpyrexia (heat stroke)
Hypothermia
Carbon monoxide
Toad poisoning
Oleander toxicity
Chocolate (theobromine) toxicity
Doxorubicin cardiotoxicity

Infectious/Inflammatory Myocardial Diseases

Bacterial (e.g., Lyme disease)
Viral (e.g., parvovirus)
Mycotic
Protozoal (e.g., trypanosomiasis)

Miscellaneous

Systemic lupus erythematosus (SLE)
Neurologic disease
Gastric dilatation-volvulus complex (GDV)
Pancreatitis
Traumatic myocarditis

---

cardiac output. Peripheral vasodilation increases tissue perfusion and decreases afterload. As blood volume increases, increased venous return to the heart and increased preload result. The combination of increased preload, increased contractility, increased heart rate, and decreased afterload results in increased cardiac output. The chronic volume overload and the high metabolic rate can result in heart failure even though the cardiac output is still greater than normal. This is referred to as high-output heart failure.

- Hypertension is a potential sequela of hyperthyroidism in cats, with a prevalence in newly diagnosed hyperthyroid cats ranging from 9% to 23% in recent reports. This result occurs despite peripheral vasodilation and probably reflects the increased stroke volume and heart rate that increases cardiac output. Blood pressure is a function of cardiac output and systemic vascular resistance. Approximately 20% of hyperthyroid cats have systemic hypertension after treatment, with median time from treatment to subsequent development of hypertension of 5.3 months. Approximately one third of these cats had a serum creatinine level greater than 2 mg/dL, and two thirds had normal kidney function. The mechanism of this posttreatment hypertension is unknown.
- The combination of volume and pressure overload alters myocardial protein synthesis and degradation, which results in myocardial

hypertrophy and chamber dilation. These changes are most notable in the left side of the heart. In rare cases, hyperthyroid cats with congestive heart failure have a cardiomyopathy of overload that resembles dilated cardiomyopathy (DCM).

KEY POINT

The net effects of hyperthyroidism on the cardiovascular system are enhanced cardiac contractility, tachycardia, cardiomegaly, left ventricular hypertrophy, high cardiac output, systemic hypertension, and occasionally high-output heart failure.

DIAGNOSIS

HISTORY AND PHYSICAL EXAMINATION

- Historical findings and clinical signs include weight loss, polyphagia, unkempt hair coat, polydipsia, diarrhea, nervousness, hyperactivity, vomiting, tremor, polyuria, lethargy, aggression, decreased appetite, weakness, episodic panting, and bulky, foul-smelling stool.
- Cardiovascular abnormalities that may be present on physical examination include tachycardia, premature heart beats, a gallop sound, an apical systolic murmur, accentuated heart sounds, forceful precordial beat, bounding

femoral pulses, jugular venous distention, and dyspnea when stressed.

- Noncardiac findings can include a low body condition score, a palpable thyroid gland, hyperactivity, dehydration, easily stressed, small kidneys, depression, weakness, and ventral flexion of the neck.

ELECTROCARDIOGRAPHY

- ECG findings in hyperthyroid cats include sinus tachycardia, right bundle branch block, tall R waves in lead II, left anterior fascicular block, ventricular premature complexes (VPCs), atrial premature complexes (APCs), atrial tachycardia, or atrial fibrillation. Ventricular tachycardia, ventricular bigeminy, ventricular preexcitation, and atrioventricular (AV) block have also been described.
- Sinus tachycardia and high R wave voltage resolve with treatment of hyperthyroidism. APCs and VPCs may decrease in frequency or disappear. Conduction disturbances may or may not resolve. If arrhythmias or R wave amplitude changes persist after hyperthyroidism is controlled, the patient should be evaluated for idiopathic cardiomyopathy or systemic hypertension.

RADIOGRAPHY

- Mild to severe cardiomegaly may be seen.
- Evidence of congestive heart failure (pulmonary edema or pleural effusion) is reported in fewer than 5% of cases.

ECHOCARDIOGRAPHY

- Common findings with hyperthyroidism include left atrial enlargement, left ventricular free wall and septal hypertrophy, hyperkinetic left ventricular free wall and septum, left ventricular dilation (eccentric hypertrophy), and increased fractional shortening.
- A dilated form of cardiomyopathy occasionally develops and is characterized by left atrial and ventricular dilation and a low fractional shortening.

CLINICAL PATHOLOGY

- Elevated serum values for alkaline phosphatase, aspartate aminotransaminase, and alanine aminotransaminase are common.
- Mild azotemia is present in approximately 34% of cases.
- The thyroxine (T_4) value is usually elevated and is the diagnostic screening test of choice; however, thyroid hormone levels fluctuate during the day and may dip into the normal range in mildly hyperthyroid animals. Additional diagnostic tests may occasionally be needed to confirm the diagnosis of hyperthyroidism in cats with normal resting T_4 values on repeated assessment. These include measuring the free T_4 level and performing a triiodothyronine (T_3) suppression test.

- Cardiac biomarkers N-terminal pro–B-type natriuretic peptide (NT-ProBNP) and troponin I (cTnI) levels are elevated in approximately one half of hyperthyroid cats. These tests cannot be used to differentiate cats with hyperthyroidism from cardiomyopathy; however, levels generally return to normal after 3 months of effective therapy for hyperthyroidism.

SPECIALIZED DIAGNOSTIC TESTS

Blood Pressure Determination

- Systemic hypertension was present in 9% to 23% of newly diagnosed hyperthyroid cats in recent reports.
- Approximately 20% of hyperthyroid cats have systemic hypertension within 6 months of initiating treatment for hyperthyroidism

Thyroid Imaging

- Thyroid imaging with radioactive technetium 99m will identify the affected gland(s). This imaging study is recommended before surgery in any hyperthyroid cat with nonpalpable thyroid glands because the thyroid glands can migrate into the chest.

KEY POINTS

Hyperthyroidism should be ruled out in older cats with elevated NT-ProBNP or cTnI levels before ascribing the elevations to cardiomyopathy. Blood pressure should be monitored for up to 6 months after initiation of antithyroid therapy.

THERAPY

MANAGEMENT OF HYPERTHYROIDISM

- Radioactive iodine is curative and does not require anesthesia or surgery. In most instances it is the safest and most effective treatment.
- Surgical treatment effectively cures the condition and eliminates the need for chronic medication. Medical management generally is instituted to stabilize the patient before surgery. The most frequent complication of surgery is transient postoperative hypocalcemia.
- Medical management generally involves administering methimazole orally or as a transdermal

formulation in pluronic lecithin organogel. Carbimazole, an alternative to methimazole, is available in Europe. These drugs inhibit the formation of thyroid hormones but do not inhibit or block the release of already formed T_3 and T_4. Thus serum thyroid levels do not drop acutely.

- Inorganic iodine therapy is rarely used. Iodine blocks thyroid hormone synthesis and release, and thyroid levels rapidly drop. Rapid reduction of thyroid levels may benefit patients with severe congestive heart failure. Preoperative use may decrease the vascularity of the thyroid gland. Administer one dose of methimazole before the iodine so that the iodine is not incorporated into new thyroid hormone.

- Sodium or calcium ipodate blocks the conversion of $T_4.T_3$. Ipodate is not effective in all cats and should be considered a treatment of last resort.

MANAGEMENT OF ARRHYTHMIAS

- The expedient way to manage tachyarrhythmias is to start methimazole therapy. Even before euthyroidism is restored, many arrhythmias improve or are abolished. In this fashion, ancillary therapy is usually unnecessary.

- Severe tachyarrhythmias (i.e., atrial tachycardia, multiform VPCs, ventricular tachycardia) in patients without heart failure are best managed with beta-adrenergic blockers such as atenolol (3.125 to 6.25 mg per cat PO q12h) or propranolol (2.5 to 7.5 mg per cat PO q8h). Higher than normal doses of beta-adrenergic blockers may be needed because of an increased rate of metabolism and elimination in hyperthyroid animals. Supraventricular arrhythmias in cats with asthma should be managed with diltiazem (7.5 mg per cat PO q8h) rather than a beta blocker.

- Supraventricular arrhythmias in patients with congestive heart failure can be managed with digoxin, beta blockers, or diltiazem. Exercise caution when using beta blockers in the presence of congestive heart failure because these agents depress cardiac contractility and may acutely exacerbate heart failure. Cats with hyperthyroidism almost always have increased contractility, so worsening of congestive heart failure with beta blockade is rare. Ideally, congestion should be treated and controlled with diuretics before a beta blocker is prescribed. Diltiazem also depresses contractility but less so than beta blockers. The vasodilative effects of diltiazem usually offset its negative inotropic effects.

MANAGEMENT OF HYPERTENSION

- Usually accomplished with control of the hyperthyroid state. The use of beta blockers (e.g., atenolol), angiotensin-converting enzyme (ACE) inhibitors (e.g., enalapril, benazepril), or amlodipine are occasionally indicated.

MANAGEMENT OF CONGESTIVE HEART FAILURE

- Diuretics are used to control pulmonary edema and pleural effusion.

- Enalapril or benazepril also may be helpful in refractory cases.

- Treat arrhythmias as discussed previously.

- Pimobendan may be useful in cases where chronic hyperthyroidism results in DCM.

PROGNOSIS

- The prognosis for remission of sinus tachycardia, voltage changes, arrhythmias, and congestive heart failure is generally favorable when the hypermetabolic state is controlled.

- Systemic hypertension develops in 20% of cats following treatment of hyperthyroidism; therefore blood pressure monitoring is recommended. Renal insufficiency can also be unmasked after control of the disease.

- The prognosis is poor if DCM has developed secondary to chronic overload of the heart (rare).

HYPOTHYROIDISM

- Hypothyroidism is a common endocrinopathy in dogs and is rarely encountered as a naturally occurring condition in cats. It is most commonly diagnosed in middle-aged dogs (22% are 2 to 3 years old; 32% are 4 to 6 years old; 22% are 7 to 9 years old). Many breeds are affected, and there appears to be a breed predilection in the Golden Retriever, Doberman Pinscher, Dachshund, Irish Setter, Miniature Schnauzer, Great Dane, Poodle, and Boxer. There is no gender predilection. Hypothyroidism is rare in cats and generally limited to postoperative cases after surgical removal of unilateral or bilateral functional thyroid tumors.

- The cardiac effects of hypothyroidism are generally the opposite of those found in hyperthyroidism. The cardiac effects of hypothyroidism rarely have severe consequences. However, hypothyroidism can aggravate heart failure and complicate the management of cardiac patients.

CARDIAC PATHOPHYSIOLOGY

- Cardiac contractility is decreased as a result of decreased Na^+, K^+-ATPase activity, decreased mitochondrial protein synthesis, and decreased synthesis of contractile properties of myosin.

- Cardiac conduction is decreased as a result of a decreased rate of sinoatrial firing, increased threshold of atrial activation, and prolonged refractory period of the conducting tissue. Enhanced vagal tone in hypothyroidism also slows the heart rate and accentuates sinus arrhythmias.
- Thyroid hormone plays an important role in lipid and cholesterol metabolism. Hypothyroidism predisposes animals to increased levels of cholesterol and, to a lesser extent, triglycerides. Although rare in dogs, hypercholesterolemia can result in atherosclerosis and myocardial infarction. Lipid abnormalities resolve with thyroid hormone supplementation.
- Hypothyroidism decreases the metabolic rate, thus lessening the required cardiac output. Correcting hypothyroidism increases the workload on the heart; remember this when treating animals in congestive heart failure.
- Hypothyroidism decreases digoxin clearance, predisposing patients to digoxin toxicity.

KEY POINT

Evaluate the thyroid status in any dog in congestive heart failure, particularly those with inappropriately slow heart rates.

DIAGNOSIS

HISTORY AND PHYSICAL EXAMINATION

- Historical findings in hypothyroid animals include alopecia and other dermatologic problems, lethargy, weakness, depression, infertility, and diarrhea.
- Cardiovascular abnormalities noted on physical examination can include muffled heart sounds, weak apex heartbeat, weak pulses, and bradycardia.
- Noncardiac physical findings can include symmetric alopecia, seborrhea, myxedema, pyoderma, hypothermia, depression, and lameness.

ELECTROCARDIOGRAPHY

- ECG changes in patients with hypothyroidism reflect decreased automaticity of pacemaker tissue and depressed conduction. Changes that reflect decreased automaticity may include sinus bradycardia, pronounced sinus arrhythmia, and atrial and ventricular arrhythmias. Changes that reflect depressed conduction may include AV block, widened QRS complexes, and inverted T waves. The most common findings reported in dogs are sinus bradycardia and inverted T waves.

- Low-voltage QRS complexes are frequently seen in hypothyroid animals.
- Atrial fibrillation in giant-breed dogs occasionally accompanies hypothyroidism, usually in association with DCM. Supplementation with thyroid hormone rarely causes conversion to sinus rhythm.

DIAGNOSTIC IMAGING

- Radiograph findings are generally normal.
- Echocardiography may reveal mild to marked decreases in indices of cardiac contractility and mild chamber enlargement. Decreased contractility is documented by an increase in left ventricular internal diameter during systole, prolongation of the preejection period (PEP), a decrease in left posterior wall thickness during systole, and a decrease in septal wall thickness during systole and diastole. There is also often a decrease in aortic root diameter, decrease in velocity of circumferential shortening, and a decrease in fractional shortening.
- Always check thyroid status when depressed contractility is noted in an animal of a breed not predisposed to DCM.

CLINICAL PATHOLOGY

- The hemogram may reveal a low-grade nonregenerative anemia.
- The most common abnormality on the serum chemistry profile is hypercholesterolemia and occasionally hypertriglyceridemia.
- A normal serum T_4 value generally is sufficient to rule out hypothyroidism. Unfortunately, a low serum T_4 does not confirm the diagnosis. Concurrent systemic ailments and numerous drugs can cause depressed serum T_4 values in animals with normal thyroid function (euthyroid sick syndrome) (Box 14.2). Making a diagnosis in these cases requires integration of the history, physical findings, and other blood test results, or confirmation by specialized diagnostic tests.
- Serum T_3 values are less reliable than T_4 values at diagnosing hypothyroidism.

SPECIALIZED DIAGNOSTIC TESTS

- The thyroid-stimulating hormone (TSH) response test has been the "gold standard" in veterinary medicine for diagnosing hypothyroidism. Animals with hypothyroidism have low baseline T_4 values and fail to increase their T_4 values above a predetermined level following administration of TSH. Animals with euthyroid sick syndrome will also have low baseline T_4 levels, but following TSH administration, their T_4 values will increase above

Box 14.2 Some Drugs and Diagnostic Agents That Can Alter Basal Serum Thyroid Hormone Concentrations in Humans and Possibly Dogs

Decrease T_4 and/or T_3	Increase T_4 and/or T_3
Amiodarone (T_3)	Amiodarone (T_4)
Androgens	Estrogens
Cholecystographic	5-Fluorouracil
agents	Halothane
Diazepam	Insulin
Dopamine	Narcotic analgesics
Flunixin	Radiopaque dyes
Furosemide	(ipodate)
Glucocorticoids	Thiazides
Heparin	
Imidazole	
Iodide	
Methimazole	
Mitotane	
Nitroprusside	
Penicillin	
Phenobarbital	
Phenothiazines	
Phenylbutazone	
Phenytoin	
Primidone	
Propranolol	
Propylthiouracil	
Radiopaque dyes	
(ipodate) (T_3)	
Salicylates	
Sulfonamides	
(sulfamethoxazole)	
Sulfonylureas	

From Feldman EC, Nelson RW: Canine and feline endocrinology and reproduction, 3rd ed, St Louis, 2004, WB Saunders.

an absolute cutoff value. Unfortunately, TSH is expensive and often difficult to obtain.

- Free T_4 by equilibrium dialysis (ED) as a diagnostic test of canine hypothyroidism has a sensitivity of 98% and specificity of 92%, compared with a total T_4 sensitivity of 90% and specificity of 90%. The free T_4 by ED should be low in a hypothyroid animal.
- As a diagnostic test for canine hypothyroidism, canine TSH levels have a sensitivity of 75% and specificity of 90%. The TSH level should be high in a hypothyroid animal.
- When the endogenous TSH is high and the free T_4 by ED is low, the diagnostic accuracy approaches 100%.

THERAPY

- Treatment of hypothyroidism with L-thyroxine is simple and inexpensive.
- Treatment in patients with congestive heart failure is more complicated. Thyroid supplementation will increase the metabolic rate and demand on the heart. If the failing heart is unable to meet these demands, heart failure will worsen. Therefore implement thyroid hormone supplementation gradually in patients with cardiac disease, especially if they are already in failure. Start with one fourth of the standard dose and increase it by one-fourth dose weekly. It should be emphasized that hypothyroidism rarely causes heart failure but may significantly worsen cardiac function in an animal with underlying heart disease.
- The risk of digoxin toxicity is increased in hypothyroid states. Monitor hypothyroid animals closely for signs of digoxin toxicity and consider assessing thyroid status in any animal with normal renal function that has digoxin toxicity while receiving reasonable doses of digoxin. Ideally the digoxin level on a sample obtained 8 hours after dose should be between 0.5 and 1 ng/mL.

PROGNOSIS

- There are few complications in the treatment of hypothyroidism.
  - Impaired myocardial function improves following thyroid supplementation.
  - Resolution of atrial fibrillation has been reported in one dog after correction of hypothyroidism. This response is rare.

HYPOADRENOCORTICISM (ADDISON DISEASE)

- Hypoadrenocorticism is a potentially life-threatening endocrinopathy that is uncommon in dogs and rare in cats. The disease is more common in female dogs and usually occurs in young to middle-aged animals. Approximately 76% of cases occur before 7 years of age with an age range of 5 weeks to 16 years.
- Primary hypoadrenocorticism (Addison disease) results from destruction of the zona glomerulosa and zona fasciculata of the adrenal gland. These areas of the adrenal gland produce aldosterone and cortisol, respectively. Destruction is generally immune mediated but also can occur secondary to infection, neoplasia, infarction, and drugs such as o,p'-dichlorodiphenyldichloroethane (o,p'-DDD, mitotane).

- Secondary hypoadrenocorticism results from decreased production or release of adrenocorticotropic hormone (ACTH) from the pituitary gland. Secondary adrenal insufficiency may occur following acute withdrawal of long-term, high-dose glucocorticoid therapy that has suppressed the hypothalamic-pituitary-adrenal axis. These patients have normal mineralocorticoid activity, so electrolyte values are normal. Cortisol values are depressed.
- Adrenal destruction occurs gradually; therefore basal hormone levels remain normal. It is only when the animal is stressed and the adrenal reserve is inadequate that signs develop. Eventually the destruction proceeds to the point that basal hormone levels are depressed and clinical signs are present without stress.

CARDIAC PATHOPHYSIOLOGY

CARDIOVASCULAR EFFECTS OF CORTISOL

- Cortisol is important in maintaining vascular integrity and responsiveness to catecholamines. Cortisol deficiency predisposes animals to hypotension.
- Cortisol has a positive inotropic effect on the heart.
- Cortisol affects the distribution and elimination of body water.
- Cortisol is important in helping the body deal with stress. This is why so many Addisonian crises follow stress and why glucocorticoid supplementation must be increased during periods of stress.

CARDIOVASCULAR EFFECTS OF ALDOSTERONE

- Aldosterone acts on the distal renal convoluted tubule and collecting duct to enhance sodium retention and potassium elimination. Aldosterone deficiency results in hyponatremia and hyperkalemia.
- Hyponatremia decreases plasma osmotic pressure causing fluid shifts out of the vascular

compartment. This contributes to hypovolemia and hypotension.
- Hyperkalemia alters cardiac conduction resulting in numerous arrhythmias. The cardiac effects of hyperkalemia are aggravated by low sodium, low calcium, and acidosis.

KEY POINT

Net cardiovascular effects of hypoadrenocorticism are hypovolemia, systemic hypotension, altered cardiac conduction, and depressed myocardial function. These changes can be fatal if not rapidly diagnosed and aggressively treated.

DIAGNOSIS

HISTORY AND PHYSICAL EXAMINATION

- A history of waxing and waning of clinical signs, with more severe signs during periods of stress, generally is present.
- Patients often have a history of anorexia, vomiting, diarrhea, depression, weakness, and cardiovascular collapse. Other signs include weight loss, polyuria, polydipsia, melena, and shivering.
- Transient improvement after intravenous (IV) fluid therapy or corticosteroid administration followed by subsequent relapse days or weeks later can occur.
- Findings on physical examination include depression, weakness, dehydration, hypothermia, slow capillary refill time, shaking, bradycardia, and weak femoral pulses.

ELECTROCARDIOGRAPHY

- ECG changes vary with the magnitude of the hyperkalemia and are aggravated by hyponatremia, hypocalcemia, and acidosis. The following ECG findings are seen with experimentally induced hyperkalemia (Figure 14.1):
  - Peaking of the T wave with a narrow base is the earliest ECG abnormality and may

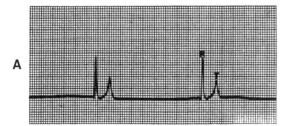
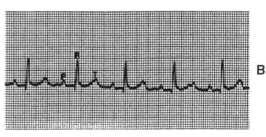

Figure 14.1 A, Hyperkalemia in a dog in cardiovascular collapse, consistent with an Addisonian crisis. P waves are absent (atrial standstill), and T waves are tall and peaked. Serum potassium was 8.4 mEq/L. **B,** After institution of therapy, P waves are present, and the T wave is of smaller amplitude. Serum potassium is now 4.8 mEq/L. (From Tilley LP: Essentials of canine and feline electrocardiography: interpretation and treatment, ed 3, Malvern, Penn, 1992, Lea & Febiger.)

be observed when serum K+ exceeds 5.7 to 6.0 mEq/L.

- P wave shape is altered, its amplitude reduced, intraatrial conduction delayed, and PR interval prolonged when serum K+ exceeds 7.0 mEq/L.
- P waves become unrecognizable (atrial standstill) at plasma K+ levels greater than 8.5 mEq/L.
- The QRS widens uniformly at plasma K+ levels greater than 9 mEq/L.
- Sinoatrial exit block or junctional rhythms with and without escape complexes may be present.
- Ventricular fibrillation and ventricular asystole may occur at plasma K+ levels greater than 10 mEq/L.
- In clinical cases, ECG changes do not correlate as closely with potassium concentrations as they do in published experimental studies.
- The rhythm with atrial standstill secondary to hyperkalemia is generally slow and may be regular or irregular. It is a sinoventricular rhythm. The sinus node continues to fire, and impulses are transmitted to the AV node and ventricles by internodal pathways. P waves are absent because atrial myocytes are not activated.

KEY POINT

Hyperkalemia is the most common cause of atrial standstill. Atrial standstill also occurs with fibrous replacement of atrial muscle cells secondary to severe atrial distention (valve disease, cardiomyopathy) in dogs and cats, with cardiac arrest, and secondary to an atrial myopathy in dogs, a condition most commonly seen in English Springer Spaniels.

RADIOGRAPHS

- Approximately 80% of untreated dogs have one or more radiographic abnormalities. Abnormalities in order of reported frequency include narrow caudal vena cava, microcardia, narrow cranial lobar pulmonary artery, and microhepatica. These changes are the result of hypovolemia and rapidly resolve with steroid and volume replacement.

CLINICAL PATHOLOGY

- A low-grade normocytic, normochromic nonregenerative anemia is present in 25% of cases but may be masked by the effects of hemoconcentration. Eosinophilia and lymphocytosis may also be present.

- A serum chemistry profile frequently reveals azotemia, hyponatremia, and hyperkalemia. A sodium/potassium ratio of less than 27 supports hypoadrenocorticism but is not pathognomonic for the disease. Hypercalcemia and hypoglycemia can also be present.
- Mild-to-moderate metabolic acidosis is common during a crisis.
- It is unusual for a dog with untreated Addison disease to have a urine specific gravity greater than 1.030, and it is often less than 1.020.
- In patients with secondary hypoadrenocorticism, sodium and potassium levels are normal. The other abnormalities described above may be present.

SPECIALIZED DIAGNOSTIC TESTS

- A tentative diagnosis is frequently obtained from the history and results of the complete blood count and serum chemistry profile. However, there are numerous causes of hyperkalemia, and acid-base and electrolyte changes associated with severe gastrointestinal disease and renal failure can cause an abnormal sodium/potassium ratio that would erroneously suggest Addison disease.
- An ACTH response test is helpful in confirming Addison disease and essential for documenting secondary hypoadrenocorticism.

THERAPY
ADDISONIAN CRISIS THERAPY

- Patients that have cardiovascular collapse and atrial standstill require aggressive therapy. Therapy is directed at rapidly correcting hypovolemia, correcting rhythm disturbances, correcting electrolyte imbalances, and replacing mineralocorticoids and glucocorticoids.
- Volume replacement, and correction of hyponatremia and hypochloremia, is initially achieved with rapid infusion of 0.9% saline at 60 to 80 mL/kg/hr for 1 to 2 hours and then at a modified rate according to patient needs. The ACTH response test can be performed while saline is being administered.
- Glucocorticoid deficiency is corrected with either methylprednisolone sodium succinate (1 to 2 mg/kg IV) or dexamethasone sodium phosphate (2 to 4 mg/kg IV) and then repeated every 2 to 6 hours. After the initial high dose of a rapidly acting, water-soluble glucocorticoid has been administered, glucocorticoid therapy can be continued with dexamethasone at a dosage of 0.05 to 0.1 mg/kg q12h added to the IV fluids. Once the patient is stable, switch to oral prednisone. It should be noted that

prednisolone interferes with cortisol assays, so ideally it should be started after the ACTH response test is performed. Dexamethasone has no mineralocorticoid effects and does not interfere with the cortisol assay.

- Mineralocorticoid deficiency is initially corrected (after the ACTH response test is performed) with desoxycorticosterone pivalate (DOCP) at 2.2 mg/kg IM or fludrocortisone acetate at 0.02 mg/kg/day PO if the dog is not vomiting.
- Hyperkalemia is corrected in several different ways:
  - Saline infusion results in rapid dilution of potassium and is often the only treatment needed.
  - Severe hyperkalemia associated with significant cardiac conduction abnormalities often requires more aggressive therapy. Treatment options include sodium bicarbonate (1 to 2 mEq/kg) given slowly IV over 5 minutes *or* a combination of regular insulin (0.5 U/kg IV) followed by dextrose added to fluids (1 g per unit insulin given). Dextrose can also be administered alone as it will stimulate endogenous insulin secretion.
  - If life-threatening cardiac arrhythmias are noted, administer calcium gluconate (10%) at 0.5 to 1.5 mL/kg IV slowly over 10 to 15 minutes. Monitor the ECG while administering calcium. Calcium will temporarily correct rhythm disturbances by countering the effect of potassium on the conduction tissue. Calcium has no effect on serum potassium levels. Calcium overdose can also cause severe cardiac disturbances; therefore careful monitoring is required.

MAINTENANCE THERAPY

- Mineralocorticoid replacement is initiated with either daily oral administration of fludrocortisone acetate or intramuscular injections of DOCP every 25 days. Doses—and dose interval for DOCP—are adjusted as needed to maintain normal electrolyte balance. Therapy must be individualized to the patient.
- Glucocorticoid replacement is achieved with either prednisone or cortisone. Some patients receiving fludrocortisone acetate or DOCP do not need glucocorticoid supplementation except during periods of stress.

PROGNOSIS

- The prognosis is excellent with therapy.
- Many dogs appear to do better with a small daily maintenance dose of prednisone or cortisone. During illness or other stressful periods, however, larger doses of glucocorticoids are necessary to avoid relapse into acute adrenal crisis.

HYPERADRENOCORTICISM (CUSHING DISEASE)

- Hyperadrenocorticism is a common endocrinopathy in older dogs and is rarely reported in cats. The syndrome is associated with excessive levels of cortisol that result from excess pituitary ACTH, or excess ACTH from ectopic nonendocrine tumors, functional adrenocortical adenoma, or carcinoma. Iatrogenic Cushing syndrome occurs with excessive glucocorticoid administration.
- Pituitary-dependent hyperadrenocorticism accounts for 80% to 85% of cases of hyperadrenocorticism. It is a disease of middle-aged and older dogs (usually older than 6 years), although a few cases have been diagnosed in dogs younger than 1 year. There is no sex predilection. Poodles, Dachshunds, and Beagles may be at increased risk.
- Dogs with functional adrenocortical tumors tend to be older, ranging from 6 to 16 years of age with a mean age of 11 years. Females are affected more frequently. German Shepherds, Toy Poodles, Dachshunds, and Terriers are most commonly affected.
- Hyperadrenocorticism rarely produces significant cardiac disease; however, signs and side effects of hyperadrenocorticism can mimic cardiac disease. Systemic effects of hyperadrenocorticism can also exacerbate underlying cardiac disease.

PATHOPHYSIOLOGY
SYSTEMIC HYPERTENSION

- Hypercortisolism increases vascular resistance by increasing smooth muscle sensitivity to catecholamines and increasing production of angiotensinogen. Mineralocorticoid properties of cortisol enhance the renal resorption of sodium, and secondary fluid retention results in an increased vascular volume. Hypertension is present in 57% to 82% of dogs with Cushing disease.
- Systemic hypertension may cause myocardial hypertrophy.
- Many affected dogs have coexisting AV valvular insufficiency and its associated cardiac changes. Hypertension might exacerbate underlying cardiac problems.

PULMONARY THROMBOEMBOLISM

- Patients with hyperadrenocorticism are predisposed to pulmonary thromboembolism, with most cases diagnosed while the animal is being treated for Cushing disease. Factors causing thromboembolism with Cushing disease include obesity, high hematocrit, hypertension, and increased levels of clotting factors.

- Pulmonary thromboembolism should be suspected in any Cushingoid patient with a history of an acute onset of dyspnea or cyanosis.

PANTING AND DYSPNEA

- Altered ventilation mechanics are often present owing to weakness in the muscles of respiration, increased thoracic fat deposition (decreasing chest wall compliance), and increased diaphragmatic abdominal pressure resulting from adipose tissue and hepatomegaly. Mild respiratory distress, or rapid respiratory rate at rest, often results.
- Many Cushingoid dogs have variable degrees of lower airway disease or pulmonary parenchymal disease.
- The triad of mitral/tricuspid insufficiency, respiratory disease, and Cushing syndrome may create intractable dyspnea caused by cardiopulmonary failure.

DIAGNOSIS

HISTORY AND PHYSICAL EXAMINATION

- The major historical features are systemic manifestations of hypercortisolism; they include polydipsia, polyuria, polyphagia, panting, alopecia, anestrus, exercise intolerance, and lethargy.
- Findings on physical examination may include abdominal enlargement, hepatomegaly, muscle weakness, testicular atrophy, symmetric alopecia, skin atrophy, hyperpigmentation, calcinosis cutis, bruising, and obesity.

ELECTROCARDIOGRAPHY

- ECGs show no characteristic changes. ECG evidence of left ventricular enlargement is often present in Cushingoid dogs with mitral valvular insufficiency.

DIAGNOSTIC IMAGING

- Hypercortisolism causes changes on thoracic radiographs that include calcification of the tracheal and bronchial rings and osteoporosis of the thoracic vertebrae. Metastatic pulmonary lesions are seen infrequently with adrenal tumors.
- Radiographic changes associated with pulmonary thromboembolism include hypoperfusion of the infarcted lung lobes, overcirculation within the normal lung lobes, pleural effusion, and blunting and thickening of the pulmonary arteries. Thoracic radiographs may have normal findings.
- Echocardiography is rarely part of the workup of Cushing disease.

CLINICAL PATHOLOGY

- Excessive production of cortisol may result in neutrophilia, lymphopenia, eosinopenia, thrombocytosis and mild erythrocytosis (females).
- Chemistry abnormalities include fasting hyperglycemia, high serum alkaline phosphatase (sometimes extremely high), high alanine aminotransferase, hypercholesterolemia, lipemia, and low blood urea nitrogen.
- Urinalysis shows specific gravity less than 1.015 and often less than 1.008. Proteinuria, glycosuria, and bacterial cystitis are sometimes noted.

SPECIALIZED DIAGNOSTIC TESTS

- A urine cortisol/creatinine ratio is a quick screening test for Cushing disease. This test has a high sensitivity but low specificity for Cushing disease.
- The low-dose dexamethasone suppression test (LDDST) is the screening test of choice unless iatrogenic hyperadrenocorticism is suspected.
- The ACTH response test is the screening test of choice if iatrogenic hyperadrenocorticism is suspected.
- If there is no suppression on a LDDST, measurement of canine ACTH (cACTH) or abdominal ultrasound is recommended to differentiate between pituitary dependent Cushing disease and an adrenal tumor.
- A high-dose dexamethasone suppression test can be considered if there is no suppression on the LDDST, and cACTH and abdominal ultrasound are not options.
- Abdominal ultrasound, computed tomography (CT) scan, and magnetic resonance imaging (MRI) can be used to try to differentiate pituitary-dependent Cushing disease from an adrenal tumor and to better characterize the extent of the disease.

THERAPY

PITUITARY-DEPENDENT HYPERADRENOCORTICISM

- Mitotane and trilostane are the two main drugs used for the treatment of pituitary-dependent hyperadrenocorticism.
- Mitotane selectively, and usually reversibly, destroys the zona fasciculata (cortisol) and zona reticularis (sex hormones) of the adrenal gland. The zona glomerulosa (aldosterone) is occasionally affected.
- Trilostane inhibits adrenal steroidogenesis through enzyme inhibition and may affect aldosterone and cortisol synthesis.

- Ketoconazole can be prescribed in animals that do not tolerate mitotane or trilostane. Ketoconazole blocks an enzymatic step that is necessary for the production of cortisol.
- Hypophysectomy is rarely performed in the United States.
- Radiation therapy can be used to treat pituitary macroadenomas.

ADRENOCORTICAL TUMOR

- Surgical removal of the affected adrenal gland(s) is recommended if possible.
- If the tumor is inoperable or metastasis is identified, mitotane is the medical therapy of choice as it has a chemotherapeutic effect. Very high doses of mitotane are usually required in patients with adrenal tumors. Trilostane can be used on dogs that do not tolerate mitotane. Many dogs with adrenal tumors respond poorly to medical management.
- Replacement steroid therapy is necessary both during and after surgery.
- Management of pulmonary embolism and systemic hypertension, if present, is undertaken through standard therapeutic protocols (see Chapters 10 and 15).

PROGNOSIS

- Excellent prognosis is confirmed with resectable, benign adrenal tumors.
- Nonresectable or metastatic adrenal adenocarcinomas have a poor prognosis.
- Therapy with mitotane or trilostane for pituitary-dependent hyperadrenocorticism has potential side effects, but most treated dogs respond well to therapy. The average survival is 2 years, with dogs living longer than 6 months usually dying of causes unrelated to hyperadrenocorticism.
- Systemic hypertension generally resolves with control of hypercortisolism.

HYPERSOMATOTROPISM (ACROMEGALY) IN CATS

- Acromegaly is a syndrome associated with high levels of growth hormone (hypersomatotropism).
- In cats, acromegaly occurs secondary to a pituitary tumor. It is an uncommon endocrinopathy that is seen in primarily male, middle-aged to old cats (mean age: 10 years; median age: 9 years; range: 4 to 17 years).
- In dogs, hypersomatotropism is associated with progestogen treatment or endogenous progestogens that are produced during diestrus. It does not cause clinically significant cardiac problems in dogs. The syndrome is seen in females and is reversible with discontinuation

of progestogen therapy or resolves spontaneously with the end of diestrus.

CARDIOVASCULAR PATHOPHYSIOLOGY

- The trophic effect of growth hormone results in generalized organomegaly, including the heart. Cardiac changes are those of myocardial hypertrophy, interstitial fibrosis, myocytolysis, and intramural arteriosclerosis. Heart failure is a common sequela of acromegaly in cats.
- Systemic hypertension is seen frequently in humans with acromegaly. Systemic hypertension is sometimes present in cats with acromegaly and is usually accompanied by evidence of renal insufficiency.

DIAGNOSIS
HISTORY AND PHYSICAL EXAMINATION

- Most cats have a history of polyuria, polydipsia, upper respiratory stridor, and weight gain.
- Cardiac abnormalities noted on physical examination may include a systolic murmur, gallop sound, and, less commonly, signs of congestive heart failure (dyspnea, cyanosis, muffled heart sounds, or crackles).
- Other abnormalities include hepatomegaly, nephromegaly, large head, arthritis, prognathism, pot belly, large tongue, and circling.

CARDIAC TESTS

- ECG abnormalities have not been observed in these patients.
- Radiographs of the thorax usually demonstrate cardiomegaly, and less commonly, pulmonary edema or pleural effusion.
- The echocardiogram generally reveals hypertrophy of the intraventricular septum and left ventricular free wall.

CLINICAL PATHOLOGY

- The hemogram is generally unremarkable, but some cats have erythrocytosis.
- All cases have hyperglycemia and glucosuria. Most cats also have hyperproteinemia, azotemia, and hyperphosphatemia. Hypercholesterolemia, high alanine aminotransferase, high serum alkaline phosphatase, and ketonuria are seen less frequently.

SPECIALIZED DIAGNOSTIC TESTS

- A commercially available validated growth hormone assay is not currently available for cats.
- Insulin-like growth factor I (IGF-1) levels are elevated in most cases. One large study

involving cats with high IGF-1 concentrations revealed that 90% of them had documented pituitary tumors evident on CT scans. This test is commercially available.
- CT can be used to identify the pituitary tumor, and in advanced cases, boney and soft tissue changes.
- Procollagen propeptide concentrations in serum are elevated in cats with hypersomatotropism.
- Blood pressure should be evaluated in any suspected or confirmed cases.

THERAPY

- Treatment options include hypophysectomy, radiation therapy, and medical management.
- Hypophysectomy has been performed successfully and resulted in remission of concurrent diabetes mellitus in 80% of treated cats. Perioperative and postoperative mortality is reported at 16%.
- Radiation therapy is difficult to obtain and effect is unpredictable.
- Medical management with common somatostatin analogues (e.g., octreotide) and dopamine agonists (e.g., bromocriptine) is generally unsuccessful. Pasireotide (a high-affinity analogue of multiple somatostatin receptor subtypes) has been shown to successfully decrease growth hormone and IGF-1 levels in cats but is expensive and requires twice daily injections.
- Supportive medical care includes high doses of insulin for insulin-resistant diabetes mellitus and diuretics for congestive heart failure.

PROGNOSIS

- Survival in cats with acromegaly ranges from 4 to 60 months (generally 1.5 to 3 years) from time of diagnosis.
- Most cats die or are euthanized owing to severe congestive heart failure, renal failure, or expanding pituitary tumor.

Note: Hypersomatotropism without acromegaly has been associated with hypertrophic cardiomyopathy in some cats. A total of 31 cats with hypertrophic cardiomyopathy were shown to have growth hormone levels that were four times the control levels. None of the cats that were examined postmortem had pituitary tumors, and none demonstrated hyperinsulinism or diabetes mellitus.

PHEOCHROMOCYTOMA

- Pheochromocytomas are catecholamine-producing tumors derived from chromaffin cells.
- These tumors of adrenal medullary origin are uncommonly detected in dogs. They are typically seen in old dogs (mean age, 11 years, with a range of 1 to 16 years) and extremely rarely in cats.

- In addition to important effects on the cardiovascular system, catecholamines have significant metabolic effects, stimulating glycogenolysis and gluconeogenesis.

CARDIAC PATHOPHYSIOLOGY

- The cardiovascular effects of pheochromocytomas result from the alpha-1, beta-1, and beta-2 effects of norepinephrine and epinephrine. Stimulation of alpha- and beta-adrenergic receptors generally causes opposite effects. The dominant effect varies with relative receptor density and activation thresholds. For example, in vascular smooth muscle, alpha-adrenergic effects predominate. Thus, hypertension results when both alpha- and beta-adrenergic receptors are stimulated.
- Beta-1 adrenergic effects include sinus tachycardia, increased cardiac conduction velocity, and increased contractility.
- Beta-2 adrenergic effects on the cardiovascular system include venous and arteriole vasodilation.
- Alpha-1 adrenergic effects on the cardiovascular system include venous and arteriole vasoconstriction. Approximately 50% of dogs with pheochromocytomas are hypertensive at the time of testing.
- Myocardial injury and coronary vasoconstriction may result from catecholamine excess. Multifocal cardiomyocyte necrosis with contraction bands, interstitial fibrosis, cardiomyocyte degeneration, myocardial hemorrhage, and lymphohistiocytic myocarditis have been reported in dogs. Cardiac lesions were detected in approximately 15% of cases examined.

DIAGNOSIS

HISTORY AND PHYSICAL EXAMINATION

- Historical observations include weakness, collapse, anorexia, vomiting, weight loss, panting, dyspnea, lethargy, diarrhea, whining, pacing, polyuria, polydipsia, shivering, and epistaxis.
- Abnormalities noted on physical examination include lethargy, tachypnea and dyspnea, arrhythmias, systolic murmur, pulmonary crackles, tachycardia, weak pulse, pale mucous membranes, and muscle wasting.
- Other physical examination findings are emaciation, peripheral edema, ascites, and abdominal mass.
- Many symptoms and physical findings are reported to be episodic because of the episodic release of catecholamines by the tumor.

ELECTROCARDIOGRAPHY

- Nonspecific ST segment and T wave changes may be noted.

- Arrhythmias can occur, especially VPCs and paroxysmal ventricular tachycardia. Complete AV block has been reported in several dogs.
- Consider 24-hour ambulatory ECG monitoring (Holter monitoring) to detect intermittent arrhythmias associated with episodic catecholamine release.

RADIOGRAPHY

- Generalized cardiomegaly and pulmonary edema can develop, probably owing to sustained chronic hypertension.
- Adrenal tumors can be identified in one third of the cases.

ECHOCARDIOGRAPHY

- Ventricular hypertrophy is usually present, most commonly the left ventricle. Both concentric and eccentric hypertrophies have been reported.

CLINICAL PATHOLOGY

- No consistent abnormalities are present on the hemogram or chemistry profile.
- Plasma catecholamines and demonstration of elevated 24-hour urinary excretion of vanillylmandelic acid, total metanephrines, and fractionated catecholamines support the diagnosis.

SPECIAL DIAGNOSTIC TESTS

- Abdominal ultrasound may be helpful as a localizing procedure. The presence of an adrenal mass on ultrasound with no evidence of Cushing disease is highly suggestive.
- Angiography can be used in some situations to evaluate adrenal masses invading the caudal vena cava.
- CT, nuclear imaging, and provocative testing to induce hypertension (with histamine, tyramine, and glucagon) or hypotension (with phentolamine) may be useful but rarely are practical or available in general practice.
- Blood pressure determination reveals systemic hypertension in approximately 50% of cases. As catecholamine release is often episodic, the patient should be rechecked several times if blood pressure is initially normal.

THERAPY

- Alpha- and beta-adrenergic blocking drugs may help control hypertension and arrhythmias, respectively. Always start with an alpha-adrenergic blocker such as phenoxybenzamine (0.2 to 1.5 mg/kg PO q12h). If a hypertensive crisis is

identified, administer phentolamine at 0.02 to 0.1 mg/kg IV, followed by IV administration (0.02 to 0.1 mg/kg IV prn). If tachyarrhythmias remain a problem, then add a beta blocker such as propranolol (0.2 to 1 mg/kg PO q8h) or atenolol (0.25 to 1 mg/kg PO q12 to 24h). The inclusion of a beta blocker without alpha blockade can result in severe hypertension.
- Surgical tumor removal is the only definitive treatment. This should be attempted after medical stabilization in patients without metastasis.

PROGNOSIS

- Dogs with inoperable lesions have a poor prognosis. Long-term alpha- and beta-adrenergic blockers may be used in these instances.

DIABETES MELLITUS

- Diabetes mellitus causes devastating cardiovascular problems in humans. Recent studies reported hypertension (defined as a pressure >160 mm Hg systolic, 100 mm Hg diastolic, and 120 mm Hg mean) in 46% of 50 dogs with diabetes. Subclinical reduction of myocardial contractility has also been reported. A retrospective case-controlled study revealed a significantly greater risk (10.4 times greater) for the development of heart failure in cats with diabetes than in normal controls.
- Hypersomatotropism (acromegaly) has been reported in cats with diabetes (prevalence estimated at 18%-32%) and could contribute to cardiovascular complications in this species.

CARDIAC PATHOPHYSIOLOGY

- Systemic hypertension in dogs with diabetes is associated with the duration of disease and an increased urine albumin to creatinine ratio. The severity of mean and diastolic hypertension is correlated with the duration of disease. In humans, the severity of hypertension correlates with degree of glycemic control. This association has not been reported in dogs. Hypertension is rarely reported in cats with diabetes. The cause of hypertension is not known but may relate to changes in vascular compliance secondary to changes in lipid profile, generalized glomerular hyperfiltration, and immune-mediated microangiopathy affecting the basement membrane.
- Cardiac autonomic neuropathy has been observed in poorly regulated dogs with diabetes; suppression of sympathetic activity was demonstrated by decreases in both plasma norepinephrine concentrations and heart rate variability (LF component).
- Diabetic cardiomyopathy occurs in humans and is associated with myocardial hypertrophy, fibrosis,

microvascular disease, and glycoprotein accumulation. Myocardial changes result in diastolic and systolic dysfunction. In the absence of coronary microvascular disease and systemic hypertension, diabetic cardiomyopathy in humans is a mild condition. In alloxan-induced diabetes in dogs, mild reductions in fractional shortening and left ventricular ejection fraction have been reported along with increased aortic stiffness and increased collagen type 1 and type 3 protein content. Diastolic changes have been mild and inconsistent. Functional coronary artery hyperemia is attenuated, and the balance between coronary blood flow and myocardial metabolism is impaired in alloxan-induced diabetic dogs.

KEY POINT

Decreased cardiac performance in dogs with diabetes mellitus is mild and unlikely to cause clinical problems unless accompanied by other forms of heart disease such as DCM.

DIAGNOSIS

HISTORY AND PHYSICAL EXAMINATION

- No cardiovascular signs associated with diabetes
- Polyuria, polydipsia, polyphagia with weight loss, cataracts (dogs)

ELECTROCARDIOGRAPHY

- No changes related to diabetes

RADIOGRAPHY

- No changes related to diabetes

CLINICAL PATHOLOGY

- Fasting hyperglycemia, hypercholesterolemia, hypertriglyceridemia, increased alanine aminotransferase activity, increased alkaline phosphatase activity
- Glucosuria, variable ketonuria; sometimes proteinuria, microalbuminuria, and bacteriuria
- High fructosamine and glycosylated hemoglobin

SPECIAL DIAGNOSTIC TESTS

- Evaluation of systemic blood pressure may reveal hypertension.
- Echocardiography may demonstrate mild reduction in fractional shortening, increase in PEP, decrease in left ventricular ejection time (LVET), and increase in PEP/LVET.

THERAPY

- Treat hypertension with an ACE inhibitor (e.g., enalapril or benazepril), amlodipine, or a beta blocker (see Chapter 15).
- Manage diabetes with insulin. Optimizing glycemic control should reduce the risk of secondary cardiovascular complications.

PROGNOSIS

- Cardiac complications with diabetes mellitus in dogs and cats are generally mild and easy to control.

METABOLIC DISTURBANCES

DISORDERS ASSOCIATED WITH HYPERKALEMIA

- More than 95% of body potassium is intracellular, with only 2% to 5% extracellular. Therefore serum potassium values are not always reliable indicators of total body potassium stores.
- Clinical causes of hyperkalemia include the following:
  - Excessive administration of oral potassium supplements or potassium supplemented fluids
  - Decreased renal elimination associated with oliguric or anuric renal failure
  - Hypoadrenocorticism (Addison disease)
  - Drugs (potassium-sparing diuretics, ACE inhibitors, beta blockers)
  - Ruptured urinary tract and urethral obstruction
  - Translocation from intracellular to extracellular space (metabolic acidosis, rapid release from tissue during severe injury such as aortic thromboembolism)
  - Pleural effusion (possibly due to aldosterone antagonism)

DIAGNOSIS, THERAPY, AND PROGNOSIS

- ECG changes caused by hyperkalemia are dependent on magnitude and also rate of development of hyperkalemia (see p. 245).

KEY POINT

Most patients with clinically significant hyperkalemia will have bradycardia, but, uncommonly, tachycardia can also develop (Figure 14.2).

- Identification and treatment of the underlying cause of hyperkalemia is essential (see the section on Hypoadrenocorticism [Addison disease]).

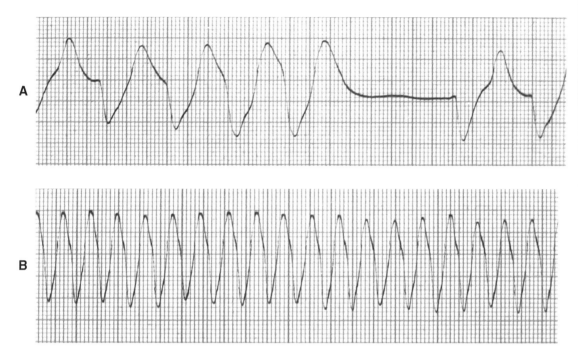

Figure 14.2 A, Hyperkalemia in cat with urinary obstruction resulting in a wide-complex bradycardia. **B**, Same cat had wide complex tachycardia as treatment with insulin and dextrose was initiated. Normal sinus rhythm developed as treatment was continued (not shown).

DISORDERS ASSOCIATED WITH HYPOKALEMIA

- When severe potassium loss has occurred, severe muscle weakness or paralysis may develop.
- Clinical causes of hypokalemia include the following:
  - Decreased intake (anorexia, especially when combined with potassium-deficient fluid administration)
  - Excessive gastrointestinal loss
    - Chronic vomiting
    - Severe diarrhea
  - Overuse of enemas, laxatives, or exchange resins
  - Excessive urinary loss
    - Renal (renal tubular acidosis, postobstructive diuresis, chronic pyelonephritis)
    - Drugs (diuretics, amphotericin B, beta agonists, theophylline)
  - Secondary hyperaldosteronism (liver failure, congestive heart failure, nephrotic syndrome)
  - Extracellular to intracellular transfer
    - Metabolic alkalosis
    - Insulin and glucose administration
    - Hyperinsulinism (insulinoma)
    - Ketoacidotic diabetes mellitus

CARDIAC PATHOPHYSIOLOGY

- Severe hypokalemia causes hyperpolarization of muscle fiber membranes and slows repolarization.

- ECG changes are manifested in delayed and abnormal repolarization, increased automaticity, and increased duration of the action potential.

DIAGNOSIS

HISTORY AND PHYSICAL EXAMINATION

- Muscle weakness may be mild or present as profound weakness and depression.
- Ventroflexion of the head is frequently seen in cats with symptoms.
- Polyuria and polydipsia may occur.

ELECTROCARDIOGRAPHY

- QT interval prolongation may occur.
- U waves may develop (usually a positive deflection immediately after the T wave).
- ST segment may become depressed (Figure 14.3) with a gradual blending of T waves and what appears to be a tall U wave.
- Ventricular and supraventricular arrhythmias may occur.
- Clinical pathology is generally reflective of the underlying disease process contributing to hypokalemia. Urine concentrating ability may be impaired.

THERAPY

- Treat the primary disease process.
- Parenteral replacement with potassium chloride is recommended when potassium loss is

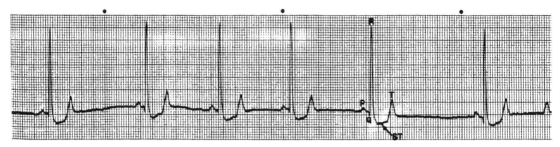

Figure 14.3 ST segment depression in a dog with hypokalemia (serum potassium 3.3 mEq/L) secondary to respiratory alkalosis. (From Tilley LP: Essentials of canine and feline electrocardiography: interpretation and treatment, ed 3, Malvern, Penn, 1992, Lea & Febiger.)

Table 14.1	Guidelines for Potassium Supplementation	
Serum Potassium (mEq/L)	mEq KCl to Add to 250 mL Fluid	Maximum Fluid Rate (mL/kg/hour)
<2.0	20	6
2.1-2.5	15	8
2.6-3.0	10	12
3.1-3.5	7	18
3.6-5.0	5	25

From Greene RW, Scott R.C.: Lower urinary tract disease. In Ettinger SJ ed: Textbook of veterinary internal medicine, Philadelphia, 1975, WB Saunders.

severe and the animal is symptomatic for hypokalemia (Table 14.1).

KEY POINT

When administering potassium chloride, do not exceed 0.5 mEq/kg/hr.

- Parenteral administration may initially decrease the serum K^+ level. This effect is minimized by avoiding dextrose-containing fluids, administering K^+ at the correct rate and concentration, and starting oral potassium gluconate supplementation early.
- Return to alimentation and treatment of the primary disease responsible for hypokalemia will replace potassium deficits. Therefore prolonged oral maintenance therapy is rarely indicated, except when ongoing excessive loss of potassium owing to diuretic administration or polyuric renal disease is present.
- Hypokalemia markedly increases the likelihood of toxicity when digitalis is being administered. Serum potassium should be promptly checked and corrected when digitalis toxicity is suspected.

- Hypokalemia increases the risk of ventricular arrhythmias and decreases the responsiveness to class I antiarrhythmic agents (lidocaine, mexiletine, procainamide, quinidine). Serum potassium should be promptly checked and corrected when refractory ventricular arrhythmias are identified.

PROGNOSIS

- The prognosis is good if the underlying condition can be corrected or managed.

DISORDERS ASSOCIATED WITH HYPERCALCEMIA

- Hypercalcemia occurs when serum calcium concentration consistently exceeds 11.5 mg/dL in mature dogs and 10.5 mg/dL in cats or when ionized calcium exceeds 1.4 mmol/L. Young, actively growing dogs may normally have calcium values of greater than 12.0 mg/dL.
- Many different conditions can cause hypercalcemia. Hypercalcemia results from calcium bone resorption, increased gastrointestinal calcium absorption, increased serum protein binding of calcium, increased calcium binding to anions, and decreased renal and intestinal calcium removal from serum.
- The following conditions are associated with hypercalcemia:
  - Young growing puppy (normal)
  - Paraneoplastic syndromes (lymphoma, anal sac apocrine gland adenocarcinoma, occasionally other soft tissue tumors, primary and metastatic bony tumors)
  - Hypoadrenocorticism
  - Renal failure
  - Skeletal lesions (septic osteomyelitis, disuse osteoporosis, hypertrophic osteodystrophy)
  - Nutritional (hypervitaminosis D, hypervitaminosis A, calcium administration)
  - Primary hyperparathyroidism
  - Other (hemoconcentration, hyperproteinemia, severe hypothermia, laboratory error)

CARDIAC PATHOPHYSIOLOGY

- Cardiovascular effects of experimentally induced acute hypercalcemia include elevated systolic and diastolic blood pressure, especially with renal failure.
- Clinically, elevated calcium levels have little, if any, direct adverse effect on cardiac function. In severe hypercalcemia, cardiac arrhythmias or arrest may occur.
- Animals with hypercalcemia may be more predisposed to complications of digitalis intoxication.
- Long-standing hypercalcemia may predispose to calcification of the myocardium, blood vessels, and other soft tissues.

DIAGNOSIS

HISTORY AND PHYSICAL EXAMINATION

- Regardless of its cause, hypercalcemia affects the kidney (renal dysfunction, polyuria, polydipsia, nocturia, nephrocalcinosis, renal failure, uremia), gastrointestinal system (anorexia, constipation, and vomiting from decreased gastrointestinal smooth muscle excitability), and nervous system (generalized skeletal muscle weakness from decreased neuromuscular activity).

RADIOGRAPHY

- Thoracic radiographs may indicate mediastinal mass(es), metastasis, abnormal bony densities, or osteolysis.
- Abdominal radiographs may show organomegaly, abnormal bone density, sublumbar masses, or sublumbar lymphadenopathy.
- Skeletal survey radiographs may exhibit isolated bony lesions that could account for hypercalcemia. Osteopenia, metastatic calcification, or focal bony lesions may be present.

ELECTROCARDIOGRAPHY

- The characteristic ECG finding is a short QT interval. In extreme cases, the ST segment may fuse with the upstroke of the T wave.

KEY POINT

ECG changes do not correlate closely with serum calcium concentration.

- With severe hypercalcemia, bradycardia may occur.
- Hypercalcemia may predispose to arrhythmias of digitalis intoxication.
- ECG changes resolve after normalization of serum calcium.

CLINICAL PATHOLOGY

- Hypercalcemia often causes diminished urinary concentrating ability. The urine is usually hyposthenuric or isosthenuric.
- Renal failure with azotemia may develop from progressive structural and functional alterations in the kidney.
- Hypophosphatemia or hyperphosphatemia may be recorded, depending on the presence or absence of renal failure and the underlying etiology of hypercalcemia.
- Serum alkaline phosphatase may be elevated if severe bone disease or concomitant hepatic disease is present.
- A hemogram may be normal, display hemoconcentration or anemia, or occasionally show evidence of leukemia (when this disease is associated with the underlying etiology).
- Bone marrow evaluation may be unremarkable or disclose evidence of lymphoma, leukemia, or multiple myeloma.

THERAPY

- Initial treatment is directed at reducing the systemic effects of hypercalcemia.
- Preexisting dehydration should be corrected and hydration maintained.
- Administration of 0.9% saline should be used to enhance the renal excretion of calcium.
- Furosemide (1 to 4 mg/kg IV, SC, PO q8 to 12h) can be used if the patient is well hydrated.
- Sodium bicarbonate (1 mEq/kg IV every 10 to 15 minutes, up to 4 mEq/L maximum dose) may also help in cases of moderate-to-severe hypercalcemia.
- Glucocorticosteroids may limit bone resorption, decrease intestinal calcium absorption, increase renal calcium excretion, and be cytolytic in certain neoplasms. Administration may interfere with a diagnosis of neoplasia.
- Dietary therapy may be of benefit in some cats with idiopathic hypercalcemia.
- Definitive treatment is directed at the underlying etiology.

PROGNOSIS

- The prognosis depends on early detection, on the ability to establish a definitive diagnosis, and on the success of treatment. The prognosis of many causes of hypercalcemia is guarded to poor.

DISORDERS ASSOCIATED WITH HYPOCALCEMIA

- Hypocalcemia, although encountered infrequently, can cause profound clinical signs. It occurs when serum calcium concentration is

less than 8 mg/dL in the dog and less than 7 mg/dL in the cat (ionized calcium less than 5 in dogs and less than 4.5 in cats).
- Serum calcium can be artificially lowered by hypoalbuminemia due to decreased protein binding.
- If hypoalbuminemia is present then calcium should be corrected before further diagnostics.
- The following conditions may be associated with hypocalcemia:
  - Renal failure
  - Eclampsia (puerperal tetany)
  - Canine acute pancreatitis
  - Primary or secondary (nutritional) hypoparathyroidism
  - Idiopathic
  - Postoperative (during bilateral thyroid surgery)
  - Ethylene glycol toxicity
  - Hyperphosphatemia
  - Excessive diuretic therapy

CARDIAC PATHOPHYSIOLOGY

- Hypocalcemia causes an excitatory effect on nerve and muscle cells. Neuromuscular irritability, tetany, and seizures may result.
- Animals with coexisting congestive heart failure may experience decreased cardiac systolic function that improves with restoration of calcium levels (owing to the augmenting effect of calcium on myocardial contractility).
- Acutely induced hypocalcemia (i.e., treatment with chelating agents) can potentially cause sharp reductions in blood pressure resulting in cardiovascular shock.

DIAGNOSIS

HISTORY AND PHYSICAL EXAMINATION

- Tetany, seizures, anorexia, vomiting, and abdominal discomfort are the predominant signs in affected animals.

- Synchronous diaphragmatic flutter has been reported in association with hypocalcemia.
- Synchronous diaphragmatic flutter is the contraction of the diaphragm in synchrony with the heart beat due to irritability of the phrenic nerve.
- Aggressive rubbing of the ears, nose, face, and eyes can also be seen.
- Handling or stress may precipitate tetany.

ELECTROCARDIOGRAPHY

- The typical ECG manifestation of hypocalcemia is QT prolongation, but QT interval duration is heart rate dependent (Figure 14.4).

CLINICAL PATHOLOGY

- Clinical pathology will reflect abnormalities associated with the underlying disease process. Hypocalcemia is usually diagnosed when low serum calcium levels are detected during clinical investigation of tetany, seizures, renal failure, pancreatitis, or other disorders through analysis of a serum biochemical profile.

THERAPY

- Severe hypocalcemia (<6 mg/dL) is a life-threatening emergency.
- Ten percent calcium gluconate is administered intravenously (0.5 to 1.5 mL/kg) slowly over a 15- to 30-minute interval.
- Calcium should be administered slowly because ECG changes do not closely conform to serum calcium levels, especially when other electrolyte and acid/base disturbances are present.
- ECG monitoring should accompany administration.
- Calcium infusion should be temporarily interrupted if QT interval shortening, ST segment elevation, or bradycardia occurs, to be reinstated at a slower rate when these changes have abated.

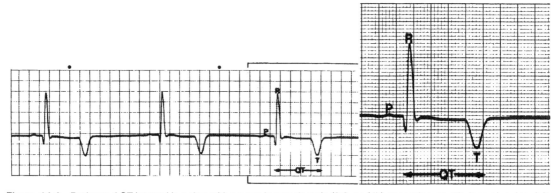

Figure 14.4 Prolonged QT interval in a dog with severe hypocalcemia (2.2 mg/dL) secondary to ethylene glycol toxicity. (From Tilley LP: Essentials of canine and feline electrocardiography: interpretation and treatment, ed 3, Malvern, Penn, 1992, Lea & Febiger.)

- Gradual QT interval shortening from its prolonged state may accompany calcium infusion.

- Subsequent IV calcium administration may be repeated every 6 to 12 hours or as needed.
- Clinical signs of hypocalcemia may abate slowly despite calcium infusion. Resolution of clinical signs may not provide a reliable guide as an endpoint of adequate calcium administration. Some hypocalcemic signs (i.e., weakness, anorexia) may persist even if cardiotoxic doses of calcium are infused.
- Vitamin D therapy may be required in some disorders to maintain control of hypocalcemia. In treatment of postoperative parathyroid insufficiency, care must be taken to detect recovery of parathyroid function to avoid vitamin D–associated hypercalcemia.

PROGNOSIS

- For most causes of hypocalcemia that are carefully managed, the prognosis is good to excellent.

DISORDERS ASSOCIATED WITH HYPOMAGNESEMIA AND HYPERMAGNESEMIA

- Abnormalities in magnesium levels rarely affect cardiac function directly, but they may potentiate problems caused by other electrolyte derangements.
- Causes of hypomagnesemia are very similar to causes of hypokalemia.

CARDIAC PATHOPHYSIOLOGY

- Abnormalities of magnesium have minimal effects on the ECG with normal calcium and potassium levels.
- Hypomagnesemia will exacerbate problems due to hypocalcemia.
- Hypomagnesemia predisposes to digitalis-induced arrhythmias.
- Hypomagnesemia prevents correction of hypokalemia.

DIAGNOSIS

- Consider hypomagnesemia with conditions that lead to hypokalemia.
- Consider hypomagnesemia when there is difficulty correcting hypokalemia.

- Consider hypomagnesemia in patients with intractable cardiac arrhythmias.

THERAPY

- Treat the underlying disease process.
- Parenteral replacement if there is evidence of cardiac complications or if there is difficulty correcting hypokalemia. Magnesium sulfate at 0.75 to 1.0 mEq/kg/day in 5% dextrose in water (D_5W) as a constant rate infusion could be considered.

HYPOGLYCEMIA

- Hypoglycemia may be caused by the following:
  - Hyperinsulinism due to a functional islet cell pancreatic carcinoma
  - Insulin overdose for the treatment of diabetes mellitus
  - Nonpancreatic tumors
  - Glycogen storage diseases
  - Neonatal/juvenile hypoglycemia
  - Septic shock
  - Addison disease
  - Hepatic disease

CARDIAC PATHOPHYSIOLOGY

- Irrespective of the etiologic factors, hypoglycemia triggers catecholamine release, which causes tachycardia, increases in myocardial oxygen demand, and potentially cardiac arrhythmias.

DIAGNOSIS

HISTORY AND PHYSICAL EXAMINATION

- Clinical manifestations of hypoglycemia range from lethargy to episodic weakness and seizures.

ELECTROCARDIOGRAPHY

- ECG changes are typically related to resultant elevated sympathetic tone, myocardial hypoxia, or concurrent electrolyte abnormalities such as hyperkalemia in Addison disease.
- ECG findings can include the following:
  - ST depression
  - T wave flattening
  - QT prolongation
  - Supraventricular or ventricular arrhythmias
  - ECG changes usually resolve with correction of hypoglycemia

LABORATORY FINDINGS

- A low blood glucose level (<60 mg/dL) is usually present. A fasting blood glucose level may be needed to confirm hypoglycemia.

- Elevated insulin levels or abnormal insulin; the insulin/glucose ratio may be increased with insulinoma.

THERAPY

- A hypoglycemic crisis regardless of cause is managed by slow, IV administration of 50% dextrose to effect. A slow IV bolus of 0.5 to 1.0 mg/kg (over 1 to 3 minutes) could be considered.
- Treat the underlying disease or improve diabetic regulation.

PROGNOSIS

- Resolution of neurologic signs due to hypoglycemia is usually abrupt and virtually complete.
- Prolonged, untreated hypoglycemia may result in cerebrocortical hypoxic damage. Lack of symptom amelioration after therapy may indicate cerebral hypoxia and edema.

UREMIA

- Uremia is generally associated with renal failure.
- Uremia is common in geriatric populations.
- Renal failure can affect cardiac function and reduce elimination of many cardiac drugs (digoxin, most ACE inhibitors, and many beta blockers).

CARDIAC PATHOPHYSIOLOGY

- Hypertensive cardiovascular disease, electrolyte imbalance, fluid overload, and anemia can contribute to the production of cardiac disturbances in uremic patients.
- Renal failure can cause elevations or reductions of potassium and calcium; associated changes may register on the ECG.
- Systemic hypertension is a common sequela of chronic renal failure in dogs and cats and is reported in 50% to 93% of dogs and 65% of cats.
- Pericardial effusion is reported as an uncommon sequela of uremia in cats and dogs. The effusion may occur secondary to uremic serositis.
- Pulmonary thromboembolism may occur associated with protein-losing glomerular nephropathy (Figure 14.5).

KEY POINT

Uremic toxins have a cardiodepressant effect.

- Uremic pneumonitis can uncommonly cause noncardiogenic pulmonary edema.

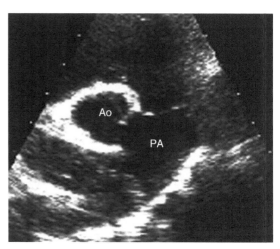

Figure 14.5 Right parasternal short-axis view at the base of the heart in a dog with protein-losing nephropathy. A well circumscribed thrombus can be seen at the bifurcation of the pulmonary artery. *Ao*, Aorta; *PA*, pulmonary artery.

DIAGNOSIS

HISTORY AND PHYSICAL EXAMINATION

- Signs that may accompany uremia include polyuria, polydipsia, depression, anorexia, lethargy, vomiting, diarrhea, and weight loss.
- Uremic pneumonitis and metabolic acidosis cause dyspnea or tachypnea that may be confused with signs of congestive heart failure.

ELECTROCARDIOGRAPHY

- Nonspecific ECG abnormalities may be attributed to hypertension, anemia, electrolyte abnormalities, and pericarditis.
- Conduction defects or arrhythmias may occur.

ECHOCARDIOGRAPHY

- Echocardiography may show changes consistent with hypertension or chronic anemia.

CLINICAL PATHOLOGY

- Clinical pathology may reveal abnormalities in the hemogram, urinalysis, and biochemistry profile consistent with uremia (increased blood urea nitrogen, creatinine, and phosphorus, nonregenerative anemia, and isosthenuria).

THERAPY

- Treatment is directed at managing uremia and its underlying causes. Therapy generally includes parenteral fluids, protein and phosphorus restriction, phosphate binders, and sometimes calcitriol and erythropoietin.

- Management of severe azotemia in patients with concurrent heart disease is extremely challenging and often frustrating.
- Azotemia identified while treating congestive heart failure may be prerenal or renal in origin.
- Rehydrate cautiously.
  - Consider low-sodium fluids (half-strength saline).
  - Consider reduced administration rates (start at a maintenance rate).
  - It may take 48 hours to see improvement in azotemia.
- Monitor clinically and radiographically for development of congestive heart failure.
- Reduce doses or avoid cardiac drugs eliminated by the kidneys. If using ACE inhibitors or digoxin, monitor kidney function and electrolytes frequently. Monitor digoxin levels periodically, particularly if there is a decrease in appetite. Pimobendan, hydralazine, or nitroglycerin can be substituted for ACE inhibitors.
- Monitor and control systemic hypertension, electrolyte, and acid-base disturbances.

PROGNOSIS

- Resolution of the uremic state may improve ECG abnormalities, but arrhythmias may persist.
- The development of congestive heart failure in the face of severe azotemia carries a poor prognosis.

ANEMIA

- Anemia is a sign of a disease, not a disease entity.
- Evaluation should emphasize history (drug or toxin exposure), clinical signs related to other disorders complicated by anemia (fever, lethargy, bleeding, and weight loss), physical examination (petechiae, lymphadenopathy), and clinical pathology.
- Symptoms of reduced cardiac reserve associated with anemia depend on the severity of anemia, rate of anemia development, and on the presence and extent of underlying cardiac disease.

CARDIAC PATHOPHYSIOLOGY

- Tissue hypoxia results in peripheral vasodilation. This in conjunction with reduced blood viscosity leads to decreased systemic vascular resistance. The body responds to decreased systemic vascular resistance by increasing sodium and water retention, resulting in an increased stroke volume and cardiac output.
- Tissue hypoxia may also result in sinus tachycardia.

- When anemia is associated with increased viscosity (multiple myeloma or macroglobulinemia), cardiac output may fail to rise.
- Physiologic consequences depend on the developmental rate of anemia.
  - With acute blood loss (i.e., hemorrhage), hypovolemic shock may predominate.
    - Acute blood loss leads to volume depletion and a resultant decrease in cardiac output. In addition, acute anemia can lead to myocardial hypoxia and resultant depressed cardiac function.
  - With chronic anemia, blood volume is maintained, but systemic vascular resistance may fall and cardiac output may rise as described previously.
    - The sodium and water retention may result in cardiac dilation and hypertrophy. Chronic anemia is usually well tolerated because of compensatory mechanisms that include increased cardiac output, redistribution of blood flow, and increased oxygen affinity of red blood cells.
    - Uncommonly the volume overload can result in congestive heart failure. In many of these cases, preexisting subclinical heart disease may be a factor.
    - Pulmonary thromboembolism may occur with autoimmune hemolytic anemia.

DIAGNOSIS

HISTORY AND PHYSICAL EXAMINATION

- Chronic anemia produces variable symptoms that may include fatigue and mild exertional dyspnea. In rare situations, chronic anemia can lead to syncope.
- Acute anemia may present with collapse, weakness, lethargy, stupor, and dyspnea.
- Physical examination may reveal that the apex beat is hyperkinetic, bounding or pistol shot arterial pulses, pale or icteric mucous membrane color, and prolonged capillary refill time.
- A soft, systolic murmur at the left apex, generally grade 1 to 3 or 4, is common with severe anemia.
- Heart sounds may be accentuated.

RADIOLOGY

- Thoracic radiographs may display cardiac enlargement, but this will vary depending on the presence and extent of previously existing heart disease.
- Uncommonly, the cardiac effects of anemia can result in congestive heart failure (evidence

of pulmonary venous congestion, pulmonary edema, or pleural effusion).

ELECTROCARDIOGRAPHY

- Sinus tachycardia is often present. The heart rate varies with the rate of onset and degree of anemia.
- VPCs may be seen.
- Evidence of left ventricular enlargement (wide QRS complex and/or tall R waves) may be present.

ECHOCARDIOGRAPHY

- It may show evidence of left ventricular, left atrial, right ventricular, or right atrial dilation.
- Hyperdynamic cardiac function (increased fractional shortening, decreased end-systolic left ventricular diameter) is usually seen in the presence of volume overload with an otherwise normal heart.
- Evidence of preexisting cardiac disease may be present.

CLINICAL PATHOLOGY

- The laboratory database varies considerably depending on the cause of anemia.

THERAPY

- Treatment of anemia depends on the underlying cause.
- Animals with congestive heart failure secondary to anemia should be given furosemide as needed. Once the anemia is controlled, chronic cardiac therapy may not be necessary.
- Animals with concurrent congestive heart failure and life-threatening anemia should be given furosemide and transfused simultaneously. Packed red blood cells may be more appropriate than whole blood owing to the smaller volume that can be administered to correct the anemia.
- Caution with fluid administration should always be exercised when cardiomegaly is present in the face of significant anemia.
- A decision as to when to transfuse a patient is based on the clinical assessment, which includes the rate of anemia development, the patient's state of compensation, and the presence of continued red blood cell loss.

PROGNOSIS

- Successful management of anemia and underlying causes confers a good short-term prognosis. Long-term prognosis depends on the cause of the anemia.

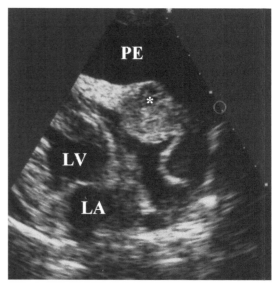

Figure 14.6 Slightly oblique right parasternal long-axis view. A large soft tissue mass effect (*) can be seen in the wall of the right atrium. Moderate pericardial effusion (*PE*) is present resulting in diastolic collapse of the right atrium. *LA,* Left atrium; *LV,* left ventricle.

NEOPLASTIC AND INFILTRATIVE HEART DISEASES

HEMANGIOSARCOMA

- This tumor originates from endothelial cells.
- It can be seen in any portion of the heart but appears to be more common in the wall of the right atrium (Figure 14.6).
- It is rare in cats.
- Average age of affected dogs is 10 years, no gender predilection, and the incidence is increased in German Shepherds.
- Metastasis is common.
- Other common sites of hemangiosarcoma include the spleen, liver, and lungs.

CHEMODECTOMA

- This tumor originates from neuroepithelial cells most commonly found in the aortic bodies.
- Masses are typically seen at the heart base. Because of the complexity of the heart base, small masses can be difficult to identify (Figure 14.7).
- It is rare in cats.
- It is more common in dogs older than 6 years, there is no gender predilection, and there is an increased incidence in Boxers and Boston Terriers.
- Metastasis is uncommon but can appear in lungs, liver, lymph nodes, and bone.

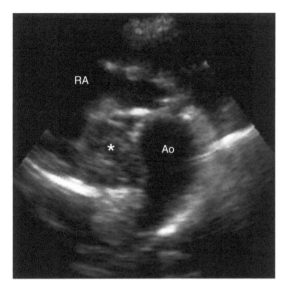

Figure 14.7 Slightly oblique right parasternal short-axis view at the heart base above the left atrium. A small, soft tissue mass effect (*) can be seen associated with the aorta (*Ao*) and above the left atrium. Mild to moderate pericardial effusion is also present. *RA,* Right atrium.

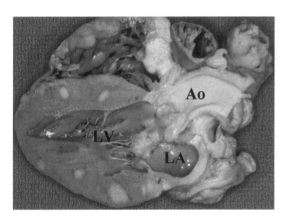

Figure 14.8 Transverse section through the heart of a dog with cardiac lymphoma. Multiple pale nodules can be seen in the left and right ventricular myocardium. *Ao,* Aorta; *LA,* left atrium; *LV,* left ventricle.

OTHER CAUSES

- Lymphoma is the most common tumor that metastasizes to the heart in cats, but it also can be seen in dogs (Figures 14.8 and 14.9).
- Ectopic thyroid carcinomas occur at the heart base and rarely in the right ventricular outflow tract.
- Cardiac myxomas are rare but are more common in the right heart (right atrial lumen) (Figure 14.10).
- Rarely, cardiac fibroma, fibrosarcoma, and rhabdomyosarcoma are diagnosed in young dogs.

- Infiltrative myocardial disease (e.g., amyloidosis, hypereosinophilic syndrome) involving nonneoplastic cells is rare in dogs and uncommon in cats.

CARDIAC PATHOPHYSIOLOGY

- Tumors from other tissues gain access to the heart by invasive growth from adjacent structures or spread by hematogenous or lymphatic vessels.
- The relative infrequency of cardiac metastasis has been attributed to metabolic peculiarities of striated muscle, rapid coronary blood flow, efferent lymphatic drainage from the heart, and the vigorous kneading action of the myocardium.
- Myocardial neoplasia may cause congestive heart failure because of diastolic dysfunction, obstruction to ventricular inflow or outflow, pericardial tamponade, or arrhythmias.

DIAGNOSIS
HISTORY AND PHYSICAL EXAMINATION

- Cardiac involvement may not always lead to clinical signs. Signs depend on the site and extent of metastasis. Resultant cardiac dysfunction may cause signs of congestive heart failure, weakness, or syncope.
- Pericardial effusion and tamponade may lead to similar clinical signs.
- Possible physical findings include muffled heart sounds on auscultation, jugular venous distention, ascites, weakness (often acute), hypokinetic pulses, tachypnea, weight loss, and pale mucous membranes.

RADIOGRAPHY

- Radiographic evidence of a cardiac mass is uncommonly seen (Figure 14.11).
- Cardiac enlargement and rounding of the cardiac silhouette may be observed if pericardial effusion is present.
- Dilation of the caudal vena cava may be present secondary to cardiac tamponade or obstruction to blood flow within the lumen of the right heart. In general, the diameter of the caudal vena cava should be less than the length of the thoracic vertebra above the carina.
- Pneumopericardiography or angiocardiography may assess the thickness and any irregularities of the pericardium, epicardium, and endocardium.
- The use of MRI or CT angiography may allow visualization of a cardiac mass, but cardiac gating is necessary.

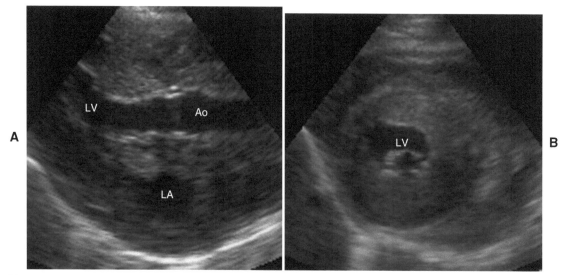

Figure 14.9 Right parasternal long-axis (**A**) and short-axis (**B**) views in a cat with cardiac lymphoma confirmed on histopathologic examination. Note the marked thickening of the left ventricular and left atrial myocardium. *Ao,* Aorta; *LA,* left atrium; *LV,* left ventricle.

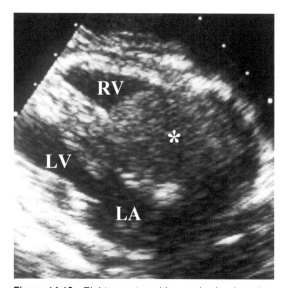

Figure 14.10 Right parasternal long-axis view in a dog. A large, well-circumscribed mass effect (*) is seen filling most of the right atrial lumen. The mass was confirmed as a myxoma on histopathologic examination. *LA,* Left atrium; *LV,* left ventricle; *RV,* right ventricle.

ELECTROCARDIOGRAPHY

- Reduced QRS voltage on the ECG and electrical alternans occur in many but not all cases with pericardial effusion.
- Atrial or ventricular arrhythmias, conduction disturbances, and complete heart block can occur.

ECHOCARDIOGRAPHY

- Echocardiographic evidence of pericardial effusion may be demonstrated. Diastolic right atrial or right ventricular collapse signifies pericardial tamponade. Dilation of the abdominal vena cava and/or hepatic veins is also typically seen with tamponade.
- Two-dimensional echocardiography may facilitate identification of cardiac neoplasia. Unfortunately, because of the elusive nature of some cardiac masses, the lack of a mass on echocardiogram does not rule out neoplasia.
- Whenever safely possible, an echocardiogram should be performed while pericardial fluid is present. The fluid can outline the borders of a mass, improving identification.
- Pericardiocentesis may uncommonly detect cytologic evidence of neoplasia. Most of the time, fluid analysis will come back as nonspecific hemorrhagic effusion.
- Biopsy of the tumor is possible without thoracotomy with techniques such as myocardial biopsy or thoracoscopy.

THERAPY

- Pericardiocentesis may offer temporary relief from cardiac tamponade.
- If recurrent pericardiocentesis is necessary, then partial pericardectomy via thoracotomy or a pericardial window via thoracoscopy could be considered.
- Surgery would likely improve the patient's quality of life but may not prolong life.

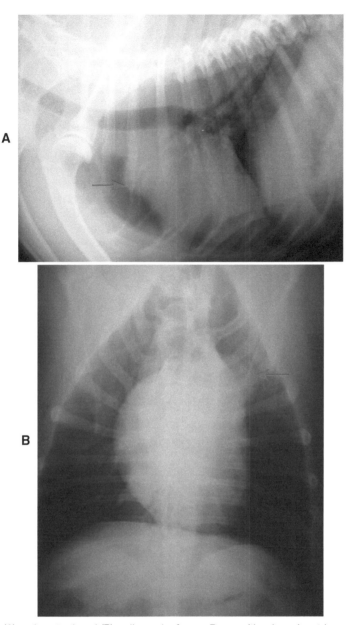

Figure 14.11 Lateral (**A**) and ventrodorsal (**B**) radiographs from a Boxer with a large heart base mass. A bulge in the area of the cranial waist (*arrow* in **A**) of the cardiac silhouette can be seen on the lateral. A similar bulge can be seen on the ventrodorsal projection at the 2 o'clock position (*arrow* in **B**) on the cardiac silhouette.

- Other than standard thoracotomy concerns and risks, the main complication with surgery is ongoing hemorrhage from the tumor. This can result in hemothorax.
- Animals with myocardial infiltration of tumors sensitive to chemotherapy or radiotherapy may respond favorably, but this is uncommon.
- Congestive heart failure and arrhythmias resulting from cardiac neoplasia can be difficult to treat.
- Surgical resection or debulking of cardiac masses is not commonly possible.

- Masses confined to the right atrial appendage can periodically be removed with resection of the appendage.
- Some intraluminal cardiac masses can be removed with cardiac bypass or inflow occlusion. Studies with long-term follow-up with such patients are not available.

PROGNOSIS

HEMANGIOSARCOMA

- Surgical resection may be possible, but distant microscopic metastasis is almost always present.

- Poor response to chemotherapy in general, although a combination of surgical resection and chemotherapy may improve the prognosis to some degree.
- Pericardectomy may improve quality of life.

CHEMODECTOMA

- In many cases, heart base tumors can be an incidental finding. Because they are often slow growing, they can be present for extended periods before clinical signs develop.
- Debulking surgery is an option, but complete resection of the tumor is rarely possible.
- Pericardectomy may improve quality of life.
- Radiation therapy may be beneficial in some cases, but general response to chemotherapy is poor.

KEY POINT

In general, long-term prognosis with cardiac cancer is poor because of difficulty in surgical resection, minimal response to chemotherapy and radiation therapy, and detrimental side effects of chemotherapy and radiation therapy on the heart.

PHYSICAL AND CHEMICAL AGENTS THAT AFFECT THE CARDIOVASCULAR SYSTEM

- Many noninfectious stimuli can cause myocardial injury. Damage can be acute and transient or chronic and lead to permanent myocardial changes. Effects are usually related to the severity, dose, and rate of exposure.

HYPERPYREXIA (HEAT STROKE)

- Hyperpyrexia is usually associated with heat stroke when the rectal temperature rises to 41° to 44° C (106° to 111° F). Experimentally, signs of heat stroke develop consistently at temperatures above 43° C (109° F) in dogs.
- Heat stroke develops in animals exposed to high environmental temperatures or during heavy activity in warm environmental temperatures. It commonly occurs in animals left in unventilated automobiles during the summer months.
- High humidity reduces evaporation of water from the oral and nasal cavities and reduces the ability of small animals to regulate their temperatures.
- Animals that are obese, have brachycephaly, are very young, are very old, or have cardiopulmonary disease are predisposed to heat stroke.

- Malignant hyperthermia is a rare but a potentially fatal abnormal response to anesthetic agents. It is characterized by an acute, rapid rise in body temperature and severe biochemical changes accompanied by muscle rigidity.

CARDIAC PATHOPHYSIOLOGY

- Heat-induced vasodilation results in hypotension and decreased organ perfusion.
- Respiratory alkalosis may result from panting.
- Dehydration with hemoconcentration may occur, in addition to mild hyperkalemia and hypophosphatemia.
- Tachyarrhythmias and cardiogenic shock can occur owing to myocardial hemorrhage, ischemia, and necrosis.
- Disseminated intravascular coagulopathy (DIC) may develop owing to destruction of clotting factors.
- Right-heart dilation may occur.
- Mechanisms suggested for myocardial injury include direct thermal effects, circulatory collapse with secondary myocardial hypoxia, decreased coronary blood flow, and secondary metabolic injury.
- Animals that recover from heat stroke may be prone to subsequent occurrences as a result of heat-induced damage to the thermoregulatory zone of the hypothalamus.

DIAGNOSIS

HISTORY AND PHYSICAL EXAMINATION

- The diagnosis is usually made on the reported history of an animal being exposed to high environmental temperatures. However, some cases have a more subtle history.
- Depending on the duration and severity of the heat stroke, clinical signs may include panting, sinus tachycardia, bright red oral mucous membranes, and hyperthermia. Extremities become hot to the touch.
- Red mucous membranes may turn pale because of diminished circulation or vasoconstriction.
- Watery diarrhea may occur, which can progress to bloody diarrhea.
- Stupor and coma with respiratory arrest can follow.
- With malignant hyperthermia, an acute, profound temperature elevation may be the first noticeable sign to the surgeon.
- If the heart rate is monitored, tachycardia may be the earliest indication.
- Skeletal muscle hypertonus may occur.
- ECG may show tachycardia, extrasystoles (especially if DIC develops), and ST segment and T wave abnormalities.

- Clinical pathologic alterations relate to the stage and severity of the hyperpyrexia.

THERAPY

- Therapy should begin with lowering body temperature. Submergence in cool water and wetting the extremities with rubbing alcohol are useful techniques. Rectal temperature should be recorded every 5 to 10 minutes. Discontinue cooling when the body temperature drops below 39.5° C (103° F), to avoid hypothermia.
- If laryngeal paralysis, laryngeal edema, or tracheal stenosis is present, it may impede heat loss through the respiratory system. If these conditions are present, then a temporary tracheotomy or endotracheal intubation may have to be performed.
- Supportive care should include isotonic fluid therapy (0.45% saline or half-strength lactated Ringer solution with 2.5% dextrose), correction of acid-base and electrolyte abnormalities, and treatment for DIC.
- Nonsteroidal antiinflammatory drugs or antipyretics (e.g., aspirin, flunixin meglumine) are contraindicated. The use of glucocorticoids remains controversial, but they are often used when cerebral edema is suspected.
- When malignant hyperthermia is anesthetic related, all inhalation agents and relaxants should be discontinued. Hyperventilation with 100% oxygen should be started.
- For malignant hyperthermia, dantrolene 2 mg/kg IV, up to 10 mg/kg IV, has been used in the dog. No proved efficacy is known. Its use is based on experience from humans, horses, and pigs. Dantrolene exhibits muscle relaxation activity by direct action on muscle.
- Administer mannitol (0.25 to 2 g/kg of a 20% solution over 15 to 20 minutes) if cerebral edema is suspected or if stupor or coma develops.
- The patient should be monitored for several days for the development of complications, such as renal failure and DIC.

PROGNOSIS

- The prognosis for heat stroke is guarded to good if detected and treated early.
- Malignant hyperthermia is rare but seems to offer a worse prognosis.
- Coagulopathy and renal failure confer a worse prognosis.

HYPOTHERMIA

- Lowering of body temperature can occur accidentally, as a result of deep cooling from external cold, drugs, or interference with thermoregulatory centers during anesthesia. Physiologic consequences of hypothermia depend on the extent and duration of exposure.

CARDIAC PATHOPHYSIOLOGY

- Cardiac dilation with epicardial and subendocardial hemorrhage can result from severe hypothermia. Microinfarcts can occur in myocardial tissue.
- Lesions may result from circulatory collapse, hemoconcentration, sludging of blood in capillaries, or decreased cellular metabolism.

DIAGNOSIS

HISTORY AND PHYSICAL EXAMINATION

- Signs vary with the degree of hypothermia (reduction in core temperature), mild (32° to 35° C or 89.6° to 95° F), moderate (28° to 32° C or 82.4° to 89.6° F), and severe (< 28° C or 82.4° F).
- Signs include lethargy, ataxia, stupor, shivering, and bradycardia. Cardiopulmonary arrest may occur with severe hypothermia.

ELECTROCARDIOGRAPHY

- Mild hypothermia results in prolongation of the PR interval, QRS duration and QT interval, APCs, and inverted T waves.
- Moderate hypothermia produces atropine-resistant bradycardia and ventricular arrhythmias.
- Severe hypothermia may cause cardiac arrest secondary to ventricular fibrillation or asystole.

THERAPY

- Treatment initially involves warming the patient.
- Active external warming with warm-water blankets is recommended for mild to moderate hypothermia. External warming causes vasodilation of skin vessels, which may initially transfer cooled blood to the body core, further lowering internal temperature. This is rarely a significant clinical complication with mild to moderate hypothermia.
  - Internal (core) warming is recommended if the rectal temperature is less than 30° C (86° F) or the cardiovascular status is unstable. This is accomplished by peritoneal dialysis with dialysate fluids warmed to 45° C (113° F).
  - Appropriate supportive care (e.g., IV fluids, ventilation) must be administered. Severe hypothermia can cause cardiopulmonary collapse. Keep these patients well oxygenated and administer warmed IV fluids.
  - Cardiac output and ECG abnormalities improve after warming.

- Evaluation of the patient for underlying systemic disorders that could have predisposed it to hypothermia should be performed once normothermia has been achieved.

CARBON MONOXIDE TOXICITY

- Carbon monoxide is a colorless, odorless, tasteless, toxic gas that has the molecular formula CO. CO is produced by the incomplete combustion of the fossil fuels: gas, oil, coal, and wood used in boilers, engines, oil burners, gas fires, water heaters, solid fuel appliances, and open fires. CO is a commercially important chemical. It is also formed in many chemical reactions and in the thermal or incomplete decomposition of many organic materials.
- Dangerous amounts of CO can accumulate when, as a result of poor installation, poor maintenance or failure, or damage to an appliance in service, fuel is not burned properly or when rooms are poorly ventilated and produced CO is unable to escape.

CARDIAC PATHOPHYSIOLOGY

- CO competes with oxygen for binding sights on hemoglobin, diminishing oxygen transport capacity. This results in myocardial hypoxia. Myocardial hemorrhage and necrosis may occur.

DIAGNOSIS
HISTORY AND PHYSICAL EXAMINATION

- The history often supports exposure to fumes from a gasoline-burning engine.
- Clinical signs are often associated with cardiac hypoxia (sudden death) or hypoxia to the brain (convulsions, disorientation, and coma).
- The physical examination is often unremarkable.
- A blood sample will be cherry red.

ELECTROCARDIOGRAPHY

- ECG abnormalities can include ST segment changes, conduction abnormalities, or arrhythmias.

SPECIALIZED DIAGNOSTIC TEST

- Carboxyhemoglobin blood levels can be measured.

TREATMENT

- One hundred percent oxygen should be administered.
- Any arrhythmias should be treated as needed.

- Supportive care should include correction of electrolyte and acid-base imbalances.

PROGNOSIS

- Clinical recovery usually occurs if the situation is detected and treated early.

TOAD POISONING

- The Colorado River toad (*Bufo alvarius*) and the marine toad (*Bufo marinas*) secrete toxins from the parotid glands that can cause profound cardiotoxicity. The parotid gland secretions contain epinephrine, norepinephrine, dopamine, serotonin, bufotenine, bufagenins, and bufotoxins. The animal does not have to ingest the toad to become poisoned. Toxic parotid secretions can be absorbed through the oral mucous membranes just holding the toad in its mouth.

CARDIAC PATHOPHYSIOLOGY

- Bufagenins and bufotoxins can have digitalis-like effects on the heart.

DIAGNOSIS
HISTORY AND PHYSICAL EXAMINATION

- The pet is often observed playing with the toad.
- Clinical signs occur within minutes and may include hypersalivation, vomiting, diarrhea, weakness, pulmonary edema, and seizures. Coma and death can occur within 30 minutes.

ELECTROCARDIOGRAPHY

- In experimental studies, the digitalis-like effect of the toxin may result in any type of arrhythmia. In natural exposure, arrhythmias are rare. The most common rhythms noted are sinus arrhythmia and sinus tachycardia.
- Severely intoxicated dogs with bradycardia, tachycardia, neurologic disability, or signs of shock should get an initial ECG. Monitoring the ECG is recommended if significant arrhythmias are noted.

THERAPY

- The patient's mouth should be rinsed immediately. Atropine may help decrease salivation but is reserved for patients with heart rates less than 50 beats/min. The inclusion of atropine to treat excess salivation in dogs with normal heart rates or tachycardia can lead to more severe arrhythmias.
- Vomiting should be induced if ingestion was recent. The venom may enter enterohepatic circulation; therefore multiple doses of

- activated charcoal should be administered. Sorbitol cathartic is advised.
- Provide supportive care, including anticonvulsive and antiarrhythmic medication, as needed.
- Pentobarbital anesthesia will control seizures.
- Propranolol is quite effective for tachyarrhythmias. In patients without asthma or preexisting heart disease, doses of 0.02 to 0.06 mg/kg can be given slowly IV, to effect.

OLEANDER TOXICITY

- Oleander (*Nerium oleander*) is an ornamental shrub found mostly in the southeast United States.

CARDIAC PATHOPHYSIOLOGY
- The toxin of oleander is a digitalis-like glycoside.

DIAGNOSIS
HISTORY AND PHYSICAL EXAMINATION

- Signs of vomiting and diarrhea occur within 2 to 3 hours.
- ECG may reveal any type of arrhythmia due to the digitalis-like compounds.

THERAPY
- Supportive care that includes fluid therapy, electrolyte replacement, and control of vomiting and diarrhea is recommended.
- Arrhythmias should be treated as needed.

CHOCOLATE TOXICITY

- Toxic effects of chocolate are due to methylxanthines, in particular theobromine and caffeine.
- The median lethal dose of theobromine and caffeine is 100 to 200 mg/kg (0.2 to 0.5 oz baking chocolate/kg). Mild signs can occur with 20 mg/kg, severe signs at 40 to 50 mg/kg, and seizures at 60 mg/kg.

CARDIAC PATHOPHYSIOLOGY
- Theobromine increases cyclic adenosine monophosphate, causes release of catecholamines, blocks adenosine receptors, and increases calcium uptake by the sarcoplasmic reticulum.
- The net effect is to increase heart rate and the force of contractions.

DIAGNOSIS
HISTORY AND PHYSICAL EXAMINATION

- Clinical signs associated with chocolate toxicity include vomiting and diarrhea, hyperactivity, ataxia, hyperthermia, muscle tremors, coma, and death.

- Tachycardia and bradycardia are frequently noted.
- ECG findings may include sinus tachycardia, sinus bradycardia, and ventricular arrhythmias.

THERAPY
- Symptomatic therapy should include prevention of absorption, increasing elimination, maintenance of life support, and control of cardiac arrhythmias and seizures.
- Vomiting should be induced if ingestion was recent. Activated charcoal (1 to 4 g/kg orally) should be administered. Because methylxanthines undergo enterohepatic recirculation, giving repeated doses of activated charcoal is usually beneficial in animals with symptoms.
- Arrhythmia management
  - Lidocaine is used for control of ventricular arrhythmias, if needed. Beta blockers can be added if additional control and maintenance therapy is required. Because propranolol hydrochloride reportedly delays renal excretion of methylxanthines, metoprolol succinate or metoprolol tartrate is the beta blocker of choice, if available.
  - Treat supraventricular tachycardia with beta blockers (i.e., propranolol, metoprolol, atenolol).
  - Seizure control can be done with diazepam or barbiturate.

DOXORUBICIN CARDIOTOXICITY

- Doxorubicin is an anthracycline antibiotic used for its antineoplastic properties. Its mechanism of action as a chemotherapeutic agent is inhibition of nucleic acid synthesis. Cardiotoxicity manifested as arrhythmias or DCM usually develops after cumulative doses of 240 mg/m^2 in dogs, but toxicity can occur at dosages as low as 130 mg/m^2 (dog range, 135 to 265 mg/m^2; cat range, 130 to 320 mg/m^2). Clinical studies in humans have shown a reduced incidence of toxic cardiomyopathy when people are treated with prolonged infusions (24 hours) of doxorubicin. Prolonged infusion therapy in dogs is still under investigation.
- Acute cardiotoxicity is manifested by arrhythmias during or shortly after administration. DCM may develop with chronic treatment. Although histologic lesions and echocardiographic changes may develop, clinical signs of congestive heart failure are uncommon in cats treated with doxorubicin.

CARDIAC PATHOPHYSIOLOGY
- The mechanism by which doxorubicin causes cardiotoxicity is unknown, but free radical

generation and lipid membrane peroxidation may be involved in the pathogenesis. The heart rate at the time of drug administration may also determine the degree of cardiac toxicity, with slower heart rates associated with less toxicity.

- Histologic lesions consist of myocyte vacuolization, myocytolysis, and occasionally, interstitial fibrosis.

DIAGNOSIS

HISTORY AND PHYSICAL EXAMINATION

- Clinical signs and physical findings are associated with DCM and include exercise intolerance, dyspnea and coughing, hepatomegaly, and ascites. Congestive heart failure usually develops acutely.

ELECTROCARDIOGRAPHY

- In dogs, ECG abnormalities include ST segment and T wave changes, decreased QRS voltages, intraventricular conduction abnormalities, and atrial and ventricular arrhythmias. ECG changes are rare in cats treated with doxorubicin.
- ECG changes can occur acutely during drug administration. In this situation, stopping the drip and then reinstituting it at a slower rate may resolve the problem.

RADIOGRAPHY

- With DCM, radiography may show cardiomegaly, pulmonary edema, pleural effusion, hepatomegaly, and ascites.

ECHOCARDIOGRAPHY

- The most consistent abnormalities with doxorubicin cardiotoxicity are increased left ventricular end-systolic internal dimensions and decreased fractional shortening. As cardiac function deteriorates, progressive left atrial enlargement can be seen.

THERAPY

- If congestive heart failure develops, the patient should be treated accordingly. Unfortunately, the therapeutic response is poor. An ECG is recommended before each doxorubicin treatment, especially in dogs. If arrhythmias develop, doxorubicin treatment should be discontinued. An echocardiogram is recommended after the third cycle in dogs or fifth cycle in cats, and every one to three cycles thereafter. Doxorubicin treatment should be

discontinued if a reduction in contractility from baseline is recognized.

- Protection from cardiomyopathy has been demonstrated with dexrazoxane.
- The mechanism for cardio protection is not understood. One suggested mechanism is dexrazoxane, which prevents the formation of free radicals and subsequent lipid peroxidation that occurs from free iron and iron associated with the doxorubicin-iron complex.
- It is approved by the Food and Drug Administration (FDA) for use in women with doxorubicin administration against metastatic breast cancer.
- It has been shown in studies to protect mice, rats, hamsters, pigs, and dogs from doxorubicin cardiac toxicity.
- Although it appears to prevent cardiotoxicity, it does not protect against other toxic effects caused by anthracyclines.
- Dexrazoxane ameliorates anthracycline extravasation lesions.
- The recommended dose ratio of dexrazoxane to doxorubicin is 10:1. It is given as an infusion over 15 minutes, 30 minutes before doxorubicin is used.
- Expense of the drug limits its routine use.

INFECTIOUS/INFLAMMATORY DISEASES

- The heart can be involved in an inflammatory process because of many infectious agents. Myocardial cells, myocardial interstitium, or cardiac vessels may be affected.

CARDIAC PATHOPHYSIOLOGY

- Myocardial injury can occur from direct myocardial invasion of an infectious agent, from a myocardial toxin produced by the agent, or from a secondary immune-mediated reaction.
- Important causes of myocardial injury in small animals include the following:
  - Bacterial myocarditis
    - Pyogenic bacteria originate in septicemic states or from other septic foci.
    - Clinical signs range from subclinical and nonspecific (weight loss, lethargy) to apparent and specific (arrhythmias, congestive heart failure).
  - Viral myocarditis has been associated with canine parvovirus and distemper virus in dogs and with suspected but not yet identified viral pathogens in cats. Clinical abnormalities include cardiomegaly, arrhythmias, and nonspecific ECG abnormalities.

The severity of the cardiac changes ranges from congestive heart failure with canine parvovirus to subclinical myocarditis with canine distemper virus.

- Fungi and algae can infect the heart secondary to a disseminated disease process, often in conjunction with reduced host defense.
- Protozoal myocarditis can occur in dogs with canine trypanosomiasis (*Trypanosoma cruzi*) or in dogs and cats with toxoplasmosis (*Toxoplasma gondii*).
  - Trypanosomiasis is discussed later.
  - Toxoplasmosis can produce signs characterized by the extent and severity of the multiorgan system involvement.

THERAPY

- Treatment is often supportive and usually focused on the most prominent systemic manifestation of the disease process.

BORRELIOSIS (LYME DISEASE)

- Borreliosis is caused by the spirochete *Borrelia burgdorferi*. Transmission is by ticks of the *Ixodes* species. The incidence of cardiac involvement is unknown in animals. In humans, 10% of patients with borreliosis have cardiac involvement. Borreliosis in animals is usually acute and cured by antibiotics. However, the prognosis may be poor if second-stage disease involving the heart, kidneys, or central nervous system (CNS) develops.

CARDIAC PATHOPHYSIOLOGY

- Spirochetes have been isolated from myocardial biopsies in humans.
- DCM has been reported in a few humans with Lyme disease. Cardiac damage may involve an immune-mediated mechanism.

DIAGNOSIS
HISTORY AND PHYSICAL EXAMINATION

- Ticks may be found on dogs, or owners may report recent exposure to ticks in endemic areas.
- Although nonspecific, clinical signs include anorexia, depression, and lameness.
- Physical examination reveals fever, joint pain, and lymphadenopathy.

ELECTROCARDIOGRAPHY

- The most common ECG finding in humans is AV block.
- Ectopic beats and ST segment abnormalities have also been reported in humans.

- AV block secondary to *B. burgdorferi* in the dog has been reported in one case.

SPECIALIZED DIAGNOSTIC TESTS

- Commercial test kits are available, but titers should be interpreted in view of the history, physical examination, and clinical signs. False-positive and false-negative titers are not uncommon.

THERAPY

- Antibiotics are the treatment of choice for borreliosis. Tetracycline, doxycycline, ampicillin, or amoxicillin appear to be the most effective first line agents.
- Humans with cardiac involvement are often treated with IV ceftriaxone or cefotaxime.
- A 5- to 7-day course of antiinflammatory doses of corticosteroids may be helpful for heart block that does not rapidly resolve with appropriate antibiotic therapy.

TRYPANOSOMIASIS (CHAGAS DISEASE)

- Trypanosomiasis is a rare disease caused by the protozoan *Trypanosoma cruzi*. It usually occurs in young dogs in the southeastern United States. Transmission is through the bite of a reduviid bug.

CARDIAC PATHOPHYSIOLOGY

- During the acute stage (2 to 4 weeks after infection), cardiac damage occurs when trypomastigotes rupture from myocardial cells. This causes myocardial failure, conduction disturbances, and arrhythmias.
- If animals survive the acute stage, they may remain symptom free for months. During this time, myocardial degeneration occurs, and DCM develops. Myocardial damage during this stage may be related to immune mechanisms or to the release of toxic parasitic products.

DIAGNOSIS
HISTORY AND PHYSICAL EXAMINATION

- Clinical signs during the acute stage are related to left-sided and (mainly) right-sided heart failure. Collapse and sudden death may be noted in a previously healthy dog. Gastrointestinal signs of anorexia and diarrhea are also common. The lymph nodes will be enlarged during the acute stage.
- Clinical manifestations during the chronic stage are associated with DCM, with signs of right-sided heart failure often predominating. Various cardiac arrhythmias also occur.

The cardiomyopathy is not curable and responds poorly to treatment.

- Physical findings associated with heart failure—pale mucous membranes, weak femoral pulses, and ascites—can be seen during acute and chronic stages.

ELECTROCARDIOGRAPHY

- Conduction disturbances, ectopic beats, and sustained arrhythmias can be seen during the acute and chronic stages.

RADIOGRAPHY

- Radiography may show cardiomegaly, pulmonary edema, pleural effusion, hepatomegaly, or ascites.

ECHOCARDIOGRAPHY

- Echocardiography is normal during the acute phase. As the disease becomes chronic, ventricular contractility and wall thickness decrease, and cardiac chambers dilate.

SPECIALIZED DIAGNOSTIC TESTS

- Trypomastigotes may be seen on a blood smear during the acute stage. The patient becomes aparasitemic 2 to 4 weeks after infection.
- Indirect fluorescent antibody, direct hemagglutination, and complement fixation tests confirm antibodies to *T. cruzi*.
- Blood cultures can be performed but are time consuming.

THERAPY

- Treatment of this disease is very unrewarding. By the time the diagnosis is made, the disease is often no longer responsive to antiprotozoal medication.
- Various therapeutic recommendations include oral benzimidazole (5 mg/kg PO q24h for 2 months), allopurinol (30 mg/kg PO q12h for 100 days), or nifurtimox (2 to 7 mg/kg PO q6h for 3 to 5 months).
- Alert owners and veterinary staff to potential zoonotic risk.

PARVOVIRUS

- Parvovirus has caused cardiac disease when it infected puppies less than 2 weeks of age. Current cases of parvoviral myocarditis are very rare.

CARDIAC PATHOPHYSIOLOGY

- Viral multiplication occurs in rapidly dividing myocardial cells, resulting in cell death and scarring.

DIAGNOSIS
HISTORY AND PHYSICAL EXAMINATION

- The cardiac form of parvovirus often results in sudden death.
- Some puppies that survived the acute phase developed heart failure weeks to months later and died from cardiac arrhythmias or DCM 6 to 12 months later.
- ECG reveals atrial or ventricular arrhythmias.

ECHOCARDIOGRAPHY

- In some infected dogs, echocardiography revealed abnormalities consistent with DCM, including decreased fractional shortening, left atrial and ventricular enlargement, and increased E-point septal separation.

THERAPY

- Heart failure is managed with diuretics, pimobendan, and ACE inhibitors.
- Arrhythmias should be treated accordingly.

MISCELLANEOUS DISEASES
SYSTEMIC LUPUS ERYTHEMATOSUS

- Cardiac disease due to systemic lupus erythematosus (SLE) is a common finding in humans, rare in dogs, and not reported in cats. Pericarditis is the most common cardiac abnormality associated with SLE in humans. Other abnormalities in humans include myocarditis, congestive heart failure, and valvular heart disease. Ventricular arrhythmias were reported in two dogs and heart failure in one dog diagnosed with SLE.

CARDIAC PATHOPHYSIOLOGY

- Pericarditis occurs secondary to vasculitis.
- Myocarditis and endocarditis can also occur.

DIAGNOSIS
HISTORY AND PHYSICAL EXAMINATION

- Clinical signs associated with heart disease are usually overshadowed by systemic signs of SLE.
- Clinical findings associated with arrhythmias or heart failure may be present.
- ECG may reveal ventricular arrhythmias.
- Echocardiographic abnormalities have not been reported in dogs or cats with SLE.

SPECIALIZED DIAGNOSTIC TESTS

- A diagnosis of SLE can be made with a positive antinuclear antibody titer in conjunction with clinical signs.

THERAPY

- Immunosuppressive doses of prednisone (2 mg/kg PO q12h) are advised. If there is no improvement after 7 days, more aggressive immunosuppressive therapy should be considered.
- Pericardiocentesis is recommended if pericardial effusion is present.

NEUROGENIC CARDIOMYOPATHY

- In client-owned animals, CNS disease has been associated with myocardial lesions in all domestic species except the cat. Experimentally, stimulation of specific areas of feline brains can cause myocardial necrosis. Most cases involve trauma to the brain or spinal cord. CNS neoplasia, infection, encephalomalacia, and ruptured intervertebral discs can also result in myocardial damage.

CARDIAC PATHOPHYSIOLOGY

- Histologic lesions include degeneration or disintegration of myocardial cells with necrosis and mineralization. Scar formation may develop. The endocardium is most frequently involved, with occasional involvement of the subepicardium.
- Myocardial necrosis may be evident as early as 3 days after the CNS damage, and generally is present within 5 to 10 days in affected animals. Cardiac arrhythmias are the most frequent clinical sequelae.
- The myocardial lesions probably occur secondary to increased sympathetic tone and release of catecholamines.

DIAGNOSIS

HISTORY AND PHYSICAL EXAMINATION

- Clinical signs are usually referable to the CNS disease and sometimes arrhythmias.

ELECTROCARDIOGRAPHY

- Atrial and ventricular arrhythmias, ST segment depression, prolonged QT interval, and T wave abnormalities have been reported.
- The diagnosis is often made on necropsy.

THERAPY

- Appropriate therapy for the CNS disease is advised. Treat arrhythmias as necessary.

GASTRIC DILATION–VOLVULUS COMPLEX

- Gastric dilation–volvulus complex (GDV) is a life-threatening emergency in the dog. It is most common in large, deep-chested dogs.

No specific etiology has been determined, but GDV is often associated with exercise following a large meal. Cardiac arrhythmias occur in up to 40% of patients with GDV. Most arrhythmias are ventricular in origin. Atrial arrhythmias have also been reported. Arrhythmias usually occur within 36 hours of admission. The presence of arrhythmias does not worsen the prognosis.

CARDIAC PATHOPHYSIOLOGY

- The exact mechanism for the arrhythmias is unknown. Theories include acid-base imbalances, autonomic imbalances, myocardial hypoxia, electrolyte imbalances, or a myocardial depressant factor.

DIAGNOSIS

HISTORY AND PHYSICAL EXAMINATION

- Clinical signs are restlessness, pacing, lethargy, weakness, attempts to vomit, and abdominal distention.
- The physical examination findings often include pale mucous membranes; rapid heart rate; weak femoral pulses; pain upon abdominal palpation; distended, tympanic stomach; and signs associated with shock.

ELECTROCARDIOGRAPHY

- The ECG may reveal ventricular and occasionally atrial arrhythmias. The most common appears to be an accelerated idioventricular rhythm (AIR). The terminology for this arrhythmia is still in dispute. Other terms for this ventricular rhythm are slow ventricular tachycardia, fast idioventricular rhythm, or idioventricular tachycardia.
- The features of AIR are a wide, bizarre complex rhythm, typically with a rate similar to the underlying sinus rate. As the sinus rate slows, the ventricular rate may "capture" the heart rhythm. Commonly, fusion beats are seen as the rhythm waxes between the sinus and the ventricular rhythm. As the underlying sinus rate slows, the ventricular rate may also slow (Figure 14.12).
- ST segment and T wave changes may be evident.

RADIOGRAPHY

- The stomach is gas-filled, distended, and often rotated.
- The cardiac silhouette may be small owing to decreased venous return.

TREATMENT

- Treatment should be directed toward gastric decompression and shock therapy.

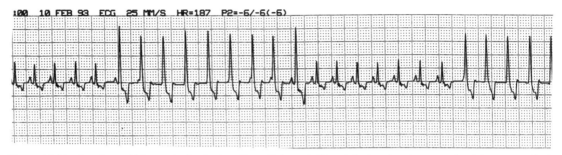

:00   10 FEB 93   ECG   25 MM/S   HR=187   P2=-6/-6(-6)

Figure 14.12   Accelerated idioventricular rhythm. Beats 7 through 13 and the last four beats on the right are ventricular in origin. These beats represent an accelerated ventricular rhythm. Beats 6 and 14 are fusion beats, a hybrid of the sinus beat and the ventricular focus.

- Any arrhythmias should be treated as needed; however, suppression of AIR is generally not necessary as long as blood pressure and perfusion are not affected by its presence.

PANCREATITIS

- Pancreatitis is a disease most frequently diagnosed in middle-aged, obese dogs and cats. Although many factors have been associated with pancreatitis, the cause is often unknown.

CARDIAC PATHOPHYSIOLOGY

- A myocardial depressant factor is released from the pancreas, which can result in decreased myocardial contractility and cardiac arrhythmias.
- Activated pancreatic enzymes may also damage the myocardium directly or play a role in thrombus formation, resulting in myocardial ischemia.
- Acid-base and electrolyte imbalances may also contribute to arrhythmias.

DIAGNOSIS
HISTORY AND PHYSICAL EXAMINATION

- Clinical signs are nonspecific and include vomiting, diarrhea, anorexia, and depression.
- Physical examination may reveal abdominal pain, fever, dehydration, and shock.
- Sudden death associated with cardiac complications can occur.

ELECTROCARDIOGRAPHY

- Atrial and ventricular arrhythmias and ST segment changes have been reported.

RADIOGRAPHY

- Abdominal radiographs may reveal an increased density, calcification, or gas in the area of the pancreas.

CLINICAL PATHOLOGY

- Leukocytosis, hyperglycemia, high liver enzymes, with high amylase and lipase in serum and peritoneal fluid are common findings in animals with pancreatitis.

THERAPY

- It is important to decrease pancreatic secretions by withholding food and water.
- Supportive care should include fluid and electrolyte replacement along with antibiotics.
- Cardiac arrhythmias should be treated as needed, although most arrhythmias will resolve spontaneously with resolution of the underlying disease.

TRAUMATIC MYOCARDITIS

- The term *traumatic myocarditis* is a catchall phrase for arrhythmias that may occur following blunt trauma. The arrhythmias seen after blunt trauma include supraventricular tachycardia, ventricular arrhythmias, or bradyarrhythmias. The trauma does not have to occur directly to the chest.

CARDIAC PATHOPHYSIOLOGY

- Blunt trauma mechanisms include the following: (1) unidirectional force; (2) bidirectional force (compressive); (3) indirect force; (4) force associated with deceleration; and (5) concussive force.
- The actual mechanism for the cause of the arrhythmias is not known. Direct damage to the heart from the trauma does not have to occur to result in the arrhythmias. Autonomic imbalance or reperfusion of ischemic tissue may have a role.

DIAGNOSIS

- Various arrhythmias, both atrial and ventricular, may be seen following trauma. The most common appears to be an AIR. The terminology for this arrhythmia is still in dispute. Other terms for this ventricular rhythm are slow ventricular tachycardia, fast idioventricular rhythm, or idio-ventricular tachycardia.

- The features of AIR are a wide, bizarre complex rhythm, typically with a rate similar to the underlying sinus rate. As the sinus rate slows, the ventricular rate may "capture" the heart rhythm. Commonly, fusion beats are seen as the rhythm waxes between the sinus and the ventricular rhythm. As the underlying sinus rate slows, the ventricular rate may also slow (see Figure 14.12).

THERAPY

- The main goal of therapy is supportive care for the underlying disease: fluid therapy, control of hemorrhage, oxygen therapy, analgesia, and correction of electrolyte imbalance.
- Therapy for the ventricular arrhythmias is necessary only if the tachycardia is persistent and the clinician feels it has a role in the patient's hypotension. Because the ventricular rate is often relatively normal, AIR does not necessitate antiarrhythmic treatment. If therapy is thought to be necessary, then lidocaine by IV route is recommended at 2 to 4 mg/kg as a bolus. The maximum dose to be given over a 10-minute period is 10 mg/kg. Lidocaine can cause nausea, vomiting, hypotension, and seizures. If this therapy suppresses the arrhythmias, then a constant-rate infusion of lidocaine can be given at 40 to 100 µg/kg/min. A repeat bolus of lidocaine may be needed once after starting the lidocaine infusion, if more than 10 minutes elapses after injection of the original test bolus. It is not unusual for the constant-rate infusion of lidocaine to lose its effect after several hours.
- If lidocaine is not effective, then procainamide may be tried. The IV dose of procainamide is 2 mg/kg over 2 to 3 minutes. The total dose given over a 20-minute period should not exceed 15 mg/kg. The constant-rate infusion for procainamide is 25 to 50 µg/kg/min. Alternatively, oral or intramuscular dosing could be initiated following the IV dose.
- Other therapies, such as other ventricular antiarrhythmics, beta blockers, or magnesium (IV), have been suggested.

PROGNOSIS

- Fortunately the arrhythmias are generally not lethal. They have a tendency to resolve over 3 to 5 days as the patient improves clinically. In general, progression of underlying disorders, and not the arrhythmia, causes the patient's demise.
- If the patient requires antiarrhythmic therapy, it is usually discontinued before discharge or within several days of discharge.

FREQUENTLY ASKED QUESTIONS

How useful is the ECG in diagnosing electrolyte disturbances, and what changes would you expect to see?

The ECG can be helpful in raising suspicion regarding the presence of some electrolyte abnormalities, most notably hyperkalemia, but it is not a very sensitive test for detecting electrolyte abnormalities. One of the reasons that the ECG is not very sensitive is that the shape of the ECG complexes is influenced by several electrolytes (e.g., sodium, potassium, calcium) and further influenced by the patient's acid-base status. As potassium levels rise above normal, T waves become peaked with a narrow base, P wave amplitude decreases, and the P-R interval prolongs. If potassium is very high, QRS complexes widen, and P waves disappear (atrial standstill), and with further elevation in potassium, conduction delays lead to ventricular fibrillation and ventricular asystole. Hypokalemia produces prolonged QT intervals, U waves, and ST segment depression, with possible ventricular and supraventricular arrhythmias. Hypocalcemia may cause QT interval prolongation, whereas hypercalcemia may shorten the QT segment, and with severe hypercalcemia, bradycardia may develop.

A patient has a ventricular arrhythmia. What systemic disturbances should be considered?

VPCs may be seen with a variety of noncardiac conditions, including pancreatitis, GDV, traumatic myocarditis, splenic disease, neoplasia, cardiac masses, hypokalemia, trypanosomiasis, shock, heat stroke, and pyrexia. Drugs and plant toxins such as doxorubicin, methylxanthines (chocolate, theophylline), digoxin, sympathomimetics, and oleander can all cause VPCs.

A dog has echocardiographic evidence of myocardial failure based on depressed indices of systolic function (stroke volume, fractional shortening). What needs to be considered in addition to idiopathic DCM?

Systolic function can be depressed secondary to several systemic diseases, nutritional deficiencies, and toxic insults. Systemic abnormalities associated with depressed myocardial function include hypothyroidism, pancreatitis, sepsis and shock, and trypanosomiasis. Taurine and L-carnitine deficiencies can lead to DCM. Adriamycin toxicity leads to myocardial failure. Note that in some animals, especially large dog breeds, fractional shortening may be slightly below normal values established for smaller breeds and represent a normal variant.

A cat has left ventricular hypertrophy on the echocardiogram. What systemic disturbances need to be considered along with idiopathic hypertrophic cardiomyopathy?

Consider the possibility of systemic hypertension, acromegaly, hyperthyroidism, or infiltrative processes such as lymphoma. Dehydration causes a reduction in the size of the left ventricular lumen and as a result can give the impression of left ventricular hypertrophy.

SUGGESTED READINGS

Appel MJ: Lyme disease in dogs and cats, Compend Cont Ed 12:617, 1990.

Atkins CE: Cardiac manifestations of systemic and metabolic disease. In Fox PR, Sisson D, Moise NS, eds: Textbook of canine and feline cardiology, Philadelphia, 1999, WB Saunders.

Barr SC: American trypanosomiasis in dogs, Compend Cont Ed 13:745, 1991.

Barnewolt BA, Walter FG, Bey TA: Metabolic effects of metaproterenol overdose: hypokalemia, hyperglycemia, and hyperlactemia, American College of Toxicologists 43:158, 2001.

Carson TL: Toxic gases. In Kirk RW, ed: Current veterinary therapy IX, Philadelphia, 1986, WB Saunders.

DiBartola SP, deMorais HSA: Disorders of potassium: hypokalemia and hyperkalemia. In DiBartola SP, ed: Fluid, electrolyte and acid-base disorders in small animal practice, ed 4, St Louis, 2012, Elsevier Saunders, pp 92–119.

Edmondson EF, Bright JM, Halsey CH, et al: Pathologic and cardiovascular characterization of pheochromocytoma-associated cardiomyopathy in dogs, Vet Pathol, May, 2014.

Feldman EC, Nelson RW, Reusch C, et al: Canine and feline endocrinology, ed 4, St. Louis, 2015, Saunders.

Hooser SB, Beasley VR: Methylxanthine poisoning (chocolate and caffeine toxicosis). In Kirk RW, ed: Current veterinary therapy IX, Philadelphia, 1986, WB Saunders.

Kienle RD, Bruyette D, Pron PO: Effects of thyroid hormone and thyroid dysfunction on the cardiovascular system, Vet Clin North Am 24:495, 1994.

King JM, Roth L, Haschek WM: Myocardial necrosis secondary to neural lesions in domestic animals, J Am Vet Med Assoc 180:144, 1982.

Kintzer PP, Peterson ME: Primary and secondary canine hypoadrenocorticism, Vet Clin North Am 27:349, 1997.

Klein I: Endocrine disorders and cardiovascular disease. In Bonow RO, Mann DL, Zipes DP, Libby P, eds: Braunwald's Heart disease, ed 9, St Louis, 2012, Elsevier Saunders.

Little CJ, Gettinby G: Heart failure is common in diabetic cats: findings from a retrospective case-controlled study in first-opinion practice, J Small Anim Pract 49:17, 2008.

Loar AS, Susaneck SJ: Doxorubicin-induced cardiotoxicity in five dogs, Semin Vet Med Surg 1:68, 1986.

Melian C, Stefanacci J, Peterson ME, Kintzer PP: Radiographic findings in dogs with naturally-occurring primary hypoadrenocorticism, J Am Anim Hosp Assoc 35:208, 1999.

Muir WM: Gastric dilatation-volvulus in the dog, with emphasis on cardiac arrhythmias, J Am Vet Med Assoc 180:739, 1982.

Niessen SJ, Petrie G, Gaudiano F, et al: Feline acromegaly: an underdiagnosed endocrinopathy? J Vet Intern Med 21:899, 2007.

Nichols R: Complications and concurrent disease associated with canine hyperadrenocorticism, Vet Clin North Am 27:309, 1997.

O'Keefe DA, Sisson DD, Gelberg HB, et al.: Systemic toxicity associated with doxorubicin administration in cats, J Vet Intern Med 7:309, 1993.

Palumbo ME, Perri SF: Toad poisoning. In Kirk RW, ed: Current veterinary therapy VIII, Philadelphia, 1983, WB Saunders.

Pirintr P, Chansaisakorn W, Trisiriroj M, et al: Heart rate variability and plasma norepinephrine concentration in diabetic dogs at rest, Vet Res Commun 36:207, 2012.

Rosenthal DS, Braunwald E: Hematologic-oncologic disorders and heart disease, In Braunwald E, ed: Heart disease, ed 4, Philadelphia, 1992, WB Saunders.

Ruslander D: Heat stroke. In Kirk RW, ed: Current veterinary therapy XI, Philadelphia, 1992, WB Saunders.

Sangster JK, Panciera DL, Abbott JA, et al.: Cardiac biomarkers in hyperthyroid cats, J Vet Intern Med 28:465, 2014.

Schenck PA, Chew DJ, Nagode LA, et al: Disorders of calcium: hypercalcemia and hypocalcemia, In DiBartola SP, ed: Fluid, electrolyte and acid-base disorders in small animal practice, St Louis, 2012, Elsevier Saunders.

Sennello KA, Schulman RL, Prosek R, Siegel AM: Systolic blood pressure in cats with diabetes mellitus, J Am Vet Med Assoc 223:198, 2003.

Struble AL, Feldman EC, Nelson RW, Kass PH: Systemic hypertension and proteinuria in dogs with diabetes mellitus, J Am Vet Med Assoc 213:822, 1998.

Tilley LP, Bond BR, Patnaik AK, Liu S-K: Cardiovascular tumors in the cat, J Am Anim Hosp Assoc 17:1009, 1981.

Yates RW, Weller RE: Have you seen the cardiopulmonary form of parvovirus infection? Vet Med April, p 380, 1988.

Systemic Hypertension

15

Scott A. Brown | Rosemary A. Henik

Hypertension may be transient, because of fear or excitement, or sustained and pathologic. Small animal patients most commonly have secondary hypertension, with an underlying disease triggering increased blood pressure (BP). Although there is no widely accepted threshold for the diagnosis of systemic hypertension in dogs and cats, it is reasonable to conclude that hypertension is present whenever reliable BP measurements demonstrate a sustained elevation of systolic (>160 mm Hg) or diastolic (>120 mm Hg) BP. The prevalence of idiopathic hypertension in dogs and cats is unknown.

POPULATION AT RISK

CATS

- Chronic kidney disease (CKD), with or without proteinuria, and hyperthyroidism are the two most common causes of hypertension in cats. Although effective resolution of hyperthyroidism may reduce BP, some cats will become hypertensive only after therapy for this endocrinopathy.
- Occasionally, hyperaldosteronism, pheochromocytoma, or other endocrine diseases may also be associated with hypertension.
- Many cats that are not hypertensive initially will become hypertensive when fluid therapy, steroids, erythropoietin, or vasoconstrictive drugs are given.
- Some clinicians are incorporating the routine measurement of BP into geriatric wellness examinations. This practice may occasionally identify a hypertensive cat with subclinical kidney disease; however, it should be realized that the risk of a false-positive result (i.e., high BP measurement) increases when the prevalence of a disease is low (as in a healthy population).
- BP measurement is advised in all cats with the following:
  - CKD
  - Endocrinopathy
  - Compatible ocular signs (e.g., hemorrhage, retinal detachment, retinal vessel tortuosity)
  - Neurologic signs (e.g., nystagmus, head tilt, other cranial nerve signs, or seizures)

- Heart murmur or gallop rhythm
- Radiographic cardiomegaly
- Echocardiographically determined left ventricular hypertrophy (although this is not a consistent change in hypertension)

DOGS

- CKD (i.e., chronic glomerular or tubulointerstitial disease associated with proteinuria) is most commonly associated with hypertension in dogs.
- Endocrine diseases including hyperadrenocorticism, diabetes mellitus, pheochromocytoma, and hyperaldosteronism may be associated with hypertension.
- Metabolic abnormalities including obesity or hypercholesterolemia may result in hypertension.
- Resolution of the endocrinopathy may not restore normal BP in dogs.
- BP measurement is advised in any dog with the following:
  - CKD
  - Endocrinopathy
  - Ocular signs or neurologic signs as described previously
  - Cardiac hypertrophy (although rare in the dog as an acquired change), which should also prompt the clinician to perform BP measurement

KEY POINT

CKD and endocrinopathies are most commonly associated with systemic hypertension in cats and dogs.

CONSEQUENCES AND CLINICAL SIGNS OF HIGH BLOOD PRESSURE

OCULAR SIGNS

- Tissue injury from persistently elevated BP is referred to as target-organ damage (TOD). Severe systemic hypertension can lead to ocular TOD. Findings associated with hypertensive injury include hemorrhage within the retina, vitreous, or anterior chamber; retinal detachment and atrophy; retinal edema; perivasculitis; retinal vessel tortuosity; and glaucoma.

- A sudden onset of blindness due to retinal hemorrhage and detachment is a common presenting complaint (Figure 15.1).

NEUROLOGIC SIGNS

- Signs consistent with cerebrovascular hemorrhage (head tilt, depression, seizures) have been seen clinically in cats and dogs with uncontrolled hypertension and are often associated with a poor prognosis.
- Cats with marked or sudden systemic hypertension (rapid rise in BP or systolic BP >280 mm Hg) may have a syndrome of progressive stupor, head pressing, or seizures that rapidly resolves with effective antihypertensive therapy. This syndrome of hypertensive encephalopathy is due to cerebral edema caused by high intracapillary hydrostatic pressure that develops once the BP exceeds the autoregulatory range.

RENAL SIGNS

- Persistent elevation of systolic BP to values >160 mm Hg is associated with progressive renal injury in dogs, and the severity of renal injury has been correlated to the degree of elevation. Potentially pathologic renal changes induced by systemic hypertension include both glomerular and tubulointerstitial changes and can result in ischemia, necrosis, atrophy, and

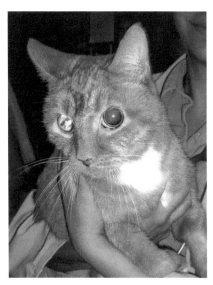

Figure 15.1 A cat with acute blindness due to systemic hypertension secondary to an aldosterone-secreting adrenal tumor. This cat had a systolic blood pressure > 300 mm Hg. There are severe ocular hemorrhages bilaterally.

exacerbation of proteinuria. These gradual and additive changes may be difficult to quantify in living animals with preexisting kidney disease, but systolic hypertension at the time of presentation (>160 mm Hg) increases the odds of uremic crisis and death in dogs with CKD. A systolic BP >160 mm Hg is also likely to be a risk factor for progressive renal damage in cats.

- Proteinuria is perhaps the best marker that high BP is injurious to the kidney. The presence of microalbuminuria or an elevated urine protein-to-creatinine ratio (>0.5 in dogs, >0.4 in cats) in a hypertensive animal (systolic BP >160 mm Hg) should be considered an indication of ongoing renal damage.

CARDIAC SIGNS

- Increased arterial pressure (i.e., afterload) increases left ventricular workload, leading to possible diastolic dysfunction, left ventricular hypertrophy, and secondary valvular insufficiency. Changes may regress with antihypertensive treatment.
- Cardiac murmurs or gallops commonly occur.
- Congestive heart failure secondary to systemic hypertension is rare.

MEASUREMENT OF BLOOD PRESSURE

PATIENT SELECTION

- Currently there is no evidence to suggest that BP should be measured in all animals.
- BP should be measured in those animals that have clinical signs attributable to high systemic arterial BP, such as blindness, hyphema, seizures, ataxia, or sudden collapse (signs compatible with cerebral vascular hemorrhage, edema, or stroke).
- Animals with CKD, hyperadrenocorticism, hyperthyroidism, pheochromocytoma, hyperaldosteronism, marked obesity, or cardiac hypertrophy should also be evaluated for hypertension.

METHODS

- BP may be measured by either direct or indirect methods. Direct BP measurement is the "gold standard," but it is technically difficult in unsedated dogs and cats and may be painful and associated with hematoma formation and other complications.
- Indirect techniques are more applicable to a clinical setting because they require less restraint and are technically easier to perform. They include the auscultatory, ultrasonic Doppler, oscillometric, and photoplethysmographic methods.

- All of the indirect techniques use an inflatable cuff wrapped around an extremity. The pressure in the cuff is measured with a manometer or pressure transducer. A squeeze bulb or automated device is used to inflate the cuff to a pressure in excess of systolic BP, thereby occluding the underlying artery. As the cuff is gradually deflated, changes in arterial flow are detected by one of several means; the value for cuff pressure at various levels of deflation is then correlated with systolic, diastolic, or mean BP. The detection method varies among different indirect methods.
- For the auscultatory method, a stethoscope is placed over the artery distal to the cuff, and the listener hears a tapping sound when the inflation pressure falls below systolic pressure. In dogs and cats, the arterial (Korotkoff) sounds are low in both amplitude and frequency, and the auscultatory technique is difficult in these species.
- Doppler flow meters detect blood flow as a change in the frequency of reflected sound (Doppler shift) caused by the motion of underlying red blood cells. BP is read by the operator from an aneroid manometer connected to the occluding cuff placed proximal to the Doppler transducer.
- Devices with the oscillometric technique detect pressure fluctuations produced in the occluding cuff resulting from the pressure pulse. Machines with the oscillometric technique generally determine systolic, diastolic, and mean BP as well as pulse rate.
- Another device for measuring BP indirectly is the photoplethysmograph, which measures arterial volume by attenuation of infrared radiation and is designed for use on the human finger. It can be used in cats and small dogs that weigh less than 10 kg (22 lb).
- The ultrasonic Doppler and oscillometric methods have been well studied in conscious dogs and cats. In both species, the oscillometric devices tend to underestimate BP by increasing amounts as pressure increases. Another problem is the excessive time required to obtain readings in cats. The major limitation of the Doppler technique is the imprecise discrimination of the sounds designating the diastolic and therefore mean BP. The Doppler method may therefore be unreliable for the routine diagnosis and surveillance of patients with diastolic hypertension.
- In general, devices with the Doppler principle have been recommended for use in cats; either the oscillometric or the Doppler devices are recommended in dogs. However, a recent study indicated that high-definition oscillometry is accurate in cats. For comparative purposes, the same device should be used each time in an individual animal.

Doppler is the most commonly used method of measurement in unsedated cats; the oscillometric technique is also used in dogs.

CUFF SIZE AND PLACEMENT

- A complete range of pediatric cuff sizes should be available for an optimal patient limb circumference to cuff width ratio.
- For dogs, a cuff width that measures 40% of the circumference of the limb should be used; for cats, a width of 30% to 40% of the limb circumference should be used. The cuff width should be noted in the medical record for future reference.
- An oversized cuff may give erroneously low recordings; an undersized cuff may give erroneously high recordings. If the ideal cuff width is midway between two available sizes, the larger cuff should be used because it will theoretically produce the least error.
- The cuff may be placed around the brachial, median, or cranial tibial artery or around the medial coccygeal artery. The "artery" arrow should be placed over the artery, with the arrow pointing in either direction.
- In general, for the Doppler technique, the cuff is placed over the median artery, and the transducer is placed between the carpal and the metacarpal pads (Figure 15.2). Clipping the hair and applying acoustic gel at the site of transducer placement may enhance the signal, but clipping the hair may increase stress artifacts.
- For the oscillometric technique, studies have demonstrated that the coccygeal or cranial tibial artery in dogs may provide more reliable values than other sites (Figure 15.3).

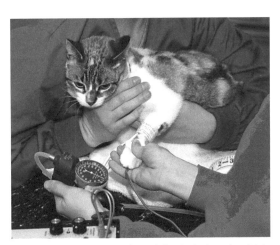

Figure 15.2 Demonstration of the technique to obtain systemic blood pressure (BP) measurements with a Doppler transducer in a cat.

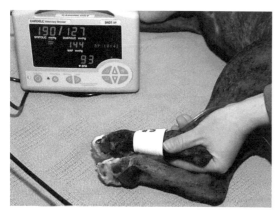

Figure 15.3 Demonstration of cuff placement over the cranial tibial artery in a dog. The oscillometric unit is most reliable in medium- and large-breed dogs.

- For comparative purposes, the same site for cuff placement should be used each time in an individual animal and recorded in the medical record.
- The cuff should be placed at the level of the aortic valve (heart base). If not, a compensation can be made for gravitational effect, with a 1.0 mm Hg rise in BP expected for each 1.3 cm of vertical distance between the level of the cuff and the level of the aortic valve. This "correction" is relevant only in large dogs.

ENVIRONMENT AND PERSONNEL

- Provide an environment that is quiet and away from other animals.
- The owner may be present to help calm the animal.
- Allow for a quiet equilibration time for the animal of 5 to 15 minutes.
- The same individual (preferably a technician) should perform all BP measurements following a standard protocol.
- Measurements should be obtained only in a patient that is calm, minimally restrained, and motionless. A blanket on the floor or table may allow the patient to be more comfortable.

RECORD KEEPING

- A standard form for recording results of the BP measurement should be developed for the medical record. The following data should always be noted, along with each measurement obtained:
  - Cuff size (30% to 40% of limb circumference in cats; 40% in dogs)
  - Limb used (including left or right)
  - Time of day
  - Time of administration of any medication(s)
  - Technique used (i.e., Doppler or oscillometric)

- Degree of agitation, restlessness, or limb movement
- Technician performing measurement
- If a different room or unusual environmental conditions exist (e.g., a long wait before BP measurement with noisy dogs present), then this should also be noted if higher than normal values are obtained.

TECHNIQUES

DOPPLER

- In cats, a Doppler flow meter or high-definition oscillometry is used most commonly, whereas dogs can be evaluated with either the Doppler or oscillometric unit. Cuff size is determined after the foreleg above the carpus is measured and the cuff is snugly wrapped around the foreleg and secured with a piece of tape.
- The patient and cuff position should be well tolerated with the cuff at, or close to, the level of the right atrium. For the Doppler flow meter, an excellent blood flow signal can usually be obtained from the median artery between the carpal and metacarpal pads by wetting down the hair with alcohol and applying coupling gel and the 10-MHz (i.e., pediatric) Doppler transducer.
- The Doppler transducer should be aligned parallel to blood flow so that the wire from the transducer is parallel with the limb (i.e., it emerges from under the paw). Unlike in the operative setting, the transducer is held in place, not taped.
- The Doppler cuff is inflated to a pressure 30 to 40 mm Hg higher than that required to obliterate the pulse, and then slowly deflated (about 2 to 5 mm Hg/sec). A slower heart rate requires a slower deflation time to accurately determine systolic pressure. A too-slow deflation time, however, will result in discomfort to the animal.
- The first sound heard as blood begins to flow through the artery is the systolic pressure. The cuff should be completely deflated before reinflation for the next measurement.
- Four to six measurements are advised over a 5- to 10-minute period because BP often falls with repeated measurements as the patient adjusts to the feel of the cuff inflating and deflating. The first measurement should be discarded and the average of three to five consecutive, consistent indirect measurements should be obtained. Any measurement obtained during limb movement should be discarded.
- If BP measurements are thought to be borderline or falsely high, the animal may be hospitalized for several hours in a quiet room to acclimate to the environment and BP measurement repeated.

OSCILLOMETRIC TECHNIQUES

- In dogs, the oscillometric method gives reliable systolic results, with the addition of diastolic and mean arterial pressures. In cats, BP measurements from high-definition oscillometry have been shown to be accurate, particularly for systolic BP. The rear limb is often preferred for the oscillometric technique in dogs, and the circumference of the metatarsus (i.e., below the hock) is measured for cuff width determination.
- Medium- and large-breed dogs are positioned on a blanket on the floor with the technician, who snugly wraps the cuff as described previously.
- The oscillometric unit is activated, and the same number of readings is obtained as described above for cats. If for any reason the oscillometric technique yields spurious results (as in very small dogs), the Doppler method is used.
- The average of all values obtained, or the average of all values obtained after the highest and lowest pressure readings are discarded, should be taken as the final value. Each measurement, in addition to the information mentioned previously in the section on record keeping, should be recorded.
- If results are borderline or inconsistent, repeat the measurement session on another day.

ANXIETY-INDUCED ARTIFACT: THE "WHITE COAT EFFECT"

A clinic visit, hospitalization, a strange environment, restraint in the examination room, clipper noise and vibration, cuff placement, cuff inflation, and other unusual stimuli may induce anxiety in an animal during BP measurement. As a consequence, a falsely elevated value for BP may be obtained secondary to catecholamine release associated with this anxiety. The magnitude of this effect may be minimized by the following:

- Obtaining BP measurements before a physical examination or other manipulations to which the animal may object
- Performing all measurements in a quiet room with a calm and reassuring manner
- Allowing the animal to acclimate to its surroundings for at least 5 minutes before obtaining BP measurements

CHOICE OF ANIMALS TO TREAT

There is a clear association between marked systemic hypertension and TOD in dogs and cats, particularly for ocular and renal injury. However, some of the other adverse effects of systemic hypertension are theorized on the basis of extrapolation from clinical studies in humans or from experimental studies in laboratory rodents.

TREATMENT GUIDELINES

- The American College of Veterinary Internal Medicine Hypertension Consensus Panel and International Renal Interest Society has recommended that treatment for high BP be based on patient classifications (Table 15.1), which depend on both reliable BP measurements and knowledge of TOD.
- We consider antihypertensive treatment to be indicated in any dog or cat with a sustained systolic

Table 15.1 Blood Pressure Staging				
	Risk of Future Target Organ Damage (Risk Levels AP0-AP3)*:			
	Minimal or no risk	Low risk	Moderate risk	High risk
	(AP0)	(AP1)	(AP2)	(AP3)
Blood pressure (mm Hg)				
Systolic	<150	150-159	160-179	≥180
Diastolic	<95	95-99	100-119	≥120
Substage				
No complications present (nc)†	AP0nc	AP1nc	AP2nc	AP3nc
Complications present (c)	AP0c	AP1c	AP2c	AP3c
Should patient be treated?				
No complications present†	No	No	±	Yes
Complications present	No	Yes	Yes	Yes

*If blood pressure is not measured, the patient is classified as risk not determined.
†Complications include any evidence of target organ damage in eyes (e.g., intraocular hemorrhage or retinal detachment), central nervous system (e.g., seizures or otherwise unexplained neurologic signs), cardiovascular system (e.g., congestive heart failure), or kidneys (e.g., azotemia or proteinuria).

BP >200 mm Hg or a diastolic BP >120 mm Hg (AP3), regardless of other clinical findings.
- In both species, any animal with clear evidence of ongoing TOD (AP3c, AP2c, AP1c) should generally be considered a candidate for antihypertensive therapy.
- There is considerable uncertainty and difficulty associated with BP measurement in dogs and cats. Thus, in animals in which the systolic/diastolic BP is classified as AP2nc (no clinical abnormalities related to systemic hypertension are identified), the rationale for therapy is less clear. Currently, some clinicians recommend treatment for animals in this range, and others do not.
- Animals with no clinical signs and mildly elevated BP (AP1nc) should not be treated.

KEY POINT

Animals with normal BP *or in which BP has not been measured* should not be treated with antihypertensive agents.

ANTIHYPERTENSIVE THERAPY

GENERAL

- Systemic arterial BP is the product of the cardiac output and the total peripheral vascular resistance; therefore antihypertensive therapy is generally aimed at reducing cardiac output, total peripheral vascular resistance, or both.
- Therapy may be loosely classified as dietary and pharmacologic.
- Treatment is generally conducted by sequential trials. In general, dosage adjustments or changes in treatment should be instituted no more frequently than every 2 weeks, unless extreme hypertension necessitating emergency treatment is present.
- When pharmacologic agents are used, a wide range of dosages should be considered, with initial dosages at the low end of the range.
- If an agent or combination of agents is incompletely effective, the dosage(s) may be increased, or additional agents may be added. Often, multiple agents are used concurrently, especially in dogs.
- It is usually not possible to restore BP to normal values when treating a hypertensive animal. It should be the veterinarian's goal to lower the BP to <150/100 mm Hg, with emphasis given to the systolic value.

DURATION OF TREATMENT

- The diagnosis of hypertension associated with CKD necessitates lifelong antihypertensive treatment, with periodic dosage adjustments based on BP measurements.

- Hypertension associated with hyperthyroidism or hyperadrenocorticism can be expected to resolve within 1 to 3 months after effective treatment of the underlying condition, unless CKD is also present. Occasionally, dogs with well-controlled hyperadrenocorticism remain hypertensive.
- In other patients, the duration of treatment cannot be predicted, but it may be a lifelong requirement. Periodic dosage adjustments based on BP measurements are indicated.

DIETARY THERAPY

- Though poorly studied, a low-sodium diet that provides <0.25% sodium on a dry-weight basis may be introduced. Dietary sodium restriction may be used as a first step if hypertension is mild (i.e., systolic BP <170 mm Hg) and there is no TOD present.
- In some animals with hypertension, it may be more important to maintain adequate caloric intake rather than insist on a low-sodium diet. Therefore drug therapy is instituted first, and when BP is stabilized, the animal may be switched to a lower sodium diet.
- Obesity can elevate BP in humans and dogs and, perhaps, in cats. Consequently, weight loss is desirable in obese, hypertensive animals.

PHARMACOLOGIC AGENTS: GENERAL

- Medical treatment of hypertension in dogs and cats has, until recently, been extrapolated from human protocols. Recommendations for medical therapy have included the following:
  - Vasodilators (e.g., angiotensin-converting enzyme [ACE] inhibitors and angiotensin receptor blockers [ARBs])
  - Dihydropyridine calcium channel blockers
  - Hydralazine
  - Phenoxybenzamine
  - Prazosin
  - Diuretics
  - Beta blockers
- These agents are often given in concert with dietary sodium restriction.
- In animals with systemic hypertension and CKD, ACE inhibitors or ARBs are the preferred initial choice in dogs, and amlodipine is the preferred initial choice in cats. Usually cats are treated with both amlodipine and an ACE inhibitor (or ARB) because amlodipine activates the renin-angiotensin-aldosterone system. In this setting, ACE inhibitors (or ARBs) are presumed to be renoprotective.

VASODILATORS

- Are considered first-line drugs for hypertension in veterinary patients

- **ACE inhibitors** (e.g., **enalapril** or **benazepril** 0.5 mg/kg PO q12h in dogs and q24h in cats) and **ARBs** (e.g., **telmisartan** 1.0 mg/kg PO q24h) may lower BP, particularly in dogs. At present, largely because of familiarity, an ACE inhibitor is generally selected rather than an ARB. In cats, the role of the renin-angiotensin-aldosterone system in the maintenance of systemic hypertension is less clear, but ACE inhibitors (or ARBs) are administered for renoprotection. Benazepril may be preferred in patients with CKD because it is eliminated by both urinary and biliary excretion (compared with only urinary excretion for enalapril). In humans, combination therapy with an ACE inhibitor plus an ARB is often used, but there are no data on which to recommend for, or against, this approach in dogs and cats.
- **Amlodipine besylate** (0.1 to 0.5 mg/kg PO q24h; typically 0.625 mg q24h in cats), a long-acting dihydropyridine calcium antagonist, reduces total peripheral resistance and has been used successfully as a single agent in hypertensive cats. Larger cats (more than 4 kg) may require 1.25 mg PO q24h. BP decreases significantly during amlodipine treatment, and significant adverse effects (i.e., hypotension, azotemia, hypokalemia, inappetence, and weight loss) are uncommon. In dogs with CKD, a dosage of 0.05 mg/kg given PO q24h lowered BP in initial pharmacokinetic trials, but in many spontaneously hypertensive dogs, amlodipine appears to be less effective particularly at this low dosage.
- Recently, concern has been raised about the potential for deleterious effects of calcium channel antagonists. These concerns arise from studies in humans and dogs with diabetes in which renal injury or proteinuria was exacerbated during therapy with calcium channel antagonists. In addition, there are theoretical rationales for use of an ACE inhibitor (or ARB) in animals with preexisting CKD. However, the coadministration of a calcium channel antagonist and an ACE inhibitor (or ARB) blocked adverse effects of calcium channel antagonism. In addition, because calcium channel antagonists are usually very effective in cats with systemic hypertension, they should be considered appropriate for use in affected cats until further information regarding long-term effects on renal function in cats becomes available.
- Direct-acting arterial vasodilators, such as **hydralazine** (0.5 to 2.0 mg/kg PO q12h), can be added to an ACE inhibitor and amlodipine for refractory hypertension. Hydralazine acts quickly, resulting in a rapid decrease in pressure, and therefore may result in clinical signs of hypotension (e.g., tachycardia, ataxia, syncope, lethargy). Hydralazine should always be started at the lower end of the dosage range, especially in those already receiving other antihypertensive agents such as an ACE inhibitor (or ARB) or amlodipine. Because the renin-angiotensin-aldosterone system is activated by hydralazine, coadministering an ACE inhibitor (or ARB) and possibly spironolactone with hydralazine is appropriate.
- **Phenoxybenzamine** (0.25 mg/kg PO q12h in dogs or 2.5 mg/cat q12h in cats), an alpha-receptor antagonist, lowers BP by lowering peripheral vascular resistance. It is indicated for animals with pheochromocytoma and is given with a beta blocker to block the effects of catecholamines on the cardiovascular system.

KEY POINT

ACE inhibitors (or ARBs) are first-line drugs for hypertensive dogs, and amlodipine is the antihypertensive of choice in cats (generally with the addition of an ACE inhibitor or ARB if CKD is present).

BETA BLOCKERS

- Beta blockers exert an antihypertensive effect by reducing cardiac output and decreasing renin release, but their efficacy in hypertensive veterinary patients is poor. In hyperthyroid, hypertensive cats, a cardioselective beta-1 antagonist, such as **atenolol,** may be given at a dosage of 6.25 mg PO q12h (or approximately 1.0 mg/kg q12h) to block the cardiotoxic effects of thyroid hormone. The addition of amlodipine, however, is generally required to lower BP effectively. Beta blockers are not used routinely in hypertensive dogs unless pheochromocytoma is present.

DIURETICS

- **Spironolactone,** an aldosterone antagonist, is both a diuretic at higher doses (1 to 2 mg/kg PO q12h) and a neurohormone blocker at lower doses. It is a potassium-sparing diuretic and limits the effects of excess aldosterone (hypokalemia, hypertension) associated with hyperaldosteronism. Aldosterone levels are generally high with ACE inhibitor treatment (so-called aldosterone escape); therefore spironolactone may limit the renal and cardiac fibrosis as well as fluid retention associated with elevated aldosterone levels.
- Loop diuretics (**furosemide,** 2 to 4 mg/kg PO q12h in dogs and 1 to 2 mg/kg PO q12h in cats) are rarely used in hypertensive animals. These

agents lower extracellular fluid volume and cardiac output. These agents, as well as the thiazide diuretics (which are commonly used as first-line drugs in humans with hypertension), may cause a significant decrease in serum potassium concentration.

- Adverse effects include dehydration, volume depletion, and worsening azotemia. Because hypokalemia may occur with either class of diuretics, plasma potassium and creatinine concentrations should be carefully monitored in all animals with CKD that are receiving a diuretic.

EMERGENCY MANAGEMENT OF HYPERTENSION

PATIENT SELECTION

- Animals with neurologic signs or severe ocular manifestations of hypertension, such as retinal detachment, warrant aggressive treatment. **Sodium nitroprusside** (1.0 to 10.0 µg/kg/min constant-rate intravenous infusion), an arterial (predominantly) and venous vasodilator acting as a donor of nitric oxide inside vascular smooth muscle cells, can be used for the initial treatment of hypertensive crisis. This drug must be given by constant-rate infusion, can be titrated very precisely according to BP response, and usually does not cause reflex tachycardia.
- If a constant rate of infusion is not available, **hydralazine** and **furosemide** can be used in combination. The hydralazine dose can be repeated after 2 hours to titrate the effect.
- If intensive monitoring is not available in a veterinary hospital, then **amlodipine** is an excellent alternative choice, especially in cats.
- Regardless of initial therapy chosen for the management of an acute hypertensive crisis, a drug of choice for long-term management of systemic hypertension should be instituted soon after presentation to facilitate the eventual transition to long-term maintenance therapy.

FOLLOW-UP CARE AND ADDITIONAL MEDICATIONS

- In all animals treated for systemic hypertension, the routine examination should include a fundic examination, evaluation of any underlying diseases, and measurement of body weight, BP, and serum concentrations of creatinine and electrolytes. The owner should be questioned for evidence of drug toxicity, which may include lethargy, increased time spent sleeping, ataxia, or anorexia. Animals undergoing multiple drug regimens are more likely to exhibit adverse effects than those receiving a single antihypertensive agent.

- Once BP is controlled, the animal should be evaluated at 3-month intervals. A complete blood count, biochemical panel, and urinalysis should be evaluated at least once every 6 months.
- Many hypertensive animals have kidney disease. Other treatments for CKD should accompany antihypertensive therapy, as appropriate. Potassium supplementation is often needed in cats with CKD. Because animals with renal dysfunction generally have an impaired ability to adapt to sudden changes in sodium input, the administration of electrolyte solutions can lead to volume overload, worsened systemic hypertension, and pleural effusion (or peripheral edema) in animals with renal azotemia. Similarly, a sudden reduction in dietary sodium intake in an animal with renal azotemia can lead to extracellular fluid volume depletion. Some treatments, such as the administration of recombinant erythropoietin to elevate hematocrit, may exacerbate systemic hypertension and should not be used until systemic hypertension is controlled.

FREQUENTLY ASKED QUESTIONS

Because dogs are often more refractory to the effects of antihypertensive treatment than cats, what is a reasonable stepwise approach to antihypertensive therapy in dogs?

Hypertensive dogs (i.e., those with a sustained systolic BP >160 mm Hg) are likely to be proteinuric given the underlying diseases associated with systemic hypertension in that species.

- ACE inhibitors (e.g., enalapril, benazepril) have been shown to decrease proteinuria and cause balanced vasodilation; therefore they are usually the starting drug in the treatment of canine hypertension. Enalapril or benazepril (0.5 mg/kg PO q12 to 24h) is given, and BP is measured after 2 weeks of treatment. An alternative approach to interfering with the renin-angiotensin-aldosterone system would be an ARB (e.g., telmisartan at 1.0 mg/kg PO q24h).
- If hypertension is still present, then amlodipine (0.1 mg/kg PO q24h) can be administered with the ACE inhibitor (or ARB). The combination of an ACE inhibitor and a calcium channel blocker may be effective; however, sustained hypertension warrants the addition of drugs that have different mechanisms of action.
- Hydralazine, a direct-acting arterial vasodilator, can be given at a starting dose of 0.5 mg/kg PO q12h, and slowly uptitrated in increments of 0.5 mg/kg to a maximum dose of 2.0 mg/kg. BP and serum creatinine should be monitored with each increase in dose.

- Regardless of therapeutic approach, increased levels of aldosterone should be expected, and the addition of spironolactone (1 to 2 mg/kg PO q12h) is advised to block the effects of aldosterone.
- If BP remains above 160 mm Hg, then amlodipine may be increased to 0.1 mg/kg q12h (or 0.2 mg/kg q24h), or a beta blocker may be added to decrease heart rate and renin release.

Cats and dogs with CKD often exhibit systemic hypertension. What is the causative factor in this relationship, and how should these animals be managed? How can you tell if hypertension is damaging the kidney?

This has often been referred to as a chicken-and-egg question, but it is more properly seen as an example of a complex positive feedback loop that complicates therapy in animals affected with both problems. High BP produces barotrauma within the microvasculature of the kidney, effectively destroying renal tissue over time (weeks to months). On the other hand, CKD produces abnormalities in body fluid volumes and can alter neurohumoral control of BP. These factors combine to make high BP relatively common (approximately 25% prevalence) in dogs and cats with CKD. Furthermore, it is still generally accepted that something has to be wrong with the kidney for sustained systemic hypertension to be present.

- Interestingly, in the short-term, high BP tends to improve glomerular filtration rate. This is why the level of azotemia should always be assessed shortly (3 to 14 days) after any changes in antihypertensive therapy.
- Furthermore, vasodilators with intrarenal effects are often preferred for antihypertensive therapy in animals with kidney disease, largely because the vasodilatory effect may help to preserve renal function.
- Typical agents to select for initial therapy when both hypertension and renal azotemia are present in dogs would be an ACE inhibitor (or ARB) such as enalapril or benazepril (0.5 mg/kg q12 to 24h) and in cats, a calcium channel blocker such as amlodipine (0.1 mg/kg PO q24h) with or without an ACE inhibitor (or ARB).
- Perhaps the best index of hypertensive damage of the kidney is proteinuria. The presence of microalbuminuria or an elevated urine protein-to-creatinine ratio (>0.5 in dogs, >0.4 in cats) is generally an indication for the use of an ACE inhibitor (e.g., enalapril or benazepril 0.5 mg/kg q24h in cats or q12 to 24h in dogs) or an ARB (e.g., telmisartan 1.0 mg/kg q24h).

SUGGESTED READINGS

Binns SH, Sisson DD, Buoscio DA, et al: Doppler ultrasonographic, oscillometric sphygmomanometric, and photoplethysmographic techniques for noninvasive blood pressure measurement in anesthetized cats, J Vet Intern Med 9:405, 1995.

Bodey AR, Michell AR, Bovee KC, et al: Comparison of direct and indirect (oscillometric) measurements of arterial blood pressure in conscious dogs, Res Vet Sci 61:17, 1996.

Brown CAJ, Munday J, Mathur S, et al: Hypertensive encephalopathy in cats with reduced renal function, Vet Pathol 42:642–649, 2005.

Brown S, Finco D, Navar L: Impaired renal autoregulatory ability in dogs with reduced renal mass, J Am Soc Nephrol 5:1768, 1995.

Brown S, Atkins C, Bagley R, et al: Guidelines for the identification, evaluation, and management of systemic hypertension in dogs and cats: ACVIM Consensus Statement, J Vet Intern Med 21:542, 2007.

Brown SA, Brown CA: Single-nephron adaptations to partial renal ablation in cats, Am J Physiol 269:R1002, 1996.

Brown SA, Finco DR, Crowell WA, et al: Single-nephron adaptations to partial renal ablation in the dog, Am J Physiol 258:F495, 1990.

Brown SA, Walton CL, Crawford P, et al: Long-term effects of antihypertensive regimens on renal hemodynamics and proteinuria, Kidney Int 43:1210, 1993.

Carter J, Irving A, Bridges J, et al: The prevalence of ocular lesions associated with hypertension in a population of geriatric cats in Auckland, New Zealand, N Z Vet J 62:21, 2014.

Chakrabarti S, Syme HM, Elliott J: Clinicopathological variables predicting progression of azotemia in cats, J Vet Intern Med 26:275, 2012.

Cowgill LDD: Systemic hypertension. In Kirk RW, ed: Current veterinary therapy IX, Philadelphia, 1986, Saunders.

Cowgill LD, Kallet AJ: Recognition and management of hypertension in the dog, In Kirk RW, ed: Current veterinary therapy VIII, Philadelphia, 1983, Saunders.

Finco DR: Association of systemic hypertension with renal injury in dogs with induced renal failure, J Vet Intern Med 18:289, 2004.

Henik R, Snyder P, Volk L: Treatment of systemic hypertension in cats with amlodipine besylate, J Am Anim Hosp Assoc 33:226, 1997.

Jacob F, Polzin DJ, Osborne CA, et al: Association between initial systolic blood pressure and risk of developing a uremic crisis or of dying in dogs with chronic renal failure, J Am Vet Med Assoc 222:322, 2003.

Jensen J, Henik RA, Brownfield M, et al: Plasma renin activity, angiotensin I and aldosterone in feline hypertension associated with chronic renal disease, Am J Vet Res 58:535, 1997.

Jepson RE, Elliott J, Brodbelt D, Syme HM: Effect of control of systolic blood pressure on survival in cats with systemic hypertension, J Vet Intern Med 21:402, 2007.

Kallet A, Cowgill L, Kass P: Comparison of blood pressure measurements in dogs by use of indirect oscillometry in a veterinary clinic versus at home, J Am Vet Med Assoc 210:651, 1997.

Labato MA, Ross LA: Diagnosis and management of hypertension. In August JR, ed: Consultations in feline internal medicine, Philadelphia, 1991, Saunders.

Leblanc N, Stepien R, Bentley E: Oculate lesions associated with systemic hypertension in dogs: 65 cases (2005-2007), J Am Vet Med Assoc 238(915), 2011.

Littman MP: Spontaneous systemic hypertension in 24 cats, J Vet Intern Med 8:79, 1994.

Littman MP, Robertson JL, Bovee KC: Spontaneous systemic hypertension in dogs: five cases (1981-1983), J Am Vet Med Assoc 193(486), 1988.

Martel E, Egner B, Brown SA, et al: Comparison of high-definition oscillometry—a non-invasive technology for arterial blood pressure measurement—with a direct invasive method using radio-telemetry in awake healthy cats, J Feline Med Surg 15:1104, 2013.

O'Neill J, Kent M, Glass EN, Platt SR: Clinicopathologic and MRI characteristics of presumptive hypertensive encephalopathy in two cats and two dogs, J Am Anim Hosp Assoc 49:412, 2013.

Ortega TM, Feldman EC, Nelson RW, et al: Systemic arterial blood pressure and urine protein/creatinine ratio in dogs with hyperadrenocorticism, J Am Vet Med Assoc 209:1724, 1996.

Remillard RL, Ross JN, Eddy JB: Variance of indirect blood pressure measurements and prevalence of hypertension in clinically normal dogs, Am J Vet Res 52:561, 1991.

Ross LA: Hypertension and chronic renal failure, Semin Vet Med Surg Small Anim 7:221, 1992.

Snyder PS, Henik RA: Feline systemic hypertension, Proc Twelfth Annual Vet Med Forum, San Francisco, 126, 1994.

Stiles J, Polzin DJ, Bistner SI: The prevalence of retinopathy in cats with systemic hypertension and chronic renal failure or hyperthyroidism, J Am Anim Hosp Assoc 30:564, 1994.

Williams TL, Elliott J, Syme HM: Renin-angiotensin-aldosterone system activity in hyperthyroid cats with and without concurrent hypertension, J Vet Intern Med 27:522, 2013.

SECTION 3

TREATMENT OF CARDIOVASCULAR DISEASE

Pathophysiology and Therapy of Heart Failure

16

Keith N. Strickland

DEFINITIONS

- Heart disease is any structural (microscopic or macroscopic) abnormality of the heart that may or may not result in heart failure.
- Heart failure is the pathophysiologic state that occurs when the heart is unable to function at a level commensurate with the requirements of the metabolizing tissues or can only do so at elevated filling pressures.
- Preload is the degree of muscle fiber stretch just before contraction. This correlates to the volume of blood within the ventricle just before contraction (cardiac preload, venous return).
- Afterload is the load against which a muscle exerts its contractile force. Cardiac afterload refers to the blood pressure the ventricle must overcome to eject blood.

OVERVIEW

- The function of the cardiovascular system is to maintain normal arterial blood pressure and flow (cardiac output) while maintaining normal venous and capillary pressures during rest and exercise. This function is necessary to provide adequate blood flow for oxygen and nutrient delivery to vital tissues (such as the brain, the heart, and the kidneys), as well as for the removal of metabolic waste products from these tissues.
- Heart failure results in a reduction in the previously described functions of the cardiovascular system. If blood pressure and cardiac output are not maintained or if venous and capillary pressures are markedly increased, then death can occur within hours to weeks (depending on the severity of the abnormality). Heart failure can be associated with systolic or diastolic dysfunction.

HEART FAILURE

PATHOPHYSIOLOGY

Our understanding of the progression from asymptomatic heart disease to symptomatic heart failure has changed from the traditional concept of biomechanical dysfunction to a concept emphasizing neuroendocrine dysfunction secondary to chronic biomechanical dysfunction.

- The current model embodies the idea that some cardiac damage or dysfunction results in chronically altered hemodynamics that lead to activation of neurohumoral mechanisms designed to promote cardiac function and tissue perfusion. Chronic activation of these compensatory mechanisms leads to progressive cardiovascular dysfunction culminating in life-threatening congestive heart failure (CHF), low-output failure, or sudden death.
- Cardiac dysfunction that leads to the clinical syndrome of heart failure can be subdivided into systolic and diastolic dysfunction. Systolic dysfunction occurs when the heart's ability to pump blood in a forward direction is impaired. Components of systolic function include myocardial contractility, valvular competence, preload, afterload, and heart rate.

PHASES OF HEART FAILURE

- Phase 1: Cardiac injury
- Phase 2: Compensatory mechanisms
- Phase 3: Cardiac failure with clinical signs of cardiac dysfunction

KEY POINT

CHF occurs when cardiac diastolic filling pressures result in elevated venous and capillary hydrostatic pressures with subsequent edema formation. Therapy for CHF is directed toward reducing cardiac diastolic filling pressures so that edema fluid can be mobilized, suppressing activated neuroendocrine systems and improving cardiac output.

- Low-output failure occurs when cardiac function does not produce adequate cardiac output to maintain blood pressure and tissue perfusion.

MYOCARDIAL FAILURE

- Impaired contractility may occur with primary heart disease (idiopathic dilated cardiomyopathy [DCM]) or secondary heart disease.
  - Chronic heart disease of varying causes may mimic primary cardiomyopathy. Systolic failure following chronic overload may be secondary to chronic valvular insufficiency and left-to-right shunting lesions, such as patent ductus arteriosus or ventricular septal defect.
  - Nutritional deficiencies, such as taurine deficiency, have been recognized as a cause of myocardial failure in the cat and have been associated with DCM in certain breeds of dogs (American Cocker Spaniels, Golden Retrievers, Dalmatians, Boxers, Welsh Corgis, Newfoundlands). Myocardial deficiency of L-carnitine has been reported in Boxers and Doberman Pinschers.
  - Metabolic cardiomyopathies include feline hyperthyroidism, canine hypothyroidism, and chronic uremia.
  - Toxic cardiomyopathy: doxorubicin-induced DCM
  - Infiltrative cardiomyopathy: neoplastic (e.g., lymphosarcoma), amyloidosis

VALVULAR INSUFFICIENCY

- Valvular insufficiency is one of the most common causes of volume overload encountered in veterinary medicine. Incompetency of an atrioventricular valve (endocardiosis, endocarditis, congenital malformation) allows retrograde ejection (regurgitation) of blood into the corresponding atrium during systole, reducing forward flow and decreasing cardiac output. Severe regurgitation also increases atrial and ventricular filling pressures, with the risk of CHF.
- Valvular insufficiency can be primary (myxomatous degeneration) or secondary (associated with other conditions that alter valvular function such as ventricular hypertrophy, ischemia, etc.).

EXCESSIVE AFTERLOAD

- Normally, an abrupt increase in afterload causes a positive inotropic effect (Anrep effect). However, when the hemodynamic overload is severe or chronic, myocardial contractility may be depressed. Chronically increased afterload leads to a reduced rate of ejection, a reduced amount of blood ejected at any given preload, and increased myocardial oxygen consumption with the risk of ischemic damage.
- Pulmonary/systemic hypertension or ventricular outflow obstructions (aortic or pulmonic stenosis) are examples of clinically significant causes of increased afterload.

INADEQUATE PRELOAD

- In cases in which inadequate preload is the primary hemodynamic abnormality (such as pericardial effusion causing cardiac tamponade), the reduction in preload decreases stroke volume and cardiac output. Normally, the reduced preload may be compensated for by systemic mechanisms that result in increased venous return and ventricular end-diastolic volume; however, significant pericardial effusion obstructs venous inflow and limits the end-diastolic volume, precluding the circulatory system from fully compensating for the reduced cardiac output.

DIASTOLIC DYSFUNCTION

- Diastolic dysfunction may result in heart failure. Indeed, most cases of overt heart failure have some degree of diastolic dysfunction. Adequate ventricular filling is dependent on several factors, such as the following:
  - Ventricular relaxation
  - Ventricular elasticity (change in muscle length for a change in force)
  - Ventricular compliance (change in ventricular volume for a given change in pressure)
- Ventricular relaxation may be decreased in several diseases or disorders (e.g., idiopathic hypertrophic cardiomyopathy [HCM], ischemia).
- Ventricular compliance may be reduced when elevated filling pressure is required. This change can be associated with:
  - Volume overloading
  - An increase in muscle mass or wall thickness, as with myocardial concentric hypertrophy
  - A decrease in ventricular distensibility (usually associated with extrinsic compression of the heart)
  - Diseases that result in myocardial fibrosis (e.g., restrictive cardiomyopathy [RCM], ischemic heart disease) also cause a decrease in ventricular compliance.
- Diastolic dysfunction may increase ventricular end-diastolic pressure, which is then transmitted to the corresponding atrium and the venous system. Elevation in venous and capillary pressures may result in interstitial and alveolar pulmonary edema or ascites through hydrostatic factors.

COMPENSATORY MECHANISMS IN CHRONIC HEART FAILURE

FRANK-STARLING MECHANISM

- The Frank-Starling mechanism is an adaptive mechanism by which an increase in preload enhances cardiac performance. Venous return and fluid status determines the preload of the ventricle. Physiologic increases in ventricular end-diastolic volume are associated with increases in myocardial fiber length. This allows the sarcomere to function near the upper limit of its maximal length (optimal length), where it is able to generate the maximal amount of force during contraction.

- To better understand the role of the Frank-Starling mechanism, consider the hemodynamic changes associated with exercise. Cardiac output is increased during exercise through the following mechanisms: (1) increased heart rate and contractility through increased sympathetic nervous system (SNS) activity, (2) increased venous return (preload) with a more vigorous contraction (Frank-Starling mechanism), and (3) reduced afterload associated with reduced peripheral vascular resistance. In this way, cardiac performance is enhanced during exercise in the absence of heart failure. In the presence of heart failure, cardiac output and ventricular performance may be maintained within normal limits at rest only because the ventricular end-diastolic fiber length and the preload are elevated (ventricular performance is maintained through the Frank-Starling mechanism).
- In the failing heart, these factors that normally help increase cardiac output during exercise are chronically active and cause increased preload and ventricular end-diastolic pressures (especially in a noncompliant, dilated ventricle), with the threat of edema formation. Exercise drives the ventricle along the flat portion of the ventricular performance curve, where increases in ventricular volume and diastolic pressure do not increase ventricular performance.

RENIN-ANGIOTENSIN-ALDOSTERONE SYSTEM

- The renin-angiotensin-aldosterone system (RAAS) is a complex neurohormonal compensatory system that functions to maintain relatively normal blood pressure and tissue perfusion when cardiac output is reduced. Reduced renal perfusion detected by renal baroreceptors results in release of renin (Figure 16.1). Other factors that cause the release of renin include decreased sodium delivery to the macula densa and SNS stimulation of beta-1 adrenoceptors in the juxtaglomerular apparatus of the kidney. Renin initiates a cascade resulting in the formation of angiotensin II, a potent vasoconstrictor. Angiotensin II also causes activation of the SNS, and it increases synthesis and release of aldosterone from the zona glomerulosa of the adrenal cortex and release of antidiuretic hormone.

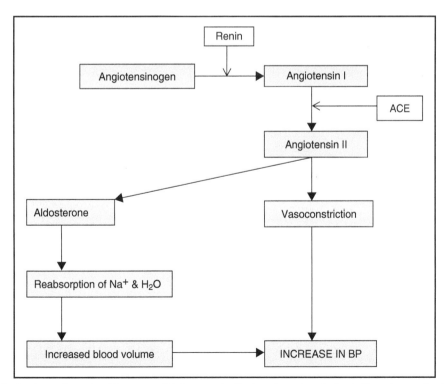

Figure 16.1 Renin-angiotensin-aldosterone (RAA) cascade. Reduced renal perfusion is the primary stimulus for renin release, which leads to activation of the angiotensin-aldosterone system. RAAS activation results in sodium and water retention and peripheral vasoconstriction. *ACE*, Angiotensin-converting enzyme; *BP*, blood pressure. (Used with permission of Dr. Walt Ingwersen, Ontario, Canada.)

- Aldosterone causes sodium retention in the distal renal tubules to promote fluid retention. Aldosterone also promotes fibrosis of the myocardium and vascular smooth muscle.
- The RAAS can be subdivided into the following:
  - Systemic or renal RAAS
  - Tissue RAAS
- The tissue RAAS (brain, vascular, and myocardial tissues) can generate angiotensin II independently of the circulating RAAS.
- Angiotensin II stimulates the release of growth factors that promote remodeling of the vessels and myocardium. Vascular remodeling (smooth muscle cell growth and hyperplasia, hypertrophy, and apoptosis; cytokine activation; myocyte and vascular wall fibrosis) results in decreased vascular responsiveness to alterations in blood flow, decreased vascular compliance, and increased afterload. Angiotensin II also causes pathologic ventricular hypertrophy and exerts cytotoxic effects, resulting in myocardial necrosis and loss of myocardial contractile mass with resultant cardiac dysfunction.

SYMPATHETIC NERVOUS SYSTEM ACTIVATION

- The autonomic nervous system plays a crucial role in the compensation of heart failure. The activity of the SNS is increased in part by baroreflex-mediated parasympathetic withdrawal, as well as by activation by the RAAS. Early activation of the SNS helps to maintain cardiac output, blood pressure, and tissue perfusion by increasing venous return to the heart (vasoconstriction of the splanchnic vessels), vasoconstriction of other various vascular beds, and positive inotropic and chronotropic cardiac effects. Activation of the SNS early in heart failure is beneficial, but it then becomes maladaptive when chronically activated (Figure 16.2).

SYMPATHETIC DESENSITIZATION

- Chronic activation of the SNS is associated with elevated levels of plasma norepinephrine (NE), cardiac NE depletion, downregulation and desensitization of beta-1 adrenergic receptors, and abnormal baroreflex function. Plasma NE levels appear to be increased because of a combination of increased release of NE from adrenergic nerve endings and reduced uptake of NE by adrenergic nerve endings. The depletion of myocardial NE (serum NE levels increase and myocardial levels decrease) probably represents the depletion of the neurotransmitter in adrenergic nerve endings.
- The downregulation of beta-1 adrenergic receptors occurs relatively soon (24 to 72 hours) after

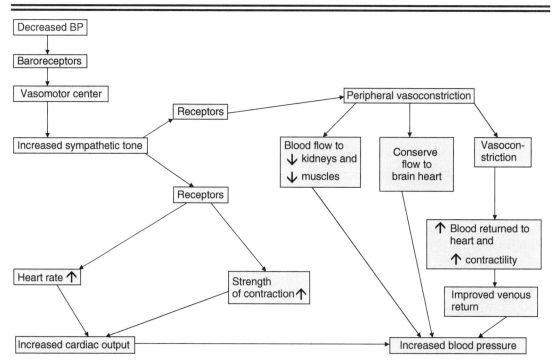

Figure 16.2 Effect of compensatory sympathetic system in response to a reduction in blood pressure (*BP*). Decreased systemic BP results in activation of the sympathetic nervous system (SNS) and a cascade of consequences that are deleterious in the long term. (Used with permission of Dr. Walt Ingwersen, Ontario, Canada.)

the initial SNS activation, making it progressively more difficult for the SNS to counter impaired contractility.
- Chronic activation of the SNS also overloads the heart by increasing venous return (to a heart that is already volume overloaded), increasing myocardial oxygen consumption (by increasing heart rate and volume overloading of the heart), and damaging the myocardium, creating a substrate for arrhythmogenesis.

MYOCARDIAL HYPERTROPHY

Myocardial hypertrophy occurs as a compensatory mechanism directed toward normalizing cardiac output, wall tension, and filling pressures. The hemodynamic load imposed on the heart (either volume or pressure overloading) determines the type of hypertrophy (eccentric or concentric). Chronic activation of the RAAS and the SNS produces pathologic changes (remodeling) within the ventricular myocardium, which contribute to cardiac dysfunction. The result can be myocardial failure with low-output signs or elevated filling pressures with the risk of CHF.

- Eccentric myocardial hypertrophy (or volume-overload hypertrophy) occurs with heart disease as a compensatory mechanism to allow the ventricle to pump a relatively normal amount of blood despite abnormal systolic function. Eccentric hypertrophy is characterized by chamber dilation, a response to the increase in blood volume and venous return associated with activation of the RAAS and SNS. More specifically, the increased venous return is secondary to sodium (aldosterone effect) and water (antidiuretic hormone/vasopressin effect) retention, as well as to venoconstriction of the splanchnic vascular bed (RAAS and SNS effect). Chronic heart failure represents a non-osmotic (mediated by SNS and RAAS, instead of osmotic hypertonic) stimulus for antidiuretic hormone release from the hypothalamus. Chronic volume overload causes an increase in diastolic wall stress, and this leads to replication of sarcomeres in series, elongation of myocytes, and ventricular dilation.
- Concentric myocardial hypertrophy (or pressure-overload hypertrophy) is characterized by thickening of the ventricular walls in response to increased systolic wall stress, and occurs as a compensatory mechanism to normalize systolic wall tension. Increased systolic wall stress stimulates the replication of sarcomeres in parallel, increasing myocardium thickness and thereby normalizing systolic wall stress (known as the Laplace relationship: wall tension = pressure × radius/wall thickness). The increase in thickness of the ventricular wall compensates for the increased systolic wall stress in a pressure-overloaded ventricle. If the compensatory concentric hypertrophy is inadequate and the systolic wall stress is increased, then afterload-mismatch and decompensation occur. When significant eccentric hypertrophy occurs in a volume-overloaded ventricle, systolic wall tension is increased secondary to the increase in ventricular diameter. Therefore both eccentric and some degree of concentric hypertrophy are present in severely volume-overloaded ventricles.

KEY POINT

In the syndrome of heart failure, changes in ventricular mass and geometry are a culmination of compensatory hypertrophy (in response to pressure or volume overload) and pathologic hypertrophy (in response to activation of the RAAS and SNS).

- These compensatory mechanisms require days to weeks to become fully activated. If the cardiac dysfunction is acute and severe, then the compensatory mechanisms do not have sufficient time to become fully activated (with the exception of the SNS, which is immediately activated).
  - For example, most dogs with idiopathic DCM have insidious, progressive cardiac dysfunction that worsens over a period of years, therefore allowing the compensatory mechanisms to become fully activated. Although these dogs have compensated heart failure chronically, at some point they may acutely decompensate, mimicking an acute disease process.
  - Conversely, a dog with a peracute disease syndrome (such as a very rapid supraventricular tachyarrhythmia like atrial fibrillation) may have heart failure without activating compensatory mechanisms other than the SNS.

ADDITIONAL COMPENSATORY MECHANISMS/NEUROENDOCRINE MECHANISMS

- Endothelins, a vasoactive family of peptides that are released from endothelial cells, play an important role in the regulation of vascular tone and blood pressure. Endothelin-1 is a strong, vasoconstrictive agent with inotropic and mitogenic actions; it is a strong stimulus for activation of the RAAS and SNS. Additionally, endothelin-1 may play an important role in the pathogenesis of pulmonary hypertension.

- Natriuretic peptides are regulators of salt and water homeostasis and blood pressure control with potential value as diagnostic and prognostic markers in patients with CHF. Natriuretic peptide levels are elevated in many disease conditions resulting in expanded fluid volume (such as DCM and chronic valvular insufficiency in dogs and cardiomyopathy in cats).
- Atrial, brain, and C-type natriuretic peptides have been identified (ANP, BNP, and CNP, respectively).
- BNP is primarily produced in the atria and is released in response to atrial stretch, resulting in natriuresis, diuresis, and balanced vasodilation.
- Natriuretic peptides antagonize the RAAS and SNS, inhibit release of antidiuretic hormone, prevent myocardial fibrosis, and modulate cell growth and myocardial hypertrophy.
- Inflammatory and immune mediators such as tumor necrosis factor alpha, interleukins (IL-1, IL-2, and IL-6), nuclear factor-kappa-B, and reactive oxygen species are thought to play a role in the progression of heart failure. The "cytokine hypothesis" suggests that heart failure progresses because cytokine pathways are activated in response to cardiac dysfunction and exert negative effects on the cardiovascular system.

COURSE OF EVENTS: COMPENSATORY MECHANISMS

- Reduced cardiac output leads to decreased tissue perfusion.
- Activation of baroreceptors in kidney, carotid arteries, aorta, and heart results in SNS activation and parasympathetic nervous system withdrawal.
- SNS activation (positive inotropic and chronotropic activity, vasoconstriction to increase venous return and maintain blood pressure, stimulation of antidiuretic hormone and renin)
- RAAS activation associated with reduced renal perfusion, decreased sodium delivery to the macula densa, and SNS activation
- Renal sodium and water retention to increase blood volume and, therefore, venous return to the heart
- Myocardial hypertrophy (dilation of the affected atrium and ventricle) to maintain relatively normal cardiac output and systolic wall tension while preventing diastolic filling pressures from rising
- Stretch-induced release of atrial natriuretic factor serves to facilitate sodium excretion. The effects of this factor are quickly negated, owing to degradation by neutral endopeptidases and the effects of overstimulation of the RAAS and SNS.

- Initially, these mechanisms allow the body to compensate for the decreased cardiac output by increasing blood volume and blood pressure. However, with chronicity, the compensatory mechanisms are maladaptive and facilitate progression of heart failure.
- Overstimulation of inflammatory/immune mediators (tumor necrosis factor-alpha, IL-1, IL-2, IL-6, reactive oxygen species) exert deleterious effects on the heart and circulation.
- The sustained effects of the SNS and RAAS continue to increase the workload of the heart by increasing blood volume and venous return to a heart that has maximized its ability to compensate by eccentric hypertrophy. Ventricular filling pressures begin to increase, with the threat of edema formation. The onset of edema formation is variable, depending on the severity and onset of ventricular dysfunction. Dogs with cardiomyopathy may have mild edema for days to weeks and only show minimal clinical signs, such as tachypnea and exercise intolerance.

TYPES OF HEART FAILURE

MYOCARDIAL FAILURE

- Myocardial failure is associated with decreases in contractility. It can be associated with the following:
  - Primary myocardial disease (idiopathic DCM); and
  - Secondary myocardial diseases (chronic congenital and valvular heart disease, thyrotoxicosis, taurine deficiency, infectious/inflammatory and infiltrative diseases).
- Myocardial failure causes systolic dysfunction and activation of compensatory mechanisms, which increase sodium and water retention to increase venous return to the heart. The ventricles must obtain a larger end-diastolic dimension to maintain a relatively normal total stroke volume (TSV). As the myocardial function deteriorates (as noted by a decrease in fractional shortening and a decrease in ejection fraction), the ventricles progressively enlarge so that the TSV is maintained, even though the percentage of blood being ejected is decreasing. Severe left ventricular dilation causes distortion and dilation of the mitral valve annulus, resulting in mitral regurgitation (MR) and further volume overloading of the left ventricle.
- Once the compensatory limits are reached, further increases in blood volume (associated with sodium and water retention) and venous return cause an increase in cardiac filling pressures, with threat of CHF development.

VOLUME OVERLOAD

- Volume overload is associated with the following two common causes of heart failure:
  - Valvular insufficiency
  - Shunts

ATRIOVENTRICULAR VALVULAR INSUFFICIENCY

- Atrioventricular valvular insufficiency can result from the following:
  - Degenerative valvular disease
  - Valvular endocarditis
  - Congenital valvular dysplasia
  - Chamber dilation
  - Valvular insufficiency may result in systolic dysfunction and activation of compensatory mechanisms that maintain cardiac output and tissue perfusion by vasoconstriction and fluid retention. As with impaired contractility, valvular insufficiency forces the ventricle to achieve larger end-diastolic dimensions to compensate for the decrease in forward stroke volume. The difference between volume overloading secondary to impaired contractility (DCM) and valvular insufficiency (MR) is associated with the changes in TSV (end-diastolic volume minus end-systolic volume). In MR without myocardial failure, TSV is increased to compensate for the amount of blood leaking through the incompetent valve. The end-diastolic volume increases, but the end-systolic volume remains normal (evidence of normal contractility), thereby resulting in an increased TSV. With impaired contractility, TSV is normal or decreased (depending on the disease stage) because both end-diastolic and end-systolic volumes have increased. End-diastolic volumes increase to compensate for the increased end-systolic volumes, reflecting impaired contractility.
- Shunts such as patent ductus arteriosus, ventricular septal defect, and arteriovenous fistula are similar to valvular leaks in that the heart increases TSV to compensate for the reduction in forward flow.

PRESSURE OVERLOAD

- Lesions that cause increased intraventricular systolic pressures usually do not cause CHF because the heart is generally able to compensate for the increased intraventricular systolic pressures with concentric hypertrophy (Laplace principle), and the ventricular systolic function remains relatively normal. When the obstruction to flow is severe (critical stenosis) or acute, however, pressure overload may result in myocardial failure and heart failure. More

commonly, CHF occurs when there is a concurrent valvular insufficiency (e.g., pulmonic stenosis with tricuspid regurgitation, subvalvular aortic stenosis with MR or aortic regurgitation, pulmonary hypertension with tricuspid regurgitation).
- Alternatively, sudden death may occur in dogs with severe (noncritical) congenital subvalvular aortic stenosis or possibly valvular pulmonic stenosis. When the ventricle is severely hypertrophied, coronary perfusion is impaired, and regions of the myocardium (especially the papillary muscles and subendocardial regions) are at risk of hypoxia. Myocardial hypoxia can result in impaired contractility as well as ventricular tachyarrhythmias, which may degenerate into ventricular fibrillation, leading to sudden cardiac death.

DECREASED VENTRICULAR COMPLIANCE OR ABNORMAL VENTRICULAR RELAXATION

- In idiopathic HCM, diastolic dysfunction typically progresses from abnormal relaxation to decreased ventricular compliance secondary to ventricular fibrosis. The abnormal myocardial architecture and energetics result in abnormal ventricular relaxation. The increase in ventricular or septal wall thickness is associated with decreased ventricular compliance (increased ventricular stiffness). Myocardial or endocardial fibrosis (RCM) can also increase ventricular stiffness.
- Decreased ventricular compliance and abnormal ventricular relaxation may result in elevated diastolic intraventricular pressures (filling pressures), even though the ventricular diastolic volume is not increased. During the course of diastole, for any increase in preload, there is an abnormal increase in intraventricular pressure. Over time, the corresponding atrium dilates to compensate for the elevated filling pressure. Once compensatory dilation of the atrium has reached its limit, further elevation of the ventricular filling pressure results in the development of edema (or pleural effusion in cats).
- Pericardial disease with cardiac tamponade is the clinical syndrome in which there is compression of the heart by fluid within the pericardial space (pericardial effusion), resulting in signs of right-sided heart failure and low-output failure. Elevation of intrapericardial pressure, progressive limitation of ventricular diastolic filling, and reduction of stroke volume and cardiac output characterize cardiac tamponade. The clinical course depends on the size and rate of accumulation of effusion and the compliance of the pericardial sac.

- **Acute tamponade** is usually associated with an acute hemorrhage from a neoplastic lesion, such as hemangiosarcoma, but it may also be associated with rupture of the left atrium secondary to chronic severe MR. As the effusion accumulates, intrapericardial pressures increase and eventually exceed the diastolic pressures in the right atrium and ventricle, thereby restricting venous inflow to the right heart. The restriction of venous return causes a reduction in right ventricular cardiac output, pulmonary blood flow, and left-sided venous return that is associated with a reduction in left ventricular stroke volume and cardiac output and signs of low-output heart failure.
- **Chronic tamponade** associated with the slow accumulation of pericardial effusion differs from acute tamponade in that the body has time to compensate for the impediment of cardiac inflow, secondary reduction in stroke volume, and cardiac output. Although compensation may somewhat normalize cardiac output, signs of right-sided CHF are often present (jugular distention and ascites).

CLINICAL DESCRIPTIONS OF HEART FAILURE

- CHF is the accumulation of fluid in tissues associated with increased capillary hydrostatic pressures and elevated diastolic intra-atrial and intraventricular pressures. Diseases that cause diastolic or systolic dysfunction are capable of increasing cardiac filling pressures, leading to CHF.
- Low-output failure can be defined as poor cardiac output, resulting in reduced tissue perfusion and inadequate tissue oxygenation. In general, the term *low-output failure* is used to describe clinical scenarios in which cardiac output is dramatically reduced by end-stage, primary, systolic dysfunction.
- Right-sided heart failure may result when the right atrium or right ventricle develops elevated filling pressures associated with valvular insufficiency, pericardial disease, outflow tract obstruction, or pulmonary hypertension. Volume and pressure overloading of the right ventricle can cause hepatic congestion accompanied by ascites, pleural effusion, and, rarely, peripheral subcutaneous edema. These diseases may also reduce the forward flow of blood into the pulmonary circulation and the left heart, resulting in reduced stroke volume, cardiac output, and, possibly, signs of low-output heart failure.
- Left-sided heart failure may result when the left side of the heart develops elevated filling pressures associated most commonly with valvular insufficiency, impaired contractility, or diastolic dysfunction. Elevated left ventricular filling pressures are transmitted to the left atrium and pulmonary venous and capillary beds, with the threat of fluid accumulation in the interstitial and alveolar spaces (pulmonary edema). In dogs, pleural effusion may develop when biventricular or right ventricular failure is present. Cats may have pleural effusion with pure left-sided heart failure apparently because the visceral pleural lymphatics drain into the pulmonary venous circulation. Pulmonary venous hypertension creates a functional obstruction, thereby restricting the ability of the lymphatics to maintain a normal amount of fluid in the pleural space.

DIAGNOSIS OF HEART FAILURE

KEY POINTS

- The diagnosis of CHF is considered to be multimodal, on the basis of a careful history, physical examination, and ancillary diagnostics including electrocardiography, thoracic radiography, and echocardiography.
- Good quality thoracic radiographs are invaluable in the diagnosis of many instances of left-sided heart failure.
- Exclude diseases that mimic CHF (e.g., chronic bronchointerstitial disease is often present in patients with cardiac disease).

HISTORY

- A complete medical history is important to establish the clinical course of the presenting complaint, as well as the presence of concurrent diseases that may complicate heart disease.
- Coughing, tachypnea, dyspnea (respiratory distress), exercise intolerance, lethargy, and weakness are common complaints of clients with pets with symptomatic heart disease or heart failure. Additionally, pets with heart failure may have a history of inappetence, weight loss, and syncope.
  - Coughing is a very common historical finding in dogs with heart failure, especially those with chronic MR. In this scenario, a cough reflex is associated with left atrial compression of the left mainstem bronchus. Alternatively, dogs with severe alveolar pulmonary edema may also cough. It is important to be cognizant that other, noncardiac diseases may also cause coughing and that coughing is not specific for heart failure. Diseases such as tracheal collapse and chronic pulmonary disease also cause coughing and may occur concurrently with heart disease.

- Tachypnea (increased respiratory rate) is a common sign of heart failure. Tachypnea can be caused by many nonpathologic mechanisms and is often overlooked by the client and the clinician. Left-sided CHF with interstitial pulmonary edema causes stimulation of receptors within the pulmonary interstitium that reflexively increase the respiratory rate. The increase in respiratory rate can occur with or without the presence of hypoxia. Because of this concept, the resting respiratory rate may be used effectively to monitor the status of patients with left-sided CHF. The normal resting respiratory rate for most small animals is usually below 30 to 35 breaths per minute. Typically, trends of increasing resting respiratory rate indicate progressive decompensation of left-sided heart failure and the need for cardiac medication adjustments (i.e., an increase in furosemide dosage or frequency of administration).
- Dyspnea (perception of difficult breathing) usually accompanies severe heart failure that has resulted in pulmonary edema or pleural effusion. Dyspnea is exacerbated by exercise in patients capable of exercising. This is a term used in human medicine describing how a person feels when trying to breathe. This term has been loosely applied to veterinary medicine to describe animals that have tachypnea with distress (that may manifest as anxiety and/or postural changes to facilitate ventilation).
- Orthopnea (difficult breathing during recumbency) may occur before dyspnea. Often, the client may recognize orthopnea because the patient is reluctant to lie down or because the patient has difficulty breathing when lying down.
- Nocturnal coughing or dyspnea typically occurs after the patient has been recumbent for some time. It is not specific for left-sided CHF.
- Exercise intolerance may be a very early sign of heart failure in animals that are active; however, it may be difficult to identify in animals that are inactive. Reduced tolerance for exercise results because cardiac function is abnormal, and the metabolic demands of tissues (especially the working muscles) are not met, leading to hypoxia, lactic acidemia, muscle weakness, and fatigue.
- Abdominal distention secondary to ascites may be associated with right-sided or biventricular failure and must be differentiated from effusions associated with other conditions, such as hypoproteinemia, liver disease, and abdominal neoplasia. Evaluation of the jugular and abdominal subcutaneous veins may aid in determining that ascites is associated with right-sided CHF. With right-sided heart failure, these vessels are often distended and engorged.
- Obesity paradox is an interesting clinical pearl in that dogs with obesity do not tend to be in CHF. The scenario in cats is different; obese cats can be in CHF.

CARDIOVASCULAR PHYSICAL EXAMINATION FINDINGS

MURMUR

- A cardiovascular murmur is a series of auditory vibrations associated with turbulent (nonlaminar) blood flow and, occasionally, with vibrating valve leaflets. When blood flow velocities are supraphysiologic (i.e., higher than normal physiologic velocities) or when blood viscosity is reduced (e.g., with anemia), blood flow tends to be nonlaminar and turbulent. Nonlaminar blood flow generates acoustic energy that vibrates the structures within the heart or the associated vessel(s). The intensity (loudness), timing in the cardiac cycle, frequency (pitch), configuration (shape), quality, duration, location, and direction of radiation of the sound created by the blood flow are important characteristics of cardiac murmurs.
  - The intensity of the murmur refers to the loudness of the murmur and is graded on a scale from 1 to 6 (1 being the least audible murmur and 6 being the loudest).
  - The timing is defined as being systolic, diastolic, or continuous.
  - The configuration of the murmur refers to the shape of the sound created by the abnormal blood flow and is described as being either a plateau (regurgitant murmur) or a crescendo-decrescendo (ejection murmur) sound.
  - A cardiac murmur is present in many dogs with heart failure, but the presence of a cardiac murmur is not specific for heart failure.

CARDIAC RHYTHM DISTURBANCES

- Arrhythmias are relatively common in animals with heart failure.
  - Atrial fibrillation is a common supraventricular arrhythmia present in some dogs with DCM and chronic MR secondary to primary valve disease, as well as in cats with cardiomyopathy.
  - Ventricular tachyarrhythmias may be present in dogs with heart failure or with extracardiac disease, such as thoracic trauma, splenic

disease, and gastric dilatation-volvulus. Ventricular arrhythmias are especially common in Boxers and Doberman Pinschers with cardiomyopathy.

- Bradyarrhythmias such as third-degree (complete) atrioventricular block may cause signs of reduced cardiac output (lethargy, weakness, and exercise intolerance) and, occasionally, CHF.
- Gallop sounds are abnormal heart sounds in dogs and cats that are often associated with heart failure. A third heart sound (S_3) gallop occurs just after the second heart sound (S_2) during the rapid diastolic phase of ventricular filling. An S_3 gallop occurs commonly in dogs with heart failure associated with volume overload, particularly dogs with DCM. During early diastolic filling, blood rushes out of the atrium into a noncompliant ventricle, which then vibrates, resulting in a low-frequency sound just after S_2. A fourth heart sound (S_4) gallop occurs just before the first heart sound (S_1) and is associated with atrial contraction. Ventricular filling in late diastole associated with atrial contraction vibrates the noncompliant ventricle, creating a low-frequency sound just before S_1 and the onset of systole. S_4 gallops are commonly auscultated in cats with hypertrophic or RCM. Summation gallops (S_3 and S_4) may occur during periods of tachycardia.

DIAGNOSTICS
BIOMARKERS
Natriuretic Peptides

- Circulating natriuretic peptides are elevated in patients with significant cardiac remodeling or ventricular dilation. These levels may be used in combination with other diagnostic tests (discussed later) to differentiate between symptoms associated with cardiac disease and symptoms associated with primary pulmonary disease. The commercially available test evaluates the N-terminal pro–B-type natriuretic peptide molecule (NT-ProBNP) because the BNP molecule is relatively labile. Normal BNP levels help rule out a diagnosis of CHF. In general, dogs with chronic valvular disease have a progressive increase in NT-ProBNP levels with a significant increase during the 3- to 6-month period before symptomatic CHF. NT-ProBNP levels can be used to identify cats with occult cardiomyopathy. It is important to note that NT-ProBNP levels can be elevated with renal insufficiency and pulmonary hypertension. To this end, NT-ProBNP levels may be helpful in monitoring the response to therapy for pulmonary hypertension.

Cardiac Troponin-I

- This regulatory protein of the contractile apparatus is released into the serum as a result of myocardial cell damage, much like alanine transferase is released in the presence of hepatocellular damage. The most common causes of increased cardiac troponin-I are myocardial ischemia, myocarditis, neoplasia, gastric dilation-volvulus, and sepsis.

ELECTROCARDIOGRAPHY

- Electrocardiography is used to detect cardiac rhythm disturbances, chamber enlargement, or conduction abnormalities that may be associated with cardiac disease. Electrocardiographic abnormalities are not specific for heart failure and therefore should not be used to determine the presence of heart failure. Furthermore, a normal electrocardiogram does not rule out the possibility of severe heart disease with secondary chamber enlargement.

THORACIC RADIOGRAPHY

- Thoracic radiography is important in the evaluation of patients with suspected heart disease or CHF. In general, with respect to heart disease and heart failure, three questions should be answered when evaluating a thoracic radiograph:
  - Is cardiomegaly present? If so, which side of the heart is affected? The vertebral heart score (VHS) is a method of evaluating the size of the heart on a lateral thoracic radiographic view. The height or long axis of the heart (measured from the carina to the apex) and the width or short axis (measured at the widest part of the heart; perpendicular to the long axis) of the heart are measured and expressed as the number of vertebral bodies beginning with T4, measured caudally (normal: dogs 9.7 ± 0.5; cats 6.7 to 8.1). This score is reliable in dogs older than 3 months of age into adulthood. There is variation between breeds (Pugs, Pomeranians, Yorkshire Terriers, Dachshunds, Bulldogs, Shih Tzus, Lhasa Apsos, Boston Terriers, Cavalier King Charles Spaniels, Boxers, and Labrador Retrievers can have increased VHS as a normal finding).
  - What is the pulmonary vascular pattern (e.g., normal, undercirculated, overcirculated, venous distention, or arterial distention)?
  - Is there evidence of heart failure (pulmonary edema, pleural effusion, or ascites)?
- With compensated left-sided heart failure, the earliest evidence of pulmonary edema formation is pulmonary venous congestion (stage I

of pulmonary edema formation). That is, the pulmonary veins are distended and larger than their respective arteries. At this time, pulmonary capillary pressures are approximately 15 to 20 mm Hg.

- As pulmonary venous and capillary pressures progressively increase with left-sided heart failure, decompensation occurs, and fluid leaks into the interstitium (interstitial edema, stage II).
- As pulmonary venous and capillary pressures continue to rise (e.g., 30 to 40 mm Hg), the alveoli are flooded with edema fluid, and stage III (alveolar edema) is present.
- Cardiogenic pulmonary edema may be primarily perihilar (centrally located) in distribution, or it may be diffuse and generalized. As the edema progressively becomes more generalized, it is commonly noted first in the right caudal lung lobe. In cats, pulmonary edema may appear as a patchy mixed interstitial-alveolar pattern that is not primarily located in the perihilar region.
- Pleural effusion may be evident in cases with biventricular or severe right-sided heart failure in dogs and may be present with left-sided or biventricular heart failure in cats.

ECHOCARDIOGRAPHY

- The three principal modalities of echocardiography are two-dimensional, M-mode, and Doppler evaluation of the heart. Because of the noninvasive nature of echocardiography, it has essentially replaced cardiac catheterization in the diagnosis of heart disease in small animals. Echocardiography enables the trained specialist to identify diseases that may cause or be associated with heart failure, such as:
  - Valvular leaks
  - Myocardial failure
  - Intracardiac or extracardiac shunts
  - Decreased ventricular compliance
  - Pericardial disease
- The combination of thoracic radiographs and echocardiography allows the clinician to define structural heart disease and identify CHF in most cases. Typically, heart failure is not present without atrial enlargement (with the exception of pericardial diseases and some other uncommon diseases). The atria are usually compliant and enlarge as filling pressures increase.

DIFFERENTIAL DIAGNOSES

- Primary pulmonary disease may mimic cardiac disease or failure because both may cause coughing, abnormal bronchovesicular sounds, and respiratory distress. The presence of pulmonary crackles, a respiratory sinus arrhythmia, and respiratory distress in a dog without

a cardiac murmur is almost always associated with pulmonary disease rather than with heart failure.
- Ascites and pleural effusion may occur secondary to diseases other than heart failure. Evaluation of the jugular veins may aid in differentiating ascites associated with heart failure from ascites associated with hypoproteinemia secondary to liver or renal disease.

THERAPY OF HEART FAILURE

- In 2009, representatives from the American College of Veterinary Internal Medicine (ACVIM) Specialty of Cardiology published a consensus statement regarding the guidelines for diagnosis and treatment of CHF in dogs with chronic valvular heart disease. They used a classification of heart failure with the goal of linking the severity of clinical signs with the appropriate treatment for that stage of the disease.
- Heart failure classification
  Stage A: Predisposed to heart disease
  Stage B: Heart disease present
    Stage B1: Heart disease present with no evidence of cardiac remodeling
    Stage B2: Heart disease present with evidence of cardiac remodeling (chamber enlargement)
  Stage C: Heart disease with clinical signs of heart failure
  Stage D: Heart disease with clinical signs of refractory heart failure
(see later for specific treatment strategies)
- The medical management of heart failure is aimed at relieving symptoms and cardiac dysfunction because, in most cases, heart disease and heart failure are not curable. In addition to relieving heart failure symptoms, heart failure therapy is directed toward increasing the patient's survival time.
- Signs of congestion can be treated with agents that reduce cardiac filling pressures (preload reducers such as diuretics and venodilators) and agents that facilitate cardiac performance (positive inotropes and arterial dilators). Modulation of the compensatory mechanisms (e.g., RAAS system, inflammatory cytokines) that exacerbate chronic heart failure is important in the therapy of heart failure.
- Monotherapy with diuretics and simply restricting dietary sodium intake are no longer accepted therapies for treating chronic heart failure. In fact, these therapies may actually promote activation of the compensatory mechanisms that are responsible for overloading the failing heart.
- It is important to note that the appropriate therapy for a given patient is determined by the clinical signs present, their severity, and the underlying disease entity.

- Combinations of angiotensin-converting enzyme (ACE) inhibitors, diuretics, and pimobendan represent the conventional therapy for chronic heart failure. In addition, modulation of aldosterone activity with spironolactone appears to have a positive effect on outcome. Adjunctive therapy in selected patients may include additional agents for heart rate control, nutritional supplementation (e.g., taurine, fish oils), or additional medications for refractory symptomatic heart failure.
  - *Occult heart disease* refers to disease that has resulted in the first detectable changes associated with heart disease (myocardial dysfunction, chamber dilation, arrhythmias). This description is usually used to describe patients with cardiomyopathy (e.g., Doberman Pinschers with idiopathic DCM). Recent studies have demonstrated that therapy with benazepril or pimobendan can delay clinical signs of CHF in Doberman Pinschers with DCM.

THERAPEUTIC STRATEGIES FOR THE MANAGEMENT OF HEART FAILURE

DIETARY MODIFICATIONS

- A reduction in dietary sodium intake can blunt the tendency to conserve sodium and to develop edema. Theoretically, the use of low-sodium diets in combination with vasodilators and ACE inhibitors may allow for less reliance on diuretics to control edema and signs of congestion. Early in the course of heart failure, dietary sodium restriction should be in the form of elimination of high-salt–containing snacks. Mild to moderate salt restriction may be helpful if CHF is present. Severe salt restriction may cause sodium conservation through the RAAS, causing further progression of heart failure. Reduced dietary sodium intake stimulates the synthesis and secretion of aldosterone. Another disadvantage is the unpalatable nature of such diets. General recommendations for dietary sodium intake levels in patients with heart disease are as follows:
  - Asymptomatic heart disease: avoid high-sodium diets (recommend <100 mg/100 kcal)
  - Early CHF: mild sodium restriction (recommend <80 mg/100 kcal)
  - Severe CHF: more aggressive sodium restriction may be beneficial

KEY POINT

The general theme regarding sodium restriction in patients with heart failure is to avoid treats or foods with excessive sodium content.

- **L-Carnitine** supplementation may be indicated in patients that have myocardial failure associated with definitive myocardial L-carnitine deficiency. Some Boxers with cardiomyopathy may respond to L-carnitine supplementation. In most cases, however, it is likely that myocardial L-carnitine deficiency is a result of the underlying disease and myocardial failure rather than the cause of the myocardial failure. The dosage for L-carnitine supplementation in dogs is 50 to 100 mg/kg PO q8h.
- Taurine supplementation (sometimes in combination with L-carnitine) has been effective in reversing some secondary DCMs associated with taurine deficiency in cats, American Cocker Spaniels, and other Spaniel breeds. The addition of taurine to feline diets after 1987 dramatically reduced the incidence of taurine deficiency–induced DCM in cats. Although DCM secondary to taurine deficiency in cats is uncommonly encountered today, it is prudent to evaluate plasma taurine levels or to supplement taurine on a trial basis in all cats with DCM. In patients with taurine deficiency–induced DCM, supplementation with taurine results in clinical and echocardiographic improvement typically within 2 to 3 months (the Multicenter Spaniel Trial [MUST]). Dosage for taurine supplementation:
  - Dogs: 500 to 1000 mg PO q12-24h.
  - Cats: 250 to 500 mg PO q12-24h.
- The n-3 polyunsaturated fatty acids levels are reduced in dogs with CHF, and fish oil supplementation can normalize these plasma fatty acid abnormalities. I currently recommend a fish oil dosage to provide 40 mg/kg/day EPA (eicosapentaenoic acid) and 25 mg/kg/day DHA (docosahexaenoic acid) for patients with heart failure; fish oil has a positive effect on appetite and reduces cardiac cachexia, particularly if started before the development of cachexia. Fish oil supplementation is associated with a decrease in ventricular ectopy in Boxers with arrhythmogenic right ventricular cardiomyopathy.

VASODILATOR THERAPY

- Indications: Arterial vasodilators are used to reduce systemic vascular resistance in patients with CHF. In doing so, cardiac function is improved. Myocardial systolic wall tension is an important determinant of myocardial oxygen consumption. By decreasing systemic vascular resistance (and, therefore, afterload and systolic wall tension), arterial vasodilators reduce myocardial oxygen consumption. In addition, the reduction in afterload results in an increase

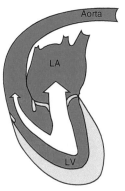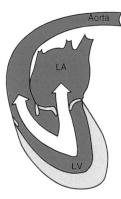

Figure 16.3 Drawings of the left side of the heart from a dog with severe mitral regurgitation (MR) before and after administration of an afterload-reducing agent. Note that forward flow (out the aorta) increases with afterload reduction because of the reduction in systemic vascular resistance. *LA*, Left atrium; *LV*, left ventricle.

in cardiac output. Arterial vasodilators decrease the volume of regurgitation across an insufficient valve and, therefore, increase forward flow in patients with mitral or aortic regurgitation (Figure 16.3). Arterial vasodilators may lessen the magnitude of left-to-right shunting in patients with ventricular septal defects. However, arterial vasodilators may exacerbate right-to-left shunting in patients with tetralogy of Fallot or with nonrestrictive ventricular septal defects.

- Indications: Venous vasodilators are used to reduce congestive symptoms by redistributing blood volume within the circulatory system (the capacitance vessels and the splanchnic veins) and reducing venous return, which results in lower filling pressures (preload).
  - Classification of vasodilators based on vessels affected
    - Arterial (e.g., hydralazine)
    - Venous (e.g., nitroglycerin, isosorbide dinitrate)
    - Mixed (e.g., nitroprusside, prazosin, ACE inhibitors, pimobendan)
  - Classification of vasodilators based on mechanism of action
    - Direct acting (e.g., nitroprusside, nitroglycerin, isosorbide dinitrate, hydralazine)
    - Alpha-adrenergic blocking agents (e.g., prazosin)
    - Calcium channel-blocking agents (e.g., amlodipine, verapamil, diltiazem)
    - ACE inhibitors (e.g., captopril, enalapril, lisinopril, benazepril)
    - Phosphodiesterase (PDE) inhibitors (e.g., pimobendan)

ANGIOTENSIN-CONVERTING ENZYME INHIBITORS

- ACE inhibitors cause mixed vasodilation by preventing the conversion of angiotensin I to angiotensin II. Angiotensin II is a potent vasoconstrictor. The decrease in angiotensin II levels results in a reduction in the level of vasoconstriction as well as decreased SNS activity. ACE inhibition also results in decreased aldosterone synthesis and secretion so that there is less sodium and water retention, among many other benefits beyond the scope of this discussion.
- Several large, multicenter clinical trials have demonstrated the safety and efficacy of ACE inhibitors in the therapy of CHF secondary to DCM and primary valve disease. ACE inhibitors significantly decrease the clinical signs of heart failure, improve the quality of life, and decrease mortality when used in combination with conventional therapy (diuretics and pimobendan). Enalapril has been extensively studied in veterinary medicine (this list is not exhaustive): Invasive Multicenter Prospective Veterinary Enalapril (IMPROVE) study, the Cooperative Veterinary Enalapril (COVE) study, the Long Term Investigation of Enalapril (LIVE), the Benazepril in Canine Heart Disease study group (BENCH and BENCH II), and many others. Enalapril is approved for use in dogs in the United States.
- In general, there is no clear indication for therapy with ACE inhibitors in patients with asymptomatic chronic valve disease. This is particularly true for dogs without left atrial enlargement. Two large, multicenter, placebo-controlled, double-blind studies (SVEP and VetPROOF) were unable to demonstrate a delay in symptomatic heart failure in patients with chronic valve disease when given enalapril. However, some clinicians initiate ACE inhibitor therapy in patients with valve disease with severe cardiomegaly, pulmonary venous hypertension, pulmonary arterial hypertension, or systemic hypertension (>150 to 160 mm Hg average systolic pressure).
- ACE inhibitors should not be used as a primary agent (monotherapy) in emergency treatment for acute CHF. Significant clinical improvement attributable to ACE inhibition may not be evident until 2 to 3 weeks after initiation of therapy.
- Side effects associated with ACE inhibitor therapy occur infrequently.
- Anorexia or inappetence, vomiting, hypotension, and azotemia are the most common side effects of ACE inhibitor therapy. Azotemia secondary to decreased renal perfusion represents

the most important clinical consideration. Azotemia and renal dysfunction secondary to a decrease in renal perfusion result from loss of protective mechanisms to maintain filtration pressures. Angiotensin II causes vasoconstriction of the renal efferent arterioles in an effort to maintain glomerular filtration pressures in the face of decreased renal perfusion. The relative decrease in angiotensin II can significantly decrease glomerular perfusion and filtration, resulting in azotemia. Furthermore, renal dysfunction is more likely to occur in patients with preexisting renal disease. As a result, renal function should be evaluated before and 5 to 7 days after instituting ACE inhibitor therapy and every 2 to 3 months thereafter, especially during concurrent diuretic therapy.

- Most complications are likely to occur shortly after beginning therapy, in association with acute cardiac decompensation or in conjunction with systemic disease that may alter the patient's hydration status (e.g., vomiting or diarrhea). Side effects are much more likely to occur with captopril than with the other commonly used ACE inhibitors.

KEY POINT

ACE inhibitors are recommended for patients with asymptomatic myocardial dysfunction; in patients with symptomatic CHF secondary to chronic valvular disease, DCM, and other causes of CHF; and in patients with systemic hypertension.

- Agents and dosages
  - **Enalapril**
    - Dogs: 0.5 mg/kg PO q12-24h
    - Cats: 0.25 to 0.5 mg/kg PO q12-24h
  - **Imidapril**
    - Dogs and Cats: 0.5 mg/kg PO q24h
  - **Benazepril**
    - Dogs: 0.25 to 0.5 mg/kg PO q12-24h
    - Cats: 0.25 to 0.5 mg/kg PO q12-24h
  - **Ramipril**
    - Dogs: 0.125 mg/kg PO q12h
    - Cats: 0.5 mg/kg PO q24h

CALCIUM CHANNEL-BLOCKING AGENTS

- Verapamil, diltiazem, nifedipine, and amlodipine are calcium channel-blocking agents. In general, they differ with regard to their antiarrhythmic effects, their vasodilating effects, and their negative inotropic effects.
- Verapamil is used primarily (intravenously) for the short-term control of supraventricular arrhythmias (negative chronotropic effect).

It possesses minimal vasodilating properties but exerts a significant and sometimes detrimental negative inotropic effect in patients with heart failure.

- Nifedipine is a more potent vasodilator with more limited direct effects on the heart than verapamil. Nifedipine is not commonly used in veterinary medicine.
- Diltiazem's vasodilating action is weaker than that of nifedipine and more pronounced than that of verapamil. Diltiazem exerts a negligible negative inotropic effect in normal, conscious dogs, but when given rapidly intravenously, it may cause a pronounced negative inotropic effect in animals with heart failure. The antiarrhythmic and negative chronotropic effects of diltiazem are similar to those of verapamil. A positive lusitropic (enhanced relaxation) effect may also be associated the administration of diltiazem to cats with HCM.
- Agents and dosages
  - **Diltiazem**
    - Dogs: 0.5 to 2.0 mg/kg PO q8-12h
    - Cats: 7.5 mg PO q8-12h or 45 to 60 mg PO every day of sustained-release formulations
  - **Amlodipine**
    - Primarily used as therapy for systemic hypertension in cats and dogs
    - Dogs: 0.05 to 0.2 mg/kg PO q12-24h
    - Cats: 0.625 to 1.25 mg PO q12-24h
- In general, I use calcium channel blockers (1) to control heart rate and to facilitate ventricular filling and relaxation in cats with HCM; (2) to supplement therapy for control of the ventricular response rate in some supraventricular tachycardias, such as atrial fibrillation, in dogs and cats; and (3) to treat systemic (amlodipine) and pulmonary (diltiazem) hypertension.

DIRECT-ACTING ARTERIAL VASODILATORS
HYDRALAZINE

- Hydralazine has been evaluated in dogs with spontaneous CHF secondary to MR.
- Hydralazine has been shown to decrease MR, increase forward flow, reduce left atrial pressures, and improve exercise capacity. Whereas these studies provide a reasonable basis for the short-term use of hydralazine in dogs with decompensated left-sided heart failure caused by MR, poor patient tolerance and lack of owner compliance limit the usefulness of hydralazine for long-term therapy.
- I currently use hydralazine only in cases with refractory heart failure associated with MR that no longer are responding well to ACE inhibitor–diuretic–pimobendan combination therapy. I do not use hydralazine in cats.

- Onset of action for orally administered hydralazine is approximately 1 hour, the peak effect is achieved within 3 hours, and the effect remains stable for several hours, with a total duration of effect of about 12 hours.
- Agents and Dosages
  - **Hydralazine:**
    - Dogs: Initial dose at 0.5 mg/kg PO; the dose is gradually increased until a clinical response is elicited or up to a maximum dose of 3.0 mg/kg BID. The endpoints of drug titration can be determined by the veterinarian by monitoring blood pressure, by observing the patient's clinical response, and by obtaining radiographic evidence that pulmonary edema has resolved.
    - Cats: 2.5 mg PO q12-24h.
  - Hydralazine may play a role in emergency therapy for severe MR secondary to ruptured chordae tendineae.
- Many side effects are associated with hydralazine and limit its usefulness
  - Hypotension
  - Gastrointestinal disturbances
  - Reflex tachycardia
  - Furthermore, there is evidence of enhanced neurohormonal activity (increased aldosterone levels) in dogs receiving hydralazine.

SODIUM NITROPRUSSIDE

- Nitroprusside is the only direct-acting mixed vasodilator available (not approved) for use in dogs with CHF. It is an extremely potent vasodilator that is primarily used to rescue dogs with severe, decompensated CHF associated with MR or DCM.
- The indications for nitroprusside therapy are short-term treatment of refractory, life-threatening CHF in dogs with MR or DCM or critical systemic hypertension. Combination therapy with dobutamine, digoxin and/or pimobendan, and diuretics provides the best effect.
- Agents and dosages
  - **Nitroprusside**
    - Dogs: Intravenous (IV) constant rate infusion at an initial rate of 1.0 µg/kg/min (following dilution in 5% dextrose), titrated to effect by monitoring blood pressure and pulmonary capillary wedge pressure to a maximum dose of 10 µg/kg/min.
  - Hypotension, tachycardia, nausea, and vomiting are the most significant adverse effects of nitroprusside administration.
  - Cyanide poisoning may also occur with chronic administration.

- Hypotension is easily managed by slowing the rate or by discontinuing the infusion (nitroprusside has a very short half-life).

VENOUS VASODILATORS (NITROGLYCERIN, ISOSORBIDE DINITRATE)

- These nitrate vasodilators are excellent preload reducers, although their efficacy in dogs and cats is controversial and unproven. The development of nitrate tolerance limits the continuous use (i.e., more than 36 hours) of these agents. Tolerance may be avoided by intermittent use (24 hours on and 24 hours off) and possibly concurrent use of ACE inhibitors.
- Agents and dosages
  - **2% nitroglycerin** paste
    - Dogs: ¼ to 2 inches cutaneously q6-8h for 24-48h.
    - Cats: ⅛ to ¼ inch cutaneously q6-8h for 24-48h.
    - Nitroglycerin paste should be applied to hairless areas such as the pinna or the axillary region. If perfusion to the ears is poor (e.g., ears are cold), the axilla or groin will provide better absorption. Because nitroglycerin is absorbed transcutaneously, gloves should be worn during administration.
  - **Isosorbide dinitrate**
    - Dogs: 0.2 to 1.0 mg/kg PO q8h

ALPHA-ADRENERGIC RECEPTOR ANTAGONISTS (PRAZOSIN)

- The use of prazosin has been reported in dogs with CHF, but neither its short-term hemodynamic nor long-term clinical effects have been documented. Current indications for its use appear to be limited to the short-term treatment of acute heart failure when other agents are ineffective or contraindicated. It is rarely used in veterinary medicine.
- Agents and dosages
  - **Prazosin,** titrated to effect
    - Small dogs and cats: 0.25 to 1 mg PO q8h
    - Medium dogs (<40 lb): 1 to 3 mg PO q8h
    - Large dogs (>40 lb): 3 to 10 mg PO q8h

DIURETIC THERAPY
LOOP DIURETICS
Furosemide

- The mechanism of action of loop diuretics is the reversible inhibition of the sodium/potassium/chloride cotransporter in the thick ascending limb of the loop of Henle.

- Furosemide is the most commonly used agent in this class of diuretics because it is potent and has a fast onset of action. The result is the obligatory loss of sodium and water into the urine. IV and intramuscular (IM) furosemide acutely increases venous capacitance secondary to release of vasodilatory prostaglandins. This vasodilatory effect occurs within the first 20 minutes after IV or IM administration, and the peak diuretic effect occurs after 30 to 45 minutes.
- Of interest to the clinician, there is a bioavailability difference between furosemide and generic oral formulations; I therefore do not recommend switching back and forth from one formulation to the other.
- The peak effect after oral administration of furosemide is 30 minutes to 2 hours.
- Agents and dosages
  - **Furosemide**
    - Chronic oral administration
      - Dogs: 2 to 3 mg/kg PO q8-12h
      - Cats: 1 to 2 mg/kg PO q12-24h
    - Parenteral administration (IM or IV)
      - Dogs: 2 to 8 mg/kg as needed to control edema
      - Cats: 1 to 2 mg/kg as needed to control edema
      - Continuous-rate infusion: 0.66 mg/kg IV bolus followed by 0.66 mg/kg/hr
- Adverse side effects of furosemide include electrolyte abnormalities, such as hypokalemia, hyponatremia, and hypochloremia (hypochloremic metabolic alkalosis).
- Typically, drug withdrawal or a dose reduction results in resolution of the alkalosis. Severe metabolic alkalosis can be treated with judicious use of half-strength saline with or without 2.5% dextrose. Overzealous diuretic therapy may cause dehydration, low cardiac output, and, possibly, circulatory collapse. Furthermore, diuretics activate systemic compensatory mechanisms, such as the RAAS and SNS.
- In the therapy of heart failure, furosemide should always be used in combination with an ACE inhibitor; chronic furosemide monotherapy is not recommended.
- Diuretic resistance: Potential mechanisms include activation of neurohormonal systems, hypertrophy of nephron segments, and increased renal solute absorption in portions of the nephron other than the loop of Henle. Diuretic resistance has been shown in dogs receiving doses of furosemide as low as 2 mg/kg and for durations as short as 14 days. Resistance could be lessened by administration of diuretics with different pharmacologic and pharmacokinetic properties. In humans, the dose of furosemide is a marker of heart failure severity and independently predicts long-term mortality. Therefore strategies to prevent diuretic resistance and minimize diuretic dose might improve long-term outcome.

Torsemide

- Although similar to furosemide, this loop diuretic is more potent (approximately 10 times the strength of furosemide) and has a longer duration, less potassium excretion in dogs, and less diuretic resistance than furosemide.
- Antialdosterone effects
- Used in patients with refractory CHF and/or furosemide resistance.
- Agents and dosages
  - **Torsemide**
    - Chronic oral administration
      - Dogs: 0.2 to 0.3 mg/kg PO q8-12h
      - Cats: 0.1 to 0.2 mg/kg PO q12-24h

THIAZIDE DIURETICS (CHLOROTHIAZIDE, HYDROCHLOROTHIAZIDE)

- Thiazide diuretics act by inhibiting distal tubule electrolyte reabsorption. These diuretics are less potent natriuretic agents and are usually not successful in controlling signs of congestion when used as a monotherapy. In general, thiazide diuretics are administered when heart failure is refractory and conventional therapy (pimobendan, ACE inhibitor, and furosemide) fails to control the clinical signs of congestion.
  - Agents and dosages
    - **Chlorothiazide:** 20 to 40 mg/kg PO q12-24h
    - **Hydrochlorothiazide:** 2 to 4 mg/kg PO q12-24h

POTASSIUM-SPARING DIURETICS

Spironolactone

- In general, the potassium-sparing diuretics are weak diuretics that are rarely used alone to control edema in heart failure patients. They are often used together with a more potent diuretic to control refractory edema. More recently, studies have demonstrated a positive effect on mortality, including a decrease in risk of cardiac-related death or worsening of CHF. Although a consensus regarding the use of spironolactone as standard therapy was not reached at the time of the 2009 ACVIM Consensus Statement, these recent findings will make spironolactone a part of standard therapy with ACE inhibitors, furosemide, and pimobendan in patients with stage C and D heart failure. They may also have a role in stage B2.
- Because of their potassium-sparing effects, they should be used with caution with concurrent ACE inhibitor therapy. This is an uncommon side effect.

- Spironolactone, an aldosterone antagonist, is usually used in conjunction with furosemide.
- Aldosterone antagonism may provide a cardio-protective effect by reversing and inhibiting myocardial and vascular fibrosis. The antialdosterone effect may prove to be an important part in the management of chronic heart failure, particularly in patients with "aldosterone escape" (a non-RAAS-associated increase in aldosterone).
- Agents and dosages
  - **Spironolactone:**
  - 1 to 2 mg/kg PO q12-24h.

- The appropriate timing for the initiation of spironolactone or other aldosterone antagonist therapy is not clear at this time. The author routinely administers spironolactone to patients with refractory heart failure.
- Administration of spironolactone may also be appropriate in patients with evidence of myocardial remodeling.
- Spironolactone may reduce the risk of hypokalemia in patients treated with chronic furosemide therapy.

DIGITALIS GLYCOSIDE THERAPY

Digoxin

- Digoxin acts by inhibiting sarcolemmal Na^+, K^+-ATPase, which causes an accumulation of sodium that is then available for exchange with extracellular calcium through the Na^+-Ca^{++} exchanger. The exchange results in increased intracellular calcium. Calcium is then available for interaction with the sarcoplasmic reticulum (calcium-induced release of sarcoplasmic reticular calcium), and therefore the release of more calcium for interaction with the contractile elements (positive inotropic effect). Digitalis glycosides shift the Frank-Starling curve upward by increasing the velocity and force of contraction of the myocardium at any given level of preload. In addition, digitalis glycosides slow conduction through the atrioventricular node by both direct and vagal effects. Digoxin may also partially restore baroreceptor reflexes that are desensitized by the chronically elevated sympathetic tone associated with CHF.
- Indications for digoxin therapy:
  - Digoxin is typically reserved for patients with supraventricular tachyarrhythmias (such as atrial fibrillation) for heart rate control and can be used in combination with either diltiazem or sotalol (a class III antiarrhythmic agent).

- Method of administration
  - Oral and IV routes of administration are available for digoxin. In most cases where indicated, digoxin can be administered orally at maintenance levels, with the desired effect occurring 3 to 5 days after initiation (depending on the patient).
- Agents and dosages
  - **Digoxin**
    - Rapid IV digoxin (not recommended)
      - Dogs: 0.0025 mg/kg IV bolus, repeat hourly 3 to 4 times (total up to 0.01 mg/kg)
      - Arrhythmias may be the first sign of toxicity with IV digoxin
    - Rapid oral digoxin (not recommended)
      - Dogs: Rapid oral digitalization can be used in animals that require therapeutic blood levels before the 72 to 92 hours required with maintenance dosage schedules; however, rapid oral digitalization (similar to IV digitalization) is usually not necessary. I typically administer digoxin at the maintenance dose instead of rapid digitalization.
    - Maintenance oral digoxin dose
      - Dogs: 0.22 mg/m² PO twice a day or 0.002 to 0.005 mg/kg PO q12h
      - Cats: One fourth of a 0.125-mg tablet PO every day or every other day (approximately 0.008 mg/kg every day or every other day). Serum digoxin levels should be determined 5 to 7 days after initiation of therapy (therapeutic serum levels = 1.0 to 2.0 ng/mL in most laboratories [8 to 12 hours after dosing]). The oral dose is then adjusted based on this trough serum level.

Initiate digoxin at a chronic oral maintenance dosage of 0.002 to 0.004 mg/kg q12h and never use other methods (IV or rapid oral) to initiate therapy. The most common indication for digoxin therapy is heart rate control in patients with supraventricular tachyarrhythmias. Digoxin can be used in patients that cannot tolerate pimobendan and need chronic inotropic support.

- There are several special tips regarding the use of digoxin. A 20-lb dog usually gets 1 mL of the 0.05 mg/mL elixir; a 10-lb dog gets 0.5 mL, and so forth. *Do not use the elixir in cats because it makes them froth at the mouth.* The elixir has a small amount of alcohol in it, which may cause gastrointestinal disturbance without drug toxicity.

Signs of digitalization include the following: slowing of the heart rate, relief of clinical signs of heart failure, increased PR interval (unreliable), and demonstration of therapeutic blood levels (a therapeutic trough level of digoxin is 1 to 2 ng/mL; animals with serum levels greater than 3 ng/mL usually demonstrate signs of toxicity).

- *Determinants of digoxin dosages*
  - Many factors (such as dosage form, electrolyte status, renal status, thyroid status, and concurrent medications) affect the serum levels attained in a particular patient receiving digoxin.
  - Digoxin elixir is more completely absorbed than the tablet form, resulting in higher blood levels at a given dosage. Do not switch patients back and forth from one to the other.
  - Hypokalemia and hypercalcemia are associated with the development of digitalis toxicity at lower digoxin doses. Electrolyte status should be monitored periodically (every 2 to 3 months) or after changes in therapy (i.e., increases in furosemide or ACE inhibitor) or in the patient's clinical status.
  - Concurrent medications such as quinidine, verapamil, and drugs that inhibit hepatic microsomal enzymes (tetracycline, chloramphenicol) may result in increased digoxin serum levels, requiring a reduction in digoxin dosage. Use an alternative to quinidine whenever possible (e.g., procainamide).
  - Hypothyroid animals often require less digoxin than euthyroid animals. Hyperthyroid animals may also require a decreased dose. Digoxin is excreted primarily by the kidneys. The presence of renal dysfunction often necessitates a reduction in digoxin dosage or frequency of administration.
  - Dosage should be based on lean body weight. Obesity, pregnancy, or the presence of ascites should be noted, and the dose should be adjusted accordingly.
- *Adverse and toxic effects of digitalis glycosides*
  - Caution must be used when administering digitalis glycosides intravenously. When given rapidly intravenously, they have direct vasoconstrictive effects.
  - The main determinants of myocardial oxygen consumption are the ventricular wall tension, heart rate, and state of contractility. Increased contractility associated with digoxin therapy results in increased myocardial oxygen consumption that is usually offset by the decrease in heart rate and ventricular size (and thus wall tension) and increased coronary perfusion.

- The signs of toxicity are variable but in general fall into one or more of three following categories:
  - Neurologic (lethargy and depression)
  - Gastrointestinal (inappetence, anorexia, diarrhea, nausea, vomiting)
  - Cardiac (arrhythmia)
- With oral administration, gastrointestinal signs almost always occur before arrhythmias. Some of the more common arrhythmias associated with digitalis toxicity are first- and second-degree atrioventricular block, accelerated junctional rhythms, ventricular premature complexes, ventricular tachycardias, and atrioventricular dissociation. A nonrespiratory sinus arrhythmia in a patient receiving digoxin may indicate high serum levels.
- The treatment of digoxin toxicosis is based on its elimination half-life, and the goal is to return digoxin serum levels to within target range (0.8 to 1.0 ng/mL). In healthy dogs, the serum half-life of digoxin is approximately 24 to 36 hours. Therefore it takes about 1½ days to decrease the serum level to half the original level.
- **CASE EXAMPLE:** If the starting serum level is 6 ng/mL and the drug is discontinued for 1½ days, the serum level should be around 3 ng/mL (still in the toxic range). If the drug is discontinued for another 1½ days, the serum level should drop from 3 ng/mL to 1.5 ng/mL. Therefore, in this example, the digoxin should be discontinued for approximately 3 to 4 days and then continued at approximately one third of the original dose to achieve serum levels in the therapeutic range. Check electrolyte status and correct hypokalemia if present. Life-threatening arrhythmias may be treated with atropine, lidocaine, or a beta blocker (depending on the arrhythmia present). Additionally, a specific antidote (Fab-antibody fragments that scavenge the free drug from the body) is available, but its use may be cost prohibitive.

PIMOBENDAN (THE "INODILATOR")

- Pimobendan, in combination with diuretics and an ACE inhibitor, is standard therapy for patients with CHF secondary to degenerative valve disease and DCM.
- Pimobendan is a benzimidazole-pyridazinone agent with PDE III inhibitor activity, resulting in positive inotropic and vasodilatory effects. The mechanism of action is an increase in cardiac levels of cyclic adenosine monophosphate (cAMP) by inhibition of PDE. Increased cAMP levels mediate increased calcium delivery to the

contractile elements of the myocyte, as well as possibly increasing calcium availability by augmenting the storage and release of calcium by the sarcoplasmic reticulum. Increases in cAMP in vascular smooth muscle result in muscular relaxation and a direct-acting arterial vasodilator effect. Furthermore, an increase in calcium sensitivity of the contractile proteins results in additional positive inotropy. Current studies have demonstrated increased survival times and improved quality of life in patients with CHF (stage C and D) secondary to DCM or chronic valve disease. Pimobendan delays the onset of clinical signs in Doberman Pinschers with occult DCM (stage B). Pimobendan is also beneficial for pulmonary hypertension secondary to chronic left-sided CHF and other disease scenarios resulting in myocardial failure, such as heartworm disease and congenital heart disease.
- Pimobendan is tolerated by cats despite the differing pharmacokinetics (longer elimination half-life and higher plasma levels); pimobendan should be avoided in hypotensive patients with obstructive HCM.
- Agent and dosages
  - **Pimobendan**
    - Dogs: Standard dosage is 0.25 mg/kg BID q12h
    - Cats: Currently unknown; empirical therapy with pimobendan (0.625 to 1.25 mg PO q12h) should be considered in normotensive cats with stage C or D CHF and myocardial failure

MISCELLANEOUS AGENTS/ADJUNCTIVE THERAPY FOR HEART FAILURE

- Bronchodilators, antitussives, sympathomimetics, positive inotropes, and sedatives/tranquilizers are all used as adjunctive therapy in the management of CHF. As monotherapy, none of these agents is capable of effectively ameliorating the signs of CHF. However, these agents may be useful in decreasing some of the signs associated with heart failure (coughing, cardiac asthma, and signs of low-output failure).

BRONCHODILATORS

- Theophylline is a bronchodilating agent that inhibits PDE. PDE is the enzyme responsible for reducing intracellular levels of cAMP. Inhibiting it results in the accumulation of AMP, which causes increased calcium influx. An increase in calcium influx in the smooth muscles of the airways results in smooth muscle relaxation and bronchodilation. In addition, the change in calcium ion movement in other tissues, such as nodal and myocardial tissue, results in a

positive chronotropic and inotropic effect. This agent may be helpful in dyspneic patients with fatigue of the muscles of respiration. Dogs and cats may experience transient gastrointestinal disturbance (usually self-limiting and resolving within the first 2 weeks of drug administration), tachycardia, and hyperexcitability and/or restlessness. Occasionally, we use theophylline in patients with complete atrioventricular block that are not candidates for permanent pacemaker implantation.
- Agents and dosages
  - **Theophylline**
    - Dogs: 10 mg/kg PO q12h
    - Cats: 25 to 50 mg/cat in the evening
  - **Aminophylline**
    - Dogs: 11 mg/kg PO q8-12h
    - Cats: 5 mg/kg PO q12h

COUGH SUPPRESSANTS

- Cough suppressants may be effective in reducing the frequency of coughing in dogs with left mainstem bronchial compression secondary to left atrial enlargement. If chronic airway disease is also present, the long-term results of antitussive therapy are often disappointing.
  - **Hydrocodone**
    - Dogs: 0.22 mg/kg PO every day up to 4 times a day
    - Cats: Do not use
  - **Butorphanol**
    - Dogs: 0.05 to 1 mg/kg PO 2 to 4 times a day
    - Cats: No established antitussive dose

SEDATIVES AND TRANQUILIZERS

- These drugs may be useful in selected cases. Respiratory distress may cause anxiety and stress in a patient with CHF. Agents with minimal cardiovascular effects should be chosen to prevent exacerbation of the CHF by causing hypotension or reduced contractility.
  - **Morphine sulfate** (reduces anxiety, decreases sympathetic tone)
    - Dogs: 0.1 to 1.0 mg/kg SQ IM
  - **Acepromazine** (reduces anxiety, vasodilator)
    - Dogs: 0.1 to 0.2 mg/kg SQ IM
  - **Butorphanol:**
    - Dogs and Cats: 0.1 to 0.3 mg/kg IV or IM

POTASSIUM SUPPLEMENTS

- Usually not necessary in most patients with CHF as long as they are eating and drinking. Dogs and especially cats may become hypokalemic as a result of inappetence/anorexia and aggressive concurrent diuretic therapy. The potassium supplement dose in cats is 2 to 6 mEq/day PO.

OXYGEN THERAPY

- Use as needed in cases with acute pulmonary edema.

POSITIVE INOTROPIC THERAPY

- The IV bipyridines amrinone and milrinone increase inotropy through inhibition of PDE (like pimobendan) and also have mild arteriolar dilating properties.
- Their use is limited to the treatment of severe refractory myocardial failure. The route of administration for amrinone and milrinone is IV. Amrinone is approved only for short-term IV administration in humans.
- Agent and dosages
  - **Amrinone**
    - Dogs: 1.0 to 3.0 mg/kg IV bolus or 10 to 80 μg/kg/min as a continuous-rate infusion
- Adverse and toxic effects associated with amrinone and milrinone have been described. Thrombocytopenia, a dose-related increased heart rate, gastrointestinal signs (diarrhea, anorexia), and hypotension (at high doses) have been reported. In addition, these agents appear to be arrhythmogenic (i.e., potentiate the development of arrhythmias) in some humans and dogs with heart failure.
- The presence of serious ventricular arrhythmias represents a contraindication for the use of these agents. Because the half-life of the parental formulations is quite short, discontinuing the medication is the treatment for toxicosis. We rarely use these agents in dogs and cats with heart failure.

SYMPATHOMIMETICS (DOBUTAMINE, DOPAMINE, AND ISOPROTERENOL)

- Sympathomimetics are agents that mimic the actions of the SNS (i.e., alpha- and beta-adrenergic receptor agonists).
- Dobutamine and dopamine are used only in the therapy of acute severe heart failure. Both dobutamine and dopamine exert a positive inotropic effect by stimulating myocardial beta-1 adrenergic receptors, which results in increased cAMP levels through adenylate cyclase stimulation. The increased levels of cAMP cause an increase in the slow inward calcium currents as well as an increase in calcium storage by the sarcoplasmic reticulum, making more calcium available to the contractile

elements. Dobutamine stimulates both beta-1 and beta-2 adrenergic receptors in the peripheral vasculature, and this combination results in no major changes in blood pressure.
- The positive chronotropic effect that is seen with dobutamine at higher doses should be avoided in most cases. The effects of dopamine are similar to dobutamine with the following exceptions:
  - Dobutamine favors blood flow to myocardial and skeletal muscle, whereas dopamine favors blood flow to the renal and mesenteric systems.
  - Dopamine infusion rates above 10 μg/kg/min may be associated with vasoconstriction.
  - Dopamine may increase diastolic intraventricular pressures.
- All sympathomimetic agents are best suited to short-term IV use. Isoproterenol stimulates beta-1 and beta-2 receptors, resulting in increased myocardial contractility, increased heart rate, and peripheral vasodilation. Isoproterenol is used mainly for the temporary control of heart rate in animals with symptomatic bradycardia. The chronotropic and arrhythmogenic effects make it unsuitable for the treatment of animals with CHF.
- Agents and dosages
  - **Isoproterenol hydrochloride**
    - Dogs: 0.04 to 0.1 μg/kg/min IV infusion following dilution in dextrose
  - **Dobutamine hydrochloride**
    - Dogs: 5 to 20 μg/kg/min IV continuous infusion diluted in 5% dextrose (monitor closely for arrhythmia)
  - **Dopamine hydrochloride**
    - Dogs: 2 to 8 μg/kg/min IV continuous infusion diluted in 5% dextrose

KEY POINT

Quick Dobutamine Drip Tip: Dilute 1 mL dobutamine (Dobutrex, 250 mg in a 20-mL vial or 12.5 mg/mL) for each 20 lb of body weight in 250 mL of 5% dextrose. Deliver by continuous-rate infusion at a rate of 1 mL/min (1 drop every 4 seconds) to obtain a dose of 5 μg/kg/min if using a Venoset delivery system.

- The adverse and toxic effects associated with sympathomimetic administration are usually dose related and may include the following:
  - Tachycardia
  - Arrhythmias
  - Gastrointestinal disturbances (anorexia, nausea)
  - Hypertension (dopamine)

- Hypotension (isoproterenol)
- Possible occurrence of phlebitis if the agent goes extravascular
- Dobutamine should not be initiated before therapy for heart rate control in patients with severe heart failure and rapid atrial fibrillation.
- The treatment for catecholamine toxicity involves stopping or slowing the administration of the drug.

Therapy with positive inotropic agents in veterinary medicine is, for the most part, limited to the use of dobutamine or dopamine in emergency scenarios, digoxin for chronic heart failure, and, more recently, pimobendan for chronic heart failure.

BETA-ADRENERGIC RECEPTOR BLOCKERS

- **Beta**-adrenergic receptor blockers (selective beta-1 agents such as atenolol and nonselective agents such as propranolol or carvedilol) are agents that in the past have primarily been used as antiarrhythmic agents in the control of the ventricular response rate to atrial fibrillation. Recent evidence has suggested that beta blockade may be effective in the therapy of mild to moderate CHF. Chronic SNS stimulation results in downregulation and desensitization of cardiac beta receptors. Beta blockers have been demonstrated to upregulate myocardial beta receptors and to improve myocardial function in dogs, using certain models of heart failure.
- However, if severe heart failure is present, beta blockade must be used very cautiously.
- Patients with pathologic concentric hypertrophy (e.g., HCM, aortic or pulmonic stenosis, and tetralogy of Fallot) theoretically benefit from administration of beta blockers. These patients may have symptoms during exercise because of myocardial ischemia or dynamic outflow tract obstruction. Marked concentric hypertrophy predisposes the myocardium to hypoxia, and tachycardia exacerbates this scenario. Beta blockers reduce myocardial oxygen consumption by reducing the heart rate. However, the use of atenolol in dogs with severe subvalvular aortic stenosis did not improve survival times in one study. In addition, the negative inotropic effects of beta blockers may reduce the dynamic outflow tract obstruction seen in some of these patients.
  - **Carvedilol**, a third-generation, nonselective beta blocker with alpha-1-blocking activity as well as antioxidative effects, can be administered to stable patients with heart failure for cardioprotective effects at a dosage of 1.56 mg PO q24h for 1 to 2 weeks, then 1.56 mg PO every 12h, and then upward titration to the maximal tolerated dosage (0.4 mg/kg PO q12h).

In general, beta blockers in patients with advanced cardiac disease should be used only under the guidance of a specialist.

NOVEL VASODILATORS (SILDENAFIL)

- Sildenafil is a PDE V inhibitor that has been shown to improve both exercise tolerance and quality of life in humans with pulmonary hypertension.
- Initial clinical reports indicate that sildenafil may also have a positive effect in dogs with acquired pulmonary hypertension secondary to chronic valve disease, congenital heart disease, chronic pulmonary disease, heartworm disease, and possibly congenital heart disease with Eisenmenger physiology (left-to-right shunt that results in pulmonary hypertension and subsequent right-to-left shunting).
- Can be used in combination with pimobendan for additional inodilator effect.
  - Dosage: **Sildenafil**: 0.5 to 1.0 mg/kg PO q8h.

TREATMENT PROTOCOLS

- The following treatment protocol for canine heart failure caused by mitral valve disease is based on the 2009 consensus statement by ACVIM Specialty of Cardiology. I have expanded these recommendations to include dogs with DCM and other forms of heart disease.
- When heart failure therapy for dogs with chronic valve disease or DCM is considered, it is helpful to think of patients with heart disease or heart failure as being on a continuum ranging from the following:
  - Stage A (risk for heart disease)
  - Stage B
    - B1: heart disease present; no evidence of cardiac remodeling
    - B2: heart disease present; evidence of cardiac remodeling
  - Stage C
    - C1: stabilized CHF
    - C2: mild to moderate CHF
    - C3: severe and/or life threatening CHF
  - Stage D (refractory CHF)

STAGE A

- These patients are at risk of having heart disease because of certain genetics, a family history of heart disease, a breed predisposition, or concurrent systemic disease with cardiovascular implications. Examples include Cavalier King Charles Spaniels (at risk of having chronic valve disease), Doberman Pinschers (at risk of having DCM), and Boxers (at risk of having arrhythmogenic right ventricular cardiomyopathy).

- No therapy is indicated for dogs in stage A
- Manage predisposing conditions
- Manage systemic hypertension, if present
- No dietary sodium modifications necessary

STAGE B

- Heart disease is present, but there are no clinical signs of CHF
  - Same as in stage A.
  - Increase the awareness of signs of CHF (tachypnea, dyspnea, coughing).
  - Periodic reevaluation for signs of disease progression and complications.
  - For patients with chronic valve disease, there is no evidence indicating that there is any beneficial effect of using an ACE inhibitor at this stage.
  - For patients with certain forms of DCM, therapy with pimobendan and benazepril can delay the onset of clinical signs (or progression to stage C).

STAGE C1

- Stabilized CHF; historical signs of CHF, but no symptoms are currently present
  - Goals are to keep clinical signs stabilized, use the minimum effective dosage of furosemide, modulate neurohormones (ACE-inhibitor, aldosterone antagonist), support contractility (pimobendan), and preserve renal and myocardial function. Additional drugs may be added at this stage for their cardioprotective effects.
  - Drugs for routine use: furosemide, ACE inhibitor, pimobendan, spironolactone.
  - Drugs for selected patients: digoxin, thiazide, amlodipine/hydralazine, or other vasodilator.
  - If possible, avoid excessive sodium intake, corticosteroids, and IV fluids (unless required for concurrent disease; requires careful monitoring of the respiratory rate trend).

KEY POINT

The dosage of furosemide should be adjusted (within a range specified by the clinician) on the basis of the resting/sleeping respiratory rate trend and other clinical signs as monitored by the owners.

STAGE C2

- Mild to moderate CHF is present.
  - Goals are to revert back to stage C1 (eliminate pulmonary edema or effusions), improve hemodynamics, and modulate neurohormonal activation.
  - In patients with chronic valve disease, the use of furosemide, an ACE inhibitor, and pimobendan is recommended. Consider therapy with spironolactone. Digoxin (usually with diltiazem) is recommended to control the ventricular response rate if atrial fibrillation is present. Beta blockers should be avoided in patients with overt CHF.
  - In patients with symptomatic DCM, furosemide, ACE inhibitor, and pimobendan are recommended. Consider therapy with spironolactone. Digoxin (usually with diltiazem) is recommended to control the ventricular response rate if atrial fibrillation is present. Beta blockers should not be introduced at this time.
  - Avoid, if possible, excessive sodium intake, beta blockers, corticosteroids, and IV fluids (unless required for concurrent disease; requires careful monitoring of the respiratory rate trend).

STAGE C3

- Severe or life-threatening CHF
  - Treat hypoxemia, increase cardiac output, continue previous cardiac drugs (see Stage C2), and stabilize the patient in hospital with IV drugs.
  - Drugs for routine use: same as for stage C2 plus oxygen, IV furosemide, nitroglycerin
  - Drugs for selected patients: dobutamine, nitroprusside

KEY POINT

Aggressive diuresis (repeated IV boluses or continuous-rate infusion of furosemide) is indicated when life-threatening CHF is present.

STAGE D

- Refractory, chronic CHF
  - Drugs for routine use: continue current cardiac medications as in stage C plus spironolactone, thiazides, digoxin, subcutaneous furosemide, repeated centesis for effusions, and moderate salt restriction.
  - Drugs for selected patients: as per stage C3
    - For chronic valve disease, consider additional vasodilation with amlodipine or hydralazine.
    - For DCM, dobutamine (continuous-rate infusion for 48 hours every 3 weeks) may be helpful.

SPECIFIC DISEASE TREATMENT

CHRONIC VALVE DISEASE: ASYMPTOMATIC (PRECLINICAL) MITRAL REGURGITATION (STAGE B)

- A majority of cardiologists consider starting ACE inhibitor therapy when there is clinical evidence that the heart disease has led to radiographic cardiomegaly and pulmonary venous congestion despite no evidence of pulmonary edema. These findings might be further supported by echocardiographic findings and evaluation of biomarkers.
- In this scenario, enalapril (0.5 mg/kg PO q12 to 24h) or some other ACE inhibitor may be initiated (with pretreatment and 1-week posttreatment renal evaluations), despite lack of clear evidence that this will delay onset of clinical signs. Left atrial enlargement can result in compression of the left mainstem bronchus, resulting in coughing in absence of CHF. Concurrent chronic bronchointerstitial disease is common.
- These cases can benefit from owner monitoring of patient resting respiratory rate and effort at home in an effort to detect signs of developing congestion. In patients with bronchial compression, cough suppression can be administered.

CHRONIC VALVE DISEASE WITH CLINICAL SIGNS OF CONGESTIVE HEART FAILURE (STAGE C2)

- Decompensated heart failure usually leads to the clinical signs of moderate CHF. The earliest signs of decompensation are usually not noticed by the pet's owner. Elevated respiratory rates during rest (tachypnea) may be mistaken for panting and are often overlooked. Tachypnea is associated with the onset of interstitial (stage II) pulmonary edema.
- In addition to tachypnea, dogs with moderate CHF may also exhibit exercise intolerance or coughing. Again, thoracic radiography can reveal the presence of interstitial pulmonary edema (increased interstitial pattern, enlarged pulmonary veins with fuzzy, indistinct borders, and concurrent left atrial and ventricular enlargement) as well as bronchial compression, if present.
- The appropriate therapy for this patient includes an ACE inhibitor (**enalapril** 0.5 mg/kg PO q12h), **furosemide** (2 to 4 mg/kg PO q12-24h), and **pimobendan** (0.25 mg/kg PO q12h).
  - Digoxin is reserved for patients with atrial fibrillation or other supraventricular tachyarrhythmias.

- The resting respiratory rate can be used to monitor the response to therapy. A trend of decreasing resting respiratory rate indicates adequate preload reduction. Once the respiratory rate has stabilized in the normal range (usually less than 30 breaths per minute), the diuretic dose is tapered down to the lowest dose that is effective in controlling the signs of CHF.
- A trend of increasing resting respiratory rate suggests the worsening of pulmonary edema and the need for higher dosages of diuretics.

CHRONIC VALVE DISEASE WITH LIFE-THREATENING SIGNS OF CONGESTIVE HEART FAILURE (STAGE C3)

- Dogs with severe CHF secondary to primary valve disease have clinical signs at rest and typically require hospitalization and aggressive therapy to control pulmonary edema. These patients typically require relatively high dosages of furosemide as well as optimized dosages of ACE inhibitor and pimobendan.
- If the patient has severe clinical signs, hospitalization is indicated to provide oxygen therapy in addition to close monitoring and parenteral administration of furosemide.
- Thoracocentesis may be necessary if pleural effusion is present.
- Furosemide (up to 6 to 8 mg/kg IV) is administered, and the respiratory rate is monitored for a decreasing rate trend. If no decline in respiratory rate is observed within 1 to 2 hours, furosemide is again administered at the same or a slightly higher dose. The respiratory rate is again monitored, and the preceding is repeated if there is no improvement. Monitor for urination. As the respiratory rate decreases, the dosage and frequency of administration are reduced to the lowest dose effective in controlling the pulmonary edema. Pretreatment evaluation of renal function and hydration status aids in selecting the appropriate furosemide dose.
- In the presence of refractory, severe, chronic CHF, the addition of spironolactone with or without a thiazide to conventional therapy may help control edema.

PRECLINICAL OR OCCULT DILATED CARDIOMYOPATHY (STAGE B)

- The presence of ventricular ectopy, chamber dilation, or evidence of myocardial failure (reduced fractional shortening percentage and increased mitral valve E-point septal separation), particularly in dogs that are predisposed to idiopathic DCM (Doberman Pinschers and others), suggests a diagnosis of occult DCM.

- Although these dogs are usually symptom free, they often have progressive heart failure. ACE inhibitor therapy (enalapril 0.5 mg PO q12h or benazepril 0.25 mg PO q12-24h) should be initiated to prolong the asymptomatic phase of the disease.
- Beta-adrenergic blocking agents may also be indicated in these patients.
- Pimobendan therapy (0.25 mg/kg PO q12h) is indicated in Doberman Pinscher patients with echocardiographic evidence of myocardial failure.
- Some Spaniel breeds (American Cocker Spaniels, Cavalier King Charles Spaniels) and other breeds (Golden Retrievers, Newfoundlands) may have DCM secondary to taurine deficiency. Therefore plasma taurine levels should be evaluated and taurine supplementation instituted (500 mg PO q12h) if indicated.

DILATED CARDIOMYOPATHY WITH CLINICAL SIGNS OF CONGESTIVE HEART FAILURE (STAGE C2)

- As heart failure progresses, filling pressures eventually become elevated and pulmonary edema may develop.
- The therapeutic protocol in this patient is essentially the same as that for a patient with moderate heart failure secondary to MR. The only difference is that pimobendan is initiated earlier in the disease course of cardiomyopathy.
- Standard therapy for patients with symptomatic heart failure consists of an ACE inhibitor, furosemide, and pimobendan. These patients frequently have cardiac rhythm disturbances that may be associated with symptoms or may be aggravating the CHF. In this scenario, antiarrhythmic therapy is indicated (e.g., digoxin with or without diltiazem to control the ventricular response to atrial fibrillation). Antiarrhythmic therapy is typically not indicated in patients with arrhythmias that are not associated with clinical signs of reduced cardiac output and poor tissue perfusion.

DILATED CARDIOMYOPATHY WITH LIFE-THREATENING SIGNS OF CONGESTIVE HEART FAILURE (STAGE C3)

- Aggressive therapy is indicated in patients with severe symptomatic heart failure. Oxygen therapy, ACE inhibitors, pimobendan, furosemide, and, possibly, dobutamine and nitroprusside may be necessary to control pulmonary edema in life-threatening heart failure.
- Furosemide (up to 6 to 8 mg/kg IV) may be given q1-2h until the resting respiratory rate is decreasing. Then administer furosemide (2 to 4 mg/kg IV) q4-8h, depending on the status of the patient. The goal is to taper the dose to the lowest effective dose and the frequency of administration to two to three times a day as quickly as possible.
- If IV dobutamine/nitroprusside therapy is necessary to control the symptoms of heart failure, the nitroprusside dose should be adjusted to decrease mean or systolic arterial blood pressure by 15 to 30 mm Hg. The long-term survival of dogs with severe, life-threatening heart failure is poor.

FELINE CARDIOMYOPATHY (DILATED CARDIOMYOPATHY, RESTRICTIVE CARDIOMYOPATHY, AND HYPERTROPHIC CARDIOMYOPATHY)

- The medical approach for the feline with cardiomyopathy is based on the type and severity of the cardiomyopathy present and the presence of clinical signs of CHF. Evaluation of the patient with electrocardiography, thoracic radiography, and echocardiography usually enables the clinician to characterize the cardiomyopathy as being associated with myocardial systolic failure (DCM and, sometimes, RCM) or diastolic dysfunction (HCM and RCM).
- In general, cats with primary systolic dysfunction have symptoms at diagnosis. They receive enalapril (1 to 2 mg PO every other day to twice a day, depending on renal status), furosemide (6.25 to 12.5 mg PO q12-24h), and pimobendan (0.625 to 1.25 mg PO q12h).
- Cardiogenic thromboembolism occurs in approximately 10% to 14% of cats with cardiomyopathy (predisposing factors include severe left atrial enlargement, spontaneous contrast during echocardiography, excessive moderator bands, and poor systolic function). In this scenario, clopidogrel (18.75 mg PO q24h) is the therapy of choice. Clopidogrel was associated with increased survival times in cats surviving an initial episode of thromboembolism. Aspirin (25 mg/kg PO every 3 days) may prevent thrombus formation in cats at risk of intracardiac thrombus formation. Low-molecular-weight heparins such as dalteparin (100 U/kg subcutaneously q24h) or enoxaparin (1 to 1.5 mg/kg subcutaneously q12-24h) may also have beneficial effects in cats at risk. However, these dosages have largely been borrowed from the human literature, and specific dosages have not

been established in cats. Warfarin is not recommended.

- Cats with HCM may be completely symptom free or may have with tachypnea and dyspnea associated with decompensated diastolic heart failure.

- There is some controversy as to which agent is the drug of choice in cats with diastolic dysfunction. Calcium channel blockers (diltiazem) and beta blockers (atenolol) facilitate diastolic function but in different ways. Beta blockers probably facilitate diastolic function only by decreasing heart rate and myocardial oxygen consumption. Calcium channel blockers facilitate diastolic function by improving myocardial relaxation through normalization of abnormal myocardial calcium currents as well as by coronary vasodilation to improve myocardial perfusion.

- In symptom-free cats with HCM, therapy is based on the presence of tachycardia, dynamic left ventricular outflow obstruction, and the severity of concentric hypertrophy and left atrial enlargement. If tachycardia (heart rate more than 200 beats/min), dynamic left ventricular outflow obstruction, and marked hypertrophy are present, beta blockade is initiated (atenolol 6.25 to 12.5 mg PO q12-24h). Beta blockers appear to be more effective than calcium channel blockers in controlling the heart rate in tachycardic cats. In addition, beta blockers are probably more effective in reducing the dynamic outflow tract obstruction seen in some cats with HCM. Beta blockers should be avoided in decompensated CHF.

- Tachycardia, CHF, and thromboembolism are considered to be negative prognostic indicators in cardiomyopathic cats.

- The number one priority when presented with a cat with CHF is to avoid stressing the patient with diagnostic tests such as radiographs or electrocardiograms. Cats with symptomatic heart failure typically have pulmonary edema or pleural effusion. If the cat is dyspneic or has life-threatening heart failure, a thoracocentesis is performed to rule out the presence of pleural effusion. Preload reducers such as furosemide (1 to 4 mg/kg IM or IV q3-4h) is effective in reducing filling pressures, therefore facilitating the resolution of pulmonary edema. The dosing frequency and dosage of furosemide are reduced once clinical improvement is noted, as evidenced by a reduction in resting/sleeping respiratory rate.

- In addition to preload reducers, an agent to improve diastolic function (beta blocker or calcium channel blocker) may be used. Caution should be exercised when administering beta blockers to patients with severe CHF and possible myocardial failure. Oxygen therapy is also indicated.

- The medical management of feline RCM is similar to that for DCM because systolic dysfunction is usually present in both. Combinations of enalapril, pimobendan, and furosemide are currently recommended.

PERICARDIAL DISEASE

- The management of chronic pericardial effusion and cardiac tamponade is straightforward. An echocardiogram is performed to confirm the diagnosis of pericardial effusion and to attempt to ascertain if the underlying cause is neoplasia. If the prognosis is favorable, pericardiocentesis is performed to relieve the compression on the heart by the elevated intrapericardial pressure. If the effusion returns more than once, a pericardectomy is recommended (see Chapter 12).

CONGESTIVE HEART FAILURE ASSOCIATED WITH CHRONIC HEARTWORM DISEASE

- The approach to dogs with CHF associated with chronic heartworm disease involves cage rest, diuretic therapy, and heartworm adulticide therapy. These patients are cage rested a minimum of 1 week before and 4 to 6 weeks after adulticide therapy (staged melarsomine adulticide protocol). Heart failure medications (ACE inhibitors, furosemide, spironolactone, pimobendan, and sildenafil) may be discontinued in some patients 4 to 8 weeks after adulticide therapy (see Chapter 11).

FREQUENTLY ASKED QUESTIONS

When is activation of the SNS maladaptive to the cardiac health of the animal? Select one

   A. In a normal animal that is in a flight or fight stress response

   B. In an animal with RAAS activation

   C. In an animal with early heart failure

   D. In an animal with chronic heart failure

(D is the correct answer.)

Rationales:

A. The activation of the SNS is essential for the animal under stress. With an increase in the heart rate, the cardiac output, and selective vasoconstriction (e.g., to gut) and vasodilation (e.g., to muscles), the animal may engage the cardiovascular system effectively to deal with an acute threat.

B. The acute activation of the SNS results in stimulation of beta-1 adrenergic receptors in the juxtaglomerular apparatus of the kidney. Angiotensin II also causes activation of the SNS, so these two systems are closely intertwined, not maladaptive.

C. Early activation of the SNS in early stages of heart failure helps to maintain:
- Blood pressure
- Tissue perfusion
- Cardiac output

(How? By increasing venous return to the heart via vasoconstriction of the splanchnic vessels, vasoconstriction of other various vascular beds, and positive inotropic and chronotropic cardiac effects)

D. This is a maladaptive situation because chronic SNS overactivity produces the following:
- Downregulation and desensitization of beta-1 adrenergic receptors
- Abnormal baroreflex function
- An overload of the heart by increasing venous return
- An increase in myocardial oxygen consumption (by increasing heart rate)
- Cardiac NE depletion and elevated plasma NE
- Damage to the myocardium, resulting in potential arrhythmogenesis

How are natriuretic peptide levels useful in the assessment of heart disease?

Though not yet widely used, these assays may be an important addition to the diagnostic toolkit for selected heart diseases. Circulating natriuretic peptide levels may be used to differentiate symptoms associated with cardiac disease from those associated with primary pulmonary disease.

Natriuretic peptides are salt and water homeostasis regulators, and they are involved in blood pressure control so changes in these parameters may help us to understand the stage of the cardiovascular condition. Their potential value is as diagnostic and prognostic markers in patients with CHF particularly.

Natriuretic peptide levels are elevated in many disease conditions resulting in expanded fluid volume (e.g., DCM, chronic valvular insufficiency in dogs, and cardiomyopathy in cats).

SUGGESTED READINGS

Atkins CE, Bongura J, Ettinger S, et al: Guidelines for the diagnosis and treatment of canine chronic valvular disease, J Vet Intern Med 23:1142, 2009.

Hamlin RL: Physiology of the failing heart. In Fox PR, Sisson D, Moise NS, eds: Textbook of canine and feline cardiology: principles and clinical practice, ed 2, Philadelphia, 1999, Saunders.

Kittleson MD: Management of heart failure. In Kittleson MD, Kienle RD, eds: Small animal cardiovascular medicine, St Louis, 1998, Mosby.

Kittleson MD: Pathophysiology of heart failure. In Kittleson MD, Kienle RD, eds: Small animal cardiovascular medicine, St Louis, 1998, Mosby.

Mann DL: Pathophysiology of heart failure. In Bonow RO, Mann DL, Zipes DP, Libby P, eds: Braunwald's heart disease: a textbook of cardiovascular medicine, ed 9, Philadelphia, 2012, Elsevier Saunders.

Sisson D, Kittleson MD: Management of heart failure: principles of treatment, therapeutic strategies, and pharmacology. In Fox PR, Sisson D, Moise NS, eds: Textbook of canine and feline cardiology: principles and clinical practice, ed 2, Philadelphia, 1999, Saunders.

Treatment of Cardiac Arrhythmias and Conduction Disturbances

17

Marc S. Kraus | Anna R. M. Gelzer

Cardiac arrhythmias are defined as variations of the cardiac rhythm from normal sinus rhythm. Some cardiac arrhythmias are benign and clinically insignificant and require no specific therapy; others may cause severe clinical signs such as syncope or degenerate into malignant arrhythmias (i.e., ventricular fibrillation [VF]), leading to cardiac arrest and sudden death. The goal of this chapter is to discuss treatment strategies for management of clinically important arrhythmias.

GENERAL REMARKS

Antiarrhythmic drugs commonly target two general areas of the heart because of their specific electrophysiologic properties:

- Sinoatrial and atrioventricular (AV) nodal tissue: Depolarization of nodal cells is calcium channel driven. For the treatment of arrhythmias that originate or encompass the sinoatrial or AV nodal tissue, calcium channel blockers (CCBs) and beta blockers (BBs) are primarily used. The most commonly prescribed CCB for these indications is diltiazem (available orally [PO] and intravenously [IV]). The beta1-selective BBs atenolol and esmolol (IV only) are the most frequently used antiarrhythmic BBs. Sotalol, a BB combined with marked potassium channel blocking characteristics, is also used for supraventricular arrhythmias involving nodal tissue. Digoxin may also be used as an antiarrhythmic agent for its vagomimetic effects, which can indirectly prolong AV node conduction time. Its antiarrhythmic application is limited to slowing the ventricular response in the treatment of atrial fibrillation (AF). For drug dosages, consult Table 17.1 and Table 17.2.
- Atrial or ventricular myocardium: Depolarization is sodium channel gated and repolarization is potassium channel dominated. For treatment of arrhythmias that originate from the atrial and ventricular myocardium, Na

channel blockers (NCBs), K channel blocker (KCBs), or combinations thereof are often used in conjunction with BBs. The NCBs used for treatment of arrhythmias in dogs are lidocaine (IV only), mexiletine, and, rarely, procainamide. The most important KCB is sotalol, which also has BB properties. We also use amiodarone, which is predominantly a KCB but also has potent NCB and some CCB and BB activity. For drug dosages, consult Table 17.1 and Table 17.2.

Even though a correct diagnosis of an arrhythmia may be obtained by a short in-hospital electrocardiogram (ECG), a 24-hour Holter recording is required in some patients with an intermittent arrhythmia to establish a definitive diagnosis. For optimal long-term management of most arrhythmias, a 24-hour Holter recording should be acquired in addition to the ECG before starting antiarrhythmic therapy.

The decision regarding how and when to treat an arrhythmia should be based on the clinical signs and urgency of intervention. Emergency management that includes IV drugs may be required before a 24-hour Holter recording can be obtained. Both diltiazem and esmolol are available in IV formulations, allowing emergency treatment of excessively rapid supraventricular arrhythmias (SVAs). Lidocaine is the most important IV drug used for life-threatening ventricular arrhythmias.

- The benefits of a 24-hour Holter recording include in-depth assessment of quantity and quality of the arrhythmia(s). The following parameters should be examined: number of abnormal beats (supraventricular or ventricular) relative to overall number of beats, duration and rate of runs of abnormal beats, average hourly and daily heart rate (HR), amount of time when the HR is >120 and <50 beats/min, and presence and length of pauses. A diary kept by the client or hospital staff with the

Table 17.1   Agents for Rate Control/Abolishing Arrhythmias in Canine Patients with Supraventricular Arrhythmias

Drug	Oral administration	Intravenous administration	Indication
Diltiazem XR	2-4 mg/kg BID (most patients require 3 mg/kg)		AF, AFL, AT, OAVRT
Diltiazem	0.5 mg/kg TID titrated up (max 1.5-2 mg/kg TID)	0.1-0.2 mg/kg bolus, then CRI 2-6 µg/kg/min	Acute AF, AFI, OAVRT
Atenolol	0.25-1 mg/kg SID to BID		AFI, AT, OAVRT
Esmolol		50-100 µg/kg bolus (repeat up to max 500 µg/kg); 50-200 µg/kg/min CRI	Acute AF, AFI, AT, OAVRT
Sotalol	1-2.5 mg/kg BID		AF, AFI, AT
Digoxin	0.003-0.005 mg/kg BID Liquid suspension available for small dogs Max dose for Dobermans: 0.25 mg BID		AF
Procainamide		10-15 mg/kg IV bolus slowly over 2 minutes; if needed start a CRI: 25-50 µg/kg/min	AT
Amiodarone	10 mg/kg BID for 1 week (loading dose)* 5 mg/kg SID (maintenance dose)*		AF, AT
Lidocaine		2 mg/kg IV bolus, repeat if needed	AF if because of narcotics

*Recommended dose range in veterinary medicine is anecdotal and variable.
AF, Atrial fibrillation; *Afl,* atrial flutter; *AT,* atrial tachycardia; *BID,* twice daily; *CRI,* continuous-rate infusion; *OAVRT,* orthodromic atrioventricular reciprocating tachycardia; *SID,* once daily; *TID,* three times daily; *VA,* ventricular arrhythmias; *VT,* ventricular tachycardia.

Table 17.2   Agents for Rate Control/Abolishing Arrhythmias in Canine Patients with Ventricular Arrhythmias

Drug	Oral administration	Intravenous administration	Indication
Sotalol	0.5-2 mg/kg BID		VA, VT
Mexiletine	4-8 mg/kg TID		VA, VT, Usually not effective as monotherapy
Amiodarone	10 mg/kg BID for 1 week (loading dose)* 5 mg/kg SID (maintenance dose)*		Refractory VA, VT
Lidocaine		2 mg/kg IV bolus, repeat 3 times, if needed start a CRI: 30-80 µg/kg/min	Life-threatening VT
Procainamide		10-15 mg/kg IV bolus slowly over 2 minutes, if needed start a CRI: 25-50 µg/kg/min	Life-threatening VT
Atenolol	0.25-2 mg/kg SID to BID		VA, VT, effective only in combination with mexiletine
Esmolol		50-100 µg/kg bolus, repeat up to max 500 µg/kg) if needed start a CRI: 50-200 µg/kg/min	Life-threatening VT

*Recommended dose range in veterinary medicine is anecdotal and variable.
BID, Twice daily; *CRI,* continuous-rate infusion; *SID,* once daily; *TID,* three times daily; *VA,* ventricular arrhythmias; *VT,* ventricular tachycardia.

sleep/wakefulness activity or observed events such as syncope or excessive anxiety or panting help correlate ECG changes on the Holter with clinical signs. These parameters are vital for a baseline evaluation of a patient's arrhythmias and needs for antiarrhythmic therapy.

- If treatment is instituted, it is critical to obtain a repeat Holter recording after 1 or 2 weeks to determine if the drugs are efficacious in suppressing the abnormal rhythms or possibly harmful by being arrhythmic (i.e., causing more arrhythmias or excessive pauses). This can only be established if a comparison to the pretherapy baseline is performed.
- If Holter monitoring shows that a drug is effective, we recommend monitoring the progression of the arrhythmia by repeat Holter recordings every 6 to 12 months. If an animal experiences recurrent syncope during that time, an immediate repeat Holter is recommended.
- In animals that need to be stabilized immediately (no time for a baseline 24-hour Holter recording before IV antiarrhythmics), a posttreatment Holter recording is still advisable to evaluate drug efficacy and possible toxicity once the dog is stabilized and receiving chronic oral antiarrhythmic therapy.

SUPRAVENTRICULAR ARRHYTHMIAS

SVAs include rhythms that originate in the sinus node, atrial tissue, and AV junction. Importantly, SVA must be differentiated from accelerated normal sinus rhythm. Physiologic sinus tachycardia can be caused by many conditions, including febrile states, anemia, heart failure, adrenergic medications, and anxiety. In these cases, management should foremost be focused on correcting the underlying cause or disease resulting in increased sympathetic tone.

- Because of the mechanism of action of antiarrhythmic drugs, it is useful to assess SVA as either AV node *independent* (does not need the AV node to sustain the rhythm) or AV node *dependent* (requires the AV node to sustain the rhythm).
- An SVA is AV node independent if the ECG contains P waves not conducted to the ventricle without termination of the SVA. Interventions such as vagal maneuvers or drugs that slow AV node conduction can help identify the underlying mechanism:
  - If the atrial activation rate is unchanged (PP interval the same) following the intervention but the ventricular rate slows because of AV block, the SVA is likely AV node independent.

- If the intervention results in abolishment of the SVA and restoration of a normal sinus rhythm (even if it is only transient), the arrhythmia is likely AV node dependent.
- Examples of AV node–independent rhythms include sinus node reentrant tachycardia, AF, atrial flutter (AFL), and ectopic atrial tachycardia. These arrhythmias can be challenging to manage because the antiarrhythmic drugs (NCBs, KCBs, or combinations thereof) are often not very efficacious for suppression of these arrhythmias. If the abnormal rhythm cannot be abolished with drugs, the secondary mode of treatment aims at controlling the ventricular response rate by slowing the AV node conduction with CCBs, BBs, or digoxin.
- AV node–dependent SVAs include AV reentrant tachycardia (accessory pathway [AP] mediated) and AV nodal reentrant tachycardia. AV node–dependent arrhythmias can usually be treated with drugs that target the AV node (CCBs and BBs).

KEY POINT

To help guide treatment of SVAs, they should be characterized as AV node dependent or independent.

ATRIAL FIBRILLATION

- Atrial fibrillation (AF) is one of the most commonly seen SVAs in veterinary practice. In dogs and cats, AF is usually a chronic arrhythmia associated with advanced stages of chronic AV valve insufficiency or cardiomyopathy. In those patients, the ventricular response rate is often markedly elevated, which contributes to the clinical signs of heart failure. AF can also occur in the absence of overt structural heart disease (lone or primary AF). In these cases, the ventricular response rate can be normal or only mildly elevated.

KEY POINT

The management of AF largely depends on the average HR. A baseline 24-hour Holter recording acquired in the home is ideal to determine the average HR of a patient.

THERAPY

AF is an AV node–independent arrhythmia, caused by multiple simultaneous intraatrial reentrant circuits. Medical conversion of AF to sinus rhythm with drugs is very difficult and rarely

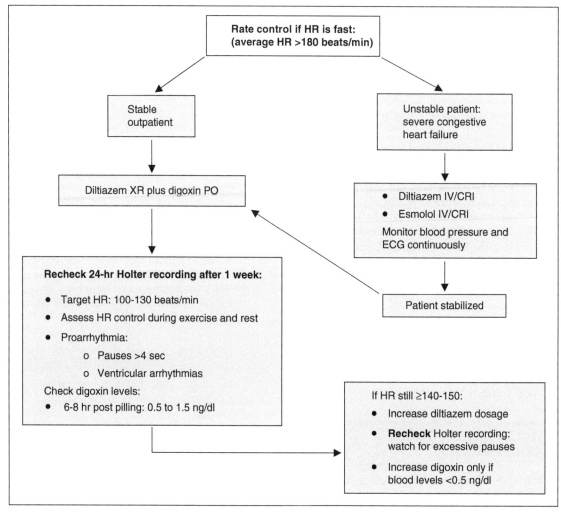

Figure 17.1 Management of dogs with atrial fibrillation (AF) and fast heart rate (*HR*) (average HR >180 beats/min). *CRI,* Constant-rate infusion.

achieved in canine patients. In most cases, ventricular rate control by the slowing of AV node conduction with diltiazem or digoxin is the goal (drug dosages are listed in Table 17.1). The veterinary literature also cites atenolol as effective for rate control of AF. We do not have much personal experience with atenolol for this purpose. The reluctance to including atenolol for rate control stems in part from the concomitant degree of advanced myocardial failure in many patients with AF. In our experience, diltiazem XR is very well tolerated even in dogs with severe systolic myocardial dysfunction.

- Dogs with normal cardiac function or only mild dysfunction and normal to moderately elevated ventricular response rates may be candidates for electric cardioversion of AF to sinus rhythm.

- Medical management varies with the initial average HR and overall condition of the dog. Figures 17.1 through 17.3 provide guidelines for treatment. Treatment can be tailored to the patient based on the approximate average HR. We prioritize treatment according to three general categories of ventricular response rate: (1) fast (Figure 17.1: average HR faster than 180 beats/min); (2) moderate (Figure 17.2: average HR 130 to 160 beats/min); and (3) slow (Figure 17.3: HR around 100 beats/min). The dosages for the drug mentioned in Figures 17.1 through 17.3 are provided in Table 17.1.

- Treatment of AF in cats is challenging. There is usually significant underlying heart disease present, resulting in markedly enlarged atria and very rapid AF. Medical management for rate control with a target HR of 130 to 150 beats/min may be achieved with either a CCB

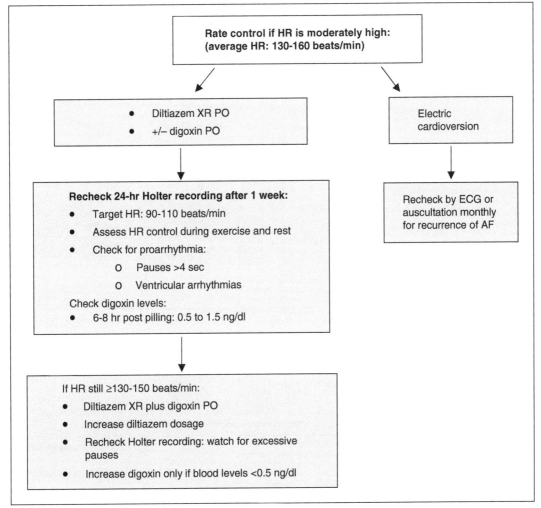

Figure 17.2 Management of dogs with atrial fibrillation (*AF*) and a moderately elevated average heart rate (*HR*) of 130 to 160 beats/min. *ECG*, electrocardiogram.

or BB (for drug dosages for antiarrhythmic drugs in cats, see Table 17.3).

- Occasionally, the administration of narcotics has been associated with the induction of AF in large dogs. This is likely caused by the increased vagal tone that occurs with narcotics. Treatment with 2 mg/kg **lidocaine** IV within 4 hours of onset has been demonstrated to restore sinus rhythm. Vagolytic drugs (atropine) should prevent onset or recurrence of AF in such cases.

KEY POINT

Digoxin monotherapy does not control the ventricular response rate adequately during times of excitement, stress, or exercise. Thus, dogs with AF and moderate to fast HRs will require combination therapy of digoxin with diltiazem or atenolol.

ELECTRIC CARDIOVERSION (RHYTHM CONTROL)

In a subgroup of canine patients with mild structural heart disease or lone AF, electric cardioversion of AF to sinus rhythm can be achieved. The goal of cardioversion is to avoid structural or functional remodeling from chronic AF, even if the HR is slow. The rate of recurrence of AF after successful cardioversion is high, and the morbidity associated with repeat transthoracic cardioversions under general anesthesia makes this management less practical. Pretreatment with sotalol, amiodarone, or angiotensin-converting enzyme inhibitors may improve the chances of cardioversion and lessen the rate of recurrence of AF; however, no studies in veterinary medicine have proven these concepts.

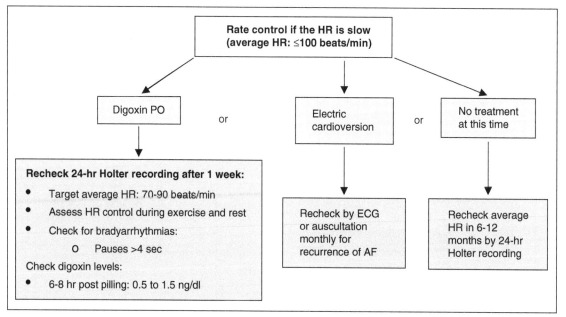

Figure 17.3 Management of dogs with atrial fibrillation (*AF*) with a low average heart rate (*HR*) (≤100 beats/min). *ECG*, electrocardiogram.

Table 17.3 Agents for Rate Control/Abolishing Arrhythmias in Feline Patients with Arrhythmias

Drug	Oral administration	Intravenous administration	Indication
Diltiazem XR	30-60 mg SID or BID (start with 30 mg SID)		AF, AT, accessory pathway
Diltiazem	10 mg/kg SID	0.1-0.2 mg/kg bolus, then CRI at 2-6 µg/kg/min	Acute AF, accessory pathway
Atenolol	6.25-12.5 mg SID or BID		AT, accessory pathway, VT
Esmolol	NA	50-100 µg/kg bolus (repeat up to max 500 µg/kg); 50-200 µg/kg/min CRI	Acute AF, AT, accessory pathway, life-threatening VT
Sotalol	1/8 of an 80-mg tablet BID*		VT
Procainamide	2-5 mg/kg BID or TID	10-15 mg/kg IV bolus slowly over 2 minutes or CRI at 25-50 µg/kg/min	AT, accessory pathway
Lidocaine	NA	0.25-1 mg/kg IV bolus (use with extreme caution in cats)	Life-threatening VT

*Recommended dosage range is anecdotal and variable.
AF, Atrial fibrillation; *AT*, atrial tachycardia; *BID*, twice daily; *CRI*, continuous-rate infusion; *NA*, not available; *SID*, once daily; *TID*, three times daily; *VT*, ventricular tachycardia.

TRANSTHORACIC ELECTRICAL CARDIOVERSION PROCEDURE

- Procedure requires a brief general anesthesia.
- "Fast Patch" electrodes are recommended instead of handheld paddles to optimize electrode position for cardioversion.
- Dog is shaved before application of the patch over the heart on both lateral sides of the thorax.
- Dog is positioned in lateral recumbency to optimally "position" the heart between the two patch electrodes.
- Defibrillator ECG cables need to record patient's ECG and synchronize to the R waves. With false synchronization to T waves (occurs if T wave is taller than the R wave), the cardioversion shock can induce VF.

- With a monophasic defibrillator
  - Start with 4 J/kg; if no cardioversion occurs, increase dose by 50 J and repeat until a maximum of 360 J.
- With a biphasic defibrillator
  - Start with 1 to 2 J/kg; if no cardioversion occurs, increase dose by 50 J and repeat until a maximum of 360 J.
  - Short, transient runs of ventricular tachycardia (VT) or sinus pauses or AV block are common following electric cardioversion.

ATRIAL FLUTTER

- Atrial flutter (AFL) is relatively uncommon in veterinary patients. Theoretically, AFL could set the stage for development of AF because of the remodeling that occurs with continuous rapid activation of the atrial myocardium. In some patients, AFL coexists with AF on a 24-hour Holter, which might represent a transition phase to chronic AF. AFL is an AV node–independent intraatrial macroreentry rhythm. The atrial activation rate (PP interval) is 300 to 600 beats/min. AFL is paroxysmal or chronic and can be associated with excessively high ventricular response rates. AV conduction usually changes between 1:1 and 3:1 or 2:1 caused by variable degrees of AV block.
- A baseline 24-hour Holter is recommended to determine if the arrhythmia is chronic or paroxysmal. If it is chronic, drug therapy is indicated.
- If it is paroxysmal and infrequent, treatment may be postponed, but a reevaluation by Holter 6 months later should be performed to check for progression from paroxysmal to chronic AFL or presence of concurrent AF.

DRUG THERAPY

- Ideally, therapy is aimed at suppressing the atrial reentry circuit using sotalol, amiodarone, or procainamide; however, abolishing the AFL with drugs is often unsuccessful. Propafenone and flecainide are used in humans with AFL, but we have had little success in dogs with these drugs. The adequate dose for dogs has not been identified. Rate control by the slowing of the AV node with CCBs or BBs is used effectively in dogs (for drug dosages, see Table 17.1). Digoxin monotherapy is ineffective for management of AFL.
- A postdrug 24-hour Holter should be obtained to determine if the drug was effective at suppressing the AFL or producing the desired AV block, thereby slowing the ventricular response adequately. It also allows survey for drug toxicity, which manifests as bradycardia or pauses secondary to excessive AV block. Pauses, if they occur only during sleep or rest, are usually of no concern.

FOCAL (ECTOPIC) ATRIAL TACHYCARDIA

- Focal atrial tachycardia (FAT) occurs when ectopic foci in the atria develop the ability to fire rapidly and spontaneously. It is an AV node–independent arrhythmia. FATs arise from a single site within the left or right atrium, in contrast to macroreentrant atrial arrhythmias (e.g., AFL) and AF, which involve multiple sites or larger circuits. FAT is often paroxysmal and may display a gradual onset and offset in HR elevation (warm-up and cool-down period). This finding suggests that the underlying mechanism involves enhanced automaticity. However, FAT may have automatic, triggered, and microreentrant origins that cannot be distinguished easily on the surface electrocardiogram. P wave morphology may be similar to that in sinus tachycardia, or vary, depending on the site of origin. The RP interval is typically longer than the PR interval. The PR interval can vary in FAT, and the HR can vary from 150 to 300 beats/min, which can cause anxiety or panting in affected dogs. Syncope is rarely reported. In cats, FAT is rare.
- A baseline 24-hour Holter should be obtained to determine what percentage of time a dog is in FAT, and how fast the HR is during the tachycardia.

THERAPY

- Ideally, suppression of the rapidly firing atrial focus is attempted by using sotalol, amiodarone, or procainamide. In people, propafenone is used for treatment of FAT, but we have not found this agent efficacious in our patients. In fact, targeting the abnormal rhythm directly with these drugs is often unsuccessful. Thus, as a second choice, therapy for FAT should be aimed at slowing AV node conduction with CCBs or BBs to reduce the ventricular response. Digoxin is ineffective for management of FAT.
- A postdrug 24-hour Holter should be obtained to determine if drugs are effective at suppressing the FAT or producing the desired AV block, thus slowing the ventricular response adequately. The Holter also allows survey for excessive AV block, which may not be desired if it occurs other than during rest or sleep.

> **KEY POINT**
>
> Although amiodarone is a potent antiarrhythmic drug, its benefits must be balanced against its slow onset to action and adverse effects, which include hepatic toxicity, gastrointestinal disturbances, and blood dyscrasias in canine patients.

ATRIOVENTRICULAR NODAL REENTRANT TACHYCARDIA

- AV nodal reentry tachycardia (AVNRT) is a form of microreentry within the AV node that gives rise to rapid, simultaneous activation of the ventricles and atria. AVNRT is AV node dependent, thus AV node–slowing medication may terminate the arrhythmia. The prevalence in dogs is likely very low, but definitive diagnosis requires intracardiac mapping studies to prove dual AV node physiology. Thus far, AVNRT has not been reported in dogs.
- For treatment of AVNRT, see the following discussion of treatment of atrioventricular reentrant tachycardia (AVRT).

ATRIOVENTRICULAR REENTRANT TACHYCARDIA

- Atrioventricular reentrant tachycardia (AVRT) is a macroreentry arrhythmia whose circuit comprises the AV node as well as an accessory (AP) that can conduct impulses from the atria to the ventricles directly, thereby bypassing the AV node and His-Purkinje system. Response to a vagal maneuver or IV drug challenge may be used to confirm its AV node–dependent properties. One-to-one AV association is a requisite of AVRT because the atria and ventricles are both integral parts of the arrhythmia circuit. If AV dissociation occurs spontaneously without termination of the SVA, AVRT can be excluded.
- AVRT may be a paroxysmal, intermittent SVA that can result in very regular, rapid HR up to 300 beats/min. In some animals it can be sustained over several hours and thus result in cardiac dysfunction (tachycardiomyopathy) and heart failure. Typically, a 24-hour Holter may be required to make a definitive diagnosis of this SVA, as well as determine its clinical significance. Animals with AVRT may be symptom free or may show signs of syncope, episodic weakness, or lethargy.
- In dogs the arrhythmia most commonly follows a pattern of orthodromic conduction through the AV node (from the atria down to the ventricles) and retrograde over the AP back up to the atria, implying that the AP is only able to conduct in one direction (concealed conduction). This form is prevalent in Labrador Retrievers and termed orthodromic AV reciprocating tachycardia (OAVRT).
- Most APs in dogs do not allow conduction in the antegrade direction (concealed conduction) and are therefore not identifiable during normal sinus rhythm. In cats with AVRT, however, the AP may conduct in both directions so

that ventricular preexcitation is present during normal sinus rhythm. Preexcitation occurs when the atrial depolarization travels through both the AV node as well as the AP, which allows rapid, early activation of the ventricles. The ECG morphology of a P wave slurring directly into the upstroke of the QRS complex (delta wave) is a distinct feature of AP. Presence of delta waves may create the appearance of wide-complex tachycardia and thus resemble VT.

THERAPY

- Treatment with oral diltiazem or atenolol is the first choice for suppression of AVRT or AVNRT in dogs and cats. For acute management, IV diltiazem or esmolol is effective. For refractory cases in dogs, sotalol, procainamide, or amiodarone may be added because any of these drugs slow conduction of the atria, APs, and ventricles.
- For a determination of whether antiarrhythmic therapy of intermittent AVRT or AVNRT is effective, a postdrug 24-hour Holter should be compared with the baseline 24-hour Holter. This also allows checking for excessive AV block, which may be undesired if it occurs other than during rest or sleep.
- Some dogs with OAVRT display antegrade conduction over the AP (preexcitation) and display a delta wave on surface ECG after antiarrhythmic drug administration.
- In severely affected dogs, drug therapy may be ineffective. In such cases, cure may be achieved with transvenous catheter ablation of the AP with radiofrequency energy. This procedure can be performed only at specialized electrophysiology laboratories, which are available at some veterinary referral centers.

BRADYARRHYTHMIAS AND CONDUCTION DISTURBANCES

The bradyarrhythmias that require treatment are usually due to sinus node dysfunction (e.g., sinus bradycardia or sick sinus syndrome [SSS]), atrial conduction disturbances causing atrial standstill, or AV node conduction abnormalities causing high-grade second- or third-degree AV block. Ventricular conduction disturbances such as left and right bundle branch block as well as left anterior fascicular block do not warrant treatment, per se.

SINUS BRADYCARDIA

- Sinus bradycardia is diagnosed when the sinus node discharge rate is low (<50 beats/min) in an awake dog. Sinus bradycardia of 45 to 60 beats/min during sleep is normal.

Sinus bradycardia can exist in the form of a pronounced sinus arrhythmia or regular sinus bradycardia. This pathologic bradycardia often persists during excitement or exercise. The bradycardia is either primary, which is a form of SSS (see next section), or secondary to an underlying systemic disease or drug toxicity (e.g., narcotics or overdosing of BBs, CCBs, or digoxin).

- Secondary sinus bradycardia is usually caused by excessive vagal tone elicited by a systemic disease. Central nervous system disease (increased intracranial or intraocular pressure or head trauma), severe pain, or respiratory or gastrointestinal disease can all cause increased vagal tone and sinus bradycardia. A vagal maneuver (e.g., carotid sinus massage) can cause transient sinus bradycardia by the same mechanism of action. Correction of the underlying condition or discontinuation of drugs will usually resolve secondary sinus bradycardia.
- Clinical signs may be absent (incidental finding) or dogs may display weakness, exercise intolerance, or syncope. A 24-hour Holter may be required to determine the severity of bradycardia and possible association of clinical signs with the slow HR. Mild exercise intolerance is often underrecognized by owners and mistakenly attributed to "old age."
- In cats, sinus rhythm at less than 120 beats/min can be considered bradycardia, and HRs below 100 beats/min are often associated with lethargy or syncope in cats.

TREATMENT

- The decision to treat sinus bradycardia should be based on clinical signs and the degree of bradycardia. In patients experiencing syncope or episodic weakness, pacemaker therapy is indicated.
- In an animal with no clinical signs, sinus bradycardia may be "waited out" with close monitoring.
- If the animal appears unstable and pacemaker therapy is not an option, medical therapy aimed at abolishing high vagal tone can be attempted for temporary support. An atropine response test may help identify patients that would benefit from such medical management. After injection of **atropine** 0.02 mg/kg (0.01 to 0.04) IM or IV, the baseline HR should increase by 50% to 100% within 5 to 10 minutes (initial worsening bradycardia caused by AV block is a normal transient response). Patients experiencing at least a partial response to atropine may be candidates for medical management of sinus bradycardia. Treatment options include either a combination of a vagolytic drug

(e.g., **propantheline bromide** 0.25 to 0.5 mg/ kg PO BID or **hyoscyamine sulfate** 0.002 to 0.004 mg/kg PO BID) or a phosphodiesterase inhibitor (e.g., **theophylline** 20 mg/kg PO BID). Alternatively, a sympathomimetic drug could be tried as well (e.g., **albuterol** 0.02 to 0.05 mg/kg PO BID or TID).
- Erratic and poor efficacy, as well as adverse effects such as anxiety, excessive panting, anorexia, or gastrointestinal signs, are significant disadvantages to these therapies.

SICK SINUS SYNDROME

- The spontaneous sinus node discharge is either slower than normal (primary sinus bradycardia) or intermittently absent (sinus arrest or exit block from the sinus node). In the latter, there are pauses of various durations without P waves or an escape rhythm. The subsidiary pacemaker tissue (AV node and Purkinje fibers) is often also abnormal, resulting in inadequate escape rhythms, such that complete asystole (pauses) can last up to 10 seconds. Miniature Schnauzers, Cocker Spaniels, West Highland White Terriers, and Dachshunds are overrepresented. Doberman Pinschers and Boxers are also reported to have syncope associated with long sinus pauses, suggestive of SSS.
- Clinical signs range from exercise intolerance and lethargy to syncope. In dogs, SSS manifests as primary sinus bradycardia, typically with only mild exercise intolerance, which is often underrecognized by owners and mistakenly attributed to "old age." SSS may be incidentally diagnosed during a routine preanesthesia workup in a geriatric dog. If these dogs are treated with a pacemaker, owners often are delighted by the return of youth and energy in their "old dogs."
- Because of the intermittent nature of the sinus pauses in some cases, a 24-hour Holter is often necessary to definitively determine the cause of clinical signs.

TREATMENT

- Pacemaker therapy is indicated for syncopal or lethargic dogs with SSS. In dogs with intact AV node function, transvenous placement of a pacing lead in the right atrium or auricle may successfully abolish the sinus pauses. However, patients with SSS often have concomitant conduction disease in subsidiary pacemaker sites and may have AVN block later in the disease. In dogs with suspected concomitant AV node dysfunction, the lead should be placed in the right ventricle or dual chamber pacing performed.

- Some cases of SSS have brady-tachy syndrome: in addition to sinus pauses, supraventricular tachyarrhythmias (e.g., atrial tachycardia, flutter, or fibrillation) are present. In such cases, a 24-hour Holter should be obtained to determine the clinical relevance of the SVA and need for antiarrhythmic therapy. Therapy for tachycardias of any nature can only be considered, once pacing is established, to avoid worsening of bradyarrhythmias. Antiarrhythmic therapy may be necessary if the SVA persists after pacemaker implantation. In many cases, however, SVA spontaneously resolves once the long sinus pauses are prevented by the pacemaker.
- If the animal does not have syncope and shows no or only mild clinical signs, medical management can be attempted (see medical treatment of sinus bradycardia). In dogs with syncope, medical management is inadequate, and pacemaker therapy is always recommended.
- Furthermore, mild forms of SSS (i.e., no syncope yet) tend to progress over weeks or months to the point of syncope, and pacemaker implantation is eventually required.

ATRIAL STANDSTILL

- Atrial standstill occurs when the atrial myocardium is not able to depolarize, and P waves cannot be identified on the surface ECG. The two main causes are (1) persistent atrial standstill or "silent atrium" caused by primary atrial muscle disease and (2) secondary atrial standstill caused by hyperkalemia (i.e., renal failure, ruptured bladder, Addison disease, or other electrolyte imbalances). Hyperkalemia alters atrial transmembrane resting potential, and the atria become inexcitable at very high plasma K+ levels. However, in this scenario, the sinus node continues to fire, albeit at a slower rate, and the ensuing rhythm is called sinoventricular rhythm. It is reversible with correction of K levels. Persistent atrial standstill is uncommon in dogs and not reversible. Initially, dogs may have a junctional escape rhythm (HR 60 to 80 beats/min). However, some dogs have progressive conduction disease (AV junction and His Purkinje system) and eventually have very severe bradycardia (ventricular escape rhythm of 20 to 40 beats/min) and also myocardial failure (cardiomyopathy). Atrial standstill is exceedingly rare in cats.

THERAPY

- If atrial muscle disease is causing atrial standstill, pacemaker therapy is required. Because the atria are structurally abnormal, the pacing lead has to be placed in the right ventricle. Unfortunately, the primary cardiac muscle disease progressively affects the ventricles. Typically within 1 to 2 years, ventricular myocardial dysfunction and significant AV valve regurgitation may develop, and pacemaker failure may ensue because of lack of capture.
- For atrial standstill secondary to hyperkalemia, emergency therapy according to the severity of the hyperkalemia and bradycardia is required. Intravenous fluids are the primary treatment. This will lower potassium values by dilution and increased excretion. Acceptable fluids include normal saline, half-strength saline with 2.5% dextrose, or 5% dextrose in water. Alternatively, potassium can be lowered by promoting entry of K ions back into the intracellular space. The dextrose in fluid therapy will lead to insulin secretion that will drive potassium back into the cells. More aggressive therapy involves IV **sodium bicarbonate** (1 to 2 mEq/kg IV slowly over 20 minutes) to drive K back into the cell. Alternatively, slow IV administration of 0.5 U/kg of regular insulin coupled with 2 g of dextrose per unit of insulin can be administered. Monitoring for hypoglycemia is required after treatment. **Calcium gluconate** (0.5 to 1.0 mL/kg of a 10% solution) may be given by very slow IV administration for refractory cases of hyperkalemia. This is "cardioprotective" because the increased extracellular Ca2+ makes more sodium channels available for activation.

ATRIOVENTRICULAR CONDUCTION ABNORMALITIES

ATRIOVENTRICULAR BLOCK, FIRST DEGREE

- Prolonged conduction time through the AV node results in an increased PR interval of greater than 0.13 second in dogs and greater than 0.09 second in cats. There are normal P waves and QRS complexes, conducting at a 1:1 ratio. No treatment is required.

ATRIOVENTRICULAR BLOCK, SECOND DEGREE

- There are normal P wave and QRS complexes with a constant PR interval, but intermittently P waves are not followed by QRS complexes. In Mobitz type I (Wenckebach) AV block, the PR interval gradually prolongs before a P wave is blocked. This form of second-degree AV block is less frequent in dogs. Mobitz type II AV block demonstrates a consistent PR interval before a blocked P wave. Mobitz type II AV block may represent a more advanced degree of conduction abnormality that occurs in the AV junction, His bundle, or below. Occasional single blocked P waves are of no clinical significance.

- In "high-grade" second-degree AV block, there are several consecutive blocked P waves. Clinical signs depend on the length of ventricular asystole. In cases with intermittent high-grade second-degree AV block, a 24-hour Holter may be required to make a definitive diagnosis. If clinical signs such as lethargy or syncope are observed, pacemaker therapy is indicated.

ATRIOVENTRICULAR BLOCK, COMPLETE OR THIRD DEGREE

- None of the P waves conduct through the AV node; thus the atrial and ventricular activities are independent. The atrial rate (PP interval) is faster than the ventricular (escape) rate, differentiating complete AV block from AV dissociation caused by accelerated idioventricular rhythms. The ventricular escape rhythm is usually regular and below 40 beats/min, whereas a low AV junctional escape rhythm has a rate of 40 to 60 beats/min in dogs. In cats with complete AV block, the ventricular escape rhythm varies from 60 to 100 beats/min.
- Complete AV block is a primary abnormality of the AV conducting system (AV node). However, it is important to evaluate the animal's electrolyte and acid-base status. Systemic diseases causing hyperkalemia such as Addison disease or urethral obstruction can cause AV block that is reversible with normalization of K levels.
- In cats, hyperthyroidism can cause significant AV node disease, which may or may not be reversible with normalization of thyroid levels. Third-degree AV block is often not as life threatening in cats as in dogs. Cats with collapse episodes may live for longer than 1 year without pacemaker implantation and often succumb to other systemic diseases or structural heart disease rather than the actual bradyarrhythmia.

TREATMENT OF COMPLETE ATRIOVENTRICULAR BLOCK

- If no underlying abnormalities are discovered, a permanent cardiac pacemaker is the only effective treatment. Ideally, pacing systems that allow sensing of P waves in the atria and subsequent pacing of the ventricles are used (i.e., dual-chamber or single-lead atrial-sensing ventricular pacing systems).

VENTRICULAR ARRHYTHMIAS

GENERAL REMARKS

Ventricular arrhythmias may occur in apparently structurally normal hearts (hereditary arrhythmias) or may be associated with myocardial abnormalities such as cardiomyopathy, significant valvular disease, or myocarditis. To date, there is no medical therapy available that is known to prevent sudden death in animals afflicted with ventricular tachyarrhythmias. However, clinical signs such as syncope or episodic weakness can be alleviated in some animals with appropriate medical therapy. Clinically important ventricular arrhythmias are most commonly identified in certain breeds such as Boxers with arrhythmogenic right ventricular cardiomyopathy (ARVC), Doberman Pinschers and Great Danes with dilated cardiomyopathy (DCM), and German Shepherds with inherited ventricular arrhythmias. Dogs with congenital heart disease, such as severe subaortic or pulmonic stenosis, are predisposed to development of ventricular arrhythmias, likely because of abnormal myocardial perfusion secondary to myocardial hypertrophy. These arrhythmias can be worse during exercise and may be exacerbated during cardiac catheterization for angiography or interventional therapy. Catheter contact with the endocardium can elicit ventricular arrhythmias and even cause VF. Other myocardial insults (i.e., myocarditis or myocardial infarcts) can result in acute, life-threatening ventricular arrhythmias and sudden death. Increased cardiac troponin I, a biomarker to monitor presence of acute myocardial injury, may suggest such underlying conditions. Antiinflammatory therapy may be recommended in these cases, in addition to antiarrhythmic therapy.

Furthermore, significant ventricular arrhythmias can be seen in any dog hit by a car (traumatic myocarditis), large-breed dogs with gastric torsion, or dogs with neoplasia involving the myocardium. In some patients with ventricular arrhythmias, a cause cannot be identified. Cats with severe forms of cardiomyopathy, hyperthyroidism, sepsis, neoplasia, or severe electrolyte imbalances may have ventricular arrhythmias. Clinical signs depend on duration and rate of the VT but may include lethargy or rarely syncope if the rate is greater than 250 beats/min. Sudden death is not uncommon in this population, presumably because of a fatal ventricular arrhythmia.

TREATMENT OF VENTRICULAR TACHYCARDIA

- Ventricular tachycardia (VT) is recognized by abnormally wide and bizarre QRS complex shape. P waves are present but not associated with QRS complexes and may be hiding in the QRS-T complexes. AV dissociation occurs because of the accelerated ventricular rate compared with the sinus rate. VT can be monomorphic (where each QRS complex is identical) or polymorphic (where the QRS complex shape varies). Rapid, polymorphic VT is considered a more unstable arrhythmia because it is more likely to degenerate into VF.

- From a treatment perspective it is also important to differentiate between "fast" VT (170 to 350 beats/min) and "slow" VT (80 to 160 beats/min).
- Fast VT causes significantly reduced cardiac output, and clinical signs depend on the duration of the episode of abnormal rhythm. Affected animals may experience syncope, weakness, sudden death, or no signs at all. It warrants antiarrhythmic therapy either to convert the arrhythmia to sinus rhythm or at least to slow down the rate of the VT or reduce the length of the runs.
- A baseline 24-hour Holter is essential before initiation of therapy of fast VT to determine the percentage of ventricular ectopic beats and the duration and rate of runs of VT as well as the possible presence and length of pauses. A diary kept by the client or hospital staff documenting the activity of the dog and the exact time of observed syncope can help correlate ECG changes on the Holter with clinical signs.
- This information is critical both to institute suitable antiarrhythmic therapy and to assess drug efficacy by comparison of the posttreatment Holter with the baseline Holter.
- Slow VT may be associated with underlying systemic disease or can occur transiently after a gastric dilatation-volvulus or hit-by-car traumatic myocarditis in patients with structurally normal hearts. Cardiac troponin I (CTnI) may be elevated, indicating acute myocardial insult, or arrhythmias may be secondary to elevated circulating catecholamine levels associated with an underlying disease. Slow VT often does not require antiarrhythmic treatment as the rate is not fast enough to cause significant hemodynamic consequences. Instead, supportive care and monitoring of the underlying condition is imperative; however, if affected animals show signs of hypotension or lethargy, then they still may benefit from treatment of slow VT.
- Single VPCs are commonly observed in cardiomyopathic cats and are usually left untreated. If syncope is unexplained by standard ECG in feline patients, 24-hour Holter monitoring can be obtained. Cats with severe ventricular arrhythmias may warrant antiarrhythmic therapy.

ACUTE INTRAVENOUS ANTIARRHYTHMIC THERAPY

- For treatment of acute life-threatening VT, IV lidocaine is the first choice. Up to 3 bolus injections can be repeated and, if effective, a continuous-rate infusion should be instituted. A lidocaine bolus causes a transient drop in blood pressure and can lead to vomiting or seizures. If serum potassium levels are too low, lidocaine may not be effective. Lidocaine should be used judiciously for life-threatening VT in cats because of their low threshold for seizures with this drug.
- If lidocaine is not successful at restoring sinus rhythm or slowing VT, then procainamide IV can be added or administered instead. Procainamide is given initially as a slow bolus, followed by a constant-rate infusion. Procainamide can lead to hypotension, so careful monitoring of the patient during the infusion is recommended.
- Intravenous esmolol may be effective, especially in cases where high catecholamine levels may be contributing to the presence of ventricular arrhythmias. In dogs developing VT while undergoing an interventional procedure (i.e., balloon valvuloplasty for pulmonic stenosis), esmolol alone or in combination with lidocaine can be effective. Combination of esmolol with procainamide may cause a significant drop in cardiac output and hypotension. Esmolol may be safer to use than lidocaine in cats with acute life-threatening VT.
- Intravenous amiodarone may be used for acute, refractory VT, but pretreatment with antihistamines or steroids is advised because they can cause anaphylactic shock in dogs. It should thus be considered a last resort therapy. See Tables 17.2 and 17.3 for drug dosages.
- Electrical cardioversion of refractory, life-threatening VT may be attempted, if drug therapies fail. However, this requires a short period of general anesthesia and an external defibrillator that can deliver shocks synchronized to the R wave.

CHRONIC ORAL ANTIARRHYTHMIC THERAPY

- The first-line oral antiarrhythmic drug for treatment of VT in most dogs is sotalol, the exception being German Shepherds, caused by proarrhythmic effects documented in this specific breed. See Tables 17.2 and 17.3 for drug dosages.
- If a dog has very advanced myocardial systolic dysfunction (fractional shortening <15%), then sotalol may not be tolerated due its beta-blocker effect.
- Alternatively, mexiletine in combination with atenolol is very effective, particularly in Boxers. The atenolol dosage can be started at the lower end, in case of poor myocardial function. A practical disadvantage of this treatment regimen is the frequency of drug administration (mexiletine is given q8h).
- For refractory VT or recurrent syncope, a combination of sotalol with mexiletine may be effective.

These drugs should be initiated in a staggered protocol (usually sotalol first, mexiletine added after 2 days) to avoid side effects such as AV block or inappetence. Because this is a treatment protocol for refractory arrhythmias, patients are usually already receiving sotalol or mexiletine, in which case addition of the second drug is quite well tolerated.

- Oral procainamide or atenolol monotherapy are usually not efficacious for treatment of VT in dogs.
- As a last resort, oral amiodarone is effective for treatment of refractory VT. It has less negative inotropic effects than sotalol or atenolol, thus can be used in dogs with end-stage myocardial failure. But caution is advised when considering amiodarone therapy because of its adverse effects. Signs of toxicity include anorexia, vomiting, lethargy, and hepatic enzymes elevation.
- Oral atenolol or sotalol may be effective for treatment for VT in cats.
- Amiodarone toxicity in dogs
  - A maintenance dosage of 200 mg PO q24h is usually well tolerated, but a maintenance dose of 400 mg q24h is consistently associated with toxicity.
  - Monitoring of serial serum chemistries is recommended because increases in liver enzymes usually precede the onset of clinical signs of amiodarone toxicity. Liver enzymes should be measured after 7 days of drug loading and once monthly during maintenance therapy. If after 3 months of maintenance therapy no enzyme elevations develop, the time interval between testing may be increased to 2 months.
  - Amiodarone hepatopathy is reversible after reduction of dosage or discontinuation of the drug. Overt clinical signs of toxicity resolve within a few days of stopping amiodarone. Hepatic enzyme activity gradually returns to normal within 3 months after amiodarone is discontinued or the dosage is reduced.
  - Doberman Pinschers have a higher prevalence of inherent hepatopathies, and thus the incidence of amiodarone toxicity is possibly increased in this breed. Preexisting liver enzyme elevations are a contraindication for amiodarone therapy in Doberman Pinschers, unless no other alternative is available.
- A posttreatment 24-hour Holter is essential both to check efficacy and assess possible proarrhythmic effects of any antiarrhythmic drug. Significant worsening of VT during sotalol therapy has been documented in Boxers and German Shepherds.

BREED-SPECIFIC ARRYHYTHMIAS

ARRHYTHMOGENIC RIGHT VENTRICULAR CARDIOMYOPATHY IN BOXERS

- Ventricular arrhythmias and DCM, both manifestations of ARVC, are a common cause of morbidity and mortality in Boxers. The clinical presentation of ARVC can be grouped into three categories: (1) isolated subclinical ventricular arrhythmias, (2) arrhythmia-associated syncope or sudden death with normal myocardial function, and (3) systolic myocardial failure with or without ventricular arrhythmias. ARVC is inherited in an autosomal dominant pattern in Boxers. There is an association with a striatin mutation with the development of DCM in Boxers. Striatin is desmosomal protein (scaffolding protein) that has been associated with ARVC in humans. In addition, the Wnt signaling pathway is now implicated in Boxers with ARVC. In brief, Wnt signaling pathways play essential roles in cell behavior, survival, and proliferation.
- The shape of VT in Boxers is characteristically positive in the ventrocaudal leads (leads II, III, and aVF), which is also called a left bundle branch block pattern, suggesting a right ventricular origin of the arrhythmia.
- Syncope is often the first clinical sign and usually, but not always, associated with rapid runs of VT. Boxers can have multiple syncopal episodes and recover. These episodes may be more common during exercise or stress.
- A subset of Boxers also has a form of SSS, wherein fainting may be caused by long pauses from sinus arrest.
- Some Boxers also have SVAs including AF, especially if they have advanced stages of DCM and congestive heart failure.

VENTRICULAR TACHYCARDIA IN BOXERS WITH ARRHYTHMOGENIC RIGHT VENTRICULAR CARDIOMYOPATHY

CHRONIC ORAL ANTIARRHYTHMIC THERAPY

- Because of the association of VT with ARVC and myocardial systolic dysfunction, an echocardiogram is recommended before specific antiarrhythmic drug recommendations are made. See Table 17.2 for drug dosages.
- Sotalol is the treatment of choice for VT in Boxers, if the myocardial function is normal or only mildly decreased. If a Boxer has significantly reduced myocardial function, sotalol administered at its most effective antiarrhythmic dosage may reduce contractility and lead to worsening of heart failure.
- In such cases, mexiletine in combination with atenolol can be used. Atenolol can be started at

a lower dose to limit the beta blocker effect on myocardial contractility.

- For refractory VT and recurrent syncope, the combination of sotalol with mexiletine is useful. If the dog is already receiving sotalol with inadequate success, addition of mexiletine is usually well tolerated.
- If VT persists or the dog does not tolerate sotalol or mexiletine/atenolol, amiodarone may be beneficial. However, amiodarone hepatopathy may occur with long-term use. Monthly monitoring of liver enzymes is recommended.

ACUTE INTRAVENOUS ANTIARRHYTHMIC THERAPY

- See the section on the treatment of VT.

VENTRICULAR ARRHYTHMIAS AND DILATED CARDIOMYOPATHY IN DOBERMAN PINSCHERS

- Ventricular arrhythmias, syncope, and sudden death associated with DCM are common in Doberman Pinschers. The DCM is characterized by a slowly progressive, clinically occult phase during which ventricular premature contractions first appear. This phase is followed by the development of left ventricular dysfunction and usually progressively more severe ventricular tachyarrhythmias. The natural outcome in cardiomyopathic patients is usually either sudden death caused by ventricular arrhythmias or end-stage congestive heart failure, often associated with AF. The incidence of sudden death before the onset of congestive heart failure is between 30% and 50%.

KEY POINTS

- VT in Doberman Pinschers has both monomorphic and polymorphic characteristics.
- Syncope or episodic weakness has been documented in Doberman Pinschers caused by VT and bradyarrhythmias such as paradoxical sinus bradycardia and cardiac asystole. Unlike Boxers with ARVC, Doberman Pinschers with VT and DCM may die suddenly during their first syncopal episode.

VENTRICULAR TACHYCARDIA IN DOBERMAN PINSCHERS WITH DILATED CARDIOMYOPATHY

CHRONIC ORAL ANTIARRHYTHMIC THERAPY

- For treatment of VT in Doberman Pinschers, sotalol is effective (see Table 17.2 for drug dosages). A combination of mexiletine with sotalol

or atenolol may be used for refractory VT. With both drug regimens, monitoring by echocardiogram is recommended to check for worsening of myocardial function because of beta blockade. In cases with only moderate VT or significantly reduced myocardial function, monotherapy with mexiletine may be beneficial because mexiletine does not affect contractility. Doberman Pinschers seem to have gastrointestinal side effects (inappetence and vomiting) from mexiletine more readily than other breeds, so the starting dose should be at the low end of the dose range.

- Amiodarone is also effective in Doberman Pinschers with significant VT and end-stage myocardial failure; however, in this particular breed, careful monitoring of liver enzyme levels is imperative because Doberman Pinschers have a high incidence of amiodarone toxicity (for more details see the section on the treatment of VT).

ACUTE INTRAVENOUS ANTIARRHYTHMIC THERAPY

- See the section on the treatment of VT.

INHERITED VENTRICULAR ARRHYTHMIAS IN YOUNG GERMAN SHEPHERDS

- Inherited ventricular arrhythmias and a propensity for sudden death occur in young German Shepherds. This disorder has a wide phenotypic spectrum where some German Shepherds have very few ventricular premature complexes and others have frequent, rapid (rates >350 beats/min) polymorphic VT and sudden death. Dogs with documented VT are at risk for sudden death. Of German Shepherds with more than 10 runs of VT per 24 hours, approximately 50% die suddenly; this represents about 10% to 15% of the total affected populations studied. The prevalence of this disorder in the general German Shepherd population is unknown. Affected dogs have electrophysiologic abnormalities in calcium cycling and altered sympathetic innervation of the heart. Ventricular arrhythmias may be initiated by calcium sparks and afterdepolarizations (early and delayed) documented in the Purkinje fibers and ventricular myocytes of these dogs.
- German Shepherds have ventricular arrhythmias at 12 to 16 weeks of age, and the frequency and severity increase until 24 to 30 weeks of age. After that time, some dogs remain severely affected, whereas others show a progressive decline in the frequency of the arrhythmias. The dogs typically do not have syncope or other clinical signs. Most dogs have a low incidence of VT. If dogs reach the age of 18 months, the probability of sudden death declines markedly.

THERAPY OF GERMAN SHEPHERDS WITH VENTRICULAR TACHYCARDIA

- Dogs with mild to moderate amounts of ventricular arrhythmias do not warrant antiarrhythmic therapy. See Table 17.2 for drug dosages.
- In dogs at high risk of sudden death (>10 runs of VT/24 hours) based on a 24-hour Holter monitoring, antiarrhythmic therapy may be administered until the dog has "survived" the vulnerable time period.
- Intravenous lidocaine is effective in eliminating the ventricular arrhythmias acutely. However, monotherapy with the oral NCB mexiletine does not suppress the ventricular arrhythmias significantly. Sotalol monotherapy has proarrhythmic effects (i.e., causes increased numbers of runs of VT) in this specific breed, probably because of the action-potential prolonging effects, which can exacerbate early after depolarization-induced triggered activity.
- Combination therapy of mexiletine and sotalol may be beneficial in reducing the incidence and rate of VT in severely affected dogs; however, it is unknown if the risk of sudden death is reduced with this treatment.
- We have not tested amiodarone therapy in this breed. There is a poor response to procainamide.

VENTRICULAR ASYSTOLE

- Ventricular asystole is characterized by the complete absence of a ventricular rhythm. P waves may be present (with complete AV block), but no QRS complexes are observed. Primary asystole occurs when the Purkinje fibers intrinsically fail to generate a ventricular depolarization. It is usually preceded by a severe bradyarrhythmia caused by complete heart block, SSS, or both.

THERAPY

- Immediate external cardiac pacing with either transthoracic, transvenous, or epicardial electrodes (temporary pacing lead) may be effective, if asystole is the result of complete AV bock. Permanent pacemaker therapy is indicated. During cardiopulmonary resuscitation, epinephrine, isoproterenol, terbutaline, or atropine can be administered IV, but little effect is to be expected.
- Secondary asystole occurs when noncardiac factors suppress the electrical conduction system, resulting in a failure to generate any electrical depolarization. Massive pulmonary embolus, hyperkalemia, hypothermia, untreated VF or VT that deteriorates to asystole, unsuccessful defibrillation, or narcotic overdoses leading to

respiratory failure can lead to secondary asystole. In such cases, the final common pathway is usually severe tissue hypoxia with metabolic acidosis.
- The prognosis is usually grave for secondary asystole because external pacing is not effective in such cases.

VENTRICULAR FIBRILLATION

- No distinctive QRS complexes are identifiable on the ECG. Instead, there is an irregularly undulating baseline of variable amplitude caused by a rapid and chaotic activation of the ventricles. The sinus node is usually discharging regularly, but P waves are buried in the VF waveform. There is no mechanical contraction of the ventricles during VF; thus blood pressure drops to zero instantaneously. The rhythm cannot convert to sinus rhythm spontaneously and causes death within a few minutes because of lack of cardiac output. VT can degenerate to VF in any of the described scenarios of VT (see the previous section). VF can also occur secondary to systemic disease (i.e., severe hyperkalemia). Dogs that have congenital heart disease and are predisposed to ventricular arrhythmias may have VF during cardiac catheterization for angiography or interventional therapy because of "catheter irritation" of the myocardium.

THERAPY

- Drug therapy is usually not effective for treatment of VF. Because there is no blood pressure or blood flow during VF, drugs administered in a peripheral vein will not reach the myocardium. Electric defibrillation is the treatment of choice for VF.
- If VF occurs secondary to electrolyte imbalances or systemic disease, then the prognosis is usually grave, despite aggressive cardiopulmonary resuscitation efforts.
- Animals with a predisposition to ventricular arrhythmias or with VF while under anesthesia for catheter treatment of heart disease (but that are otherwise relatively healthy) may be successfully cardioverted. It is imperative that defibrillation occurs within a very short time after onset of VF (within about 3 minutes).
- VF has a grave prognosis if not corrected within the first 3 minutes of onset. Development of myocardial ischemia during VF contributes to worsening prognosis as time goes by. Cardiopulmonary resuscitation with chest compression should be performed briefly before defibrillation to provide some blood flow to the myocardium and increase chances of successful defibrillation.

TRANSTHORACIC ELECTRICAL DEFIBRILLATION PROCEDURE

- Dogs in VF become unconscious within 10 seconds because of the lack of blood flow to the brain.
- Defibrillation should be attempted using transthoracic hand-held paddles or "Fast Patch" electrodes.
- Animals should be placed in dorsal recumbency, and copious contact gel should be applied to the thorax if handheld paddles are used. For optimal current flow, the chest should be shaved first, but that may not be feasible in the interest of time. The dorsal recumbent position is safest for the operator but may not be optimal for defibrillation success in deep-chested dogs. If patch electrodes are available, dogs can also be placed in lateral recumbency, which might allow the defibrillation electrodes to be closer to the heart.
- Defibrillator ECG cables or the handheld paddles placed on the thorax should be used to ascertain presence of VF before defibrillation.
- With a monophasic defibrillator
  - Start with 6 J/kg.
  - If VF persists, increase the dose by 50 J and repeat until a maximum of 360 J.
- With a biphasic defibrillator
  - Start with 3 J/kg.
  - If VF persists, increase the dose by 50 J and repeat until a maximum of 360 J.
- Short, transient runs of VT, sinus pauses, or AV block are common following defibrillation.

FREQUENTLY ASKED QUESTIONS

What are idioventricular rhythms, and should they be treated?

An idioventricular rhythm is a form of ventricular arrhythmia characterized by a rate that is slow or comparable to the sinus rates (60 to 150 beats/min in dogs and >100 beats/min in cats). The ventricular rate usually remains within 10 to 15 beats/min of the sinus rate, and the cardiac rhythm "switches" back and forth between the two competing pacemaker sites. This arrhythmia may occur for several reasons, including systemic diseases (e.g., anemia, splenic hemangiosarcoma), drugs (e.g., digoxin, opioids), and electrolyte abnormalities (e.g., hypokalemia). In general, no clinical signs are associated with idioventricular rhythms. If clinical signs are present, they are often associated with the underlying process. Idioventricular rhythms usually do not require treatment. Management of the underlying cardiac disease or metabolic abnormality is required.

What are the advantages of rate control compared with rhythm control in the management of atrial fibrillation?

Management is relatively simple because it can be achieved in the home with oral medication. Rate control successfully achieves improved left ventricular function, reduction in clinical signs, limited hospitalizations, and prevention of tachycardiomyopathy.

What are the disadvantages of rate control?

Optimal HR for dogs with atrial fibrillation is unknown. Rate control strives to improve cardiac output by lowering the ventricular response and yet not limit exercise capacity. However, it is not "perfect" compared with sinus rhythm, and the optimal HR may vary according to disease severity. Side effects from antiarrhythmic medication can occur (gastrointestinal signs, hypotension, worsening of heart failure, or arrhythmias). In addition, owner compliance and cost for lifelong therapy must be taken into consideration. Rate control can only be monitored with periodic Holter recordings acquired in the home (stress-free) environment. This increases the cost of the therapy.

What are the advantages of cardioversion (electrical or pharmacologic)?

Cardioversion has similar advantages to adequate rate control in that tachycardiomyopathy is avoided and reduction in clinical signs and improved exercise tolerance can be achieved. The most important advantage is that the patient has a "normal" physiologic sinus rhythm compared with "slow" AF. AV synchrony provides optimal cardiac output, especially in face of myocardial failure. Furthermore, sinus rhythm allows adequate changes in HR according to blood pressure and autonomic tone.

What are the disadvantages of cardioversion (electrical or pharmacologic)?

The main disadvantages of electrical cardioversion are that it requires general anesthesia, hospitalization, and expensive equipment and that it has a risk of cardiac arrest from "shocking." Pharmacologic cardioversion's main disadvantage includes side effects from drug administration; owner compliance can be of concern because of the daily need to administer drugs. There is a big risk of recurrence of AF even after successful cardioversion with either method of cardioversion.

Most patients with AF secondary to myocardial disease are treated very effectively with rate control (see Figures 17.1, 17.2, and 17.3).

SUGGESTED READINGS

Bright JM, zumBrunnen J: Chronicity of atrial fibrillation affects duration of sinus rhythm after transthoracic cardioversion of dogs with naturally occurring atrial fibrillation, J Vet Intern Med 222(1):114–119, 2008.

Gelzer ARM, Kraus MS, Moise NS, et al: Assessment of anti-arrhythmic drug efficacy to control heart rate in dogs with atrial fibrillation using 24-hour ambulatory electrocardiographic (Holter) recordings, J Vet Intern Med 18(5):779, 2004.

Gelzer ARM, Moise NS, Koller ML: Defibrillation of German shepherds with inherited ventricular arrhythmias and sudden death, J Vet Cardiol 7(2):97–107, 2005.

Gelzer AR, Kraus MS, Rishniw M, et al: Combination therapy with mexiletine and sotalol suppresses inherited ventricular arrhythmias in German shepherd dogs better than mexiletine or sotalol monotherapy: a randomized cross-over study, J Vet Intern Med 24(6):1388, 2010.

Gelzer RM, Kraus MS: Management of atrial fibrillation, Vet Clin North Am Small Anim Pract 34:1127–1144, 2004.

Jacobs G, Calvert C, Kraus M: Hepatopathy in 4 dogs treated with amiodarone, J Vet Intern Med 14(1):96–99, 2000.

Jesty SA, Jung SW, Cordeiro JM, et al.: Cardiomyocyte calcium cycling in a naturally occurring German shepherd dog model of inherited ventricular arrhythmia and sudden cardiac death, J Vet Cardiol 15(1):5–14, 2013.

Kraus MS, Moise NS, Rishniw M: Morphology of ventricular tachycardia in the Boxer and pace mapping comparison, J Vet Intern Med 16:153–158, 2002.

Kraus MS, Ridge LG, Gelzer ARM, et al: Toxicity in Doberman pinscher dogs with ventricular arrhythmias treated with amiodarone, J Vet Intern Med 19(3):407, 2005.

Meurs KM, Spier AW, Wright NA, et al: Comparison of the effects of four antiarrhythmic treatments for familial ventricular arrhythmias in Boxers, J Am Vet Med Assoc 221(4):522–527, 2002.

Meurs KM, Stern JA, Sisson DD, et al: Association of dilated cardiomyopathy with the striatin mutation genotype in boxer dogs, J Vet Intern Med 27(6):1437–1440, 2013.

Moise NS, Gilmour RF Jr, Riccio ML, Flahive WF Jr: Diagnosis of inherited ventricular tachycardia in German Shepherd dogs, J Am Vet Med Assoc 210(3):403–410, 1997.

Oxford EM, Danko CG, Fox PR, et al: Change in β-catenin localization suggests involvement of the canonical Wnt pathway in Boxer dogs with arrhythmogenic right ventricular cardiomyopathy, J Vet Intern Med 28(1):92–101, 2014.

Santilli RA, Perego M, Crosara S, et al: Utility of 12-lead electrocardiogram for differentiating paroxysmal supraventricular tachycardias in dogs, J Vet Intern Med 22(4):915–923, 2008.

18

Cardiopulmonary Arrest and Resuscitation

Vincent J. Thawley | Kenneth J. Drobatz

Cardiopulmonary resuscitation (CPR) describes a set of techniques to provide circulatory and ventilatory support following cardiopulmonary arrest (CPA). CPR encompasses both basic and advanced life support. Basic life support includes the ABCs of resuscitation and involves establishing an **ai**rway, providing manual ventilation (**b**reathing), and performing external chest **c**ompressions or internal cardiac compressions to generate forward blood flow. Advanced life support includes the Ds and Es of resuscitation, including **d**rug therapy, **d**efibrillation, and **e**lectrocardiogram (ECG) analysis during resuscitation. The goal of CPR is to maximize blood flow and oxygen delivery to the heart and brain until return of spontaneous circulation (ROSC) is achieved and the underlying cause of the arrest may be addressed.

- *CPA* is defined as the cessation of spontaneous circulation and ventilation. Causes of CPA include primary myocardial disease (although this is rare in veterinary patients), hypotension (secondary to hypovolemia, sepsis, or drug administration), hypoxemia (secondary to hypoventilation or lung disease), metabolic derangements (e.g., severe metabolic acidosis), or electrolyte abnormalities (e.g., hyperkalemia). Recognizing that these predisposing causes of arrest may be associated with either reversible or irreversible underlying disease processes is important.
- The prognosis for patients requiring CPR is guarded, and long-term survival is generally less than 10%. The likelihood of a successful outcome is improved when an arrest is rapidly recognized and a reversible cause is identified and addressed.
- CPR is most likely to be successful when the team is prepared, the techniques are practiced, the communication is clear, and the resuscitation takes place in a well-equipped area within the hospital.

BASIC LIFE SUPPORT

AIRWAY

- Establishing an airway is the first step in performing basic life support. Orotracheal intubation is generally performed in a routine fashion, and this may be facilitated by the use of a laryngoscope or a stylet for the endotracheal tube as well as an assistant to exteriorize the tongue. Have suction available if secretions or blood obscure visualization of the glottis. In situations where the glottis cannot be visualized, the larynx may be directly palpated and the endotracheal tube may be guided by feel. Intubation performed with the patient in lateral recumbency is suggested as this positioning allows for concurrent initiation of chest compressions.
- In rare situations, an emergency tracheostomy is required. This technique may be performed in less than 30 seconds after rapidly clipping and prepping the ventral cervical region. A midline incision is performed and sharp dissection is used to expose the trachea. Care is taken during dissection to remain on midline (between the sternothyroideus muscles) to avoid vascular structures. Once the trachea has been isolated, a transverse incision is made between cervical rings (approximately 50% of the diameter) and a cuffed tracheostomy tube is inserted. A standard endotracheal tube may also be used in this situation.
- Once an airway is established, it is important to confirm correct tube placement. This may be done by direct visualization, cervical palpation, auscultation of lung sounds, and observing chest wall movement. The use of end-tidal carbon dioxide ($ETCO_2$) monitoring in this situation is also useful because tracheal gas is always higher in CO_2 than esophageal gas; however, lack of detectable $ETCO_2$ does not preclude endotracheal intubation because delivery of carbon dioxide to the lungs is compromised in the setting of cardiopulmonary arrest. Once placement is confirmed, it is vital to secure the endotracheal tube, as inadvertent tube dislodgement is very common in an arrest situation.

During the resuscitation attempt, endotracheal tube placement should be assessed periodically to ensure that it has not become dislodged.
- Airway problems during an arrest (i.e., inability to auscult lung sounds, chest wall not moving with ventilation) should prompt rapid reevaluation of endotracheal tube placement. It is also important to ensure that the cuff has been inflated because this is often the source of problems. If airway problems have been ruled out, difficulty ventilating the lungs during an arrest suggests severe pleural space, airway, or parenchymal disease.

BREATHING

- The patients' lungs should be manually ventilated with 100% oxygen. Methods for providing positive pressure ventilation in an arrest situation include the use of an Ambu-bag or an anesthesia machine.
- Respiratory rate should be approximately 10 breaths per minute with an inspiratory time of 1 second. It should be noted that excessive ventilation often occurs during CPR and should be avoided. It has been shown in animal models that faster respiratory rates, long inspiratory time, and high tidal volumes result in a higher mean intrathoracic pressure, decreased myocardial perfusion pressure, and decreased survival.
- Normal chest wall motion should be observed and peak pressure of less than 20 cm H_2O should be maintained if possible to reduce the risk of pulmonary barotrauma. Problems causing decreased pulmonary compliance or diminished chest wall motion may include airway obstruction, severe parenchymal disease, or pleural space disease (e.g., pneumothorax, pleural effusion, diaphragmatic hernia, mass lesions).

CIRCULATION

- Artificial circulation during CPR may be provided by performing external chest compressions or internal cardiac massage. The goal of either technique is to maximize blood flow to the coronary and cerebral vasculature.
- Myocardial perfusion pressure (MPP) is the best predictor of ROSC in human patients and animal models of CPR, and it is represented by the following equation: MPP = aortic diastolic pressure – central venous pressure.
- Cerebral perfusion pressure (CPP) drives cerebral blood flow and is represented by the following equation: CPP = mean arterial pressure – intracranial pressure.
- There are two theories describing the mechanism of blood flow during external chest compressions. The cardiac pump theory describes actual compression of the heart through the chest wall and is likely to occur in small patients (<15 kg). The thoracic pump theory describes blood flow as a result of phasic increases in intrathoracic pressure and has been documented in larger animals (>15 kg).
- External chest compressions should be performed with the patient positioned in lateral recumbency with its dorsum toward the compressor. The chest may be compressed circumferentially or directly over the heart in small patients (<15 kg) and at the widest point of the chest in larger patients (>15 kg). Sternal compressions with the patient positioned in dorsal recumbency may be considered for barrel-chested breeds such as English Bulldogs.
- The rate of chest compressions should be 100 to 120 per minute with a ratio of compression to relaxation of 50:50. Although higher compression rates have been shown to generate greater cardiac output, it is difficult to sustain higher rates for extended periods of time during CPR. Compressions should be given with enough force to decrease the diameter of the chest wall by approximately 33% to 50%. Full elastic recoil of the chest should be permitted between each compression as this will allow for improved venous return during the decompression phase.
- Chest compressions should be initiated as soon as possible after diagnosing cardiopulmonary arrest and performed in 2-minute cycles with minimal interruptions. Experimental animal models have shown that peak CPP is only achieved after approximately 60 seconds of uninterrupted chest compressions and that there is a rapid decrease in CPP whenever compressions are stopped.
- If a sufficient number of rescuers are present, the person performing chest compressions should be rotated every 2 minutes to prevent the development of fatigue because this has been shown to negatively affect the quality of the resuscitation effort. The brief pause in compressions as rescuers are rotated is an appropriate time to assess the patient for ROSC and assess the cardiac rhythm should a continuous ECG be employed.
- Interposed abdominal compression (IAC) may be used to improve the efficacy of external chest compressions. With this technique, the abdomen is compressed during "diastole" (relaxation phase of chest compression) to increase the pressure gradient favoring blood return to the chest, thereby improving cardiac output, blood pressure, and myocardial and cerebral perfusion pressure.

- Even optimal external chest compression produces approximately 25% of normal cardiac output. Open-chest CPR and internal cardiac compression may produce 100% of normal cardiac output, with dramatic increases in blood flow to the heart and brain. Indications for open-chest CPR include pleural space disease (e.g., pneumothorax, pleural effusions, diaphragmatic hernia), pericardial effusion, penetrating wounds, chest wall trauma, intraoperative arrests, hemoperitoneum, large dogs in which closed-chest compressions are unlikely to generate effective blood flow, or prolonged resuscitations (>2 to 5 minutes without ROSC).
- For open-chest CPR to be performed, the heart may be accessed via a left lateral thoracotomy (or transdiaphragmatically in patients undergoing abdominal surgery). After a rapid clip and preparation of the left chest, an emergency thoracotomy may be performed in approximately 30 seconds. A skin incision is made in the fourth or fifth intercostal space and is extended through the chest wall musculature. Ventilation is temporarily suspended, and the pleural space is accessed. A rib spreader is used to retract the ribs. Once the heart is exposed, the ventricles may be compressed with one or two hands depending upon the size of the patient. A rate of 100 to 120 compressions per minute is recommended. It is often easier to perform direct cardiac compression once an incision has been made in the pericardium (below the level of the phrenic nerve). The pericardium should be incised before cardiac compressions are initiated if pericardial effusion with tamponade is encountered.
- Open-chest CPR allows for compression or cross-clamping of the descending aorta to direct blood flow to the heart and brain and avoids additional volume loss in cases of abdominal hemorrhage. In the absence of an atraumatic vascular clamp, the aorta may be manually compressed, or a Penrose drain or red rubber catheter may be tightened around the aorta. When appropriate, aortic flow may be gradually restored (over 5 to 10 minutes).
- Open-chest CPR requires that appropriate facilities and expertise be available for postresuscitation care and management of the emergency thoracotomy.

ADVANCED LIFE SUPPORT

ESTABLISHING ACCESS FOR DRUG AND FLUID THERAPY

- Rapid access to the circulation is vital in CPR. Central venous access (e.g., jugular vein) is ideal because drug circulation times are significantly lower when compared with peripheral venous sites. Because of the low-flow state that occurs during CPR, large flush volumes (at least 5 to 10 mL of 0.9% NaCl) are necessary, especially when peripheral catheters are used. Short, large-bore catheters are ideal, as these provide the highest flow rates for drug and fluid administration.
- Surgical cutdown should be performed immediately if the initial attempt at percutaneous vascular access is not successful. Surgical cutdown involves making a skin incision adjacent and parallel to the long axis of the vein (usually jugular, cephalic, or saphenous) to be isolated. Blunt dissection with a hemostat is used to expose the vein, and an intravenous catheter is introduced. Cut-down catheters should be secured with sutures and bandaged appropriately.
- Intraosseous (IO) access is an alternative to peripheral venous access, especially in small puppies, kittens, and exotic species. The intertrochanteric fossa of the femur, proximal humerus, and proximal tibia are readily accessible sites to obtain IO access.
- Intratracheal (IT) administration is an excellent method to deliver drugs when intravenous access is not available. Most drugs used in CPR (with the exception of sodium bicarbonate) can be delivered by this route. When drugs are delivered intratracheally, the dose is doubled, the medication is diluted to 2 to 5 mL (depending on patient size), and the drug is delivered through a red rubber catheter placed through and beyond the tip of the endotracheal tube (at the level of the carina). Air may be used to flush the catheter.
- Intracardiac drug administration is not recommended in CPR because there is a risk for inadvertent laceration of the lung or coronary vasculature, as well as the potential for intramyocardial drug administration (which may exacerbate arrhythmias or ischemia in the case of epinephrine).

ELECTROCARDIOGRAPHY

- ECG monitoring is integral to providing advanced life support. The course of action taken during CPR depends on the cardiac rhythm that is present. Changes in the cardiac rhythm during the course of an arrest often dictate changes in therapy (Figure 18.1).

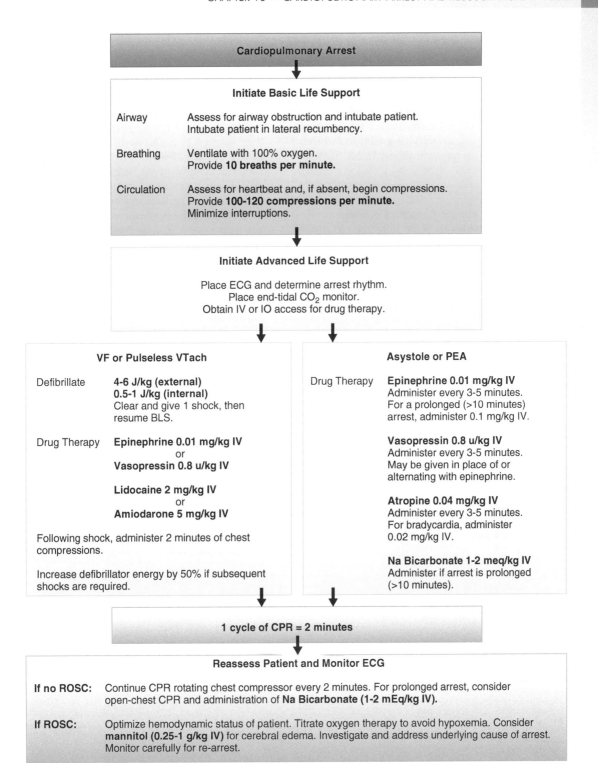

Figure 18.1 Algorithm for performing cardiopulmonary resuscitation (CPR) in veterinary patients. *BLS,* Basic life support; *CO₂,* carbon dioxide; *ECG,* electrocardiogram; *IO,* intraosseous; *IV,* intravenous; *PEA,* pulseless electrical activity; *VF,* ventricular fibrillation; *VTach,* ventricular tachycardia. (Adapted from Fletcher DJ, Boller M, Brainard BM, et al: RECOVER evidence and knowledge gap analysis on veterinary CPR. Part 7: Clinical guidelines, J Vet Emerg Crit Care 22:S2102-S131, 2012.)

- A retrospective study of veterinary patients undergoing CPR has shown that common cardiac rhythms during initial arrest include pulseless electrical activity, asystole, ventricular fibrillation, and sinus bradycardia.
- Although ventricular fibrillation is most responsive to treatment (defibrillation), a recent study of veterinary patients surviving CPR found that asystole was the most common initial rhythm identified.

DRUG THERAPY

- See Table 18.1 for drug therapy guidelines.
- **Intravenous fluids** can be administered in shock doses (90 mL/kg in dogs and 60 mL/kg in cats, given in aliquots to effect) to patients that are hypovolemic. Intravenous fluids may also be useful to help flush drugs from peripheral sites into the central circulation. It should be noted, however, that myocardial perfusion pressure may be reduced by significant increases in central venous pressure and that bolus fluid therapy may be counterproductive in patients that are euvolemic or volume-overloaded at the time of arrest.

- **Atropine** is a vagolytic drug that abolishes parasympathetic tone. It is indicated in patients with bradycardias (as may occur in vagal events), as well as in pulseless electrical activity and asystole. It should be noted that high doses of atropine may cause a profound tachycardia in patients with perfusing rhythms, and that the dose is often reduced by 50% to 75% in these situations. The dose of atropine is 0.04 mg/kg (dogs and cats) and can be given by intravenous (IV), IT, or IO routes. Atropine is available in a concentration of 0.54 mg/mL, and a shortcut to determine the dose is 1 mL/10 kg. The dose may be repeated at 3- to 5-minute intervals.
- **Epinephrine** is a potent alpha and beta catecholamine receptor agonist. Experimental studies have shown that it is the alpha (vasoconstrictor) effects rather than the beta (chronotropic/inotropic) effects that are most important in achieving ROSC. The benefit is due to the increased peripheral resistance created by adrenergic stimulation and the resultant increase in aortic pressure that leads to an increase in myocardial perfusion pressure and

Table 18.1   Guidelines for Drug Therapy and Initial Defibrillator Settings (Monophasic Waveform Defibrillators) During CPR

Weight (lb)		5	10	20	30	40	50	60	70	80	90	100
Weight (kg)		2.5	5	10	15	20	25	30	35	40	45	50
Drug (conc.)	Dose	mL										
Epi low (1:1,000)	0.01 mg/kg	0.025	0.05	0.1	0.15	0.2	0.25	0.3	0.35	0.4	0.45	0.5
Epi high (1:1,000)	0.1 mg/kg	0.25	0.5	1	1.5	2	2.5	3	3.5	4	4.5	5
Atropine (0.54 mg/mL)	0.04 mg/kg	0.2	0.5	1	1.5	2	2.5	3	3.5	4	4.5	5
Lidocaine (20 mg/mL)	2 mg/kg	0.25	0.5	1	1.5	2	2.5	3	3.5	4	4.5	5
Sodium bicarbonate (1 mEq/mL)	1 mEq/kg	2.5	5	10	15	20	25	30	35	40	45	50
Calcium gluconate (100 mg/mL)	50 mg/kg	1	2.5	5	7.5	10	12.5	15	17.5	20	22.5	25
Magnesium sulfate (4 mEq/mL)	0.2 mEq/kg	0.1	0.25	0.5	0.75	1	1.25	1.5	1.75	2	2.25	2.5
Vasopressin (20 units/mL)	0.8 unit/kg	0.1	0.2	0.4	0.6	0.8	1	1.2	1.4	1.6	1.8	2
Amiodarone (50 mg/mL)	5 mg/kg	0.25	0.5	1	1.5	2	2.5	3	3.5	4	4.5	5
Naloxone (0.4 mg/mL)	0.04 mg/kg	0.25	0.5	1	1.5	2	2.5	3	3.5	4	4.5	5
Flumazenil (0.1 mg/mL)	0.02 mg/mL	0.5	1	2	3	4	5	6	7	8	9	10
External defibrillation	4-6 J/kg	10	20	40	60	80	100	120	140	160	180	200
Internal defibrillation	0.5-1 J/kg	2	3	5	8	10	15	15	20	20	20	25

CPR, Cardiopulmonary resuscitation.

Adapted from Fletcher DJ, Boller M, Brainard BM, et al: RECOVER evidence and knowledge gap analysis on veterinary CPR. Part 7: Clinical guidelines, J Vet Emerg Crit Care 22:S102-S131, 2012.

a more successful resuscitation. Epinephrine is indicated in all cardiac arrest situations. There are both high- and low-dose recommendations for epinephrine in CPR. Current guidelines in both the veterinary and human literature suggest the use of epinephrine at the low dose (0.01 mg/kg) because high-dose therapy has not been associated with increased survival to discharge and may in fact have deleterious side effects due to adrenergic overstimulation. High-dose epinephrine (0.1 mg/kg) may be considered if ROSC is not achieved with low-dose therapy. Epinephrine can be given IV, IT, or IO, and a shortcut to calculate low-dose epinephrine volume for administration is 0.1mL/10 kg. The dose may be repeated at 3- to 5-minute intervals.

- **Vasopressin** is a noncatecholamine vasopressor drug that has recently been included in human CPR guidelines. Potential advantages of vasopressin (compared with epinephrine) include efficacy in the presence of acidosis, lack of potentially harmful beta effects, and a longer half-life. The role of vasopressin in CPR is still being investigated; however, there is evidence that this drug may be equivalent to or even superior to epinephrine in some situations. The dose of vasopressin is 0.8 units/kg (dogs and cats), and the dose may be repeated at 3- to 5-minute intervals.
- **Lidocaine** is indicated in ventricular fibrillation or pulseless ventricular tachycardia that is not responsive to initial defibrillation attempts. Like other antiarrhythmic drugs, lidocaine may increase the defibrillation threshold. In addition, lidocaine must be used with care in the postarrest period, as it may suppress a functional ventricular escape rhythm. The dose of lidocaine is 2 mg/kg (dogs, IV, IO, IT), and a shortcut to calculate the dose for the 2% (20 mg/mL) solution is 1 mL/10 kg.
- **Amiodarone** has been incorporated into human CPR guidelines and has been favorably compared with lidocaine when treating ventricular fibrillation that is refractory to defibrillation. There is limited experience with amiodarone in the context of CPR in veterinary patients. The dose of amiodarone is 5 to 10 mg/kg (dogs, IV), and it is diluted in 5% dextrose before administration. Hypotension is a common occurrence during amiodarone administration.
- **Sodium bicarbonate** is not recommended for use in *all* arrest situations. It is indicated, however, in patients with a preexisting metabolic acidosis, patients with hyperkalemia, and in prolonged (>10 minute) arrest scenarios. The dose for sodium bicarbonate is 1 to 2 mEq/kg

(dogs and cats, IV, IO). A shortcut to calculate the dose is 1 mL/kg of a standard 1mEq/mL solution. Sodium bicarbonate should not be given intratracheally, as it will inactivate surfactant and have deleterious effects on pulmonary function. Administration of sodium bicarbonate to a patient that is not appropriately ventilated during CPR may lead to hypercapnia and respiratory acidosis. Sodium bicarbonate should not be used in patients with known hypoventilation.

- **Calcium gluconate** is also not routinely recommended in every arrest situation because its use may exacerbate ischemia-reperfusion injury. It is indicated in patients with symptomatic hyperkalemia or hypermagnesemia, in patients with known hypocalcemia, and for treatment of calcium channel blocker toxicity. The dose of calcium gluconate is 50 to 100 mg/kg (dogs and cats, IV, IO).
- **Magnesium sulfate** is indicated in patients with known hypomagnesemia and in some ventricular arrhythmias (e.g., torsade de pointes). The dose of magnesium sulfate is 30 mg/kg (dogs and cats, IV, IO).
- Charts with guidelines for drug dosing during CPR are available from the Veterinary Emergency and Critical Care Society (www.veccs.org).

DEFIBRILLATION

- See Table 18.1 for defibrillation guidelines.
- Electrical defibrillation is the only effective method to convert ventricular fibrillation to a perfusing cardiac rhythm. Defibrillation is also indicated in patients with pulseless ventricular tachycardia.
- The defibrillator must be used properly to minimize risks to members of the resuscitation team. It is strongly recommended that the patient be placed in lateral recumbency for both CPR and defibrillation. Attempting to defibrillate a patient in dorsal recumbency may allow the patient's limb to contact a team member, which could lead to the unintentional delivery of current to a staff member and a potentially harmful situation. Most defibrillators have attachments for an accessory flat paddle (often called a posterior paddle) that may be placed under the patient, with the handheld paddle placed over the heart on opposite sides of the chest wall.
- Use large amounts of contact gel and press the paddles firmly onto the patient's thorax so that the current is delivered through the chest rather than "arcing" across the surface of the skin. Arcing of current is inefficient and may be dangerous, especially if alcohol has been placed on the patient. The smell of burning

hair should alert the clinician that the current is likely arcing; applying more contact gel and repositioning the paddles are warranted before administering another shock. Because of the risk of combustion during defibrillation, alcohol (to increase ECG contact) should not be used during CPR. ECG contact gel is a much safer alternative.

- Clear communication during defibrillation is also important to ensure safety. The operator must inform the other resuscitation team members of an impending defibrillation attempt and confirm that no member of the team is in contact with the patient or table before delivering a shock. Because of the safety concern, a standard protocol is followed for each defibrillation. This protocol is as follows: (1) confirm ventricular fibrillation or pulseless ventricular tachycardia, (2) apply contact gel, (3) confirm current to be delivered and charge defibrillator, (4) halt ongoing CPR, (5) call "Clear," (6) confirm that all personnel are clear of the patient (especially limbs) and table, (7) deliver current, and (8) monitor success of defibrillation.

- Immediate defibrillation is recommended only when the duration of cardiopulmonary arrest caused by ventricular fibrillation is 4 minutes or less; otherwise, a 2-minute cycle of chest compressions before defibrillation is recommended. The dose of energy for initial defibrillation is 2 to 4 J/kg (biphasic defibrillator) or 4 to 6 J/kg (monophasic defibrillator).

- If an initial shock is not successful, CPR is resumed for 2 minutes before defibrillation is attempted again. A 50% escalation in the energy delivered may be considered for subsequent defibrillation attempts.

- Mechanical defibrillation via a precordial thump can be attempted if electrical defibrillation is not available; however, this technique is thought to be of little benefit in most situations.

MONITORING CARDIOPULMONARY RESUSCITATION EFFORTS

- Patient monitoring during CPR can be difficult, and some standard techniques can be potentially misleading in an arrest situation.

- Palpation of femoral pulses during chest compression is an encouraging finding; however, the presence of pulses (and a discernible pulse pressure) does not necessarily correspond to adequate arterial blood pressure or perfusion pressures. Direct arterial pressure measurement is ideal, although this is generally only feasible in patients with a previously placed arterial line.

- As mentioned earlier, ECG monitoring is vital during CPR because this often dictates the type and timing of intervention. ECG findings must always be interpreted in the light of physical examination parameters. This is especially important when an apparent escape rhythm is present. The presence of auscultable heart sounds and palpable pulses indicates ROSC. Without these findings, the rhythm represents pulseless electrical activity, and CPR should be continued.

- $ETCO_2$ monitoring is an easily applied and extremely useful monitoring tool in CPR. If ventilation is constant, $ETCO_2$ is linearly related to pulmonary blood flow and, by extension, cardiac output. As with myocardial perfusion pressure, higher $ETCO_2$ during CPR has been shown to correlate with increased likelihood of successful resuscitation. In addition, because $ETCO_2$ is a surrogate marker for pulmonary blood flow, marked increases in this parameter serves as a useful indicator of ROSC.

- Blood gas analysis may be misleading during CPR. Despite the low-flow state and global tissue ischemia that occurs, arterial blood gas results may appear relatively normal after equilibration with alveolar gas (especially with the hyperventilation that frequently occurs during CPR). On the other hand, venous blood gas results reflect the metabolic and respiratory acidosis that characterizes the local tissue environment in the face of hypoperfusion and decreased clearance of metabolic byproducts. Therefore venous blood gas results are more useful in the monitoring of CPR. It should be noted, however, that elevated venous CO_2 may result from inadequate blood flow and local tissue hypoperfusion rather than true hypoventilation.

KEY POINT

Advanced life support techniques include the implementation of drug therapy and defibrillation. These interventions are based on the circumstances unique to each arrest and provide options to augment the effectiveness of basic life support.

SPECIAL SITUATIONS

ANESTHETIC ARRESTS

- In general, anesthetic-related arrests are rare; however, arrests that occur in conjunction with anesthesia are usually rapidly recognized, and some retrospective veterinary studies demonstrate that these patients are the most likely to be successfully resuscitated.

- Steps to take in an anesthetic-related arrest include turning off gas anesthesia and flushing the anesthetic circuit, opening the pop-off valve if it is closed, reversing injectable anesthetic agents with naloxone (for opioids) at 0.02 to 0.04 mg/kg (dogs and cats, IV), flumazenil (for benzodiazepines) at 0.02 to 0.04 mg/kg (dogs and cats, IV), or yohimbine/atipamenzole (for alpha-2 agonists) at 0.1 to 0.2 mg/kg (dogs and cats, IV), and instituting standard CPR.
- Immediate open-chest CPR should be performed in patients undergoing thoracotomy and should be considered in patients undergoing celiotomy (via a transdiaphragmatic approach).
- Possible underlying causes such as hypoventilation, hypoxemia, hypotension, or cardiac arrhythmias should be investigated and corrected immediately.

VAGAL EVENTS

- Vagal events, characterized by bradycardia, hypotension, and collapse, may occur in critically ill patients, especially in conjunction with coughing, retching, vomiting, or straining to defecate. In extreme cases, bradycardia may be profound and lead to asystole.
- **Atropine** is the treatment of choice in patients with symptomatic bradycardia, and it should be noted that significant (although transient) tachycardia is often seen in patients with perfusing rhythms given a full arrest dose (dogs and cats, 0.04 mg/kg IV, IM, IT). Because of this effect, the atropine dose can be reduced to one fourth to half of the arrest dose (dogs and cats, 0.01 to 0.02 mg/kg IV, IM, IT) in patients with palpable pulses.
- Respiratory arrest may accompany these events, and prompt intubation and manual ventilation are indicated.
- Most patients with a witnessed vagal arrest respond remarkably well to prompt intubation, ventilation, and atropine administration. Full CPR should be instituted if no response to initial therapy occurs.

POSTRESUSCITATION CARE

PREVENTING REARREST

- Many patients that are initially resuscitated have an additional episode of CPA within the first few hours, and often the first few minutes, after ROSC.
- A rapid search for underlying causes of the arrest must be undertaken, and these should be addressed immediately. Special emphasis should be placed on finding reversible disease processes, such as drug-induced hypotension, hypovolemia, hypoventilation, anemia, or electrolyte abnormalities, because these situations are most likely to result in successful outcomes when appropriately treated.

CEREBRAL PROTECTION

- Cerebral ischemia (and subsequent reperfusion) may lead to long-term neurologic dysfunction in patients with CPA and subsequent resuscitation. This process has led to the creation of the acronym *CPCR*, which stands for *cardiopulmonary cerebral resuscitation*, and reflects the importance of neurologic outcome when the success of resuscitation is assessed.
- One measure to limit progressive neurologic injury in post-CPA patients is head elevation to 30 degrees. This elevation should be accomplished by elevating the entire chest, neck, and head to avoid acute kinking of the neck and possible jugular vein compression.
- **Mannitol** can be given at a dose of 0.25 to 1.0 g/kg IV (dogs and cats) over 20 minutes to treat cerebral edema, improve cerebral microvascular flow, and provide free radical scavenging effects. The diuretic effect of mannitol should not be overlooked and may lead to inadvertent hypotension if appropriate IV fluid therapy is not provided.
- Strategies to optimize the hemodynamic status of the patient, including judicious use of IV fluids, vasopressors, or positive inotropes, should be used and titrated to maintain normotension and to achieve resolution of lactic acidosis.
- Ventilatory status should be evaluated either by $ETCO_2$ or ideally by blood gas analysis, and normocapnia should be maintained. This monitoring helps control increases in intracranial pressure created by hypercapnia-induced cerebral vasodilation and prevents hypocapnia-related cerebral vasoconstriction and diminished cerebral blood flow. Many patients that have protracted periods of CPA do not ventilate effectively in the immediate (<24 hours) postarrest period and require mechanical ventilation to maintain normocapnia.
- Induced hypothermia has been shown to be beneficial in improving neurologic outcome following CPR in humans. Although this is difficult to translate to clinical veterinary patients, overzealous rewarming of mildly hypothermic patients is not recommended.

INTENSIVE CARE

- Patients resuscitated from CPA may have a range of postresuscitation syndromes affecting multiple organ systems. The severity of these abnormalities depends on the duration of the arrest and the condition of the patient before the episode.

- In addition to neurologic dysfunction, postarrest patients often have significant cardiovascular (arrhythmia, myocardial dysfunction,
impaired myocardial contractility, hypotension),
renal (acute kidney injury), and gastrointestinal
(shock gut) sequelae. The low-flow state during
CPA and CPR creates global ischemia followed
by subsequent reperfusion, which may result in
systemic inflammation (systemic inflammatory
response syndrome), activation of the coagulation cascade, and disseminated intravascular
coagulation. There is also the possibility that
CPR has created iatrogenic injury (rib fractures,
pulmonary contusion) or has resulted in additional management concerns (postthoracotomy
or posttracheostomy patients).
- Intensive monitoring and supportive care are
required to address these conditions, as well as
conditions underlying the arrest. It is common
for post-CPA patients to require pressor therapy, mechanical ventilation, or other advanced
therapy to survive the postarrest period and be
discharged from the hospital.

KEY POINT

Postresuscitation care is essential to the ultimate
success of CPR. Intensive monitoring and
supportive care are necessary to identify
and address the underlying cause of CPA as well
as to manage post-resuscitation syndromes.

FREQUENTLY ASKED QUESTIONS

When should CPR not be performed?

The decision to perform CPR can be difficult, especially when this decision needs to be made in a crisis situation. Retrospective studies have shown that
survival to discharge is generally less than 10% for
patients with a full CPA. In general, the greatest
chance for a successful outcome involves a patient in
which a cause for the arrest can be rapidly identified
and treated. This is not often the case for patients
with advanced or multisystemic diseases. Although
many of these patients can be initially resuscitated,
survival to discharge is extraordinarily unlikely.
Speaking to an owner about a resuscitation code
(full CPR, limited CPR, or Do Not Resuscitate) is
recommended whenever a critically ill patient with
an advanced disease is admitted to the hospital. In
this way, futile resuscitation efforts can be avoided,
and appropriate end-of-life decisions can be made.

What is the neurologic outcome of veterinary patients surviving CPA?

As mentioned previously, the survival of patients with
CPA is poor. In addition, many veterinarians have
concerns about the potential for neurologic dysfunction in those patients that do survive to hospital
discharge. Although this is a major concern in people that have received CPR, a recent retrospective
study demonstrated that 16 of 18 veterinary patients
that survived CPA were neurologically normal at the
time of hospital discharge and that 1 of the remaining 2 patients was normal within 2 months.

SUGGESTED READINGS

Cole SG, Otto CM, Hughes D: Cardiopulmonary cerebral
resuscitation in small animals: a clinical practice review,
part I, J Vet Emerg Crit Care 12:261, 2002.
Cole SG, Otto CM, Hughes D: Cardiopulmonary cerebral
resuscitation in small animals: a clinical practice review,
Part II, J Vet Emerg Crit Care 13:13, 2002.
Fletcher DJ, Boller M, Brainard BM, et al: RECOVER evidence and knowledge gap analysis on veterinary CPR.
Part 7: Clinical guidelines, J Vet Emerg Crit Care 22:S102,
2012.
Hofmeister EH, Brainard BM, Egger CM, et al: Prognostic
indicators for dogs and cats with cardiopulmonary arrest
treated by cardiopulmonary cerebral resuscitation at a
university teaching hospital, J Am Vet Med Assoc 235:50,
2009.
Kass PH, Haskins SC: Survival following cardiopulmonary
resuscitation in dogs and cats, J Vet Emerg Crit Care 2:57,
1992.
Lehman TL, Manning AM: Postarrest syndrome and the
respiratory and cardiovascular systems in postarrest
patients, Compend Contin Ed Practic Vet 25:492, 2003.
Lehman TL, Manning AM: Renal, central nervous, and
gastrointestinal systems in postarrest patients, Compend
Contin Ed Practic Vet 25:504, 2003.
Waldrop JE, Rozanski EA, Swanke ED, et al: Causes of cardiopulmonary arrest, resuscitation management, and
functional outcome in dogs and cats surviving cardiopulmonary arrest, J Vet Emerg Crit Care 14:22, 2004.
Wingfield WE, Van Pelt DR: Respiratory and cardiopulmonary arrest in dogs and cats: 265 cases (1986-1991), J Am
Vet Med Assoc 200:1993, 1992.

19

Emergency Management and Critical Care

Kari Santoro-Beer | Kenneth J. Drobatz

In general, cardiac emergencies may be divided into three groups.

HEART FAILURE

- Congestive heart failure (CHF) (commonly regarded as "backward" failure)
  - Patients with CHF generally show respiratory signs (caused by pleural effusion or pulmonary edema) or abdominal distension (caused by ascites).
- Low output failure (commonly regarded as "forward" failure)
  - Animals with low-output heart failure have adequate intravascular volume but reduced cardiac output and most commonly have signs of weakness or collapse that are typically caused by dilated cardiomyopathy or pericardial effusion.
  - The term *myocardial failure* is used to denote the presence of reduced myocardial contractility (e.g., dilated cardiomyopathy).

CARDIAC RHYTHM DISTURBANCES

- The most common cardiac arrhythmias causing emergency presentations are severe brady-arrhythmias (third-degree heart block, sick sinus syndrome) and tachyarrhythmias. These animals generally show low output failure and signs of weakness or collapse.

THROMBOEMBOLISM

- Thromboembolic disease typically presents with acute dysfunction of the area of compromised blood supply. In cats with cardiomyopathy, this is most often the hind limbs because of an aortic saddle thrombus, although other limbs can also be affected. Pulmonary thromboembolism may be an acute cause of respiratory distress and low output heart failure in dogs with a variety of underlying diseases. Thromboembolic disease is also encountered in animals with infectious endocarditis.

> **KEY POINT**
>
> The ultimate cardiac emergency is cardiopulmonary arrest. The management of cardiopulmonary arrest and strategies for cardiopulmonary resuscitation in small animals are covered separately (see Chapter 18).

ASSESSING CARDIOVASCULAR FUNCTION IN THE EMERGENCY PATIENT

PHYSICAL EXAMINATION

- Historical complaints that support a primary cardiac emergency are variable and include weakness, lethargy, collapse or syncope, as well as cough, tachypnea, or respiratory distress. Additional complaints such as anorexia, vomiting, and diarrhea are not uncommon because primary cardiovascular problems may have wide-ranging effects on all major organ systems.
- Physical examination findings consistent with primary cardiac emergencies are variable depending on the specific condition.
  - Mucous membranes may be pale secondary to vasoconstriction or cyanotic secondary to hypoxemia. Capillary refill time is commonly prolonged because of diminished cardiac output and hypoperfusion. Decreased tissue perfusion is more commonly seen in instances of low output failure compared with congestive failure.
  - Many cases of canine and feline heart failure are accompanied by an audible murmur or gallop. Diminished heart sounds can occur in cases of pericardial or pleural effusion or severe myocardial failure, but they can also occur with severe hypovolemia.
  - Bradyarrhythmias or tachyarrhythmias are common and often associated with irregular rhythms and diminished pulse quality or pulse deficits.
  - Pulsus paradoxus, where pulse strength gets weaker on inspiration, is detected in less than 50% of patients with pericardial effusion.

- Tachypnea and respiratory distress are often present. In cases of pulmonary edema, auscultation will commonly reveal harsh lung sounds or crackles. In cases of pleural effusion, lung sounds are commonly diminished ventrally.
- Animals with low output failure often have a low body temperature and depressed mentation caused by poor oxygen delivery (cardiogenic shock).
- Jugular pulses or distension is commonly detected in animals with right-sided heart failure, including pericardial effusion.

DIAGNOSTIC TESTS

- Diagnostic tests include electrocardiography (ECG), pulse oximetry, blood pressure measurement, chest radiographs, and echocardiography. In special cases, cardiac output monitoring, including the measurement of pulmonary artery occlusion pressures, can be considered.
- A lead II ECG is usually sufficient for the rapid diagnosis of most cardiac rhythm disturbances.
- Pulse oximetry provides a useful estimate of hemoglobin saturation and arterial oxygen content, findings that may be further evaluated by arterial blood gas analysis.
- Blood pressure measurement may be accomplished with Doppler, oscillometric, or invasive techniques and reflects cardiac output and vasomotor tone. It is useful in the recognition of shock states and in monitoring therapeutic interventions.
- Chest radiography is the ideal method to assess size and shape of the cardiac silhouette, pulmonary vasculature, pulmonary parenchyma, and pleural space. It is the gold standard for documenting CHF in the form of pulmonary edema or pleural effusion.
- Echocardiography provides information about cardiac structure and function. It is typically used to confirm a suspected diagnosis, determine severity of disease, assess myocardial contractility, and detect intracardiac or proximal pulmonary artery thrombi. Echocardiography is particularly useful in assessing patients with pericardial effusion for cardiac neoplasia.
- Recent evidence has shown that some cardiac biomarkers, including natriuretic peptides and cardiac troponins, may be helpful in differentiating dyspnea caused by cardiac compared with respiratory disease, or in cases of specific cardiomyopathies.

KEY POINT

Animals with emergency problems related to heart disease are often not stable enough for prolonged diagnostic tests. Empiric therapy for the most likely cardiac problem based on signalment, history, physical examination, and chest radiographs is often given. In many cases, appropriate therapy can be instituted without the need for an immediate echocardiographic examination.

EMERGENCY TREATMENT OF HEART FAILURE

- Treatment of heart failure involves the following:
  - Identification and remediation of underlying causes
  - Elimination of aggravating conditions (i.e., cardiac depressants, hypertension, arrhythmias)
  - Control of congestion
  - Improvement of myocardial contractility
  - Improvement of myocardial relaxation
  - Reduction of cardiac work
  - Reduction of pathologic remodeling and neurohormonal activation

CONGESTIVE HEART FAILURE

- CHF results from elevated cardiac filling pressures that cause pulmonary or systemic venous hypertension and extravasation of fluid into the interstitial space or a body cavity.
- The location of this fluid is dependent on the failing ventricle (left-sided, right-sided, or biventricular failure), and the subsequent signs of CHF relate to the magnitude of fluid accumulation.
- CHF is the result of many cardiac diseases including chronic valvular disease, cardiomyopathies, infectious endocarditis, myocarditis, pericardial effusion, persistent arrhythmia, or congenital cardiovascular anomalies.

LEFT-SIDED CONGESTIVE HEART FAILURE

- Left-sided congestive heart failure (LCHF) results from elevated left atrial pressure. Elevated left atrial pressure may result from mitral valve insufficiency, mitral valve stenosis, or systolic or diastolic dysfunction of the left ventricle. In dogs, LCHF causes pulmonary edema; in cats it may be associated with either or both pulmonary edema and pleural effusion.
- Clinical signs
  - Clinical signs of LCHF result from pulmonary compromise and include tachypnea, respiratory distress, lethargy, and exercise intolerance. Dogs with pulmonary edema frequently have a cough; however, cough is rare in cats with heart failure.
  - Physical examination findings include harsh lung sounds and crackles in patients with pulmonary edema. Cats with pleural effusion

usually have dull lung sounds in the ventral lung fields, especially when compared with the degree of respiratory effort. Severely compromised patients will have respiratory distress, and cyanosis is not uncommon. Most patients with LCHF will be tachycardic and usually have abnormalities on auscultation such as a heart murmur, gallop rhythm, or an arrhythmia; cats can exhibit bradycardia.

DIAGNOSTICS

- Confirmation of LCHF is made with chest radiographs to document the presence and severity of pulmonary edema or pleural effusion.
- In dogs, pulmonary edema tends to be most evident at the perihilar region, although all lung lobes may be affected in severe cases. Pulmonary edema in cats does not follow this pattern, and the location of affected lung tissue is variable. Pleural effusion in cats may be found either with or without concurrent pulmonary edema. Other changes supportive of LCHF include cardiomegaly, evidence of left atrial enlargement, and dilated pulmonary vasculature, particularly of the pulmonary veins.
- ECG analysis can show a variety of changes, including prolongation of P wave duration (P mitrale), increased R wave amplitude or duration, left axis shift, bundle branch block, supraventricular or ventricular premature complexes or tachycardia, or atrial fibrillation.
- Echocardiography provides definitive information regarding the size of the cardiac chambers as well as information on systolic and diastolic cardiac function.
- Many patients that have LCHF have severe respiratory distress and cannot tolerate a full diagnostic workup. Because of this, therapy is often instituted before obtaining radiographs or an echocardiogram. In these cases, the decision to treat CHF is based on the history, clinical signs, and physical examination findings at presentation. If access to a portable ultrasound machine is available, additional information may be obtained from a brief screening examination of the thorax for the presence of pleural effusion or grossly recognizable changes in cardiac structure (e.g., dilated left atrium, myocardial chamber dimension, or wall thickness) or function (e.g., markedly diminished fractional shortening).

TREATMENT

- Emergency treatment of LCHF involves the use of diuretics, vasodilators, and, in some cases, inotropic agents. In addition, oxygen therapy is vital in patients with compromised pulmonary function, and some patients may benefit from the judicious use of anxiolytic drugs. Cats with significant pleural effusion require therapeutic thoracocentesis.

Diuretic Therapy

- The goal of diuretic therapy in the treatment of LCHF is to reduce the circulating blood volume, thereby reducing the preload of the left ventricle and left atrial pressure. The primary diuretic used in the acute management of CHF is furosemide.
- **Furosemide** should be administered intravenously if possible, although the intramuscular route may be used in patients without vascular access. The subcutaneous route is not recommended because of likely hypoperfusion and decreased absorption.
- The dose is dependent upon the severity of clinical signs and patient response. In dogs, an initial dose of 2 to 4 mg/kg intravenously (IV) or intramuscularly (IM) may be followed by additional doses q1-2h until the respiratory character improves. After improvement, additional doses of 2 mg/kg are typically given at 6- to 12-hour intervals dependent on clinical status. Cats tend to be more sensitive to furosemide therapy, and initial doses of 1 to 2 mg/kg IV or IM q12h followed by 1 to 2 mg/kg q8-12h are recommended after initial clinical response. Alternatively a CRI of 0.66 mg/kg/hr may be used and potentially can produce greater diuresis and less potassium loss.
- Side effects of furosemide include dehydration, azotemia, hypokalemia, metabolic alkalosis, and, potentially, volume depletion.

Vasodilator Therapy

- Vasodilator therapy has two purposes. First, venodilation decreases preload by providing additional vascular capacitance. Second, arterial vasodilation reduces left ventricular afterload, thereby reducing myocardial work and promoting forward flow.
- **Sodium nitroprusside** (dogs: 0.5 to 10 μg/kg/min constant-rate infusion [CRI]) increases the concentration of nitric oxide, a potent vasodilator, and is considered to be a balanced vasodilator providing both venous and arterial dilation. Combined with aggressive diuretic therapy, sodium nitroprusside is very effective in resolving severe pulmonary edema. Because of its potency and the potential for excessive vasodilation and secondary hypotension, blood pressure should be monitored closely during infusion.
  - In all cases, the initial dose should be at the low end of the range, and the dose increased

based on clinical response and blood pressure. In general, mean arterial pressure should be maintained above 60 mm Hg, whereas systolic pressures should be maintained above 90 mm Hg.

- Sodium nitroprusside is light sensitive and may induce precipitation of coadministered IV drugs. Thus, it is ideally administered through a separate, light-protected IV set and catheter.
- Long-term nitroprusside therapy is limited by the production of molecular cyanide, although toxic doses are not usually reached until 36 to 48 hours after onset of therapy.

- **Nitroglycerin ointment (2%)** is a commonly used venodilator in small animal emergency patients. The ointment is applied topically to a clipped area on either the pinna or inguinal region and is dosed according to body size. A ⅛-inch strip is used in cats and small dogs (<10 kg), a ¼-inch strip in medium dogs (10 to 25 kg), and a ½-inch strip in large dogs (>25 kg). The ointment may be applied q12h for the first 24 to 36 hours of treatment and should be handled with gloves because it may be absorbed transdermally. It is important to remember that continuous use results in tolerance after 48 to 72 hours.
  - Although the use of nitroglycerin ointment is common, it should be noted that topically applied therapy is limited in severe CHF, especially given the profound peripheral vasoconstriction that exists in these patients, and efficacy is questionable.
- **Hydralazine** (dogs: 0.25 to 2 mg/kg subcutaneously [SQ] or IM, 2 mg/kg IV, or 0.1 to 0.3 mg/kg/hr) is an arterial dilator that causes a marked reduction in afterload and is useful in cases of severe mitral regurgitation. As with other arterial dilators, hydralazine may be associated with hypotension and reflex tachycardia in the face of decreased peripheral resistance.

Positive Inotropic Agents

- Positive inotropic agents are indicated in managing LCHF associated with systolic dysfunction of the left ventricle. These drugs are administered in conjunction with diuretic and vasodilator therapy. Dilated cardiomyopathy is the most common disease producing this condition; however, myocardial failure secondary to advanced chronic valvular disease, systemic inflammatory response syndrome, sepsis, or end-stage forms of other cardiomyopathies may also result in severe systolic dysfunction.
  - **Dobutamine** (dogs, 2.5 to 20 µg/kg/min CRI; cats, 2 to 10 µg/kg/min CRI) is a beta-adrenergic sympathomimetic. Side effects

of dobutamine may include tachycardia and ventricular arrhythmias. Cats may have gastrointestinal or neurologic signs associated with administration.
- **Dopamine** (dogs and cats, 2 to 10 µg/kg/min CRI) should be used with caution because it has alpha-adrenergic effects at higher doses and may cause deleterious vasoconstriction and tachycardia in the face of diminished myocardial function.
- **Pimobendan** (0.25 to 0.3 mg/kg, PO q12h) is a phosphodiesterase inhibitor with both positive inotropic and vasodilatory effects ("inodilator") that may be useful in LCHF once patients can tolerate oral medication.
- **Digoxin** (0.003 to 0.005 mg/kg q12h, up to a maximum of 0.375 mg in dogs; 0.007 mg/kg PO every other day initially in cats) is a cardiac glycoside that increases contractility and decreases heart rate. It has a very narrow therapeutic range and can result in toxicity, which generally manifests as cardiac arrhythmias or gastrointestinal signs. The positive inotropic effect is mild. Digoxin has largely been supplanted by pimobendan for inotropic support.
- Additional options for inotropic support include phosphodiesterase inhibitors such as milrinone. **Milrinone** (dogs, 50 µg/kg slow IV bolus followed by 0.40 to 0.75 µg/kg/min CRI) is a drug that has both positive inotropic and vasodilatory properties, similar to a combination of dobutamine and sodium nitroprusside. Experience with clinical use in emergency patients is limited, but milrinone may be an effective agent for the short-term management of LCHF associated with systolic dysfunction.

Oxygen Therapy

- Oxygen therapy (40% to 60% fraction of inspired oxygen) helps to maintain the arterial oxygen content in the face of pulmonary dysfunction (in the form of ventilation-perfusion mismatch) induced by pulmonary edema. Oxygen therapy may also reduce pulmonary vascular resistance by ameliorating hypoxic pulmonary vasoconstriction.
  - An oxygen cage is often the most effective method to administer supplemental oxygen to patients with heart failure, although other alternatives (such as nasal, mask, flow-by, hood, or intratracheal oxygen supplementation) exist. Although an oxygen cage provides a quiet environment that can achieve high concentrations of oxygen, these concentrations decrease rapidly when the cage is opened. In addition, patient monitoring can

be impaired for patients in an oxygen cage. Thus, an oxygen cage is less effective when patients require frequent treatments or physical examination.

- Patients should receive oxygen supplementation until their respiratory rate and effort have improved or objective measurements of pulmonary function (i.e., pulse oximetry or arterial blood gas) have returned to normal. If possible, the fraction of inspired oxygen should be tapered over 6 to 12 hours to allow the patient to adjust to breathing room air.
- For patients with fulminant LCHF and massive pulmonary edema, standard oxygen supplementation may not be sufficient to prevent either respiratory or ventilatory failure. In these cases, only early intubation and mechanical ventilation will provide the respiratory support necessary to sustain life. Mechanical ventilation is a significant commitment for both the owner and clinician; however, in many cases, mechanical ventilation may be weaned after only a short period (1 to 2 days) following aggressive medical management of CHF.
- The use of anxiolytic agents in the treatment of CHF is common in human medicine and can also be useful in veterinary patients. Low-dose **morphine** (dogs, 0.1 mg/kg IV q4-6h as needed), **butorphanol** (dogs and cats, 0.1 to 0.2 mg/kg IV q4h), **diazepam** or **midazolam** (dogs and cats, 0.1 to 0.3 mg/kg IV q4h), or low-dose **acepromazine** (dogs and cats, 0.005 to 0.05 mg/kg IV q6-8h) can be administered.

Therapeutic Thoracocentesis

- Cats with significant pleural effusion associated with LCHF will experience considerable benefit from therapeutic thoracocentesis. Some cats will tolerate this procedure with minimal restraint, although many cats require some degree of sedation (butorphanol 0.1 to 0.2 mg/kg IV in combination with diazepam or midazolam 0.1 to 0.3 mg/kg IV).
  - Thoracocentesis is generally performed between the seventh and ninth intercostal spaces at the level of the costochondral junction, taking care to avoid the internal thoracic arteries. Ultrasound guidance should be used if possible. The area is clipped and aseptically prepared before the procedure is initiated. Thoracocentesis in cats is generally performed with a 21-gauge butterfly catheter attached to a three-way stopcock and a 10- or 20-mL syringe. In extremely obese cats, a 22-gauge needle and extension set is used in place of the butterfly catheter. In larger dogs,

an 18- or 20-gauge catheter or needle with a 60-mL syringe may be used.
  - The needle should be introduced just cranial to a rib to avoid the intercostal vessels and nerves and advanced into the pleural space. The needle should be redirected or the procedure terminated once lung tissue is felt at the tip of the needle or fluid is no longer able to be aspirated. Both sides of the chest should be aspirated because bilateral fluid accumulation is found in most cats with pleural effusion secondary to CHF. It is not uncommon to remove 200 to 300 mL of fluid from the thorax of cats with severe pleural effusion.

RIGHT-SIDED CONGESTIVE HEART FAILURE

- Right-sided congestive heart failure (RCHF) is much less common in patients that are seen in the emergency department. An exception is pericardial effusion and cardiac tamponade (see the section on pericardial effusion). RCHF results from elevated right atrial and central venous pressures (CVPs). Conditions that may result in elevated CVP include tricuspid valve insufficiency or stenosis, pulmonic valve insufficiency or stenosis, pulmonary hypertension, and right ventricular systolic or diastolic dysfunction. Rarely, right-sided intracardiac masses, massive pulmonary thromboembolism, and heartworm disease with caval syndrome can also induce RCHF.
- Clinical signs of RCHF are related to the presence of pleural effusion, ascites, or peripheral edema that results from increased right atrial pressure. Patients with large volume pleural effusion may have respiratory distress with dull lung sounds. Patients with ascites will have a distended abdomen and may have respiratory compromise. Additional indications of RCHF are the presence of distended jugular veins and prominent jugular pulses, as well as the presence of a heart murmur (particularly with a maximal intensity at the left heart base or the right side of the chest). Other changes such as a split S_2 sound or gallop sound are variable and depend on the underlying disease.
- Emergency therapy for RCHF consists of thoracocentesis for large volume pleural effusions (see the previous section).
- In animals with tense ascites, abdominocentesis can be performed to reduce pressure on the diaphragm and improve ventilation. Abdominocentesis can be performed with equipment similar to thoracocentesis.
  - The procedure may be performed with the patient standing or in left lateral recumbency, which reduces the likelihood of lacerating the spleen. An area caudal to the umbilicus

is clipped and prepared aseptically, and the needle or catheter is induced on or just lateral to the midline. An alternative technique uses two or more short 16- to 18-gauge catheters placed just caudal and to either side of the umbilicus. The animal remains standing during the procedure and fluid is allowed to drain passively. Debate exists about the volume of fluid that can be removed safely from an animal with ascites. Most dogs will tolerate the removal of 50 to 100 mL/kg of ascites without untoward effects.

PERICARDIAL EFFUSION

- Pericardial effusion typically results from an underlying neoplasia, such as hemangiosarcoma, heart base tumors, lymphoma, or mesothelioma. Other causes of pericardial effusion include inflammatory or infectious pericarditis, restrictive pericarditis, coagulopathy, atrial rupture secondary to chronic dilation, and blunt or penetrating thoracic trauma. Small volume pericardial effusions associated with CHF may also occur, and this phenomenon is relatively common in cats.
- Clinical signs result from cardiac tamponade and RCHF and may include abdominal distension from ascites, tachypnea from pleural effusion, weakness, lethargy, or collapse.
- Physical examination findings include tachycardia and dull heart sounds on auscultation. In some cases, pulsus paradoxus (decrement of pulse strength that occurs during the inspiratory phase of the respiratory cycle) may be recognized. Additional physical examination findings may include jugular distension and prominent jugular pulses, abdominal distension with a palpable fluid wave, and dull ventral lung sounds if pleural effusion is present. Depressed mentation and delayed capillary refill are suggestive of cardiovascular collapse and hypoperfusion in severe cases.
- Diagnostic test results consistent with pericardial effusion and cardiac tamponade include sinus tachycardia with diminished complex size on the ECG, with or without the presence of electrical alternans. Electrical alternans describes an alternation in the height of the R wave of the QRS complex and results from beat-to-beat changes in the mean electrical axis as the heart moves within the fluid-filled pericardium. Chest radiographs may demonstrate an enlarged cardiac silhouette as well as distension of the caudal vena cava. Pleural effusion or evidence of metastatic lung disease may be present. The cardiac silhouette often has a classic "globoid" appearance; however, this may not be true in cases of acute pericardial effusion and can also be seen with other cardiac diseases. A brief echocardiographic examination can generally confirm the presence of pericardial effusion.

KEY POINT

The differentiation of pericardial effusion from pleural effusion on echocardiographic examination can be challenging. Pericardial effusion is recognized by the circular appearance of hypoechoic fluid surrounding the heart. This fluid is bordered by the hyperechoic pericardium. Cardiac tamponade is recognized as diastolic collapse of the right atrium; in some cases, an underlying cause for the effusion is seen, such as a mass involving the right atrium or atrioventricular groove. In patients with pleural but not pericardial effusion, the fluid does not encircle the heart, and lung tissue as well as mediastinal tissue may be seen within the effusion.

- Although blood tests are not often a primary diagnostic tool in the diagnosis of pericardial effusion, documenting the presence of a coagulopathy is vital in the management of those patients in which this is a primary cause of the pericardial effusion. In addition, it should be recognized that patients with more chronic pericardial effusions can develop hyponatremia and hyperkalemia. These pseudo-Addisonian electrolyte changes result from the enhanced antidiuretic hormone secretion and decreased renal perfusion that occurs secondary to decreased effective circulating volume in these patients. These abnormalities rapidly resolve with the resolution of cardiac tamponade.
- The emergency treatment of symptomatic pericardial effusion and cardiac tamponade involves volume expansion and pericardiocentesis.
  - Volume expansion using partial shock doses (30 to 45 mL/kg) of an isotonic crystalloid transiently increases right atrial pressure. This may improve stroke volume and cardiac output and often results in clinical improvement while steps are taken to perform pericardiocentesis.
  - Pericardiocentesis is the treatment of choice for the initial management of cardiac tamponade and is a life-saving procedure in many cases. For pericardiocentesis to be performed, the patient is placed in lateral or sternal recumbency. Sedation may be required in some patients, and conservative doses of an opioid in combination with a benzodiazepine

are generally well tolerated. Other patients require only local anesthesia.

- An area from the third to the seventh intercostal spaces is clipped and prepared aseptically, and a local anesthetic is infiltrated over the apex beat, generally at the fifth intercostal space at the level of the costochondral junction. A small stab incision is made in the skin, and a catheter is advanced through the chest wall, just cranial to the sixth rib. In large dogs, a 14-gauge, 12-cm over-the-needle catheter is used, whereas a 16-gauge, 8-cm over-the-needle catheter is used in smaller dogs. In very small dogs or in cats, an 18-gauge, 2-inch over-the-needle catheter may be used.

- The catheter is slowly advanced toward the pericardium. Pleural fluid may be encountered first (usually straw colored). Entrance into the pericardium is accompanied by a loss of resistance and the presence of fluid flashing back into the catheter hub. This may be recognized sooner if a syringe is attached to the needle and a slight negative pressure is applied as it is advanced or if the needle has been filled with sterile saline before the procedure.

- Once the pericardium has been punctured, the catheter is advanced off the stylet and attached to an extension set with a three-way stopcock and syringe. The pericardial fluid is aspirated, and fluid should be immediately placed into an activated clotting time tube. This allows pericardial fluid, which should not clot, to be differentiated from peripheral blood, which should clot. The development of a clot in the sample should prompt rapid removal of the catheter system. As the pericardium is drained, additional samples should be obtained for fluid analysis and cytology.

- The ECG should be monitored during the procedure for the presence of ventricular arrhythmias that occur when the catheter contacts the epicardium. If present, these arrhythmias may be treated by slightly withdrawing the catheter or with a bolus of lidocaine (dogs, 2 mg/kg IV). The ECG is also useful to confirm the effectiveness of the procedure because the heart rate often returns to the normal range and electrical alternans disappears as the heart is decompressed.

- Once fluid can no longer be aspirated, the catheter is withdrawn. Confirmation of a successful pericardiocentesis may be obtained with a brief recheck echocardiogram. After the procedure, the patient should be monitored for recurrent effusion. Further

management of pericardial effusion involves a complete echocardiogram and the consideration of more definitive therapy such as a subtotal pericardectomy or a thoracoscopic pericardial window.

- Potential complications of pericardiocentesis include arrhythmias, coronary artery laceration, and lung laceration.

KEY POINT

In clinically stable patients, a complete echocardiographic examination is preferentially performed before pericardiocentesis because the presence of effusion supplies useful echocardiographic contrast in the attempt to identify cardiac neoplasms. In addition, performing thoracic radiographs before pericardiocentesis (if the patient is stable) allows for better visualization of the pulmonary parenchyma to screen for metastatic disease. Pericardial fluid inevitably leaks into the pleural space after centesis and may obscure the pulmonary parenchyma.

FORWARD (LOW-OUTPUT) HEART FAILURE

- Forward heart failure is the result of impaired myocardial function and results in diminished cardiac output and cardiogenic shock. Common causes of forward heart failure include dilated cardiomyopathy and myocardial failure secondary to end-stage chronic valvular disease, systemic inflammatory response syndrome, sepsis, or doxorubicin toxicity. Significant tachyarrhythmias and bradyarrhythmias may also result in a form of forward heart failure.

- Clinical signs of cardiogenic shock include weakness, lethargy, and collapse. Respiratory signs may be seen if CHF is also present. Physical examination findings associated with forward heart failure include hypothermia, pallor, delayed capillary refill time, tachycardia, and poor pulse quality. Heart sounds may be diminished or a heart murmur and/or gallop rhythm may be heard. The presence of pulmonary edema or pleural effusion will produce characteristic changes on auscultation.

- The clinical diagnosis of forward heart failure is made by finding evidence of decreased myocardial function in combination with hypotension and clinical signs of hypoperfusion. Decreased systolic function is documented using echocardiography and is evidenced by a diminished fractional shortening, increased left ventricular end-systolic dimension, increased E-point to septal separation, and decreased aortic and pulmonic flows. Chest radiographs may document the presence and severity of concurrent CHF, and a lead II ECG will help identify significant rhythm disturbances.

- Treatment of forward heart failure involves efforts to improve myocardial performance and cardiac output. This may be accomplished by ensuring that adequate preload is present and by providing inotropic support.
  - Clinical estimates of preload may be obtained by measuring left and right ventricular filling pressures.
    - Right ventricular filling pressures may be assessed by placing a central venous catheter and measuring the CVP. Normal CVP ranges between 0 and 8 cm H_2O, although wide variability exists among patients, especially those with cardiac disease.
    - Left ventricular filling pressures may be assessed by placing a pulmonary artery catheter and measuring pulmonary capillary wedge (occlusion) pressure (PCWP). Normal PCWP ranges between 5 and 14 cm H_2O. In animals with low CVP or PCWP, judicious fluid therapy may be used to increase preload and cardiac output. If the CVP or PCWP is normal or high, fluid therapy is not likely to be of benefit and may precipitate CHF. In human medicine, controversy exists regarding the benefit of pulmonary artery catheters; this technique is not commonly used in veterinary medicine.
  - Inotropic support is indicated in cases of cardiogenic shock secondary to myocardial systolic dysfunction.
    - **Dobutamine** (dogs, 2.5 to 20 µg/kg/min; cats, 2 to 10 µg/kg/min CRI) is generally the first-line agent in dogs because of its ability to increase contractility without significantly increasing heart rate. Dobutamine may also be used in cats, although gastrointestinal and neurologic side effects usually limit utility.
    - **Dopamine** (dogs and cats, 2 to 10 µg/kg/min) may also be used. Dopamine should be used with caution, however, because it has alpha-adrenergic effects at higher doses and may increase afterload and negatively affect cardiac output. In patients with a pulmonary artery catheter, cardiac output can be measured by the thermodilution method. Combined with measurements of direct arterial blood pressure and calculation of systemic vascular resistance, these techniques allow for the most effective clinical assessment of hemodynamics and the response to therapy.
    - Oral **pimobendan** therapy (0.25 to 0.3 mg/kg PO q12h) should be considered if intravenous therapy is not possible. Alternatively, digoxin therapy can also be considered, although toxicity is possible because of the narrow therapeutic range, and it is a much weaker positive inotrope than pimobendan.
- See Chapter 16 for further discussion.

CARDIAC RHYTHM DISTURBANCES

- Cardiac arrhythmias are common in emergency patients and may be associated with alterations in autonomic tone or responsiveness, drug exposure, electrolyte abnormalities, impaired myocardial oxygen delivery, myocardial trauma or inflammation, or primary myocardial disease.
- In many situations, these cardiac rhythm disturbances represent the cardiac effects of a systemic disease and do not require specific treatment. In other cases, aggressive intervention is required to address unstable rhythms or life-threatening perfusion deficits.
- Physical examination findings consistent with a cardiac rhythm disturbance include bradycardia or tachycardia, an irregular rhythm on auscultation, and the identification of pulse deficits. Depressed mentation or collapse may also be encountered, and syncope may be observed in cases of acute, arrhythmia-induced decreases in cerebral perfusion.
- Confirmation of cardiac rhythm disturbances is achieved by ECG. Obtaining a lead II rhythm strip is often sufficient to diagnose most rhythm disturbances. However, a 6- or 10-lead ECG may be helpful to accurately identify and characterize complex arrhythmias.

KEY POINT

Cardiac rhythm disorders may be intermittent and may not be noted on a single lead II ECG. Detection of rhythm disorders sometimes requires 24-hour telemetric, Holter, or event monitoring.

BRADYARRHYTHMIAS

- Bradycardia is a relatively uncommon finding in patients seen in the emergency department.
- Clinical signs associated with bradyarrhythmias include weakness, lethargy, depression, and syncope.
- Causes of symptomatic bradyarrhythmias in emergency patients include increased vagal tone, electrolyte abnormalities, hypothermia, drug toxicities, and significant disturbances of the cardiac conduction system.

- ECG rhythms seen in patients with bradycardia include sinus bradycardia, atrial standstill, sinus arrest, and high-grade second- or third-degree AV block.

SINUS BRADYCARDIA

- In emergency patients, sinus bradycardia is most often seen with increased vagal tone.
  - Increased vagal tone may result from intraabdominal or intrathoracic diseases, or from coughing, vomiting, retching, or straining to urinate or defecate. The Cushing reflex, which occurs secondary to head trauma or other causes of elevated intracranial pressure, also produces sinus bradycardia. In this situation, massive sympathetic discharge from the vasomotor center results in systemic hypertension and reflex bradycardia.
- Other causes of sinus bradycardia include absolute or relative drug overdoses, especially of anesthetic agents such as opioids, benzodiazepines, or alpha-2 adrenergic agonists. Cardiac or vasoactive medications, including calcium channel blockers, beta-adrenergic blockers, digoxin, and cholinergic agents may also produce sinus bradycardia either by increasing vagal tone or by reducing sympathetic tone. Hypocortisolemia, as with hypoadrenocorticism, can cause bradycardia, as can severe pulmonary parenchymal disease, likely secondary to J-receptor stimulation.
- Sinus bradycardia may also be associated with hypothermia or severe hypoglycemia (blood glucose <50 mg/dL).
- Management of symptomatic sinus bradycardia generally centers on the identification and treatment of underlying factors. In cases of hypothermia or hypoglycemia, the heart rate and clinical signs often improve markedly once these factors are identified and addressed. Hypothermia is best managed by the use of an indirect heating method such as a warm air blanket. This approach minimizes overheating or detrimental vasodilation that may occur with direct heat sources such as heating pads or hot water bottles. Intravenous fluids that have been warmed to body temperature are also appropriate in patients without contraindications to fluid therapy.
- Although neurologic signs usually predominate over bradycardia, symptomatic hypoglycemia may be treated with a bolus of 0.25 to 1 g/kg of 50% dextrose that has been diluted 50:50 with 0.9% saline. Additional dextrose bolus therapy or a dextrose infusion may be necessary while causes of hypoglycemia (such as insulin overdose, hypoadrenocorticism, paraneoplastic syndrome, systemic inflammatory response syndrome, or sepsis) are investigated.
- Increased vagal tone secondary to intrathoracic disease, intraabdominal disease, coughing, gagging, retching, or straining may cause severe sinus bradycardia that results in cardiovascular collapse or syncope. In these situations, immediate administration of a parasympatholytic agent is necessary. Because of its rapid onset of action and short half-life, atropine is preferred over other agents such as glycopyrrolate. Although the cardiac arrest dose of atropine is 0.04 mg/kg, lower doses (0.005 to 0.01 mg/kg) are often effective in patients with bradycardia, and these doses are less likely to be associated with rebound sinus tachycardia. Intravenous administration is ideal (rarely, a brief centrally induced exacerbation of bradycardia may occur with this route), although atropine may also be administered via intratracheal, intraosseous, or intramuscular routes. In addition to atropine administration, efforts to identify and correct the underlying cause of the increased vagal tone are necessary.
- Atropine is also indicated in treating sinus bradycardia associated with anesthetic agents, as are measures to decrease the depth of anesthesia and to administer specific drug-reversal agents. Opioids may be reversed with naloxone (0.02 mg/kg IV, IM, or SQ) and benzodiazepines may be reversed with flumazenil (0.02 mg/kg IV, IM, or SQ). Dexmedetomidine should be reversed with atipamezole (volume equal to that of the dexmedetomidine given, IM); atropine is not recommended. However, sinus bradycardia associated with the administration of parasympathomimetic agents is also atropine responsive. There are specific recommendations for the management of patients receiving overdoses of cardiac medications such as digoxin, calcium channel blockers, or beta-adrenergic blockers. These guidelines are discussed later.

SECOND- AND THIRD-DEGREE ATRIOVENTRICULAR BLOCK

- High-grade second- and third-degree AV block represent severe disruptions of the normal cardiac conduction system. Although structural heart diseases, such as myocardial fibrosis, inflammation, or infiltration, are thought to be responsible for most cases of severe AV block, these rhythms may also be seen in patients with systemic disease or drug toxicities. Drugs associated with second- and third-degree AV block include digoxin, calcium channel blockers, and beta-adrenergic blockers.

- Most emergency patients with high-grade second- and third-degree AV block will have clinical signs relating to decreased cardiac output, such as lethargy, depressed mentation, and syncope, which is common. Rarely, these rhythms will be documented in an otherwise asymptomatic patient. These symptom-free patients (generally cats) often have third-degree AV block with a relatively high ventricular escape rate supporting an adequate cardiac output.
- Medical management of high-grade second- and third-degree AV block consists of initial parasympatholytic therapy followed by sympathomimetic drugs.
  - Initially, **atropine** may be given at the full vagolytic dose of 0.04 mg/kg IV. This is often effective in elevating the rate of discharge of the sinus node but is only rarely effective in improving the AV block in these patients.
  - Alternate therapy consists of beta-1 agonist drugs given in an effort to accelerate the ventricular escape rate. **Isoproterenol** (dogs, 0.04 to 0.09 µg/kg/min CRI) is commonly used in this situation, although this drug can cause hypotension secondary to vasodilation. An alternative drug is dopamine (dogs and cats, 5 to 10 µg/kg/min) at the beta agonist dose. Dobutamine is another beta-1 agonist; however, it has less of a positive chronotropic effect than dopamine.
    - Beta-1 agonists are also indicated in the treatment of beta-adrenergic blocker overdose. Although these drugs may be effective in some cases, an alternative therapy involves the use of **glucagon.** A bolus of 0.15 mg/kg IV may increase cardiac rate and contractility in dogs. If a response is noted following the bolus, then glucagon can be continued as a CRI (dogs, 0.05 to 0.1 mg/kg/hr). Glucagon may be used in dogs with calcium channel blocker overdose at a similar dosage.
- When medical management is ineffective, artificial pacemaker therapy is indicated in the treatment of symptomatic AV block (see Chapter 22).
- Temporary transthoracic or transvenous pacing is considered emergency treatment to stabilize a patient until diagnostic tests are performed and/or definitive therapy is planned. If no underlying cause, such as a drug overdose or toxicity, is identified, patients with symptomatic AV block require the placement of a permanent pacemaker.

SINUS ARREST

- The most common cause of symptomatic sinus arrest is sick sinus syndrome (SSS), a condition characterized by periods of supraventricular tachycardia interspersed with periods of sinus arrest. Although this condition may occur in a number of breeds, it is seen most often in Miniature Schnauzers. Management is similar to patients with symptomatic AV block.

HYPERKALEMIC CARDIOTOXICITY

- Although not a primary cardiac abnormality, hyperkalemic cardiotoxicity is a frequent cause of symptomatic bradycardia in emergency patients. It is most common in cats with urethral obstruction, but it also occurs in cases of acute renal failure, uroperitoneum, hypoadrenocorticism, and reperfusion injury.
- Hyperkalemia produces a characteristic set of changes on the ECG; however, the concentration at which these changes are noted is variable. Changes rarely occur if K+ is less than 6 mmol/L. The sequence of changes involves tented/spiked T waves, flattening of the P waves, prolongation of the P-R interval, bradycardia, loss of P waves (atrial standstill), prolongation of the QRS complex, merging of the QRS and T wave complexes to form a "sine wave" pattern, and, finally, ventricular flutter, fibrillation, or asystole.
- The management of life-threatening hyperkalemia involves three phases: immediate cardioprotection, redistribution of serum potassium, and removal of potassium from the body.
  - Immediate cardioprotection is achieved through the use of intravenous **calcium gluconate** (dogs and cats, 50 to 100 mg/kg as a slow [3- to 5-minute] IV bolus) while the ECG is monitored. Overly rapid administration results in worsening bradycardia and potentially severe ventricular arrhythmias. The onset of action of calcium gluconate is usually rapid (within 5 minutes). The duration of effect is limited, however, and hyperkalemic ECG changes will recur unless steps are taken to reduce the serum potassium level.
  - Serum potassium may be transiently lowered by redistribution into the intracellular space with **regular insulin** (dogs and cats, 0.25 units/kg accompanied by dextrose bolus of 0.5 g/kg to help prevent iatrogenic hypoglycemia). Dextrose supplementation is continued in intravenous fluid therapy for 6 to 12 hours to prevent a decrease in blood glucose later in the course of treatment.
    - Alternatives or adjuncts to regular insulin therapy include **sodium bicarbonate** (dogs and cats, 1 to 2 mEq/kg given over 10 to 15 minutes) or **terbutaline** (dogs and cats, 0.01 mg/kg IV slowly).

- Definitive management involves removing potassium from the body. This is generally accomplished by establishing urine flow (relieving urethral obstruction, placing a peritoneal drainage catheter) and fluid diuresis. If adequate urine flow is unable to be achieved, patients are considered candidates for either peritoneal dialysis or hemodialysis.

TACHYARRHYTHMIAS

- Tachyarrhythmias are common in emergency patients. Clinical signs associated with pathologic tachyarrhythmias include weakness, lethargy, and collapse. On rare occasions, tachyarrhythmias may result in sudden death. Causes of symptomatic tachyarrhythmias include increased sympathetic tone, toxicities, electrolyte abnormalities, myocardial disease or ischemia, and reentrant circuits within the myocardium. Although isolated or infrequent supraventricular or ventricular premature complexes are often seen in the emergency department, most patients with symptoms have sustained tachyarrhythmias. These rhythms include sinus tachycardia, supraventricular tachycardia (including atrial or junctional tachycardia, and atrial fibrillation), and ventricular tachycardia.

SINUS TACHYCARDIA

- Sinus tachycardia is associated with increased sympathetic tone. Common causes of sinus tachycardia in emergency patients include hypovolemia, hypotension, anemia, hypoxemia, pain, stress, fear, and excitement. No specific treatment is usually required, and treatment is generally contraindicated as it may suppress a life-saving compensatory response. Rather, the heart rate responds when the underlying cause of the tachycardia is identified and addressed. In patients with sinus tachycardia associated with anxiety, anxiolytics may result in a decrease in heart rate.
- The use of beta-adrenergic blockers, such as **esmolol** (dogs and cats, 0.1 to 0.5 mg/kg IV slowly, followed by 50 to 200 µg/kg/min CRI) or **propranolol** (dogs and cats, slow IV boluses of 0.02 mg/kg up to 0.1 mg/kg), is indicated in cases of sinus tachycardia secondary to drug or toxin exposures or in cases where all other underlying causes of tachycardia (hypovolemia, hypoxemia, anxiety) have been addressed. Side effects of beta-adrenergic blockers include bradycardia, negative inotropy, and hypotension.

SUPRAVENTRICULAR TACHYCARDIA

- Supraventricular tachycardias may be atrial or junctional in origin. Atrial fibrillation is also considered to be an atrial tachycardia. Junctional tachycardias originate from within the AV node or involve reentrant circuits within the AV node. Supraventricular tachycardias are also known as *narrow-complex tachycardias*, as the QRS complex resembles the QRS associated with normal sinus complexes. In rare instances, a wide-complex tachycardia may result from a supraventricular focus because of the presence of bundle branch block in the specialized conduction system.
- Supraventricular tachycardia results from abnormalities within the atrial or junctional myocardial tissue. This may occur because of grossly identifiable diseases, such as atrial dilation in the presence of elevated filling pressures or volume overload, myocardial fibrosis in the presence of cardiomyopathy, or infiltrative diseases such as cardiac neoplasia. In other cases, including most patients with reentrant circuits, supraventricular tachycardia occurs in a heart that appears to be structurally normal. This is also the case in patients where supraventricular tachycardia is caused by electrolyte abnormalities or pharmacologic causes. Common agents that can result in supraventricular tachycardia include digoxin, caffeine, chocolate, and amphetamines or other illicit drugs.
- Patients with supraventricular tachycardia usually have symptoms such as weakness, lethargy, or collapse. Pulse quality is variable but often diminished. In cases of stimulant toxicosis, supraventricular tachycardia may be associated with excitement, hyperesthesia, or seizure activity.
- Treatment of supraventricular tachycardia involves attempting to identify and specifically treat any underlying cause of the tachycardia, such as an electrolyte abnormality or digoxin overdose. In addition, variations in sympathetic tone may affect conduction through the AV node, and possible causes of increased sympathetic tone should be investigated. If no underlying cause of the tachycardia can be determined, a vagal maneuver may be attempted.
  - Vagal maneuvers include firm ocular pressure or carotid massage and are undertaken in an attempt to slow conduction through the AV node. In some instances, vagal maneuvers may temporarily terminate a supraventricular tachycardia.
- Pharmacologic therapy of supraventricular tachycardia in an emergency situation involves the use of injectable antiarrhythmic agents. Initial choices for antiarrhythmic therapy include beta-adrenergic blockers, which limit the rate of spontaneous depolarization in ectopic pacemakers, and calcium channel blockers, which slow conduction through the AV node. Both

classes of drug have potent negative chronotropic effects and may also have profound negative inotropic properties. These negative inotropic effects are more pronounced when the drugs are given rapidly, in high doses, or in combination with other agents that impair contractility. This consideration is especially important in patients with significant structural heart disease and limited cardiovascular reserve.

- **Esmolol** (see the dose listed earlier) is generally preferred to other beta-blocking agents, such as propranolol, because of its short half-life that allows rapid titration of effect.
- The use of a calcium channel blocker is an alternative to beta-blocking agents. **Diltiazem** (dogs and cats, 0.1 to 0.25 mg/kg slowly followed by 5 to 20 µg/kg/min CRI) has a less pronounced negative inotropic effect than equivalent doses of esmolol.
- Other choices for antiarrhythmic therapy of supraventricular tachycardia include procainamide and amiodarone.
  - **Procainamide** (dogs, 6 to 8 mg/kg slowly, followed by 20 to 50 µg/kg/min CRI) is a fast sodium channel blocker and can be used for both supraventricular and ventricular arrhythmias.
  - **Amiodarone** (dogs, slow [20 to 30 minute] bolus of 5 to 10 mg/kg diluted in 5% dextrose in water) acts to prolong the action potential. Amiodarone may cause significant hypotension, vasodilation, and pruritus during IV administration, and long-term use may be associated with hepatic dysfunction in dogs. Its use is generally precluded by its potential adverse effects and the availability of safer, more effective medications as noted above.

VENTRICULAR TACHYCARDIA

- Ventricular arrhythmias are very common in emergency patients, and ventricular complexes are recognized by a wide and bizarre QRS shape. In many cases, such as isolated ventricular premature complexes, these rhythm disturbances do not require treatment. However, treatment is recommended if there are frequent or multifocal ventricular premature complexes; if the coupling interval is very rapid, creating an R-on-T shape; or if there is sustained ventricular tachycardia (rates greater than 180 beats/min) with clinical or hemodynamic sequelae.
  - An accelerated idioventricular rhythm is very common in patients with noncardiac disease. This rhythm is recognized as a regular, monomorphic ventricular rhythm that is very similar in rate to the underlying sinus rhythm, and fusion complexes may be recognized

during transitions between the ventricular and sinus rhythms. In general, this rhythm does not produce significant hemodynamic abnormalities and does not require therapy.

- Ventricular tachycardias result from abnormalities within the ventricular myocardium and are caused by abnormal automaticity, triggered activity, or reentrant circuits. Ventricular arrhythmias may occur because of primary cardiac disease, such as dilated cardiomyopathy, arrhythmogenic cardiomyopathy, hypertrophic cardiomyopathy, chronic valvular disease, aortic or pulmonic stenosis, myocarditis, or cardiac neoplasia. Ventricular arrhythmias may also be seen in a variety of noncardiac conditions, especially in patients with elevated sympathetic tone or inflammatory mediators, and with electrolyte disturbances such as hypocalcemia and hypokalemia.
- As with supraventricular tachycardia, long-standing ventricular tachycardia may produce myocardial failure in patients with otherwise normal hearts. This tachycardia-induced cardiomyopathy results in chamber dilation and diminished systolic function and can result in CHF.
- Patients with symptomatic ventricular tachycardia usually have symptoms such as weakness, lethargy, or collapse. Paroxysmal ventricular tachycardia may result in syncope or episodes of near-syncope.
- Treatment of ventricular tachycardia should involve attempting to identify and specifically treat any underlying cause of the tachycardia.
  - In many patients, ventricular arrhythmias respond to interventions such as fluid resuscitation in patients with hypovolemia, the administration of blood products in anemic animals, the implementation of oxygen therapy in hypoxemic patients, correction of electrolyte and acid-base abnormalities, and the use of analgesics in painful patients.
- Pharmacologic therapy of ventricular tachycardia in an emergency situation involves the use of injectable antiarrhythmic agents. Initial choices for antiarrhythmic therapy include class 1 agents such as lidocaine or procainamide. Alternatives include beta-adrenergic blockers or class III agents such as amiodarone.
  - **Lidocaine** (dogs, 2 mg/kg IV bolus up to 8 mg/kg and followed by 25 to 80 µg/kg/min CRI) is generally a first line choice in dogs. Cats are much more likely to have adverse effects (gastrointestinal signs, neurologic signs including seizures), and the dose is significantly decreased to prevent these signs (cats, 0.25 to 0.75 mg/kg IV bolus followed by 10 to 20 µg/kg/min CRI).

- **Procainamide** (dogs, 6 to 8 mg/kg slow IV bolus followed by 20 to 50 µg/kg/min) may also be used to treat ventricular tachycardia, particularly if lidocaine is ineffective. Rapid administration may cause significant hypotension.
- **Esmolol** (see the dose listed earlier) is generally preferred to other beta-adrenergic blockers because of its short half-life. As with procainamide, esmolol may cause hypotension, which is secondary to its potent negative inotropic effect.
- **Amiodarone** (see the dose listed earlier) may also be used for the treatment of symptomatic ventricular tachycardia; however, vasodilation and systemic hypotension are common during administration in dogs, and amiodarone is generally only used in cases where the previously listed agents are ineffective.
- As mentioned previously, in rare cases, a wide-complex tachycardia may result from a supraventricular focus with concurrent bundle branch block in the specialized conduction system. Lidocaine is unlikely to be effective in this scenario, whereas procainamide, beta-adrenergic blockers, or calcium channel blockers are more likely to be useful in the diagnosis and management of these patients.

THROMBOEMBOLIC DISEASE

- See Chapters 9 and 10 for additional discussion.
- Cardiac emergencies associated with thromboembolic disease may either be the cause or the result of severe cardiac disease. Massive pulmonary thromboembolism may cause heart disease by significantly increasing right ventricular afterload. This process results in severe pulmonary hypertension and may precipitate acute right-sided heart failure and cardiogenic shock. This disease occurs more commonly in dogs than cats and is generally associated with an underlying hypercoagulable state that results in pathologic clot formation. Conditions associated with pulmonary thromboembolism include hyperadrenocorticism, immune-mediated hemolytic anemia, sepsis, disseminated intravascular coagulation, protein-losing nephropathy and enteropathy, heartworm disease, and neoplasia.
- More commonly, emergency patients have thromboembolic disease resulting from cardiac disease. This is especially common in cats with cardiomyopathy and associated left atrial enlargement. These patients are prone to the development of blood clots that subsequently embolize the systemic arterial tree. This condition, known as *feline aortic thromboembolism*, often causes acute limb paresis and subsequent tissue ischemia secondary to obstruction of arterial blood flow.
- Cats most commonly display paraparesis but may also have unilateral hindlimb or forelimb paresis. Cats may also embolize other organs, such as the brain, kidneys, or gastrointestinal tract. CHF may be present, although arterial embolization may occur alone. All affected cats benefit from analgesia and treatment of any concurrent heart failure while in the emergency room. Thrombolytic agents such as streptokinase or tissue plasminogen activator may accelerate clot dissolution; however, their use has not provided definitive evidence of benefit in clinical trials. In addition, these agents may cause significant complications, including severe hemorrhage and fatal reperfusion syndromes.
- Conservative therapy involves the provision of supportive care and analgesia, and some cats will reestablish arterial blood flow and regain function in ischemic limbs within 2 to 3 days. Patients with CHF, more than one limb affected, or low rectal temperatures have a worse prognosis for return of perfusion and limb function. The risk of recurrence is high, with 17% to 50% of patients experiencing a repeat episode.
  - Analgesia in the form of **fentanyl** (cats, 2 to 5 µg/kg/hr CRI for 12 to 18 hours as a fentanyl patch takes effect), **butorphanol** (cats, 0.1 to 0.3 mg/kg/hr CRI or 0.1 to 0.3 mg/kg IV q4h), or **buprenorphine** (cats, 0.005 to 0.015 mg/kg IV q6-8h) is recommended. Other opioids such as hydromorphone, oxymorphone, or morphine may also be used.
  - Anticoagulation with unfractionated or low-molecular-weight heparin may be useful to help reduce clot propagation and is generally well tolerated by cats. **Unfractionated heparin** (cats, 150 to 250 units/kg SQ q6-8h or as a CRI of 20 to 50 units/kg/hr at a low fluid rate) or **low-molecular-weight heparin** (e.g., dalteparin, cats, 100 to 150 units/kg SQ q12-24h) is used. Unfractionated heparin will cause prolongation of the partial thromboplastin time (PTT), and a clinical target is to achieve a PTT 1.5 to 2.5 times the normal value. Low-molecular-weight heparin activity is typically monitored via a factor Xa assay. In addition, the PTT will be prolonged in

patients at risk for hemorrhage secondary to low-molecular-weight heparin administration. All heparinized patients should be monitored for signs of clinical bleeding and should not have jugular venipuncture or cystocentesis performed.

- Antiplatelet therapy with **aspirin** (5 mg/kg PO q72h) or **clopidogrel** (18.75 mg/cat PO q24h) may also decrease the risk of clot formation. Recent evidence suggests that clopidogrel is superior to aspirin for preventing repeat episodes in cats.
- In addition, all cats that present to the emergency department with feline aortic thromboembolism should be monitored for hyperkalemia, azotemia, hypotension, cardiac arrhythmias, and signs of cardiovascular collapse that may accompany reperfusion injury.

FREQUENTLY ASKED QUESTIONS

Why do animals with pericardial effusion not have LCHF and pulmonary edema?

Pericardial effusion results in preload reduction to the heart. The pressure that develops around the heart due to effusion prevents the heart chambers from being able to accommodate venous return to the heart. This effect is most pronounced on the right side because it is the "low pressure" side of the heart. Therefore, with severe pericardial effusion, the right side cannot fill adequately because the pericardial fluid accumulation compresses that side more readily than the left side, and right-sided heart failure develops.

What is the purpose of oxygen supplementation and sedative drugs in the treatment of CHF with pulmonary edema?

When an animal has severe pulmonary edema, hypoxemia can result. The fluid accumulation within the lung and the hypoxemia stimulate ventilation. The hypoxemia and the fluid accumulation within the lung cause anxiety and decreased lung compliance of the lung, resulting in tachycardia, increased work of breathing because of poor lung compliance, and increased oxygen demand. Oxygen helps relieve the hypoxemia, which can in turn decrease anxiety, helping slow the heart rate. Sedative drugs help relieve anxiety, which decreases another stimulus for tachycardia. This combination of therapies will ultimately increase oxygenation of the blood, slow the heart rate, and decrease oxygen demand by the respiratory muscles, all of which are favorable effects for an ailing heart.

SUGGESTED READINGS

Bonagura JD: Electrical alternans associated with pericardial effusion in the dog, J Am Vet Med Assoc 178:574, 1981.

Cote E: Cardiogenic shock and cardiac arrest, Vet Clin North Am 31:1129, 2001.

DeFrancesco TC, Hansen BD, Atkins CE, et al.: Noninvasive transthoracic temporary cardiac pacing in dogs, J Vet Intern Med 17:663, 2003.

Fuentes VL: Arterial thromboembolism: risks, realities and a rational first-line approach, J Fel Med Surg 14:459, 2012.

Kittleson MD: Management of heart failure, In Kittleson MD, Kienle RD, eds: Small animal cardiovascular medicine, St Louis, 1998, Mosby.

Laste NL: Cardiovascular pharmacotherapy: hemodynamic drugs and antiarrhythmic agents, Vet Clin North Am 31:1231, 2001.

Moise NS: Diagnosis and management of canine arrhythmias, In Fox PR, Sisson D, Moise NS, eds: Textbook of canine and feline cardiology: principles and clinical practice, ed 2, Philadelphia, 1999, Saunders.

Moise NS: Diagnosis and management of feline arrhythmias, In Fox PR, Sisson D, Moise NS, eds: Textbook of canine and feline cardiology: principles and clinical practice, ed 2, Philadelphia, 1999, Saunders.

Oyama MA, Rush JE, Rozanski EA, et al: Assessment of serum N-terminal pro-B-type natriuretic peptide concentration for differentiation of congestive heart failure from primary respiratory tract disease as the cause of respiratory signs in dogs, J Am Vet Med Assoc 235:1319, 2009.

Smith SA, Tobias AH, Jacob KA, et al: Arterial thromboembolism in cats: acute crisis in 127 cases (1992-2001) and long-term management with low-dose aspirin in 24 cases, J Vet Intern Med 17:73, 2003.

Anesthesia of the Cardiac Patient

20

Thomas K. Day

Anesthesia of the patient with heart disease can be a challenge. Most veterinary patients with heart disease that are presented for sedation or anesthesia do not have clinical signs of heart failure. Anesthetic protocols that are routinely used for normal patients without heart disease can result in acute decompensation in patients with heart disease. Differences between dogs and cats in the response to anesthetic and analgesic drugs can compound the complex nature of cardiac anesthesia. In addition, most patients with heart disease may be treated with a variety of cardiac drugs that may interact with anesthetic drugs. This chapter provides a general view of anesthetic drugs that are indicated and contraindicated in dogs and cats with heart disease. Anesthetic considerations for specific cardiac diseases are also presented.

> **KEY POINT**
>
> Suggested anesthetic protocols for dogs and cats are presented on the basis of the functional classes of heart failure.

GENERAL PRINCIPLES

- The veterinary anesthetist must understand and recognize several factors to provide safe and effective sedation or anesthesia, including the hemodynamic changes produced by heart disease, the possible interactions between cardiac and anesthetic drugs, the presence of arrhythmias, and the potential for anesthetic drugs to predispose to the production of arrhythmias.
- Knowledge of the length of sedation or anesthesia that is desired and recognition of the need for analgesia are also important.
- Virtually all anesthetic drugs directly depress cardiac function, alter vascular tone, or modify normal cardiovascular regulatory mechanisms.

- One "magic bullet" anesthetic protocol that will safely anesthetize any dog or cat with heart disease does not exist.
- Each patient and each origin of cardiac disease should be considered on an individual basis to provide the safest sedation, analgesic, or anesthetic protocol.

> **KEY POINT**
>
> The general rule of thumb is to devise an anesthetic plan that provides minimal cardiopulmonary depression and returns the patient to preanesthetic status as soon and as safely as possible.

PREANESTHETIC CONSIDERATIONS

DIAGNOSIS OF THE ETIOLOGY OF HEART DISEASE

- The decision on which sedation or anesthetic protocol to administer to a patient with heart disease should be made primarily on the specific cause. Once the cause of heart disease has been determined, specific recommendations can be provided on the choice of sedation or anesthesia.

FUNCTIONAL CLASSIFICATION OF HEART FAILURE

- Three functional classifications of heart failure are based on clinical signs. The decision on whether to immediately sedate or anesthetize a patient with heart disease should begin with placing the patient in one of the three classifications.
- The first classification describes the symptom-free patient that has confirmed heart disease yet is not exhibiting clinical signs of heart failure. Patients that fulfill criteria for this classification can be safely anesthetized without further stabilization.

- The second classification describes when mild to moderate clinical signs of heart failure are evident at rest or with mild exercise. Stabilization of clinical signs and lack of clinical signs for several days with drug therapy are recommended before sedation or anesthesia. Patients with this classification that require life-saving emergency surgery should have cardiac drug therapy instituted immediately by parenteral administration and clinical signs controlled as much as possible before anesthesia. Continuous and aggressive monitoring will be required for this classification of patient during and immediately after sedation or anesthesia. Cardiac drug therapy should continue during anesthesia and surgery and in the immediate postoperative period.
- The third classification describes when advanced clinical signs of heart failure are immediately obvious. Patients severely affected can have cardiogenic shock, and death or severe debilitation is likely without therapy.

- Anesthesia is contraindicated in this third category of patients until clinical signs are immediately stabilized with aggressive drug therapy.
- Clients should be advised of the increased risk of death or severe debilitation during or immediately after anesthesia if patients in this third category of heart failure are anesthetized following aggressive cardiac drug therapy.

ANESTHETIC RISK CLASSIFICATION

- The anesthetic risk of a patient can be determined on the basis of physical status.
- Five categories of physical status have been developed for veterinary patients, and they parallel the classification scheme adopted in human medicine by the American Society of Anesthesiologists (ASA) (Table 20.1).
- Most clinically stable cardiac patients will be ASA I or III, depending on the presence of any other underlying disorders.

- Unstable patients with clinical signs of cardiac decompensation and heart failure that fulfill the criteria of ASA IV should not be anesthetized until the cardiac disease has been stabilized.
- There may be patients that are seen in the ASA V category, especially those with a long history of heart disease that is currently refractory to all cardiac drugs. Stabilization of the signs of heart failure may not be possible, and death during anesthesia is likely.

TABLE 20.1 Classification of Physical Status for Anesthetized Patients

ASA Category	Description of Physical Status	Example
I	Normal, healthy	No cardiac disease, elective surgery (spay, castration)
II	Mild systemic disease	Compensated heart disease (no cardiac medications), fracture without shock
III	Severe systemic disease	Compensated heart disease (cardiac medications), anemia, fever, compensated renal disease, dehydration
IV	Severe systemic disease and a constant threat to life	Decompensated heart disease, electrolyte imbalance, uncontrolled internal hemorrhage
V	Moribund patient not expected to live with or without surgery	Decompensated heart disease refractory to cardiac drugs, terminal malignancy

Adapted from the ASA Physical Status Classification System, © 1995–2014, American Society of Anesthesiologists (ASA).

PREANESTHETIC DIAGNOSTIC EVALUATION AND LABORATORY TESTS

- The patient with heart disease should have a complete diagnostic cardiac evaluation.
- All patients should have the following diagnostic and laboratory tests before sedation or anesthesia.

PHYSICAL EXAMINATION

- Particular attention should be paid to thoracic auscultation of the heart and lungs. The character of the peripheral pulse, jugular veins, mucous membranes, and capillary refill time should be noted, and the peripheral pulse should be palpated simultaneously with thoracic auscultation of the heart sounds to detect pulse deficits.

Remember that about 30% of cats with significant heart disease do not have heart murmurs. Any cat with a heart murmur should not be anesthetized without further workup.

ADDITIONAL TESTS

- Thoracic radiography and an electrocardiogram (ECG) should be performed as well. If a complete cardiac diagnostic evaluation has been performed less than 1 to 2 weeks previous to anesthesia and the patient's physical status has not changed, a physical examination and ECG are the only diagnostic tests that require repetition. Complete blood count and serum chemistries should be performed at the discretion of the veterinarian, with particular attention to renal values and electrolytes.

CARDIAC DRUGS AND POTENTIAL ANESTHETIC DRUG INTERACTIONS

DIURETICS

- The loop diuretic furosemide is the most commonly used diuretic in patients with heart disease. The most common electrolyte disturbance produced by furosemide is hypokalemia. Hypokalemia can result in tachyarrhythmias or predispose to digoxin toxicity. Furosemide may promote dehydration and predispose the patient to hypotension during sedation or anesthesia.
- The potassium-sparing diuretic spironolactone can result in hyperkalemia if used alone for extended periods of time. Hyperkalemia may result in arrhythmias, with equal likelihood of tachyarrhythmias or bradyarrhythmias.
- The thiazide diuretic chlorothiazide has similar side effects as the loop diuretics with long-term use. Hypokalemia and hypomagnesemia may produce or predispose to tachyarrhythmias.

ANGIOTENSIN-CONVERTING ENZYME INHIBITORS

- Enalapril and benazepril are the most commonly used angiotensin-converting enzyme (ACE) inhibitors. Each results in arterial vasodilation that can be enhanced by acepromazine, isoflurane, and sevoflurane, predisposing to arterial hypotension. Arterial blood pressure should be monitored closely during sedation protocols involving acepromazine and during isoflurane and sevoflurane anesthesia.

> **KEY POINT**
>
> All patients receiving ACE inhibitors should be monitored with direct or indirect blood pressure during inhalation anesthesia.

DIGITALIS GLYCOSIDES

- A common side effect of digoxin administration is ventricular arrhythmias. There is the possibility of an increase in arrhythmogenesis with concurrent use of sympathomimetics (dopamine, dobutamine, norepinephrine, epinephrine) during anesthesia. Isoflurane, sevoflurane, and opioids have not been associated with increased incidence of arrhythmias secondary to digitalis.
- Hypokalemia, most commonly caused by long-term use of loop diuretics, can exacerbate digitalis toxicity. Acute onset of hypokalemia can occur during anesthesia as a result of hyperventilation (hypocarbia and concurrent respiratory alkalosis) and can exacerbate preexisting hypokalemia caused by diuretics.

> **KEY POINT**
>
> Always obtain a blood digitalis level before anesthesia.

VASODILATORS

- Hydralazine is an arteriodilator that can cause reflex tachycardia and fluid and water retention. Tachycardia secondary to use of sympathomimetics (dopamine, dobutamine, norepinephrine, epinephrine) during anesthesia can be exacerbated by hydralazine. Fluid administration must be minimized and monitored closely. Acepromazine, isoflurane, and sevoflurane may exacerbate arteriodilation and predispose to arterial hypotension.
- Prazosin causes arterial and venodilation by alpha-1 adrenergic blockade. Acepromazine is contraindicated, as arteriodilation may be excessive and produce severe hypotension. Isoflurane may exacerbate arteriodilation and may predispose to arterial hypotension.

CALCIUM CHANNEL BLOCKERS

- Diltiazem is used to treat supraventricular arrhythmias and to improve diastolic function in cats with hypertrophic cardiomyopathy (HCM). Potential side effects include vasodilation, bradycardia, and decreased myocardial contractility. Concurrent use of acepromazine, isoflurane, and sevoflurane may exacerbate vasodilation and produce hypotension. Concurrent use of opioids and inhalation anesthetics (isoflurane and sevoflurane) may exacerbate bradycardia. Decreased myocardial contractility may be exacerbated by propofol.

INODILATOR

- Pimobendan is an inodilator that is becoming more and more popular to treat mitral valve disease in dogs. The primary use for pimobendan in dogs with mitral disease is after the dog has shown signs of congestive heart failure.

Pimobendan is one of the primary cardiac drugs used to treat dilated cardiomyopathy. There is a potential for hypotension when isoflurane or sevoflurane is used because of their vasodilatory effects when combined with the mild vasodilation caused by pimobendan.

ANTIARRHYTHMIC AGENTS

- The beta-adrenergic blocking agents propranolol and atenolol are commonly used to treat arrhythmias in dogs and cats and for treatment of HCM in cats. Potential side effects include bradycardia and decreased myocardial contractile function. Bradycardia may be exacerbated with use of opioids and inhalation anesthetics. Decreased myocardial contractility may cause hypotension during anesthesia, may be less responsive to sympathomimetics (dopamine and dobutamine), and may be exacerbated by propofol.

CLASS I ANTIARRHYTHMIC AGENTS

- Procainamide and tocainide can have side effects, including decreased myocardial contractility and possible bradycardia. Decreased myocardial contractility may be exacerbated by propofol.

NONSTEROIDAL ANTIINFLAMMATORY DRUGS

- Cats with heart disease may be prescribed aspirin to potentially prevent thromboembolic disease. Aspirin impairs platelet function. Acepromazine should be avoided in cats receiving aspirin that are presented for surgery, as acepromazine also impairs platelet function. Clopidogrel has the same anesthetic concerns (impaired platelet function) as aspirin.

COMBINATION DRUG THERAPY

- Most patients with heart disease are administered more than one cardiac drug. The potential side effects of each drug must first be considered individually. Potential side effects of the combination of drugs should be considered next. The addition of anesthetic drugs may introduce a greater possibility of side effects. For example, a dog with compensated mitral insufficiency could have been prescribed digoxin, furosemide, and enalapril. There is a great potential for hypotension produced by excessive arteriodilation, bradycardia, or decreased myocardial contractility based on the combined side effects of each drug. Isoflurane and sevoflurane, which minimally decrease myocardial contractility and cardiac output, could produce severe hypotension in this patient secondary to peripheral vasodilation. Inhalation anesthesia should not be considered the primary anesthetic of choice in this dog.

ANESTHETIC DRUG SELECTION AND SUPPORTIVE CARE

CHOICE OF EITHER SEDATION OR GENERAL ANESTHESIA

- The definition of general anesthesia is the administration of injectable anesthetics, inhalation anesthetics, or a combination to produce hypnosis (sleep), analgesia, and muscle relaxation. General anesthesia is not solely produced by the administration of inhalation anesthetics. Many useful and safe general anesthetic protocols for cardiac patients are combinations of injectable anesthetic agents.

OXYGENATION AND VENTILATORY SUPPORT

- All cardiac patients that are sedated or anesthetized should have oxygen administered in some form. Sedated patients should have oxygen delivered by mask at an insufflation rate of no less than 5 L/min. All intubated patients should be attached to an anesthetic machine to deliver 100% oxygen, regardless of whether an inhalation anesthetic is delivered.
- All cardiac patients anesthetized and maintained with isoflurane, sevoflurane, or injectable anesthetics should have ventilatory support provided. Isoflurane and sevoflurane are both potent respiratory depressants and can predispose the patient to hypoxemia or hypercarbia. Hypoxemia and hypercarbia can result in the production or worsening of arrhythmias. All intubated patients should also have ventilation supported. The general rule is that four to six breaths should be delivered each minute. Expired carbon dioxide can be monitored with a capnometer (see the section on monitoring and supportive care during sedation and anesthesia) to ensure adequate ventilation.

ANESTHETIC DRUGS THAT ARE CONTRAINDICATED IN PATIENTS WITH CARDIAC DISEASE

- The following sedatives and anesthetic drugs are contraindicated in patients with heart disease, regardless of origin. The benefits of convenience, effectiveness, ease of administration, and lower cost do not justify the use of these drugs because of the profound cardiopulmonary depression, the increased possibility of arrhythmia production, and the length of recovery time.

ALPHA-2 ADRENERGIC DRUGS

- Xylazine and dexmedetomidine are potent respiratory and cardiac depressants. Decreased heart rate is usually responsive to anticholinergics.

Xylazine and dexmedetomidine can also decrease heart rate by a central mechanism of decreased sympathetic outflow that will not be responsive to anticholinergics. Xylazine decreases myocardial contractility, resulting in decreased cardiac output and hypotension. Dexmedetomidine results in intense vasoconstriction and decreased cardiac output. Decreased heart rate is usually a result of intense vasoconstriction. Administration of an anticholinergic will greatly increase cardiac work.

INHALATION ANESTHETICS

- Mask induction with isoflurane or sevoflurane is not recommended in cardiac patients. Most animals become very excited during mask induction, even with adequate preanesthetic medication, which could predispose to arrhythmias and increased myocardial work secondary to the stress response. Isoflurane has a very pungent odor and may result in laryngospasm, especially in cats, though sevoflurane is less pungent. Environmental contamination when isoflurane and sevoflurane is administered by mask is a very important consideration for the safety of all personnel.

ANESTHETIC DRUGS THAT SHOULD BE USED WITH CAUTION

PREANESTHETIC MEDICATION

TRANQUILIZERS

- The phenothiazine acepromazine is considered a major tranquilizer because of the high reliability of producing mental calming. It is also the most commonly used tranquilizer in small animals. The primary cardiovascular effect is dose-dependent peripheral vasodilation, with minimal effects on contractility and respiration. Hypotension can occur and is primarily treated with intravenous fluids and, in severe cases, peripheral vasoconstriction agents (phenylephrine, norepinephrine). The sedative and cardiovascular effects are of long duration (4 to 6 hours), and the effects are not reversible. Acepromazine can be used effectively and safely at very low dosages in otherwise healthy cardiac patients

ANTICHOLINERGICS

- Atropine and glycopyrrolate are primarily used to maintain heart rate during anesthesia or sedation and are generally not recommended for routine use unless used with anesthetic drugs that are likely to lower heart rate (opioids) through increased parasympathetic tone.

The potential side effects include the production of tachyarrhythmias (ventricular or supraventricular). The increase in myocardial oxygen consumption produced by an increase in heart rate above normal values may predispose the patient with heart disease to focal ischemia and possibly arrhythmias. There is little difference between atropine and glycopyrrolate in the effectiveness of producing an increase in heart rate, though glycopyrrolate will likely have a longer duration.

INTRAVENOUS INDUCTION AGENTS

PROPOFOL

- Propofol has cardiovascular effects similar to the barbiturates (no longer used clinically) but with less likelihood of arrhythmia production. Apnea can be profound and is closely related to speed of injection. Propofol is rapidly redistributed, resulting in very rapid recovery.

DISSOCIATIVES

- Ketamine and the combination of tiletamine and zolazepam are usually very safe and effective in cardiac patients. Transient increases in heart rate can predispose to arrhythmias, so these drugs are not recommended in patients with preexisting arrhythmias. Increased heart rate is less severe if administered after preanesthetic medication. Ketamine should not be used as the sole anesthetic agent in cats with HCM. Acute fulminate congestive heart failure has been reported in cats with HCM administered ketamine and combinations of ketamine/diazepam as the sole anesthetic.

INHALATION ANESTHETICS

- Inhalation anesthetics used as the sole anesthetic agent to induce (mask induction) and maintain anesthesia must be used with extreme caution. Both isoflurane and sevoflurane are potent vasodilators that could lead to hypotension and increased cardiac work. Both isoflurane and sevoflurane are potent respiratory depressants.

USEFUL ANESTHETIC DRUGS

PREANESTHETIC MEDICATION

- The benefits of preanesthetic medication in patients with heart disease include reducing preoperative anxiety and stress, providing preemptive analgesia, lowering the requirement for intravenous induction agents and inhalation anesthetics, and ensuring a smooth recovery. Preanesthetic medication can be administered intramuscularly, subcutaneously, or intravenously. In most cardiac patients, I recommend intramuscular administration of preanesthetic medications.

TRANQUILIZERS

BENZODIAZEPINES

- Diazepam and midazolam are considered minor tranquilizers because when used alone, benzodiazepines do not produce profound sedation in the normally mentated patient. Benzodiazepines may produce a profound effect on patients with advanced age or disease. The most common use is in combination with an opioid (neuroleptanalgesia). Both drugs minimally depress cardiopulmonary function. Both diazepam and midazolam are effectively absorbed after intramuscular administration, though diazepam may produce more pain on injection (it is propylene glycol based). Clinical effects of midazolam compared with diazepam are identical in dogs and cats, though midazolam is more expensive. The benzodiazepine antagonist flumazenil is available, though the effects of benzodiazepines rarely require antagonism.

OPIOIDS

- The primary use of opioids in veterinary anesthesia is to provide analgesia. Most opioids do not possess profound sedative effects when administered alone; however, when used in combination with tranquilizers for neuroleptanalgesia (see following), adequate sedation can be achieved. Opioids do not affect myocardial contractility or vascular tone, which makes them very attractive for use in patients with heart disease. All effects produced by opioids can be antagonized by administration of naloxone, though repeat administration will likely be required as naloxone has a very short duration of action.

MORPHINE

- Minimal sedation is produced when used alone in normal patients, though profound sedation can occur in compromised patients. Primary side effects are vomiting and bradycardia. Bradycardia is usually anticholinergic-responsive. Depression of respiration is dose dependent.

HYDROMORPHONE

- Opioid agonists have similar clinical effects and are analgesics that are 10 times more potent compared with morphine. They are usually more effective than morphine in producing sedation when used alone, though even more

effective in a neuroleptanalgesic combination. They have a potential for decreased heart rate (parasympathomimetic) but have less respiratory depression than morphine. Vomiting is likely, though less likely than with morphine. Opioid agonists can also be used as an induction agent in compromised patients.

BUTORPHANOL

- Butorphanol is an opioid agonist/antagonist that is usually less effective than hydromorphone in producing sedation alone or in a neuroleptanalgesic combination. There is minimal cardiopulmonary depression, and it is unlikely to produce bradycardia. A "ceiling effect" occurs regarding sedation and analgesia. This means that higher doses beyond the recommended maximum dose (approximately 0.8 mg/kg) do not produce more sedation or analgesia. Vomiting is a rare side effect. It is a very poor analgesic for moderate to severe pain.

BUPRENORPHINE

- Buprenorphine is a partial opioid agonist that is 20 times more potent in producing analgesia compared with morphine. It is generally a poor sedative when used alone, though slightly more effective in a neuroleptanalgesia combination. There is minimal cardiopulmonary depression, and a ceiling effect occurs similar to butorphanol. The onset of action is 20 to 30 minutes, and there is a long duration of effect. Repeat injections of naloxone are required to maintain antagonism of effects, if required.

FENTANYL

- Fentanyl is an opioid agonist that is 100 times more potent in producing analgesia when compared with morphine. The onset of action is very rapid, and it can be used as an intravenous induction agent in dogs. The duration of action is extremely short, making fentanyl an ideal agent for a continuous-rate infusion (CRI) to maintain general anesthesia. Bradycardia is more likely to occur and responds to anticholinergic administration (preferred) or a decrease in the rate of infusion.

NEUROLEPTANALGESIA

- *Neuroleptanalgesia* is defined as the effect produced by the combination of a tranquilizer and an opioid. The neuroleptanalgesia combinations that are recommended for patients with heart disease include any combination of a benzodiazepine and an opioid. Intravenous or intramuscular administration may be used to produce an effect.

OPIOID-DIAZEPAM COMBINATIONS

- The preferred neuroleptanalgesia for patients with heart disease is the combination of an opioid and a benzodiazepine. The most reliable sedation occurs with an opioid agonist (morphine, hydromorphone/oxymorphone, fentanyl) compared with an opioid agonist/ antagonist (butorphanol) and partial opioid agonist (buprenorphine) combinations. Intramuscular administration produces effects within 15 minutes. Panting is a prominent feature when opioid agonists are used in dogs (not cats), and respiratory depression can be pronounced. Bradycardia is more likely with opioid agonist combinations and is responsive to anticholinergics.

KEY POINT

A neuroleptanalgesia combination including acepromazine will produce the most profound sedative effect; however acepromazine has a long duration of effect, including vasodilation, and it has no reversal agent. Neuroleptanalgesia combinations including benzodiazepines may be much less effective in excited or nervous dogs and cats. The clinician must weigh the risks and benefits of including acepromazine.

INTRAVENOUS INDUCTION AGENTS

DISSOCIATIVES

- Ketamine is used commonly as an induction agent in patients with heart disease, but it should not be used alone. Always combine ketamine with diazepam or midazolam to minimize adverse effects of rigidity and possible seizures. Induction with ketamine and diazepam results in a rapid induction of anesthesia. The combination will increase heart rate, maintain arterial blood pressure, and have minimal effects on respiration, although apnea has been reported with ketamine-diazepam combination. Potential side effects include myoclonus activity and rough recovery. Cats with HCM should not be administered ketamine or ketamine-diazepam as sole agents. Administration of ketamine or ketamine-diazepam after neuroleptanalgesia may decrease untoward cardiovascular effects related to dissociatives.

TILETAMINE AND ZOLAZEPAM

- The effects are similar to ketamine-diazepam when administered as an intravenous bolus for induction. There is less myoclonus activity and a generally smoother induction. There are longer and potentially rougher recoveries than ketamine-diazepam when used as a sole agent without preanesthetic medication. Preanesthetic medication is highly recommended before use of tiletamine-zolazepam. Higher doses will be required if no preanesthetic medication is administered, and there is a potential for longer recoveries. There are likely the same considerations in cats with HCM as with ketamine combinations.

NONBARBITURATES

PROPOFOL

- Propofol is classified as a phenolic compound unrelated to opioids, barbiturates, or steroid anesthetics. Propofol induction is characterized as a very rapid and smooth induction with a very rapid and smooth recovery. Noncumulative effects make propofol an ideal drug for CRIs. Transient decreases in arterial blood pressure occur and are produced by a decrease in myocardial contractility. A reflex increase in heart rate is likely. Apnea can be profound, and it is closely associated with speed of injection. Use of preanesthetic medication greatly reduces the dose of propofol required for induction of anesthesia and reduces the possibility of decreases in blood pressure.

ETOMIDATE

- Etomidate is an imidazole derivative unrelated to barbiturates and opioids. Etomidate induction is characterized as a very rapid induction with a very rapid and smooth recovery. Induction with etomidate results in a much less desirable induction and recovery if administered alone without preanesthetic medication. Severe myoclonus activity can occur when used alone. Minimal cardiopulmonary depression and minimal effect on cardiac electrical activity make etomidate an ideal intravenous induction agent for the less stable patient with heart disease after appropriate preanesthetic medication. Etomidate is prepared in a propylene glycol base and has a high osmolality. Intermittent bolus or CRI is not recommended owing to possibility of acute red blood cell lysis.

MAINTENANCE OF ANESTHESIA

INHALATION ANESTHETICS

ISOFLURANE AND SEVOFLURANE

- Each inhalation anesthetic has a very similar clinical effect of rapid induction and recovery. Minimal effects on cardiac rhythm and contractility result in minimal decreases in cardiac output. The main cardiovascular effect is dose-dependent peripheral vasodilation, which is the primary mechanism of hypotension induced by isoflurane and sevoflurane. A general rule is to administer the lowest effective concentration of isoflurane or sevoflurane that will maintain a surgical depth of anesthesia. The use of preanesthetic medications and intravenous induction agents is highly recommended and will lower the amount of isoflurane necessary to maintain a surgical depth of anesthesia. Each are potent respiratory depressants that can be additive with opioids, and manual ventilation is mandatory to prevent hypoxemia and hypercarbia.

NITROUS OXIDE

- Nitrous oxide used in combination with oxygen cannot alone produce anesthesia. Therefore it is used as an adjunct to inhalation anesthesia only. Use of nitrous oxide can lower the inhalation anesthetic requirement. Safety considerations (life-threatening hypoxemia) prevent widespread use of nitrous oxide.

KEY POINT

Only experienced anesthetists should use nitrous oxide. The advent of injectable opioids such as fentanyl render the use of nitrous oxide obsolete.

INJECTABLE GENERAL ANESTHESIA

- Injectable anesthetics can be used to maintain a surgical plane of general anesthesia. The definition of general anesthesia is the production of sleep, muscle relaxation, and analgesia. All three criteria can be met effectively and safely with injectable anesthetics. Specific examples will be offered at the end of this chapter, though general concepts of using all injectable agents are offered below.

PREANESTHETIC MEDICATION AND PROPOFOL

- The neuroleptanalgesic combination of an opioid and a benzodiazepine is administered intramuscularly.
- The induction and CRI of propofol consist of an initial induction dose of 1 to 5 mg/kg IV, followed by a CRI administered by syringe pump or drip at a rate of 0.14 to 0.4 mg/kg/min IV, depending on other anesthetic drugs used as preanesthetic medication and the achieved effect. Higher infusion rates are required to maintain surgical plane of anesthesia and to maintain an endotracheal tube.

- Intermittent boluses of propofol can be used instead of a CRI. Administer propofol by slow bolus at a dosage of 0.5 to 1.0 mg/kg IV following initial induction dose, depending on other anesthetic drugs used as preanesthetic medication.

PREANESTHETIC MEDICATION AND KETAMINE-DIAZEPAM

- The neuroleptanalgesic combination of an opioid and a benzodiazepine is administered intramuscularly.
- The induction dose of ketamine and diazepam is 1 mL/10 kg of a 50:50 mixture. In general, one fourth to one third of the initial induction dose can be administered as an intermittent bolus, depending on other anesthetic drugs used as preanesthetic medication.

PREANESTHETIC MEDICATION AND FENTANYL

- The neuroleptanalgesic combination of an opioid and a benzodiazepine is administered intramuscularly.
- The induction dose of fentanyl is 2 to 5 µg/kg IV followed by a CRI of 10 to 30 µg/kg/hr. This would be a preferred technique for injectable general anesthesia. A ventilator will be required to maintain respirations as fentanyl is a potent respiratory depressant.

SPECIES DIFFERENCES (DOG COMPARED WITH CAT) IN ANESTHETIC DRUG EFFECTS

TRANQUILIZERS

- Compared with dogs, cats are less responsive to the mental calming effects of an equivalent dose of acepromazine when used alone.

OPIOIDS

- Cats are more likely to become excited from the effects of opioids and, at times, to neuroleptanalgesic combinations of diazepam and an opioid.
- Cats do not have as profound sedative effects from neuroleptanalgesic combinations. Some dogs become laterally recumbent after certain neuroleptanalgesic combinations, whereas cats rarely respond in the same manner. The general rule is that an effective neuroleptanalgesia in cats occurs when the cat assumes sternal recumbency, is very amenable to mild restraint, and has mydriasis.
- Vomiting occurs less frequently in cats with the neuroleptanalgesia combination, though it occurs frequently with hydromorphone used alone.
- Dogs have miosis when an opioid is administered, and cats have mydriasis.

DISSOCIATIVES

- The dissociatives are the primary class of anesthetic drugs recommended for chemical restraint in cats. The dissociatives are used primarily as intravenous induction agents in dogs. Ketamine should never be used as a sole anesthetic in the dog. Ketamine can be used alone in the cat, though muscle rigidity and salivation can be profound.
- Tiletamine and zolazepam are metabolized differently in cats and dogs, which can explain the general recovery characteristics. Tiletamine is metabolized at a more rapid rate than zolazepam in cats, and recoveries tend to be smooth. The reverse occurs in dogs, where zolazepam is metabolized at a more rapid rate, and recoveries tend to be rough. Use alone with extreme caution in cats with HCM. Anecdotal reports of pulmonary edema have been reported in cats.

PROPOFOL

- There is evidence that multiple exposures (consecutive days) of cats to propofol can result in oxidative injury to feline red blood cells. One anesthetic episode of propofol (induction, CRI, or intermittent boluses) will not produce oxidative injury to feline red blood cells. Propofol should not be used as an anesthetic technique for consecutive, multiple-use therapy as in radiation therapy or bandage care in cats.

ADJUNCT TECHNIQUES

LOCAL AND REGIONAL ANESTHESIA/ ANALGESIA

- Local and regional anesthesia/analgesia techniques are highly effective at reducing the amount of inhalation anesthetic required to maintain anesthesia. Many techniques are available, and the specific technique is dependent on the location of the surgical procedure. Please refer to specific anesthesia and analgesia texts for description of the available techniques.

LOCAL ANESTHETIC DRUGS

- Lidocaine (2%) and bupivacaine (0.25%) are the most commonly used local anesthetics. Lidocaine has a rapid onset (5 minutes) and short duration (60 minutes) of action. Bupivacaine has a longer onset (15 to 20 minutes) and duration (2 to 4 hours) of action. All nerve types are blocked with local anesthetics. Therefore, regional analgesia techniques such as lumbosacral anesthesia will result in temporary rear limb paralysis.

OPIOIDS

- Morphine can be used in lumbosacral epidural techniques for prolonged analgesia. However, morphine should not be used alone to provide surgical anesthesia because morphine blocks nerves that conduct pain pathways only and is meant for postoperative analgesia. The onset of action is up to 1 hour, and analgesia has been reported to be up to 12 to 24 hours. Movement of limbs is maintained because motor nerves are not affected by morphine.

INFILTRATION TECHNIQUES

- Lidocaine (2%) can be infiltrated subcutaneously to a maximum dose of 10 mg/kg in dogs and cats. Lidocaine can be diluted to 1% to obtain more total volume to block a larger area. Bupivacaine is not recommended as a sole agent for infiltration because of a long onset of action.

REGIONAL TECHNIQUES

LUMBOSACRAL EPIDURAL: DOGS

- Anesthesia or analgesia is produced caudal to the umbilicus.
- **Morphine** used as a sole agent is administered at 0.1 mL/kg diluted with 1 mL/4.5 kg sterile saline. A morphine epidural must be administered before the surgical procedure. Analgesic effects should be expected primarily during the postoperative period and should not be relied on during surgery. There is no sensory or motor blockade produced by epidural administration of opioids. Effects are limited to long-acting analgesia without effects on motor activity.
- **Lidocaine (2%)** used as a sole agent is administered at 1 mL/4.5 kg before surgery. Minimal residual analgesia occurs following surgery caused by the short duration of action.
- **Bupivacaine (0.25%)** used as a sole agent is not recommended for surgery, unless 15 to 20 minutes of time is allotted before surgery to permit maximum effect of bupivacaine. A dose of 1 mL/4.5 kg is administered.
- A combination of **morphine, lidocaine (2%), and bupivacaine (0.5%)** can be used to provide immediate and postoperative analgesia. Morphine (0.1 mg/kg) is diluted with a 50:50 mixture of lidocaine (2%) and bupivacaine (0.5%) at a dose of 1 mL/4.5 kg. The end concentration of bupivacaine is 0.25% because 0.5% bupivacaine is contraindicated in the epidural space.
- Occasionally, an epidural technique in dogs results in the appearance of cerebrospinal fluid in the spinal needle. There is no cerebrospinal fluid within the epidural space; therefore the spinal needle has entered the subarachnoid space. Either the anesthetist can remove the spinal needle and attempt the procedure again

or half the agents can be administered in the subarachnoid space. Administration of local anesthesia in the subarachnoid space is called *spinal anesthesia.*

- A common complication of epidural anesthesia is inadvertent needle puncture of a blood vessel. The local anesthetic combination should not be administered if blood enters the spinal needle.

LUMBOSACRAL EPIDURAL: CATS

- A major anatomic difference in cats compared with dogs is that the spinal cord terminates in the sacral vertebral segments in cats compared with the caudal lumbar (L4-5) in dogs. Epidural techniques are more difficult in cats and the chance of entering the subarachnoid space is more likely in cats. Administer half the volume of local anesthetic if cerebrospinal fluid is obtained in the spinal needle. Administration of local anesthesia in the subarachnoid space is called spinal anesthesia and is a reliable method of regional analgesia when compared with epidural analgesia, which has a 10% rate of ineffectiveness. There is also the possibility of spinal cord injury in cats.
- The combinations of local anesthetics and opioids used in dogs are the same for cats.

INTERCOSTAL NERVE BLOCKS

- Regional anesthesia for a lateral thoracotomy can be obtained by placing the local anesthetic at the dorsal-most aspect of the intercostal nerves at the site of incision and two intercostals spaces cranial and caudal. The maximum dose of lidocaine (10 mg/kg) should not be exceeded.

INTRAPLEURAL ANALGESIA

- Regional anesthesia for a lateral thoracotomy can be obtained by placing the local anesthetic within the pleural space after surgery. **Bupivacaine** (0.25%; 1.5 mg/kg undiluted) is administered through a thoracostomy tube or by a pleurocentesis puncture, and the patient is then placed surgery side down for 15 to 20 minutes to permit the adequate onset of action of bupivacaine.

KEY POINT

Intrapleural administration of bupivacaine is painful in the nonanesthetized patient and should be administered with extreme caution in conscious patients.

NONDEPOLARIZING MUSCLE-RELAXANT DRUGS

- Nondepolarizing muscle relaxant drugs (NMRDs) block effects of acetylcholine at the neuromuscular junction, resulting in complete paralysis of all skeletal muscle when administered at recommended doses. Use of NMRDs is reserved for specific instances during anesthesia and surgery when the patient has poor blood pressure and there is gross purposeful movement. NMRDs will permit lack of movement to complete the procedure. Ventilatory support and use of anesthetic drugs to produce sleep are mandatory when using NMRDs.
- **Atracurium** (0.25 mg/kg IV initially and 0.1 mg/kg IV for repeated administration) is a short-acting NMRD with a duration of action from 20 to 25 minutes. Atracurium is metabolized by Hoffman degradation in plasma and does not require hepatic metabolism or renal excretion. Hypothermia and acidosis will prolong the effect of atracurium.
- **Pancuronium** (0.02 to 0.04 mg/kg IV initially and 0.01 to 0.02 mg/kg IV for repeated administration) has a longer duration of action (30 to 40 minutes). Hepatic metabolism and renal excretion are required for elimination. A mild increase in heart rate can occur after initial administration because of parasympatholytic action.
- All NMRDs should be reversed at the end of anesthesia. Reversal is accomplished with neostigmine (0.02 mg/kg IV) and atropine (0.02 mg/kg IV) combined in the same syringe. Occasionally, a second dose is required using half of the original dose of both neostigmine and atropine.

MONITORING AND SUPPORTIVE CARE DURING SEDATION AND ANESTHESIA

- There are two aspects of monitoring during anesthesia: anesthetic depth and cardiopulmonary parameters. Anesthetic depth is best monitored by assessment of jaw tone. An adequately anesthetized patient has moderate jaw tone. A deeply anesthetized patient has extremely loose or no jaw tone. The only true sign of inadequate anesthetic depth is gross, purposeful movement. Heart rate, respiratory rate, and jaw tone can all increase before movement and should be monitored continuously. The use of monitoring devices to assess cardiopulmonary parameters is highly dependent on several factors, including the severity of cardiac disease, the length of anesthesia, and the procedure being performed. Minimal equipment will be required for sedation and short procedures compared to anesthesia for major surgical procedures, both cardiac and noncardiac. The physical parameters of heart rate, respiratory rate, mucous membrane color, capillary refill time, and pulse character should be monitored at regular intervals of no more than 5 minutes during anesthesia and sedation of any duration, even if monitoring equipment is used.

NONINVASIVE MONITORING
ELECTROCARDIOGRAPHY

- Continuous ECG monitoring should be performed in all patients with heart disease during sedation and anesthesia of any duration. The decision to continue ECG monitoring during the postoperative period should be determined based on the procedure and the status of the patient. The ECG can be monitored via an esophageal monitor during general anesthesia.

ARTERIAL BLOOD PRESSURE MEASUREMENT

- Indirect methods are less accurate than direct measurements (see later). However, monitoring the trends of indirect arterial blood pressure can provide valuable information. The two indirect methods are Doppler ultrasound and oscillometric.

DOPPLER ULTRASOUND METHOD

- Systolic arterial blood pressure can be consistently obtained by means of the Doppler method, and diastolic values can be determined in some patients. Doppler is easier to perform in small dogs and cats. Accuracy of obtained values is highly dependent on several factors (cuff size, skin thickness, contact of crystal, positioning of limb, vasoconstriction); therefore trends in blood pressure are monitored. The advantage of Doppler ultrasound is that active arterial blood flow can be heard at all times. There is evidence that the Doppler method to measure blood pressure represents the mean arterial blood pressure in cats.

OSCILLOMETRIC METHOD

- Systolic, diastolic, and mean arterial blood pressure and heart rate are determined. Systolic pressure is the most accurate, though values can be underestimated. Accuracy of obtained values is highly dependent on several factors (cuff size, skin thickness, contact, or positioning of cuff in relation to the artery, choice of artery, positioning of limb, vasoconstriction); therefore trends in blood pressure are monitored. Oscillometric blood pressure monitoring is extremely inaccurate in small dogs, cats, and animals in states of hypotension, despite advances in technology.

PULSE OXIMETRY

- Pulse oximetry provides indirect determination of arterial oxygenation. Active pulsation of an arterial bed is required to determine oxygenation. Pulse oximetry is inaccurate in states of hypotension and peripheral vasoconstriction (hypothermia, pain). It is most accurate when placed on the tongue; therefore heavy sedation or general anesthesia is required. Pulse oximetry can be very accurate in the ideal circumstance. However, falsely low readings may not equate to pulmonary dysfunction, especially under general anesthesia after an extended period of time. Factors that will decrease the pulse oximetry reading include a cold, dry tongue during general anesthesia, pressure exerted by the endotracheal tube on the tongue, and interference from room light. Any question about low pulse oximetry readings should be confirmed with an arterial blood gas sample.

CAPNOMETRY

- Capnometry determines the partial pressure of exhaled carbon dioxide, which is closely related to arterial partial pressure of carbon dioxide. It indirectly provides information on cardiac output. Exhaled carbon dioxide is dependent on adequate perfusion of the lungs (delivery of carbon dioxide to the lungs). Hypoventilation (increased partial pressure of carbon dioxide in arterial blood) can be detected on a breath-by-breath basis. Capnometry requires intubation in most cases for the most accurate values, though tight-fitting facemasks can provide the environment to obtain information on ventilatory status.

INVASIVE MONITORING

- The more invasive and complicated surgical procedures should incur more invasive monitoring techniques. Whereas the noninvasive techniques can provide general trends, invasive monitoring can provide more accurate data concerning cardiovascular function. Direct monitoring is less likely to provide false-negative values and is less likely to fail during anesthesia.

DIRECT ARTERIAL BLOOD PRESSURE MEASUREMENT

- A catheter placed in a peripheral artery (dorsal pedal most common) requires fairly expensive equipment, although refurbished units are affordable and very useful. It is technically more difficult to place a catheter in a peripheral artery, especially in cats and small dogs (< 5 kg). The femoral artery is much larger and less difficult to place a catheter in, although maintaining the catheter is much more difficult. It is not recommended to place a catheter in the lingual artery because of the possible complication of a hematoma that could cause postoperative airway obstruction.

KEY POINT

Technologic advances in multiparameter monitoring devices have provided veterinarians the ability to perform invasive, accurate blood pressure monitoring.

CENTRAL VENOUS PRESSURE

- The central venous pressure (CVP) monitors right-sided heart function and is the most clinically reliable indicator of intravascular volume. CVP uses a properly placed jugular catheter with the tip in the thoracic cavity. Inexpensive equipment (manometers) can be used to measure CVP, though the same device used to monitor direct arterial blood pressure can be used to monitor CVP. CVP can be a valuable tool during anesthesia or in the postoperative period to detect early cardiac failure or fluid overload.

ARTERIAL AND VENOUS BLOOD GAS

- Arterial blood gas monitoring provides information on ventilation ($PaCO_2$) and oxygenation (PaO_2). Venous blood gas monitoring from a central vein (jugular, cranial vena cava, pulmonary artery) provides indirect information on perfusion of tissues and cardiac output. Arterial and venous blood gas monitoring combined with cardiac output information can be used to calculate oxygen delivery variables (see later). Devices used for blood gas analysis are affordable and are commonly being used in clinical practice. The lingual vein can be used during general anesthesia to collect blood for analysis. Though venous, the values

are closely related to arterial values because of the close association with capillary beds.

ADVANCED CARDIOVASCULAR MONITORING: CARDIAC OUTPUT

- Cardiac output monitoring requires pulmonary artery catheterization to obtain cardiovascular values that can provide information regarding ventricular function (see Table 20.1). Cardiac output computers remain extremely high-cost expenditures. Methods to measure cardiac output via peripheral vessels show promise as a clinically useful tool.

KEY POINTS

- Cardiac output is not synonymous with arterial blood pressure. In Table 20.1, cardiac output is a determinant of the calculation for blood pressure.
- An advance in cardiac output monitoring that may become clinically available for dogs and cats is lithium dilution cardiac output.

FLUID THERAPY

- Most patients with heart disease that are anesthetized with inhalation anesthetics will require intravenous fluid support. The fluid of choice for the patient with heart disease is usually a sodium-restricted crystalloid fluid (0.45% NaCl/2.5% dextrose or 0.45% NaCl). The rate of fluid therapy administration, however, is far more important than the type of fluid administered. The rate should be less than the recommended fluid rate during anesthesia of normal, healthy patients (5 to 10 mL/kg/hr). A general rule would be to decrease the fluid rate to approximately one fourth to one third of the rate for a normal patient, yielding a rate of 2 to 3 mL/kg/hr. Routine procedures that require less than 1 hour of general anesthesia may not require IV fluid support. Less stable patients with heart disease and patients anesthetized for emergency surgery with signs of heart failure should have CVP measured to aid in monitoring fluid therapy. Colloid fluids should be used with caution in patients with heart disease, especially if a bolus of colloids is to be administered.

AFTERCARE

BASIC NURSING CARE

- Maintain body temperature by means of external warming devices such as warm water bottle, incubators, or other devices that will raise the external temperature.

- Reduce stress and anxiety by providing a quiet, dry, comfortable environment.

OXYGEN THERAPY

- Some patients may require oxygen by facemask, nasal cannula, oxygen cage, or incubator until completely recovered from anesthesia or sedation to maximize oxygen delivery parameters.

ELECTROCARDIOGRAPHIC MONITORING

- Monitor cardiac rate and rhythm continuously until the patient is completely recovered from anesthesia or sedation. Some anesthetic drugs (ketamine and inhalation anesthetics) can predispose to cardiac arrhythmias.

CARDIOVASCULAR MONITORING

- The decision to monitor blood pressure and CVP during the postoperative period should be determined by the severity of heart disease, the patient's stability, the reason for surgical intervention, and the cardiovascular status during anesthesia and surgery. Some patients will not require further monitoring, although some patients, such as a dog with dilated cardiomyopathy undergoing surgery to correct gastric dilatation-volvulus, may require all available monitoring. Invasive postoperative monitoring may be required in some patients.

ANALGESIA

- Always provide analgesia if an invasive procedure or surgery was performed. Preemptive analgesia should be practiced at all times. Preemptive analgesia is defined as analgesic techniques that are applied before surgical stimulation. Incorporating analgesic agents (opioids) in the preanesthetic medication is the easiest method of preemptive analgesia. Analgesia should be performed on a predetermined schedule (intermittent administration) or by continuous administration techniques for at least 12 to 24 hours after surgery. More invasive surgeries, such as fracture repairs, will require analgesia for a longer period of time.

OPIOID ANALGESIA TECHNIQUES
TRANSDERMAL FENTANYL

- Transdermal fentanyl is very effective in providing postoperative analgesia. Transdermal fentanyl patches are available in various sizes based on the delivery of fentanyl: 12.5, 25, 50, 75, and 100 µg/hr. Patches should be applied 12 to 24 hours before surgery for dogs and 8 to 12 hours before surgery for cats.

- The weight of the dog will determine which patch or patches to be applied. Cats and dogs weighing <3 kg can have a 12.5 µg/hr patch applied. Dogs weighing between 3 and 10 kg can have 25 µg/hr applied. Dogs weighing 10 to 20 kg can have a 50 µg/hr patch applied. Dogs weighing 20 to 30 kg will require 75 µg/hr (one each of a 25 and 50 µg/hr patch) applied simultaneously. Finally, dogs weighing >30 kg will require 100 µg/hr (two 50 µg/hr patches) applied simultaneously.

CONTINUOUS-RATE INFUSION OF OPIOIDS AND OPIOID COMBINATIONS

- Opioids alone or in combination with the local anesthetic lidocaine and the dissociative drug ketamine can be used to provide analgesia in the postoperative period in dogs and cats. Many combinations exist, and it is the decision of the clinician as to which CRI to administer. Decisions can be made based on severity of postoperative pain and clinician experience.

OPIOIDS

- Both morphine and fentanyl can be used alone to provide postoperative analgesia. The administration rate of morphine is 0.12 mg/kg/hr and the rate of fentanyl is 2 to 10 µg/kg/hr.

OPIOID COMBINATIONS: DOGS
Morphine-Lidocaine-Ketamine

- The following drugs are administered to a 1-L bag of 0.45% NaCl or 0.45% NaCl and 2.5% dextrose: morphine (15 mg/mL; 1.8 mL), lidocaine (2%; 20 mg/mL; 15 mL), and ketamine (100 mg/mL; 0.6 mL). The initial intraoperative administration is typically the anesthesia rate of fluids (10 mL/kg/hr). However, many cardiac patients will require a limited rate of fluids (2.5 mL/kg/hr) that may delay the onset of action of this combination. The postoperative administration rate will be 2.5 mL/kg/hr regardless of the intraoperative administration rate.

Fentanyl-Lidocaine-Ketamine

- The following drugs are administered to a 1-L bag of 0.45% NaCl or 0.45% NaCl and 2.5% dextrose: lidocaine (2%; 20 mg/mL; 15 mL) and ketamine (100 mg/mL; 0.6 mL). The volume of fentanyl (50 µg/mL) will vary based on the rate of fluid administration. A volume to provide a CRI of 3 µg/kg/hr should be prepared for intraoperative and postoperative administration. The fluid rates are similar to those used for morphine-lidocaine-ketamine preparations.

Some operations will require a higher dose of fentanyl. An alternative to combining all three drugs in the same bag of fluids is to combine the lidocaine and ketamine as described previously and provide a CRI of fentanyl in a separate syringe pump to deliver the higher dose of fentanyl as desired by the clinician.

OPIOID COMBINATIONS: CATS

- CRIs of opioid combinations for cats are prepared and administered differently than for dogs. Cats tend to be more likely to have side effects from lidocaine. Therefore lidocaine is not used in the combinations. Cats can become excited or show signs of dysphoria from the opioid combinations. Tranquilizers such as acepromazine (0.025 mg/kg IV) can be used to decrease any side effects caused by opioids.

KEY POINT

Opioid agonists should not be avoided because of possible side effects of excitement or dysphoria in cats.

Morphine-Ketamine

- The following drugs are administered to a 1-L bag of 0.45% NaCl or 0.45% NaCl and 2.5% dextrose: morphine (15 mg/mL; 1.8 mL) and ketamine (100 mg/mL; 0.6 mL). The initial intraoperative administration is typically the anesthesia rate of fluids (10 mL/kg/hr). However, many cardiac patients will require a limited rate of fluids (2.5 mL/kg/hr) that may delay the onset of action of this combination. The postoperative administration rate will be 2.5 mL/kg/hr regardless of the intraoperative administration rate.

Fentanyl-Ketamine

- Ketamine (100 mg/mL; 0.6 mL) is added to a 1-L bag of 0.45% NaCl or 0.45% NaCl and 2.5% dextrose. The volume of fentanyl (50 µg/mL) will vary based on the rate of fluid administration. A volume to provide a CRI of 3 µg/kg/hr should be prepared for intraoperative and postoperative administration. The fluid rates are similar to those used for morphine-ketamine preparations.

ANESTHETIC CONSIDERATIONS FOR SPECIFIC CARDIAC DISEASES AND RECOMMENDED ANESTHETIC PROTOCOLS

RECOMMENDED FOR ALL PATIENTS

- Preoxygenation with 5 L/min oxygen with facemask or "blow by" method before induction of anesthesia is used to maximize arterial oxygenation and oxygen delivery before administration of induction drugs. ECG monitoring before induction of anesthesia is also recommended. Ventilatory support should be provided to all patients maintained with inhalation anesthesia to reduce adverse effects of hypoventilation with either an anesthesia ventilator or continuous manual ventilation with close monitoring of the end-tidal carbon dioxide concentration in the expired air ($ETCO_2$).

ANESTHETIC PROTOCOLS IN DOGS AND CATS

- The choice of anesthetic protocol should be based on the patient's ASA classification (see previously) and not the specific cardiac disease. There are several differences to be noted regarding specific cardiac diseases, anesthetic drug effects, and cardiovascular support. Therefore a short discussion of the specific cardiac disease is followed by the choice of anesthetic protocol based on the ASA classification. Anesthetic techniques (including injectable techniques) for medical and minor surgical procedures are also discussed, followed by techniques for major surgical procedures within each ASA classification.

COMMON CARDIAC DISEASES AND ANESTHESIA TECHNIQUES FOR DOGS

MITRAL VALVE INSUFFICIENCY

- Mild arterial vasodilation from anesthetic drugs can result in a decrease in the regurgitant fraction across the mitral valve and maximum cardiac output.
- Supraventricular and ventricular arrhythmias are common sequelae to mitral regurgitation, and the ECG should be monitored at all times. Extremes in heart rate (bradycardia or tachycardia) can result in decreased cardiac output.

DILATED CARDIOMYOPATHY

- Inotropic support with dobutamine or dopamine is recommended for any major surgery regardless of ASA status if the dog is not receiving pimobendan. Dogs receiving pimobendan may not need inotropic support, although if hypotension persists, dobutamine or dopamine may be needed. Tachycardia may predispose to ventricular arrhythmias, and the judicious use of atropine or glycopyrrolate is not recommended. Mild arterial vasodilation can maximize cardiac output.

CONGENITAL DEFECTS

Aortic and Pulmonic Stenosis

- Cardiac output is highly dependent on heart rate, and inotropic agents contribute little to no increase in cardiac output. Tachycardia may predispose to ventricular arrhythmias, and the judicious use of atropine or glycopyrrolate is not recommended. The dose of atropine or glycopyrrolate should be decreased by half. Bradycardia can result in severe decreases in cardiac output.

Patent Ductus Arteriosus and Ventricular Septal Defect

- Pulmonary overcirculation results in a rapid uptake of inhalation anesthetic and a more rapid inhalation anesthetic induction. There may be a delay in distribution of intravenous anesthetics, although a clinical effect is likely not evident. Mild arterial vasodilation may reduce the amount of blood flow across the patent ductus arteriosus or the ventricular septal defect.

ASA II PATIENTS: MEDICAL PROCEDURE OR MINOR, MINIMALLY INVASIVE SURGICAL PROCEDURES

INJECTABLE ANESTHESIA TECHNIQUE

- The preanesthetic medication of choice would be a neuroleptanalgesic combination of **acepromazine** (0.025 mg/kg IM) and **butorphanol** (0.4 mg/kg IM). Prophylactic use of atropine is not recommended to minimize production of tachyarrhythmias.
- Induction can be achieved by means of **ketamine-diazepam** (1 mL/10 kg of a 50:50 mixture IV), and anesthesia can be maintained by means of intermittent boluses of a third to a fourth the initial dose of ketamine-diazepam if additional anesthesia time is required. Alternatively, induction and maintenance of anesthesia can be achieved by means of **propofol** (2 to 6 mg/kg IV) for induction followed by either CRI (0.14 to 0.4 mg/kg/min) or intermittent bolus (0.5 to 1.0 mg/kg IV).
- Physical parameters, ECG, and Doppler blood pressure can be used for monitoring during the procedure.

INHALATION ANESTHESIA TECHNIQUE

- Preanesthetic medication and induction are as previously described. Ketamine-diazepam is preferred over propofol because of a longer duration of action, which will require less inhalation anesthetic.
- Isoflurane or sevoflurane in oxygen at the lowest effective dose can be used to maintain anesthesia, using opioids intraoperatively as needed. Ventilation should be provided at all times during anesthesia and surgery.
- Physical parameters, ECG, Doppler blood pressure, and capnometry can be used for monitoring during the procedure.

Potent opioid agonists are usually not required for these types of minor procedures.

ASA II PATIENTS: MAJOR SURGERY

- An injectable anesthesia technique to maintain anesthesia is usually not required. These patients are considered very stable before anesthesia and surgery and should be able to tolerate inhalation anesthetics as the primary technique to maintain anesthesia.

INHALATION ANESTHESIA TECHNIQUE

- A neuroleptanalgesic combination of **acepromazine** (0.025 mg/kg IM) or **diazepam** (0.4 mg/kg IM) and **hydromorphone** (0.2 mg/kg IM) can be used for preanesthetic medication. **Atropine** (0.22 mg/kg IM) is recommended for smaller dogs (<5 kg) only.

- Potent opioid agonists are preferred over opioid agonist/antagonists to provide adequate preemptive analgesia.
- Ketamine-diazepam (1 mL/10 kg of a 50:50 mixture IV) is preferred over propofol (2 to 6 mg/kg IV) to induce anesthesia because of a longer duration of action that will initially reduce the dose of inhalation anesthetic.
- Adjuncts to general anesthesia can be used to minimize use of inhalation anesthetics. A CRI of morphine-lidocaine-ketamine or fentanyl-lidocaine-ketamine should commence at the beginning of surgery at the anesthetic rate of fluid administration (5 mL/kg/hr). An epidural injection of a combination of lidocaine-bupivacaine-morphine should be administered before the beginning of surgery for all abdominal procedures. Other local anesthetic techniques can be dictated by the surgery site. An intermittent bolus of opioid agonists may also be necessary during surgery. NMRDs can be used if blood pressure is low and the patient is not adequately anesthetized. Pancuronium (0.02 to 0.04 mg/kg IV) has a longer duration of action than atracurium (0.25 mg/kg IV) or vecuronium (0.1 to 0.2 mg/kg IV). Ventilation should be provided at all times during anesthesia and surgery.

ASA III OR IV PATIENTS: MEDICAL PROCEDURE OR MINOR, MINIMALLY INVASIVE SURGICAL PROCEDURES

INJECTABLE ANESTHESIA TECHNIQUE

- A neuroleptanalgesic combination of **diazepam** (0.4 mg/kg IM) and **butorphanol** (0.4 mg/kg IM) is administered as the preanesthetic medication. Atropine is not recommended to minimize production of tachyarrhythmias.
- Induction can be achieved with **ketamine-diazepam** (1 mL/10 kg of a 50:50 mixture IV), and anesthesia can be maintained with intermittent boluses of one third to one fourth the initial dose of ketamine-diazepam if additional anesthesia time is required. Alternatively, induction and maintenance of anesthesia can be achieved with **propofol** (2 to 6 mg/kg IV) for induction followed by either CRI (0.14 to 0.4 mg/kg/min) of intermittent bolus (0.5 to 1.0 mg/kg IV). **Etomidate** (1 to 2 mg/kg IV) should be used as the induction agent if cardiac arrhythmias are present. Multiple administrations and CRI are not recommended because etomidate may cause lysis of red blood cells. Endotracheal intubation may be necessary but is not required. Supplemental oxygen should be administered with this technique.
- Physical parameters, ECG, and Doppler blood pressure can be used for monitoring during the procedure.

KEY POINT

An inhalation anesthetic technique for a medical or minor surgical procedure is not indicated for ASA III-IV cardiac patients.

ASA III OR IV PATIENTS: MAJOR SURGERY

- An injectable anesthetic technique with low-dose inhalation, only if necessary, is recommended over a technique that relies on an inhalation anesthetic to maintain anesthesia.

KEY POINTS

- Anesthesia of ASA III or IV patients for major surgery will require intensive monitoring of anesthesia, cardiovascular parameters, and the patient.
- Neuroleptanalgesic combination of diazepam (0.2 mg/kg IV) and fentanyl (1 µg/kg IV) should be administered as preanesthetic

medication. Atropine (0.22 mg/kg IV) may be necessary if bradycardia occurs.
- Fentanyl (5 to 10 µg/kg) is recommended for induction of anesthesia. Induction with fentanyl is not considered a rapid induction and may take 30 to 60 seconds or more. Alternative induction with etomidate (1 to 2 mg/kg IV) should be administered for induction if arrhythmias are present.
- A CRI of fentanyl (10 to 30 µg/kg/hr) administered by a dedicated syringe pump is recommended to maintain a surgical plane of anesthesia.
- Ventilation should be provided at all times during anesthesia and surgery. Lidocaine and ketamine can be administered for analgesia in a separate bag of fluids. Epidural analgesia for abdominal procedures is recommended. Other local anesthetic techniques are dictated by the location of surgery. NMRDs can be used if blood pressure is low and the patient is not adequately anesthetized. Pancuronium (0.02 to 0.04 mg/kg IV) has a longer duration of action than atracurium (0.25 mg/kg IV) or vecuronium (0.1 to 0.2 mg/kg IV).
- Blood pressure (direct is preferred over indirect measurement methods), ECG, capnometry, pulse oximetry, and physical parameters are continuously monitored.

CANINE PERICARDIAL DISEASE: PERICARDIOCENTESIS

ASA I OR II DOGS THAT REQUIRE PERICARDIOCENTESIS

- Dogs not showing signs of pericardial tamponade may only require an infiltration of local anesthetic (lidocaine) in the skin and intercostals musculature at the site of needle puncture for pericardiocentesis.
- Sedation techniques for dogs not compliant to local anesthesia only include a neuroleptanalgesia combination of **diazepam** (0.2 to 0.4 mg/kg IV) and **hydromorphone** (0.1 mg/kg IV). Atropine should only be used if bradycardia occurs.

ASA IV DOGS: EMERGENCY PERICARDIOCENTESIS

- Dogs that require an emergency pericardiocentesis typically have signs of collapse, right-sided heart failure, or ventricular arrhythmias all related to pericardial tamponade. Most dogs will require only an infiltration of local anesthetic (lidocaine) in the skin and intercostals musculature at the site of needle puncture for pericardiocentesis. Occasionally, dogs will require sedation in addition to local anesthesia. The neuroleptanalgesia combination of **diazepam** (0.2 to 0.4 mg/kg IV) and **butorphanol** (0.2 mg/kg IV) is recommended. Cardiac output is highly dependent on heart rate during pericardial tamponade, and butorphanol is least likely to decrease heart rate. Atropine is not recommended. An induction agent may be necessary in addition to sedation in some instances. **Etomidate** (1 to 2 mg/kg IV) is the drug of choice as there are minimal to no cardiopulmonary effects. Multiple administrations and CRI are not recommended because etomidate may cause lysis of red blood cells.

COMMON CARDIAC DISEASES AND ANESTHESIA TECHNIQUES FOR CATS

HYPERTROPHIC CARDIOMYOPATHY

- The most common cardiac disease in cats is HCM, which is characterized primarily as diastolic dysfunction with normal ventricular contraction. Increases in heart rate and ventricular tachyarrhythmias caused by anesthetic drugs are best avoided.

ASA I AND II CATS WITH HYPERTROPHIC CARDIOMYOPATHY: MEDICAL PROCEDURE OR MINOR, MINIMALLY INVASIVE SURGICAL PROCEDURES

INJECTABLE ANESTHESIA TECHNIQUE

- A neuroleptanalgesic combination of **acepromazine** (0.025 mg/kg IM) and **hydromorphone** (0.2 mg/kg IM) is administered as preanesthetic medication. **Ketamine** (6 to 10 mg/kg IM) is administered 10 to 15 minutes after the neuroleptanalgesic combination. This three-drug combination may be all that is required to perform the procedure.
- **Propofol** (1 to 3 mg/kg IV) can be administered if additional anesthesia is required. Propofol administered as either a CRI (0.14 to 0.4 mg/kg/min) or an intermittent bolus (0.5 mg/kg IV) can be used for longer procedures.
- Physical parameters, ECG, and Doppler blood pressure can be used for monitoring during the procedure.

INHALATION ANESTHESIA TECHNIQUE

- Preanesthetic medication and induction are done as described previously.
- Isoflurane or sevoflurane in oxygen is administered at the lowest effective dose.
- The three-drug preanesthetic will greatly reduce the inhalation anesthetic requirement.

KEY POINTS

- Ventilation will be required during surgery in all cats that receive the three-drug preanesthetic combinations and inhalation anesthesia.
- Physical parameters, ECG, Doppler blood pressure, and capnometry can be monitored during the procedure.
- Buprenorphine is not potent enough to produce the level of sedation required.

ASA II PATIENTS: MAJOR SURGERY

- Injectable anesthesia is usually not required because patients are considered very stable before anesthesia and surgery and should be able to tolerate inhalation anesthetics as the primary technique to maintain anesthesia.

INHALATION ANESTHESIA TECHNIQUE

- A neuroleptanalgesic combination of **acepromazine** (0.025 mg/kg IM) and **hydromorphone** (0.2 mg/kg IM) is followed 10 to 15 minutes later by **ketamine** (6 to 10 mg/kg IM) for preanesthetic medication.

KEY POINTS

- Potent opioid agonists are preferred over opioid agonist/antagonists to provide adequate preemptive analgesia.
- Some cats may be able to be intubated without use of an induction agent. Propofol (1 to 2 mg/kg IV) can be used to effect to permit intubation.
- Ventilation should be provided at all times during anesthesia and surgery. A CRI of morphine-ketamine is recommended to provide analgesia and minimize use of inhalation anesthetics.
- Lumbosacral epidural analgesia for abdominal procedures is recommended.
- NMRDs can be used if blood pressure is low and the patient is not adequately anesthetized. **Pancuronium** (0.02 to 0.04 mg/kg IV) has a longer duration of action than **atracurium** (0.25 mg/kg IV).

ASA III OR IV PATIENTS: MEDICAL PROCEDURE OR MINOR, MINIMALLY INVASIVE SURGICAL PROCEDURES

INJECTABLE ANESTHESIA TECHNIQUE

- A neuroleptanalgesic combination of **diazepam** (0.2 to 0.4 mg/kg IV) and **hydromorphone** (0.1 mg/kg IV) is administered as preanesthetic medication.
- **Propofol** (2 to 4 mg/kg IV) is used for induction. Propofol administered as either a CRI

(0.14 to 0.4 mg/kg/min) or an intermittent bolus (0.5 to 1.0 mg/kg IV) can be used if additional time is required. **Etomidate** (1 to 2 mg/kg IV) should be used as the induction agent if cardiac arrhythmias are present. Multiple administrations and CRI are not recommended because etomidate may cause lysis of red blood cells. Endotracheal intubation may be necessary but is not required. Supplemental oxygen should be administered with this technique.

- Physical parameters, ECG, and Doppler blood pressure can be monitored during the procedure.

KEY POINT

An inhalation anesthetic technique for a medical or minor surgical procedure is not indicated for ASA III-IV cardiac patients.

ASA III OR IV PATIENTS: MAJOR SURGERY

- An injectable anesthetic technique with low-dose inhalation, only if necessary, is recommended over a technique that relies on an inhalation anesthetic to maintain anesthesia.

KEY POINTS

- Anesthesia of ASA III or IV patients for major surgery will require intensive monitoring of anesthesia and the patient.
- A neuroleptanalgesic combination of diazepam (0.4 mg/kg IM) and hydromorphone (0.2 mg/kg IM) is followed 10 to 15 minutes later by ketamine (6 to 10 mg/kg) for preanesthetic medication.
- Propofol (2 to 4 mg/kg IV) may be used if needed. Etomidate (1 to 2 mg/kg IV) should be used as the induction agent if cardiac arrhythmias are present. Multiple administrations and CRI are not recommended as etomidate may cause lysis of red blood cells
- A CRI of fentanyl (10 to 20 µg/kg/hr) administered by a dedicated syringe pump is recommended to maintain a surgical plane of anesthesia.
- Ventilation should be provided at all times during anesthesia and surgery. Ketamine can be administered for analgesia in a separate 1-L bag of fluids. Epidural analgesia for abdominal procedures is recommended.
- NMRDs can be used if blood pressure is low and the patient is not adequately anesthetized. Pancuronium (0.02 to 0.04 mg/kg IV) has a longer duration of action than atracurium (0.25 mg/kg IV).
- Blood pressure (direct is preferred over indirect measurement methods), ECG, capnometry, pulse oximetry, and physical parameters should be monitored during surgery.

FREQUENTLY ASKED QUESTIONS

Why should isoflurane and sevoflurane be used with caution to maintain anesthesia in patients with cardiac disease?

Isoflurane can certainly support cardiac output and heart rate, but it is a potent arterial vasodilator. Severe hypoperfusion and hypotension can occur during anesthesia if isoflurane or sevoflurane is used as the sole anesthetic agent to maintain anesthesia. Hypoperfusion and hypotension can be worse if the dog or cat is receiving an ACE inhibitor such as enalapril or benazepril or the inodilator pimobendan. The less isoflurane or sevoflurane used, the less likely it is that adverse cardiovascular effects will occur.

Why are the main differences in the clinical effects of opioids in dogs and cats important?

We learned long ago in our profession that cats were not small dogs. The extreme popularity of opioids for anesthesia in dogs and the advent of advanced analgesia techniques including CRIs of opioids have led to extension of opioid use to cats. However, many clinicians have been disappointed because cats do not respond in the same way to the drugs as dogs, and opioids are possibly detrimental to cats, producing hyperexcitability, opioid-related hyperthermia, and dysphoria. These effects usually cause the clinician to discontinue the opioid. Hyperexcitability and dysphoria can be treated with acepromazine and the hyperthermia will subside when the opioid is discontinued. The clinician must weigh management of clinical side effects with removing the source of adequate analgesia. Opioid use in cats is essential to prevent the untoward effects of higher doses of ketamine in cats with HCM. Opioids are extremely safe in cats with HCM, as the myocardial contractility is not affected and the heart rate is reduced. The most effective use of opioids in cats is with the concurrent use of tranquilizers. The more potent the tranquilizer, the better the clinical effect. Cats administered acepromazine with an opioid are better sedated than when a benzodiazepine is administered. The combination of a benzodiazepine and opioid in a cat could result in excitement. Clinicians should realize that cats will not be as heavily sedated (compared with dogs), and recoveries could be rough as well. Again, overall, the safety of opioids should outweigh these concerns.

What would be the most important cardiopulmonary side effect of anesthesia for the patient with cardiac disease?

By far, the most important aspect of anesthetizing a dog or cat with heart disease is respiratory depression. The opioids, dissociatives, and inhalation anesthetics are all respiratory depressants. Severe respiratory depression will occur if all three of these anesthetic classes of drugs are used in the same anesthetic protocol. The most common cause of anesthetic death is respiratory arrest. Dogs and cats with cardiac disease undergoing anesthesia should have ventilation maintained either manually or with an anesthesia ventilator to eliminate the effects of respiratory depression. Monitoring with techniques such as capnometry and pulse oximetry will lead to early diagnosis and treatment of respiratory depression. The use of NMRDs dictates the use of ventilation.

SUGGESTED READINGS

Branson KR: Injectable and alternative anesthetics, In Tranquilli WJ, Thurmon JC, Grimm KA, eds: Lumb and Jones' veterinary anesthesia, ed 4, Ames, Iowa, 2007, Blackwell.

Cornick-Seahorn JL: Anesthetic management of patients with cardiovascular disease, Comp Cont Ed 16:1121, 1994.

Day TK: Intravenous anesthetic techniques for emergency and critical care procedures, In Bonagura JD, ed: Kirk's current veterinary therapy XIII, Philadelphia, 2000, Saunders.

Day TK: Intravenous anesthetic techniques for emergency and critical care procedures: an update, In Bonagura JD, ed: Kirk's current veterinary therapy XIII, Philadelphia, 2008, Saunders.

Harvey RC, Ettinger SJ: Anesthesia and analgesia of patients with specific disease: cardiovascular disease, In Tranquilli WJ, Thurmon JC, Grimm KA, eds: Lumb and Jones' veterinary anesthesia, ed 4, Ames, Iowa, 2007, Blackwell.

Hellyer PW: Anesthesia in patients with cardiovascular disease, In Kirk RW, Bonagura JD, eds: Current veterinary therapy XI, Philadelphia, 1992, Saunders.

Lamont LA, Mathews KA: Opioid, nonsteroidal and analgesic adjuncts, In Tranquilli WJ, Thurmon JC, Grimm KA, eds: Lumb and Jones' veterinary anesthesia, ed 4, Ames, Iowa, 2007, Blackwell.

Martinez EA, Keegan RD: Muscle relaxants and neuromuscular blockade, In Tranquilli WJ, Thurmon JC, Grimm KA, eds: Lumb and Jones' veterinary anesthesia, ed 4, Ames, Iowa, 2007, Blackwell.

Mason DE, Hubbell JAE: Anesthesia and the heart, In Fox PR, Sisson D, Moise NS, eds: Textbook of canine and feline cardiology, Philadelphia, 1999, Saunders.

Muir WW, Hubbell JAE, Skarda RT, Bednarski RM, eds: Drugs used for preanesthetic medication, ed 4, Handbook of veterinary anesthesia, St. Louis, 2007, Mosby.

Robertson SA: Pain Management in the cat, In Gaynor JS, Muir WW, eds: Handbook of veterinary pain management, ed 2, St. Louis, 2009, Elsevier.

Skarda RT, Tranquilli WJ: Selected anesthetic and analgesic techniques: local and regional anesthetic techniques: dogs and cats, In Tranquilli WJ, Thurmon JC, Grimm KA, eds: Lumb and Jones' veterinary anesthesia, ed 4, Ames, Iowa, 2007, Blackwell.

21

Cardiac Surgery

E. Christopher Orton

Cardiac surgery is an option for management of a variety of congenital and acquired cardiac conditions in animals. Some cardiac surgeries are performed with curative intent, whereas others are considered palliative only. It is important that all parties (surgical team, primary care veterinarian, and animal owner) have a clear understanding of the expectations and risks of cardiac surgery. Increasingly, image-guided interventions are available to treat cardiac conditions in animals. Often these interventions offer an alternative to classic cardiac surgery and should be part of the discussion when formulating a treatment plan. Hybrid procedures that combine image-guided catheter techniques with transcardiac minimally invasive surgical approaches are emerging as an additional option, particularly for smaller animals. Factors to consider when weighing treatment options include relative invasiveness, operating time, experience of the operator, availability of specialized equipment, size of the patient, outcome and risk, and cost. Rigid adherence to one type of treatment intervention is generally not in the best interest of the patient or client. Cardiac surgeries include closed cardiac surgeries performed on the beating heart, brief circulatory arrest cardiac surgeries performed during inflow occlusion, and open cardiac surgeries performed during cardiopulmonary bypass.

CLOSED CARDIAC SURGERY

PATENT DUCTUS ARTERIOSUS LIGATION

With few exceptions, closure of patent ductus arteriosus (PDA) is indicated in all small animals with this defect. Closure can be accomplished by imaged-guided transcatheter occlusion methods or surgical ligation. Although each has theoretical advantages, both approaches are successful in the hands of an experienced operator, and neither approach should be regarded as always superior or preferred over the other. Choosing an approach depends on several factors, including client preference, availability of equipment and expertise, and urgency of the procedure. PDA

closure is curative when performed early in life before the onset of severe ventricular remodeling, systolic dysfunction, or functional mitral regurgitation MR. Surgical ligation of PDA can be accomplished with minimal operative mortality when performed by experienced surgeons.

PDA ligation is undertaken through a left fourth thoracotomy in the dog and a left fifth thoracotomy in a cat (Figure 21.1). The most frequent surgical complication is hemorrhage during dissection and isolation of the ductus. If significant hemorrhage occurs during dissection, the ductus should be closed with pledget-buttressed mattress sutures with or without division of the ductus.

PULMONIC VALVE DILATION

Pulmonic stenosis (PS) is a relatively common congenital heart defect in dogs. The natural history of PS in dogs is not well documented. Dogs with moderate PS may tolerate the defect relatively well for many years. Transvalvular pressure gradients greater than 100 mm Hg are considered an indication for intervention, especially if animals are exhibiting activity intolerance, syncope, or have concurrent tricuspid regurgitation (TR). Gradient reduction by valve dilation is considered to be palliative for dogs with moderate to severe PS.

Catheter balloon valvuloplasty is generally preferred to surgical valve dilation of PS because it is less invasive. Surgical valve dilation of PS is indicated for animals that fail balloon-catheter placement across the PS, or when equipment for cardiac catheterization is not available. Surgical valve dilation of PS is performed through a left fourth thoracotomy (Figure 21.2). A dilating instrument or balloon catheter is passed through a controlling purse-string suture in the right ventricle and across the pulmonic valve to dilate the stenosis.

PULMONARY ARTERY BANDING

Pulmonary artery banding is a palliative surgery for ventricular septal defect (VSD) that consists of placement of a constricting band around

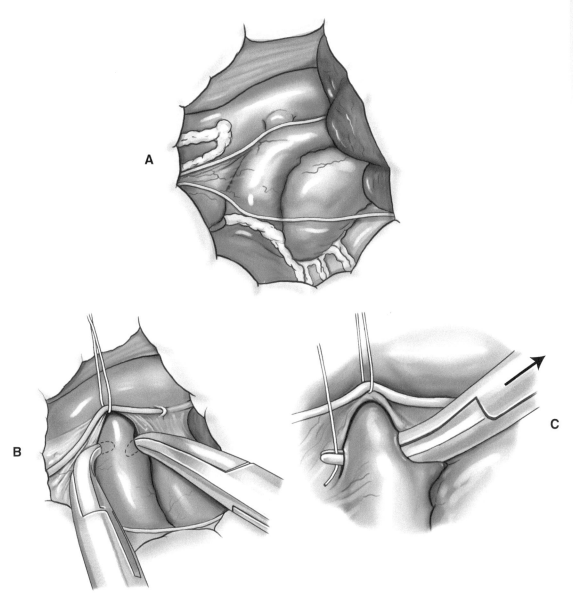

Figure 21.1   Patent ductus arteriosus (PDA) ligation. **A,** The vagus nerve courses over the ductus arteriosus and serves as an anatomic landmark for identification of the ductus arteriosus. **B,** The vagus nerve is isolated at the level of the ductus and gently retracted with one or two sutures. Occasionally, a persistent left cranial vena cava may overlie the ductus arteriosus. In this case, the vein should be carefully isolated and retracted with the vagus nerve. The ductus arteriosus is isolated by blunt dissection without opening the pericardium. Dissection of the caudal aspect of the ductus is accomplished by passing right-angled forceps behind the ductus parallel to the transverse plane. Dissection of the cranial aspect of the ductus is accomplished by angling the forceps caudally at approximately a 45-degree angle. **C,** Dissection is completed by passing the forceps medial to the ductus from a caudal to cranial direction. Two heavy silk ligatures are passed around the ductus by grasping the ligature with right-angled forceps. The ductus arteriosus is closed by slowly tightening and tying the ligature. (Redrawn from Orton, EC: Small animal thoracic surgery, Baltimore, 1995, Williams & Wilkins.)

the pulmonary artery. The intent is to increase right ventricular systolic pressure and thereby decrease the driving pressure gradient for shunt flow across the defect. The procedure provides protection against development of heart failure or progressive pulmonary hypertension that can reverse shunt flow across the defect. Pulmonary artery banding is a viable option for both cats and dogs with hemodynamically significant VSD. Diagnostic parameters that suggest the anomaly is a hemodynamically significant VSD include radiographic evidence of pulmonary over circulation, echocardiographic evidence of left ventricular dilation (increased left ventricular

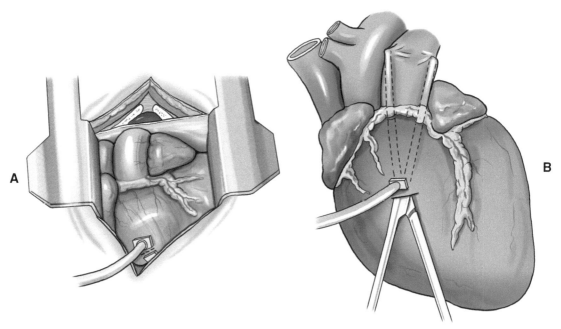

Figure 21.2 Pulmonary valve dilation. The pericardium over the right outflow tract is opened and sutured to the thoracotomy incision. **A,** A buttressed mattress suture is placed in the right ventricular outflow tract and passed through a tourniquet. A stab incision is made in the ventricle within the confines of the mattress suture. **B,** A dilating instrument is passed into the right ventricular outflow tract and across the pulmonic valve. The pulmonic valve is dilated several times. The ventricular incision is closed by tying the mattress suture. (Redrawn from Orton, EC: Small animal thoracic surgery, Baltimore, 1995, Williams & Wilkins.)

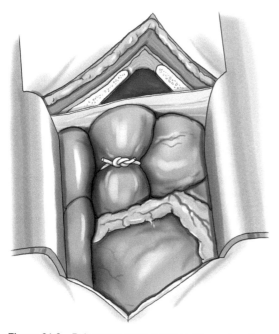

Figure 21.3 Pulmonary artery banding. The pericardium is opened and sutured to the thoracotomy incision. The pulmonary artery is separated from the aorta by sharp and blunt dissection. A large cotton or Teflon tape is passed around the pulmonary artery just distal to the pulmonic valve. The tape is tightened to reduce circumference of the pulmonary artery. (Redrawn from Orton, EC: Small animal thoracic surgery, Baltimore, 1995, Williams & Wilkins.)

diastolic diameter, left ventricular diastolic volume index [LVDVI] >150 ml/m^2), Doppler-measured shunt flow velocity <3.5 m/sec, or pulmonic flow velocity >2.5 m/sec. Evidence of progressive pulmonary hypertension is also a reason to consider surgery. Long-term palliation of VSD for several years is possible with this procedure. Complications of pulmonary artery banding include over-tightening of the band or late-term progressive constriction of the band leading to reversal of shunt flow. Worsening of concurrent TR is also a possible adverse outcome.

Pulmonary artery banding is performed through a left fourth thoracotomy (Figure 21.3). The appropriate degree of pulmonic constriction is based on pulmonary artery pressure distal to the band and systemic arterial pressures. Pulmonary artery pressure is measured during surgery by a catheter introduced into the distal pulmonary artery through a small purse-string suture in the pulmonary artery. Optimal banding is where pulmonary artery pressure distal to the band is decreased to less than 30 mm Hg (assuming significant pulmonary vascular remodeling is not present), and when the increase in systemic arterial pressure just begins to plateau. As a general rule, optimal banding requires a two-thirds reduction in the diameter of the pulmonary artery, although this

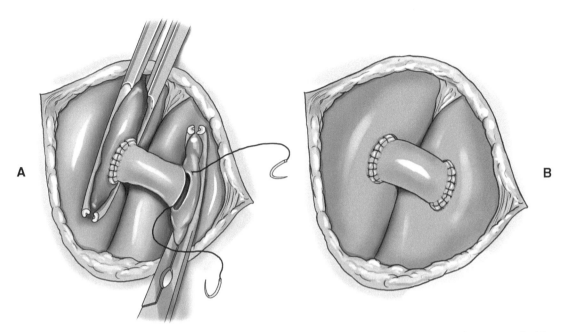

Figure 21.4 Systemic-to-pulmonary artery shunt. The pericardium is opened and sutured to the thoracotomy incision. **A,** Tangential vascular clamps are placed on the pulmonary artery and ascending aorta, and incisions are made in each vessel. The autogenous or synthetic graft is interposed between the aorta and pulmonary artery by two end-to-side anastomoses using simple continuous suture patterns with polypropylene or polytetrafluoroethylene (PTFE) suture. **B,** The vascular clamps on the pulmonary artery and aorta are released. (Redrawn from Orton, EC: Small animal thoracic surgery, Baltimore, 1995, Williams & Wilkins.)

will vary depending on the degree of pulmonary artery dilation.

SYSTEMIC-TO-PULMONARY ARTERY SHUNT

Creation of a systemic-to-pulmonary artery shunt is a palliative treatment option for tetralogy of Fallot. The functional goal of a systemic-to-pulmonary artery shunt is to increase pulmonary blood flow without creating an overwhelming left-to-right shunt. The desired result is an increase in pulmonary blood flow that lessens hypoxemia by decreasing the shunt-to-pulmonary flow ratio. Systemic-to-pulmonary shunt is indicated for animals with resting cyanosis, debilitating activity intolerance or persistent polycythemia (PCV >70%) that requires frequent phlebotomy. Most veterinary experience is based on various modifications of the classic Blalock-Taussig shunt. The original Blalock-Taussig shunt consisted of dividing the left subclavian artery and performing an end-to-side anastomosis of the distal end of the divided artery to a pulmonary artery. In animals, the left subclavian artery generally does not have sufficient length to reach the pulmonary artery without kinking. Several modifications of the classic procedure have been devised, including placement of a synthetic vascular graft matched in size to the subclavian artery, harvesting the left subclavian artery as a free autogenous graft, or using the autogenous jugular vein. Animals can receive significant palliation from any of the above methods as long as pulmonary blood flow is increased to an appropriate degree.

A modified Blalock-Taussig shunt is performed through a left fourth thoracotomy (Figure 21.4). End-to-side anastomoses are performed between the graft and the pulmonary artery and ascending aorta with the aid of side-biting vascular clamps. Hypoxemia should be lessened immediately after surgery.

PERICARDIECTOMY

Pericardial disease can result from neoplasia, bacterial or mycotic infection, foreign body, or idiopathic causes. Pericardial disease can take the form of acute or chronic pericardial effusion, constrictive pericarditis, or constrictive-effusive pericarditis. These conditions can result in pathophysiologic syndromes of acute cardiac tamponade, chronic cardiac tamponade, or pericardial constriction. Pericardiectomy is indicated for the management of chronic pericardial effusions, particularly when the effusion recurs after pericardiocentesis. Pericardiectomy is either palliative or curative depending on the underlying cause of pericardial effusion. Pericardiectomy is the only viable treatment for animals with constrictive or constrictive-effusive pericarditis.

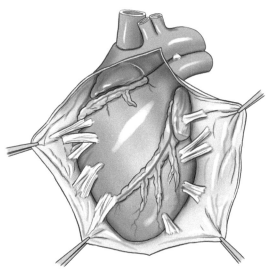

Figure 21.5 Pericardiectomy. Pericardiectomy may be performed by median sternotomy to provide access to both ventricles without extensive cardiac manipulation. In animals with constrictive pericarditis, adhesions may be present between the pericardium and epicardium.

Pericardiectomy can be performed by either a right or left thoracotomy or a median sternotomy. Median sternotomy offers the advantages of providing access to both ventricles and requiring less cardiac manipulation and thus is preferred by many surgeons (Figure 21.5). Excision of the pericardium ventral to the phrenic nerves (i.e. subphrenic pericardiectomy) is adequate in most cases. In animals with constrictive pericarditis, the pericardium may have to be separated from the epicardium by blunt and sharp dissection. In addition, epicardial decortication may be necessary to relieve constrictive physiology in animals with pericarditis. Epicardial decortication entails careful separation of the abnormal epicardial fibrous layer from the underlying myocardium by sharp dissection. Decortication should not be attempted over the atria or portions of the ventricles containing major coronary vessels.

ATRIAL APPENDECTOMY

Atrial appendectomy is occasionally indicated for palliative removal of a right atrial hemangiosarcoma, or for thrombosis of the right or left atrial appendage associated with atrial fibrillation. In the case of hemangiosarcoma, atrial appendectomy is often combined with pericardiectomy and is performed by a median sternotomy. Atrial appendectomy for atrial thrombosis is performed by a fifth thoracotomy on the right or left side (Figure 21.6). The atrial appendage is occluded with a vascular clamp, excised, and oversewn with a continuous mattress suture pattern.

CARDIAC SURGERY WITH INFLOW OCCLUSION

Inflow occlusion is a strategy for performing open cardiac surgery that consists of a brief interruption of venous inflow to the heart and complete circulatory arrest. It is indicated for cardiac surgeries that require only a limited period when the heart is open. Its principal advantages are its simplicity, lack of need for specialized equipment, and minimal cardiopulmonary, metabolic, and hematological derangements after surgery. The principal disadvantages of inflow occlusion are the limited time available to perform cardiac surgery (2 to 4 minutes), motion of the surgical field, and the lack of a fallback or rescue strategy should something delay completion of surgery. As a result, cardiac surgery performed during inflow occlusion must be meticulously planned and executed.

Circulatory arrest in a normothermic patient should be 2 minutes or less to minimize the risk of cerebral injury and ventricular fibrillation. Circulatory arrest time can be extended up to 4 minutes with mild whole body hypothermia (32° C to 34° C); however, the risk for ventricular fibrillation increases with the duration of circulatory arrest. Mild hypothermia is achieved readily in small animals through avoidance of measures that keep the animal warm, or surface cooling, with ice packs, may be necessary depending on the size of the animal. Inflow occlusion requires careful and balanced anesthetic techniques that minimize inhalation anesthetic agents. Animals should be well ventilated, and acid-base balance should be optimized before inflow occlusion. Ventilation is discontinued during inflow occlusion to prevent flooding of the field when the heart is open, and then immediately resumed when the heart is closed. De-airing of the heart is critically important just before closing the heart to prevent fatal air embolism. This process is accomplished with simultaneous positive pressure ventilation (Valsalva maneuver) and release of a venous tourniquet just as the cardiotomy site is closed with a vascular clamp. Drugs and equipment for full cardiac resuscitation must be immediately available after inflow occlusion. Gentle cardiac massage may be necessary after inflow occlusion to reestablish cardiac function. Digital occlusion of the descending aorta during this period helps direct cardiac output to the heart and brain.

Inflow occlusion can be accomplished from a left or right fifth thoracotomy or a median sternotomy depending on the cardiac surgery being performed. Direct access to the cranial and caudal vena cava and azygous vein for inflow occlusion

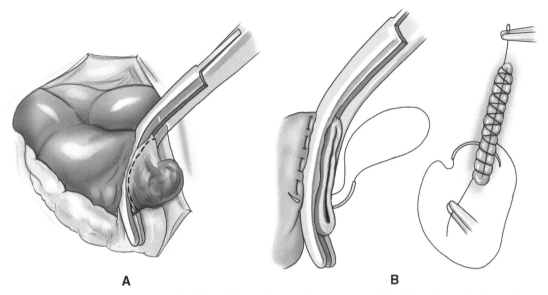

Figure 21.6 Atrial appendectomy. **A,** Excision of the atrial appendage is accomplished by placement of a continuous mattress suture pattern across the base of the atrial appendage with the aid of a vascular clamp. **B,** The atrial appendage is excised, and the atriotomy incision is oversewn with a continuous suture pattern. (Redrawn from Orton, EC: Small animal thoracic surgery, Baltimore, 1995, Williams & Wilkins.)

is obtained readily from a right thoracotomy or median sternotomy. The vena cavae and azygous vein are accessed by dissecting through the mediastinum from a left thoracotomy. Tape tourniquets are passed around the vena cavae and azygous vein for inflow occlusion. The right phrenic nerve should be excluded from the tourniquets to avoid nerve injury.

PULMONARY PATCH GRAFT

Pulmonary patch graft can be considered for dogs with severe PS who are exhibiting activity intolerance or are considered at risk for having heart failure or sudden cardiac death. Because of the inherent risk associated with this surgery, the threshold for performing this surgery should be fairly high. Pulmonic patch graft generally is undertaken in dogs who have failed to be adequately palliated by less invasive balloon-dilation valvuloplasty. Dogs with severe PS characterized by valve dysplasia or dynamic outflow obstruction, or both, are more likely to need a patch graft. Several surgical techniques for applying a patch graft to the right ventricular outflow tract during brief inflow occlusion have been described. A well-executed patch graft generally results in more effective and more sustained pressure gradient reduction compared to valve dilation techniques. Occasionally, dogs will have right-sided congestive heart failure as a late sequela to pulmonary patch graft despite good pressure gradient reduction. The cause of this late failure is not entirely clear and may be multifactorial. Contributing causes could include

TR, right ventricular systolic dysfunction, and pulmonic insufficiency. Pulmonic insufficiency is an expected consequence of the patch graft procedure and may not be as well tolerated as previously thought. English Bulldogs and Boxers with PS must be evaluated for the presence of an anomalous left coronary artery. If present, this anomaly precludes pulmonic patch graft. Patch graft correction of the PS by inflow occlusion is performed through a left fifth thoracotomy (Figure 21.7). A partial thickness incision is made in the right ventricle and a patch is presutured to the ventricular incision and pulmonary artery. A transvalvular full-thickness incision is completed during venous inflow occlusion.

COR TRIATRIATUM REPAIR

Cor triatriatum is an uncommon congenital defect in companion animals that results from persistence of an embryonic membrane that divides the atrium into two chambers. The separation can occur in either the right atrium (cor triatriatum dexter) or left atrium (cor triatriatum sinister).

Surgical correction of cor triatriatum dexter is by membranectomy through a right atriotomy during brief inflow occlusion. The surgery is performed by a right fifth thoracotomy. Tapes are placed around the cranial and caudal vena cavae and azygous vein for inflow occlusion. The pericardium is opened ventral to the phrenic nerve. The location of the membrane is often apparent by an indentation in the atrial wall. Stay sutures are placed in the lateral atrial wall to control the atriotomy incision during inflow occlusion. The atrium is opened transversely

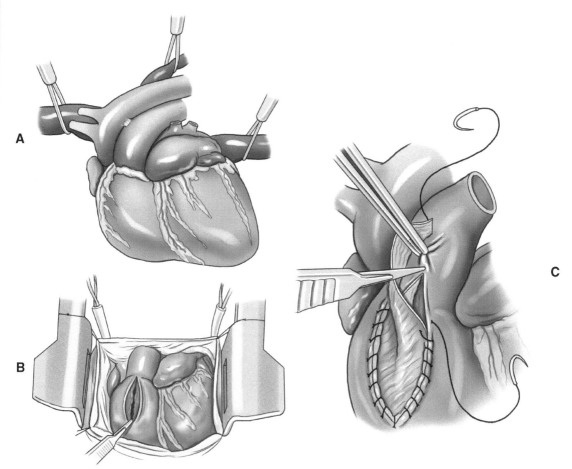

Figure 21.7 Pulmonary patch graft. **A,** Tape tourniquets are passed around the vena cavae and azygous vein for inflow occlusion. Access to the azygous vein is obtained by dissection dorsal to the descending aorta. **B,** A partial thickness incision is made in the right ventricular outflow tract. **C,** An oval-shaped expanded polytetrafluoroethylene (ePTFE) patch graft is sutured to the ventriculotomy incision and the cranial aspect of the pulmonary artery. After initiation of venous inflow occlusion, an incision is made in the pulmonary artery beneath the patch and extended full thickness across the pulmonic valve annulus and previously made partial-thickness incision in the right ventricle. The unsutured portion of the patch graft is closed with a tangential vascular clamp to minimize circulatory arrest time. Inflow occlusion is discontinued, and the heart is resuscitated as necessary. The unsutured portion of the patch graft is then closed, and the vascular clamp removed. (Redrawn from Orton, EC: Small animal thoracic surgery, Baltimore, 1995, Williams & Wilkins.)

across the defect during inflow occlusion. The abnormal membrane is excised. A tangential vascular clamp is used to close the atriotomy as inflow occlusion is discontinued. Venous blood should flow from the atriotomy as the clamp is placed to remove air from the heart. The atriotomy is closed with a continuous horizontal mattress pattern oversewn with a simple continuous pattern.

Successful surgical correction of cor triatriatum sinister with resolution of pulmonary edema by closed dilation of the atrial septum is reported in a cat.

INTRACARDIAC MASSES AND FOREIGN BODIES

Intracardiac masses can include benign and malignant neoplasias, atrial or ventricular thrombi, and penetrating foreign bodies. These intracardiac masses and foreign bodies can, under certain circumstances, be removed from the heart with the aid of inflow occlusion. Most cardiac neoplasms in dogs are malignant, and attempts at surgical excision of these tumors are rarely rewarding. Myxomas are an exception to this general rule. These benign pediculated cardiac tumors can become large enough to obstruct cardiac flow and are amendable to excision during inflow occlusion. Intracardiac thrombi can be considered for surgical removal when they are not associated with severe underlying cardiomyopathy. Penetrating foreign bodies such as pellets or bullets can be removed if they lodge within a cardiac chamber. Frequently, these foreign bodies are surrounded by large amounts of hair that cause complications if not removed. Whenever possible, intracardiac masses should be removed by an atriotomy rather than a ventriculotomy. Tumors in the right ventricular outflow tract can be removed by a right ventriculotomy.

CARDIAC SURGERY WITH CARDIOPULMONARY BYPASS

Cardiopulmonary bypass (CPB) is a procedure that provides flow of oxygenated blood to the patient by diverting flow away from the heart and lungs through an extracorporeal circuit. Cardiopulmonary bypass provides a motionless and bloodless operative field, and time to perform complex cardiac repairs. The disadvantages of CPB are its cost and considerable associated cardiopulmonary, metabolic, hematologic, and systemic inflammatory derangements.

CPB in dogs is described in more detail elsewhere. CPB is performed by a team consisting of the surgeon, perfusionist, anesthesiologist, and their assistants. A principal role of the surgical team is to perform a series of cannulations to connect the animal to the CPB circuit. Before cannulation, the patient is completely anticoagulated with sodium heparin (300 units/kg intravenously [IV]). Arterial cannulation for the return of oxygenated blood to the patient is accomplished by a single cannula placed in a femoral artery. Blood is diverted from the right heart to the CBP circuit by means of venous cannulae. Venous cannulation is accomplished by one of two strategies depending on the cardiac approach. Bicaval venous cannulation uses two angled cannulae, one in each vena cava, and is required whenever the cardiac approach is through the right atrium. Atriocaval cannulation uses a single two-stage cannula introduced into the right atrium and caudal vena cava by way of the right atrial appendage. Lastly, a cannula is placed in the ascending aorta for administration of cardioplegia solution and to vent the left heart during discontinuation of CBP. During the open cardiac repair, the aorta is cross-clamped and cardioplegia solution is administered to arrest and cool the myocardium.

VENTRICULAR SEPTAL DEFECT REPAIR

Definitive repair of a large hemodynamically significant VSD in dogs can be undertaken with the aid of CPB. Definitive VSD repair, like PDA closure, is curative as long as it is undertaken before severe myocardial dysfunction or pulmonary hypertension develops.

Open repair of a perimembranous VSD is accomplished through a right fifth thoracotomy. Venous cannulation is bicaval to allow complete isolation of the right atrium. The defect is approached through a right atriotomy. The septal leaflet of the tricuspid valve is retracted to expose the defect. The defect is closed with a Dacron or polytetrafluoroethylene (PTFE) patch secured with pledget-buttressed mattress sutures. Mattress sutures should be placed with partial thickness bites from the right side to avoid injury to atrioventricular conduction.

ATRIAL AND ATRIOVENTRICULAR SEPTAL DEFECT REPAIR

Various forms of atrial septal defect (ASD) and atrioventricular septal defect (AVSD) have been described in small animals. As with VSD, surgical closure of ASD can be undertaken with the aid of CPB with curative intent. Indications for surgery include cardiomegaly, the size of the defect on echocardiography, pulmonary overcirculation on radiographs, hepatic venous congestion on ultrasound, and a Doppler-measured transatrial septal flow velocity greater than 0.45 m/sec. Surgical correction of ASD under CBP is similar to VSD and has been described.

TETRALOGY OF FALLOT REPAIR

Definitive repair of tetralogy of Fallot under CPB can be undertaken in dogs with curative intent. Indications for surgery are the same as described previously for systemic-to-pulmonary artery shunt. The repair is accomplished by a median sternotomy and involves closure of the VSD and correction of PS by way of a right ventriculotomy.

DOUBLE-CHAMBERED RIGHT VENTRICLE REPAIR

Double-chambered right ventricle (DCRV) is an uncommon congenital heart defect of dogs characterized by a fibromuscular diaphragm at the junction of the inflow and outflow portions of the right ventricle. The defect obstructs flow through the mid-portion of the ventricle and causes hypertrophy of the proximal portion of the right ventricle, giving it a "double-chambered" appearance. The pathophysiologic features and natural history of DCRV are presumed to be similar to PS. Indications for surgery are essentially the same as for PS, although dogs with DCRV may tolerate less of a pressure gradient compared to dogs with PS.

Surgical correction for DCRV is undertaken with the aid of cardiopulmonary bypass and has been described. The pulmonic valve is preserved. Surgical correction can be expected to improve exercise capacity and reduce the risk of developing heart failure.

MITRAL VALVE REPLACEMENT

MR is the most common cause of cardiac disability and death in dogs. Causes of MR include degenerative mitral valve disease, congenital mitral valve dysplasia, and functional MR secondary to dilated cardiomyopathy. Mitral valve replacement can be performed in dogs to correct severe MR secondary to acquired mitral valve disease or congenital mitral dysplasia. Indications for considering mitral valve replacement are diuretic-dependent congestive heart failure, or severe left ventricular or atrial dilation (LVDVI >180 ml/m^2), or both. Relative contraindications for mitral valve surgery are very severe left ventricular dilation (LVDVI >300 ml/m^2) or severe secondary systolic dysfunction (LVSVI >90 ml/m^2). Atrial fibrillation is not a contraindication for surgery, but it does complicate the management after surgery. Serious systemic or noncardiac diseases are strong contraindications for the surgery.

Mitral valve replacement is one surgical option for most dogs with severe MR and heart failure. The advantages of mitral valve replacement are perfect correction of MR and a less technically demanding surgery. Disadvantages of mitral valve replacement are the need for a prosthesis (expense, limitations on patient size) and for anticoagulation therapy after surgery. Options for mitral valve replacement are mechanical valves or glutaraldehyde-fixed tissue valves. Glutaraldehyde-fixed tissue valves include porcine aortic valves and bovine pericardial valves. Mechanical valves have infinite durability but require lifelong anticoagulation therapy to prevent valve thrombosis. Despite low operative mortality and excellent short-term results, valve replacement with a mechanical prostheses is not recommended in dogs because of a high incidence of late-term thrombosis despite anticoagulation therapy. Tissue valves have a finite lifespan (about 7 to 15 years in human patients) but are less susceptible to thrombosis; and thrombosis is less catastrophic when it occurs. Other mechanisms of tissue valve prosthetic failure are structural tearing of leaflets, leaflet calcification, or an exuberant inflammatory response known as pannus. Anticoagulation therapy with warfarin is required for 3 months after valve replacement with a tissue valve. The long-term durability of glutaraldehyde-fixed tissue valves in dogs has not been established; the short-term results have been encouraging. The procedure is limited to dogs with a lean body weight of about 10 kg, and by the size of the smallest available valve prosthesis (19 mm). Mitral valve replacement is considered a palliative therapy because the consequences of a diseased native valve are replaced with the inherent management and potential complications of having a valve prosthesis. Successful mitral valve replacement generally reverses congestive heart failure as long as secondary changes in the myocardium are not too advanced at the time of surgery. Mitral valve replacement can be expected to remain curative for heart failure as long as the prosthesis remains functional. The surgical procedure for mitral valve replacement under cardiopulmonary bypass in the dog has been described.

MITRAL VALVE REPAIR

Mitral valve repair can be undertaken for dogs with moderate-to-severe MR caused by acquired degenerative mitral valve disease. Dogs with congenital mitral valve dysplasia are generally not amendable to valve repair. The principle advantages of mitral valve repair are the avoidance of anticoagulation after surgery and the lack of a need for an expensive prosthesis. The disadvantage of mitral valve repair is a less predictable outcome compared to valve replacement. Mitral valve repair is best undertaken in dogs that have structural defects isolated to one valve leaflet before or soon after the onset of congestive heart failure. Mitral valve repair employs a variety of surgical techniques to address the fundamental causes of MR. Surgical techniques and outcomes for mitral valve repair in the dog have been described.

TRICUSPID VALVE REPLACEMENT

Congenital tricuspid dysplasia is a malformation of the tricuspid valve that occurs in several large breeds of dog including Labrador Retrievers, Golden Retrievers, and German Shepherds. TR is the most common hemodynamic manifestation, although tricuspid stenosis is possible. Tricuspid valve replacement can be considered for dogs with severe TR because of congenital tricuspid dysplasia. Tricuspid valve replacement must be undertaken sooner during the course of disease than mitral valve replacement. General indications for tricuspid valve replacement are severe TR resulting in severe or progressive cardiomegaly, or hepatic venous enlargement, or both. Dogs with medically refractory congestive heart failure should not undergo tricuspid valve replacement. Atrial fibrillation is a complicating factor but not an absolute contraindication for surgery. As with mitral valve replacement, glutaraldehyde-fixed tissue valves are currently recommended over mechanical valves. Three months of anticoagulation therapy is required after tricuspid valve replacement with a tissue valve. Dramatic reductions in heart size and resolution of heart failure can be expected so long as the valve prosthesis remains functional. Tricuspid valve replacement is performed through a right fifth thoracotomy. Bicaval venous cannulation is used to isolate the right atrium. The approach to the tricuspid valve is through the right atrium. The surgical technique and outcome for tricuspid valve replacement for tricuspid dysplasia has been described.

HYBRID CARDIAC SURGERY

Hybrid cardiac procedures are emerging as an appealing alternative to classic cardiac surgery in humans and animals. Hybrid cardiac procedures combine image-guided catheter-based interventions with direct transcardiac (transatrial, transventricular, transapical) surgical approaches to the heart. Surgical access to the heart can often be achieved through minimally invasive thoracic approaches. Hybrid procedures are performed in an operating room equipped with imaging modalities that include C-arm fluoroscopy and transesophageal echocardiography (TEE) or intracardiac echocardiography (ICE). Hybrid procedures have the advantage over classic open cardiac surgery of being performed on the beating heart with much shorter operating times and without the need for CPB or circulatory arrest. An advantage of hybrid procedures over percutaneous transvascular interventions is more direct access to the heart. The latter can particularly be an advantage in small patients where vascular access might be difficult, or with more complex devices where the delivery system is large (e.g. transcatheter valve replacement). Hybrid cardiac procedures combine the skillsets of a surgeon and interventional cardiologist, making the formation of a hybrid cardiac team desirable to achieve optimal results.

Hybrid cardiac procedures have been reported in animals, including correction of cor triatriatum sinister and closure of an ASD and a VSD. Hybrid procedures for transcatheter mitral valve replacement and repair are in early clinical trials in dogs.

SUGGESTED READINGS

Arai S, Griffiths LG, Mama K, Hackett TB, et al: Bioprosthesis valve replacement in dogs with congenital tricuspid valve dysplasia: technique and outcome, J Vet Cardiol 13:91, 2011.

Bureau S, Monnet E, Orton EC: Evaluation of survival rate and prognostic indicators for surgical treatment of left-to-right patent ductus arteriosus in dogs: 52 cases (1995-2003), J Am Vet Med Assoc 227:1794, 2005.

Gordon SG, Nelson DA, Achen SE, Miller MW, et al: Open heart closure of an atrial septal defect by use of an atrial septal occluder in a dog, J Am Vet Med Assoc 236:434, 2010.

Griffiths LG, Boon J, Orton EC: Evaluation of techniques and outcomes of mitral valve repair in dogs, J Am Vet Med Assoc 224:1941, 2004.

Martin J, Orton EC, Boon J, Mama K, et al: Surgical correction of double-chambered right ventricle in dogs, J Am Vet Med Assoc 220:770, 2002.

Monnet E, Orton EC, Gaynor J, Boon J, et al: Partial atrioventricular septal defect: diagnosis and surgical repair in two dogs, J Am Vet Med Assoc 211:569–572, 1997.

Orton EC: Cardiac surgery, In Tobias KM, Johnston SA, eds: Veterinary surgery: small animal, St Louis, 2012, Elsevier Saunders, pp 1820–1825.

Orton EC, Hackett TA, Mama K, Boon JA: Technique and outcome of mitral valve replacement in dogs, J Am Vet Med Assoc 226:1508, 2005.

Orton EC, Mama K, Hellyer P, Hackett TB: Open surgical repair of tetralogy of Fallot in two dogs, J Am Vet Med Assoc 219:1089, 2001.

Saunders AB, Carlson JA, Nelson DA, Gordon SG, et al: Hybrid technique for ventricular septal defect closure in a dog using an Amplatzer Duct Occluder II, J Vet Cardiol 15:217, 2013.

Stern JA, Tou SP, Barker PCA, Hill KD, et al: Hybrid cutting balloon dilatation for treatment of cor triatriatum sinister in a cat, J Vet Cardiol 15:205, 2013.

Uechi M, Mizukoshi T, Mizuno T, et al: Mitral valve repair under cardiopulmonary bypass in small-breed dogs: 48 cases (2006-2009), J Am Vet Med Assoc 240:1994, 2012.

Wander KW, Monnet E, Orton EC: Surgical correction of cor triatriatum sinister in a kitten, J Am Anim Hosp Assoc 34:383, 1998.

22 Pacemaker Therapy

Janice McIntosh Bright

"It struck me how easily excitable the myocardium is. You just touch it and it gives you a run of extra beats—so why should the heart that is so sensitive . . . die because there's nothing there to stimulate the chest?"

PAUL M. ZOLL, INVENTOR OF THE FIRST CLINICALLY SUCCESSFUL
EXTERNAL PACEMAKER. JEFFREY K: CARDIAC PACING AND ELECTROPHYSIOLOGY
AT MILLENNIUM'S END: HISTORICAL NOTES AND OBSERVATIONS. PACE 22;1713, 1999.

Pacemaker therapy has become a common method of treating symptomatic bradycardia in dogs and cats. Pharmacologic therapy may provide temporary chronotropic support for patients with bradycardia, but successful long-term management usually requires implantation of a permanent pacemaker. The ultimate objective of cardiac pacing is to normalize cardiac function by providing optimal heart rate and rhythm chronically.

INDICATIONS FOR PACING

- Permanent pacemaker implantation is indicated for treatment of patients with chronic symptomatic bradyarrhythmias. In dogs the most frequent clinical manifestations of bradycardia are syncope, collapse, exercise intolerance, or lethargy. Less commonly, bradyarrhythmia results in congestive heart failure or seizures. In cats the most frequent complaint associated with bradycardia is syncope.
- The most common bradyarrhythmia necessitating pacemaker therapy in dogs and cats is advanced (high-grade second- or third-degree) atrioventricular (AV) block. Antibradycardia pacing is also indicated in dogs with sinus node dysfunction (sick sinus syndrome) and permanent atrial standstill. Less often permanent pacing is used to prevent vasovagal syncope.
- Most dogs needing pacemaker therapy have little to no underlying structural heart disease; however, older dogs may have some degree of degenerative mitral valve disease. In cats AV conduction block is frequently associated with underlying myocardial disease.

PREIMPLANTATION EVALUATION

- A standard electrocardiogram (ECG) should be obtained for definitive diagnosis of the arrhythmia. If it is unclear whether a patient's clinical signs are due to bradyarrhythmia, correlation of the clinical signs with the arrhythmia should be obtained with some form of ambulatory electrocardiographic monitoring (Holter monitoring or event recording). Ambulatory ECG monitoring allows the ECG to be recorded over a longer period of time, either continuously for 24 to 48 hours (Holter monitoring) or intermittently during weeks to months (event recording). Ambulatory ECG may also be needed to confirm intermittent bradycardia.
- After confirmation that an indication for permanent cardiac pacing exists, the most appropriate pacing system and pacing mode for the patient should be determined. Factors to be considered for this determination include specific underlying rhythm disturbance, overall physical condition, presence of associated medical problems including structural heart disease, and exercise requirements of the patient.
- Therefore all patients needing implantation of a permanent pacemaker should receive a thorough medical and cardiovascular evaluation before implantation to identify presence and severity of structural heart diseases or noncardiac diseases. Certain coexisting conditions may require additional medical treatment. Furthermore, these conditions often affect the type and programming of the pacing system used.

COMPONENTS AND TYPES OF PACING SYSTEMS

- A permanent artificial cardiac pacing system consists of a pulse generator (pacemaker) and one or more pacing leads. The pulse generator contains electronic circuitry and a lithium-iodide power cell (battery) sealed within a metal case with a connector block into which the lead(s) is (are) inserted. A pacing lead consists of an insulated wire or set of wires to

382

conduct electrical impulses from the generator to the myocardium, but the lead also enables the generator to detect or sense native (endogenous) cardiac electrical activity.

- Modern cardiac pacemakers have sophisticated electronic circuitry capable of discharging pacing impulses of varying duration and voltage, sensing intracardiac signals, filtering signals, providing rate response functions, and storing rhythm data. Data retrieval and generator programming are done by means of telemetry with a pacemaker programmer. The programmer is also used to display real-time ECG and intracardiac electrograms and to test battery life, lead impedance, retrograde ventriculoatrial conduction, and pacing thresholds.

- The heart can be paced by epicardial lead(s) placed surgically (or thoracoscopically) or by permanent endocardial pacing lead(s) placed transvenously. Permanent transvenous pacing has largely replaced epicardial pacing because of its ease and safety. However, epicardial leads remain available and may be preferred when venous access is limited or when there is an associated condition that would increase likelihood of bacteremia, thrombosis, or embolism with a permanent transvenous lead (e.g., a focus of sepsis or a hypercoagulable state). Epicardial leads are often used in feline patients.

- Permanent transvenous pacing leads use either active or passive fixation for attachment of the lead tip to the endomyocardium. A passive fixation transvenous lead has a "collar" of tines encircling the distal tip, which anchor the lead by becoming enmeshed in the trabeculae of the right ventricle or right atrium (Figure 22.1). An active fixation lead has a small metal helix that exits the tip of the lead to penetrate the endomyocardium (see Figure 22.1). Although the type of fixation of a transvenous lead does not appear to affect the incidence of lead dislodgement, it is wise to avoid use of passive fixation in animals with significant right ventricular (RV) dilation.

- Another consideration for selection of the pacing system is whether a unipolar or bipolar system is desired. A unipolar pacing system uses the lead tip as the cathode (negative pole) of the electrical circuit and the metal case of the pulse generator as the anode (positive pole). The impulse travels from generator to myocardium via the lead and returns to the generator via the soft tissues. A major disadvantage of unipolar pacing is the proximity of the electrical circuit to skeletal muscle, which may result in skeletal muscle twitching. Advantages of unipolar pacing include smaller diameter of the pacing lead, a single attachment site of the lead to the epicardium when epicardial pacing is used,

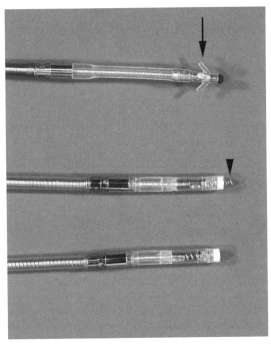

Figure 22.1 The distal ends of several transvenous (endocardial) pacing leads are shown. The lead at the top is a passive fixation lead. Note the collar of tines (*arrow*), which become trapped within trabeculae to anchor the tip of the lead to the right ventricular (RV) endocardium. At the bottom are two active fixation leads, one showing the helix retracted into the lead for placement and the other showing the helix extruded, as it would be for attachment into the endomyocardium (*arrowhead*).

and superior sensing of endogenous cardiac potentials. The increased sensitivity of unipolar sensing may be, however, a double-edged sword in that this sensing modality will also create a greater likelihood of electromagnetic interference (EMI). Bipolar pacing systems have two closely spaced electrodes located distally on a transvenous lead or closely adjacent at two ends of an epicardial lead (Figure 22.2). One electrode (usually the distal electrode on a transvenous bipolar lead) is the cathode, and the other is the anode. Electrical impulses travel to the cathode from the pulse generator and return to the anode to complete the circuit. In the majority of cases, a bipolar pacing system is preferred because there is less potential for EMI with bipolar pacing and because of absence of skeletal muscle stimulation.

- Although lead length should be given consideration before pacemaker implantation, length is often determined by availability. Most leads are longer than necessary, and excess length can be accommodated within the generator pocket. However, in large or giant breed dogs, adequate lead length may become an important factor.

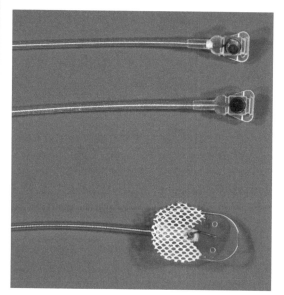

Figure 22.2 The distal tips of two epicardial pacing leads are shown. The lead at the bottom of the photo is a unipolar lead with a single electrode (cathode), which has an epicardial stab-in fixation mechanism. The lead at the top of the photo (both sides of lead are shown) is a bipolar lead with two suture-on electrodes (cathode and anode).

KEY POINT

> When a permanent pacing lead is selected, it is imperative that the lead be compatible with the pacing site selected (epicardial or endocardial, atrial or ventricular), that the lead and generator be of compatible size (typically IS-1), that the lead's polarity matches the generator's polarity, and that the lead is of sufficient length.

PACING WITH CHRONOTROPIC COMPETENCE (RATE RESPONSIVENESS)

- Initially, permanent cardiac pacing systems used in people and in dogs had a single lead that paced the ventricles at a constant rate. Later, rate-responsive pacing generators became available, which allowed the paced rate to vary depending on the activity of the patient.
- Rate response is achieved through use of sensors in the pacemaker, often motion sensors or minute ventilation sensors, which adjust the paced rate between programmed upper and lower limits to match changing metabolic requirements. Thus, rate-responsive pacing better mimics the normal physiologic response of the heart to exercise.

SINGLE-CHAMBER PACING COMPARED WITH DUAL-CHAMBER PACING

- The original goal of permanent cardiac pacing was to alleviate hemodynamic instability resulting from an abnormally low ventricular rate,

and this remains the primary goal of pacemaker therapy in most veterinary patients. However, it is now recognized that cardiac output is dependent, not only on ventricular rate but also on the physiologic heart rate variation, synchrony between atrial and ventricular contraction, and ventricular activation sequence. Modern cardiac pacing has evolved in people from single-chamber to dual-chamber ventricular pacing (atrial and ventricular sensing and pacing) primarily to provide pacing with AV synchrony.

- AV synchrony is attained either by pacing the atrium or by sensing intrinsic atrial activity and tracking this activity. Either a paced atrial depolarization or an endogenous atrial depolarization triggers an AV delay, programmable in length, after which the ventricle is paced (if intrinsic ventricular activity is not sensed). Atrial synchronous pacing provides not only AV synchrony but also physiologic heart rate variation (see the discussion of pacing modes later).
- While AV synchrony may not be clinically important for many dogs and cats needing chronotropic support, pacing that provides AV synchrony will provide higher systemic pressure and lower ventricular filling pressures than single-chamber ventricular pacing. Therefore dual-chamber pacing to provide AV synchrony is likely to be important in animals with significant underlying structural heart disease or in working animals such as military dogs and agility dogs.
- Dual-chamber pacing is becoming increasingly used in veterinary medicine as a means of providing both heart rate response and AV synchrony. Disadvantages of dual-chamber pacing include its more complex programming, increased expense (when two leads are used), increased implantation procedural time, and the technical challenge of placing atrial sensing/pacing leads in small patients.
- Normalization of the left ventricular activation sequence may be achieved by means of site-specific pacing within the right atrium and right ventricle.

SITE SPECIFIC AND BIVENTRICULAR PACING

- The typical site for transvenous ventricular lead placement is at the RV apex because of the ease of placement and the security of passive lead fixation at this site. However, long-term pacing from the RV apex produces asynchronous ventricular contraction, impaired cardiac performance, and deleterious myocardial remodeling. Therefore pacing at alternate sites within the right ventricle (such as direct His bundle pacing) and combined left and RV pacing (biventricular pacing) have evolved.

Table 22.1   Pacemaker Nomenclature for Antibradycardia Pacing

Position	I	II	III	IV	V
	Chamber(s) paced	Chamber(s) sensed	Response to sensing	Rate modulation	Multisite pacing
	O = None A = Atrium V = Ventricle D = Dual (A + V)	O = None A = Atrium V = Ventricle D = Dual (A + V)	O = None T = Triggered I = Inhibited D = Dual (T + I)	O = None R = Rate responsive	O = None A = Atrium V = Ventricle D = Dual (A + V)

From Bernstein AD, Daubert JC, Fletcher RD, et al.: North American Society of Pacing and Electrophysiology/British Pacing and Electrophysiology Group: the revised NASPE/BPEG generic code for antibradycardia, adaptive-rate, and multisite pacing, Pacing Clin Electrophysiol 25:260-264, 2002.

Manufacturers' designation only: S = Single (A or V).

- Transvenous biventricular pacing systems are feasible to implant in most medium- to large-breed dogs and should be considered for those with an expected long duration of pacing, significant structural heart disease, or heart failure.

PACEMAKER NOMENCLATURE

- Pacing nomenclature was established in 1974 and updated in 2002 for use in human medicine. This nomenclature also applies to veterinary pacemaker therapy, and awareness of it is important for understanding cardiac pacing. Pacing nomenclature classifies pacing based on the site and mode of both pacing and sensing using a series of 3 to 5 letters (Table 22.1).
- The first letter (position I) indicates the cardiac chamber or chambers in which pacing occurs: A = atrium; V = ventricle; D = dual chamber (both A and V); O = none.
- The second letter (position II) indicates the chamber or chambers in which sensing of electrical activity occurs. The letters are the same as those for the first position. (Some pacemaker manufacturers use the letter "S" in both the first and the second positions to indicate that a generator is capable of pacing or sensing only a single cardiac chamber.)
- The third letter (position III) refers to the mode of response to sensed electrical activity. In this position the letter "I" indicates that a sensed electrical event inhibits the output pulse and causes the generator to recycle for one or more timing cycles. The letter "T" indicates that an output pulse is triggered in response to a sensed electrical event. A letter "D" in this position indicates that both "I" and "T" responses can occur, and this designation is limited to dual-chambered systems.
- The fourth letter (position IV) of the pacemaker nomenclature code refers to presence or absence of rate modulation. A letter "R" in this

position designates that the generator has one or more sensors (such as a motion sensor or a minute ventilation sensor) to adjust the paced heart rate independently of intrinsic cardiac activity.
- The fifth letter (position V) of the code is used to indicate whether multisite pacing is present in A = one or both atria; V = one or both ventricles; D = any combination of the atria and ventricles; O = none of the cardiac chambers. For example, a patient with a dual-chamber rate-responsive pacemaker with biventricular stimulation would be designated as having a DDDRV pacing system. The fifth letter is often omitted when describing pacing of veterinary patients because multisite pacing within the atria and ventricles is uncommon at this time.

PACING MODES

- Currently, the most commonly used pacing mode in veterinary patients and in human patients worldwide is single-chamber, ventricular-inhibited synchronous pacing either with (VVIR) or without (VVI) rate response. In this mode the artificial pacing stimulus is delivered to the ventricle (the right ventricle if transvenous), and ventricular sensing allows sensed endogenous ventricular events to inhibit the pacemaker output. Inhibition of the output in response to endogenous ventricular activity is an important feature that prevents competitive rhythms and potentially fatal consequences of an electrical stimulus delivered during the vulnerable period of the cardiac cycle. A VVI (or VVIR) pacemaker is refractory for a specified, programmable interval after either a paced or sensed ventricular depolarization. This interval is the ventricular refractory period (VRP), and ventricular events occurring within the VRP will not reset the ventricular timing. However, an endogenous ventricular depolarization occurring after the VRP

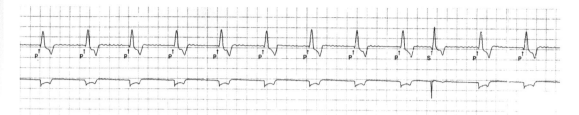

Figure 22.3 A lead II electrocardiogram (ECG) rhythm strip (*top*) and a simultaneous intracardiac electrogram (*bottom*) recorded from the pacing lead of a canine patient with complete atrioventricular (AV) block and a bipolar VVIR pacemaker. Small arrows labeled *P* indicate pacing stimuli, and each small pacing stimulus artifact results in a paced QRS complex. The tenth QRS complex is an endogenous ventricular depolarization that is sensed by the generator, resulting in brief interruption of the paced rhythm. The sensed intrinsic activity resets the timing of the next paced beat (25 mm/sec).

will be sensed, the generator output inhibited, and the timing cycle restarted from the intrinsic QRS complex. Thus, the cardiac rhythm may be irregular on auscultation in patients with VVI or VVIR pacing, and RR intervals may vary on the ECG if there is intrinsic ventricular activity (Figure 22.3).

- Single-chamber, atrial-inhibited pacing (AAI or AAIR) is identical to VVI pacing with the obvious difference that pacing and sensing occur from the atrium, and pacemaker output is inhibited by sensed atrial events. The importance of maintaining both AV synchrony and synchronous ventricular contraction makes this pacing mode attractive for dogs with sinus node dysfunction (sick sinus syndrome), particularly those with degenerative valve disease. The obvious disadvantage of atrial-based pacing is lack of ventricular depolarization should AV block occur. Therefore, despite the observation that AV block occurs infrequently in dogs with sinus node dysfunction, 24-hour ambulatory ECG monitoring before pacemaker implantation and Wenckebach testing (see later) of AV conduction at the time of implantation are recommended before permanent AAI pacing.

- Atrial synchronous pacing (VDD) is becoming increasingly popular for use in dogs with AV block. With this mode pacing occurs only in the ventricle, sensing occurs in both chambers, and ventricular output is inhibited by intrinsic ventricular activity but stimulated by ventricular tracking of sensed atrial activity. In other words, there is ventricular pacing in response to endogenous P waves. A single pacing lead with a pair of sensing electrodes located on the intraatrial portion of the lead is typically used (Figure 22.4). However, VDD pacing can also be accomplished using separate atrial and ventricular leads. In the VDD pacing mode, sensed atrial events initiate an AV delay. If an endogenous ventricular depolarization occurs during the AV delay, ventricular stimulation is inhibited, and the timing cycle is reset. If no endogenous ventricular activity

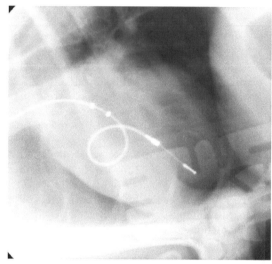

Figure 22.4 Lateral radiograph obtained from a canine patient with a transvenous VDD pacing system. The ventricular electrodes are within the right ventricle with the cathode at the ventricular apex. The atrial-sensing electrodes, located more proximally on the lead, are within the right atrium.

occurs, then a paced ventricular beat occurs at the end of the AV delay, resetting the timing cycle. If no atrial event occurs, the pacemaker escapes with a paced ventricular depolarization at the lower rate. In other words, with VDD pacing the patient will be paced VVI in absence of sensed atrial activity. VDD pacing is appropriate only for animals with AV block and normal sinus node function. If a single VDD pacing lead is to be used, the patient must be large enough for the atrial-sensing electrodes (located 11.5, 13.5, or 15.5 cm from the ventricular electrodes) to be placed in a stable position within or closely adjacent to the right atrium. Figure 22.5 shows an ECG recorded from a dog with a VDD pacing system.

- Dual-chamber pacing and sensing with inhibition and tracking (DDD) is a common mode of antibradycardia pacing in man. The primary

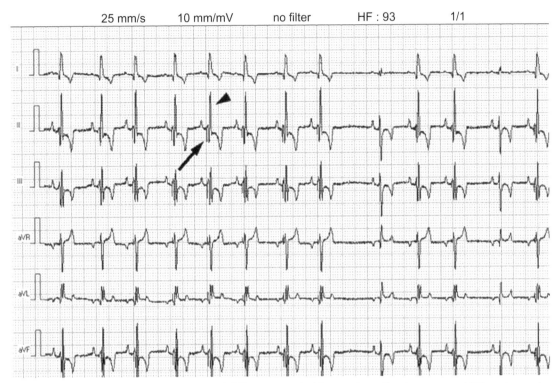

Figure 22.5 This six-lead electrocardiogram (ECG) was recorded from a dog with a transvenous VDD pacing system implanted because of high-grade second-degree atrioventricular (AV) block. The dog has normal sinus node function, resulting in normal appearing P waves with sinus arrhythmia. The P waves are sensed by the generator, and after a delay of 120 ms, there are pacing stimulus artifacts (*arrow*) followed immediately by paced QRS complexes that have left bundle branch block shape (*arrowhead*). The ninth and twelfth complexes are endogenous QRS complexes resulting from conduction of the P waves through the AV node. These QRS complexes have right bundle branch block shape (25 mm/sec).

difference between this mode and VDD mode is that in DDD mode, when there is absence of sensed intrinsic atrial activity, the atrium is paced and the atrial-paced beat is tracked by ventricular pacing. Thus, with the exception of ectopic endogenous ventricular depolarizations, AV synchrony is continuously present. This mode of pacing is important in humans with both sinus node dysfunction and AV block. However, most dogs with complete AV block have a normal sinus node, making atrial pacing unnecessary. Furthermore, DDD pacing alone does not provide rate response during AV sequential pacing (DDDR is required).

PACEMAKER IMPLANTATION

- The rate of complications associated with pacemaker implantation is inversely related to the experience of the implanter. Therefore only highly experienced, well-qualified veterinarians should attempt pacemaker implantation.
- Whereas transvenous pacemaker implantation is generally done with sedation and local anesthesia in human patients, general anesthesia is used for nearly all veterinary patients to maintain aseptic technique during the implantation.
- Application of a temporary external pacing system before induction of anesthesia is strongly recommended because a rapid and profound decrease in heart rate may occur unpredictably at any time after induction of anesthesia.
- Regardless of the type of pacing lead used, specific measurements of lead impedance, amplitude, slew rate of intrinsic cardiac electrical events (measured through the lead), and pacing threshold(s) should be obtained using a pacemaker system analyzer at the time of implantation. These measurements assure optimal placement of the lead for pacing and sensing. Atrial pacing to determine the Wenckebach point (the heart rate producing progressive prolongation of AV nodal conduction followed by second-degree AV block) is also recommended if use of a permanent atrial-based pacing system is being considered.
- Radiographs should be obtained immediately after implantation to document final lead position(s).
- A permanent transvenous ventricular pacing lead is typically inserted into the right external

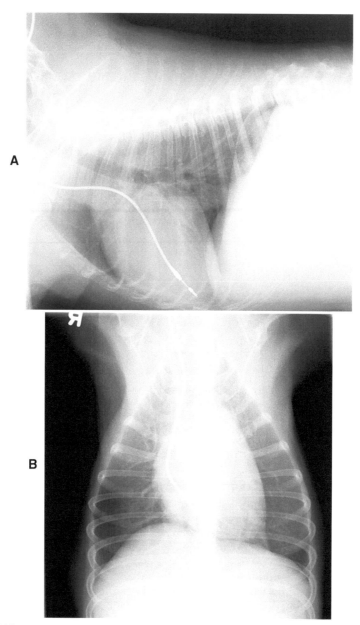

Figure 22.6   Lateral (**A**) and ventrodorsal (**B**) thoracic radiographs showing typical placement of a transvenous pacing lead in a dog. The lead tip is at the right ventricular (RV) apex.

jugular vein and advanced fluoroscopically into the ventricle, leaving the lead tip in the most apical portion of the right ventricle angled toward the diaphragm (Figure 22.6). The rare exception would be site-specific placement of a transvenous ventricular lead in the RV outflow tract or at the His bundle, in an attempt to reduce mitral regurgitation and deleterious cardiac remodeling in patients with valvular disease or dilated cardiomyopathy.

- A permanent, transvenous atrial pacing lead with straight stylet is typically inserted into the right external jugular vein and advanced

fluoroscopically until the lead tip is at the junction of the right atrium and caudal vena cava. The straight stylet is then replaced with a J-shaped stylet and the lead retracted to move the lead tip into the right auricle (Figure 22.7, *A*). In small dogs (≤10 kg), lead placement in the body of the right atrium rather than the auricle, with attachment to the atrial septum, may be necessary (Figure 22.7, *B*). If both a ventricular and an atrial lead are used, the ventricular lead is placed initially, followed by placement of the atrial lead.

- Right jugular venipuncture should not be attempted after pacemaker implantation, and a

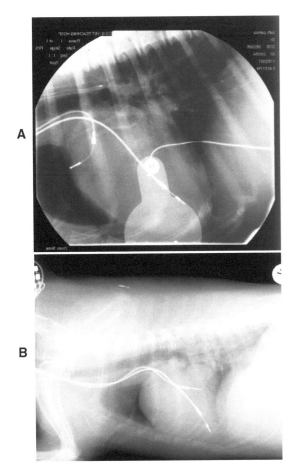

Figure 22.7 Lateral thoracic radiographs from two dogs with transvenous atrial and ventricular pacing leads. **A,** In this dog, the atrial lead was placed in the right auricle. **B,** However, this dog was too small to accommodate a lead in the auricle; therefore the atrial lead was attached to the interatrial septum.

halter or gentle leader should be used instead of a neck lead to avoid damaging transvenous pacing wires.
- When a transvenous pacing system is used, the generator is usually placed into a subcutaneous pocket made on the dorsolateral region of the neck. If a unipolar system has been used, skeletal muscle twitching in the area of the generator pocket may occur with each paced beat.
- Perioperative antibiotics are generally administered intravenously 20 minutes before beginning the implantation and repeated every 90 minutes until completion.

PACEMAKER COMPLICATIONS

- Permanent artificial cardiac pacing, whether endocardial or epicardial, is relatively safe but not completely innocuous. A 5-year retrospective study of 154 dogs receiving permanent cardiac

pacemakers showed that 84 (55%) had complications. Furthermore, the complications were life-threatening in 51 dogs (33%). There was no significant difference in the rate of major complications between epicardial and transvenous pacing systems. Similarly, a study comparing major and minor complication rates of single-chamber pacing compared with dual-chamber pacing in dogs showed no significant differences.
- The most frequent major complication in dogs with artificial cardiac pacemakers is lead malfunction because of lead dislodgement. Lead dislodgement occurs more often with transvenous leads than with epicardial leads but is equally likely to occur with either active or passive fixation leads. Surprisingly, this complication does not appear to be affected by the experience of the implanter, and it may be either acute or chronic (hours to months after implantation). There is some evidence to suggest that lead dislodgement is more common with atrial-based pacing than with ventricular pacing. Lead dislodgement may be radiographically apparent (macrodislodgement) or not radiographically apparent (microdislodgement), and radiographs showing lead position should be compared with radiographs taken at the time of implantation (Figures 22.6 and 22.8). Lead dislodgement often necessitates a second procedure to reposition the lead. Occasionally, programming the generator to higher output or changing the pacing mode from bipolar to unipolar can reestablish effective pacing without repositioning of the lead.
- Another potential cause of lead malfunction is intermittent or complete failure of pacing because of a loose connection at the interface of the lead and the connector block of the generator. This problem is usually the result of inadequate securing of the lead at the time of implantation. When connection of the lead to the generator is loose, manipulation of the generator or generator pocket may induce the pacing malfunction. The poor connection may also be apparent radiographically (Figure 22.9). A second operative procedure to secure the lead pin into the generator connector block is needed to restore reliable pacemaker function.
- Lead fracture or lead insulation breaks are causes of pacemaker malfunction occasionally encountered in veterinary patients. Fractures or insulation breaks may cause impaired sensing, impaired pacing, or both. These complications may result from biting injuries, venipuncture, excessive repetitive lead motion, or traction with a neck leash. Lead fracture or lead insulation breaks are often identified by unacceptably high or low lead impedance measurements.

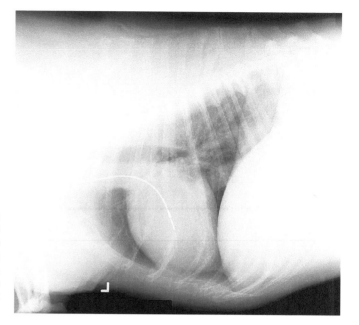

Figure 22.8 Lateral thoracic radiograph obtained from the same dog as in Figure 22.6 after dislodgement of the lead. Note that the distal tip of the lead is now located at the level of the tricuspid valve rather than at the apex. This radiograph was taken after recurrence of bradycardia caused by lack of contact between the cathode and the myocardium.

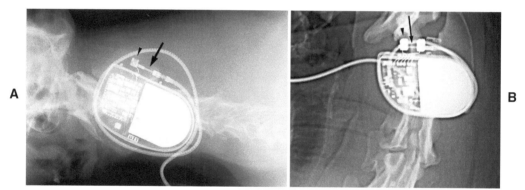

Figure 22.9   A, This radiograph was obtained from a dog with intermittent failure to pace caused by a loose connection at the interface of the unipolar lead and the connector block. The loose connection occurred because the lead pin was not adequately secured at the time of pacemaker implantation. Note that the connector pin (*arrow*) has withdrawn from the block (*arrowhead*) and is not passing all of the way through the block screw. **B,** For comparison, this radiograph shows an appropriately engaged connector pin from a patient with a bipolar pacing lead. The connector pin (*arrow*) is visible beyond the connection block screw (*arrowhead*).

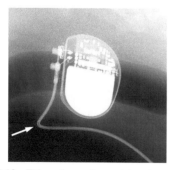

Figure 22.10   This radiograph was taken from a dog that experienced failure of a pacemaker system because of lead fracture. The fracture is visible at the tip of the arrow.

Lead fractures may also be identified radiographically (Figure 22.10).

- Exit block refers to failure of the pacing stimulus to depolarize the myocardium (failure to capture), a complication often caused by development of fibrous tissue at the electrode cardiac interface. Fibrosis is frequently secondary to inflammation incited at the time of implantation, and use of leads with steroid eluting tips is likely to minimize or prevent this problem. However, exit block may also occur from progression of underlying myocardial disease.
- Perforation of the right atrial or RV wall by a transvenous pacing lead is a rare complication that may occur at implantation or chronically. This complication may result in acute, fatal

hemorrhage or loss of effective cardiac pacing caused by failure to capture.

- Pacemaker infections may involve the pocket, lead, or both and may cause fatal septicemia or endocarditis. In dogs, most pacemaker infections occur within 3 months after implantation. With very few exceptions, treatment of an infected pacemaker or lead should consist of removal and replacement of the entire system. However, removal of a chronically implanted transvenous pacing lead is often difficult and may result in a heart wall tear, air embolism, or cardiovascular avulsion.
- Other potentially lethal pacemaker complications reported in dogs and cats include generator failure; significant arrhythmias such as ventricular asystole, atrial fibrillation, ventricular tachycardia, and ventricular fibrillation; development of congestive heart failure; cranial vena cava syndrome; and chylothorax. Extensive thrombosis and thromboembolism may also occur.
- Minor complications associated with pacemaker implantation include formation of hematomas and seromas at the generator or cervical lead site, skeletal muscle twitching at the generator site, transient or minor arrhythmias, and suture line dehiscence. For contamination or lead damage to be avoided, needle aspiration or other forms of mechanical drainage of seromas or hematomas should not be used; conservative management with pressure, warm compresses, and prophylactic antibiotics is recommended.
- EMI is a pacemaker complication that occurs when any signal, either biologic or nonbiologic, originating outside of the heart is detected by the sensing circuitry of the pacemaker. EMI can result in inappropriate inhibition of pacing, asynchronous pacing (cardiac pacing in which impulse generation by the pacemaker occurs at a fixed rate, independent of underlying cardiac activity), damage to the generator or myocardium, or reprogramming of the pacing parameters. Sources of EMI include electrocautery, electrical cardioversion or defibrillation, magnetic resonance imaging, and electroshock therapy.

PACEMAKER PROGRAMMING AND FOLLOW-UP

- State of the art pacemakers have programmable parameters that can be evaluated and altered to optimize and monitor function of the pacing system. Although there is some variation between generators, typical data obtained during a pacemaker programming and evaluating session would include output current, output voltage, lead impedance, battery status, sensitivity (sensing parameters), event records,

ECG monitoring, pacing histogram, and pacing thresholds. A real-time intracardiac electrogram can be displayed with a simultaneous surface ECG to show timing of pacing and sensing on the monitor, and a hard copy tracing may also be obtained (see Figure 22.3).

- Output programming, referring to programming of the pulse width and voltage amplitude of the pacing signals, is the most important aspect of programming that should be done routinely. Output should be high enough to provide an adequate pacing margin of safety, while also maintaining output as low as possible to maximize battery longevity. Although there is no consensus regarding the best way to program output parameters, acceptable methods include doubling the threshold voltage amplitude, tripling the pulse width at threshold, and plotting strength duration curves. Because capture threshold usually increases immediately after pacemaker implantation as healing occurs, energy output should be set relatively high at implantation and then reprogrammed after healing (approximately 8 weeks after implant).
- Sensing parameters also need to be programmed and checked. Appropriate sensing of intrinsic cardiac activity is extremely important for proper pacemaker function, whether the patient has a single- or dual-chamber pacing system. Oversensing of T waves in canine patients is a common programming error. This problem can usually be corrected with an increase in the sensing threshold.
- Appropriate programming of the refractory period is also essential for correct pacemaker function. If the refractory period is too long, intrinsic QRS complexes may cause multiple restarting of the refractory period, causing the generator to switch to asynchronous pacing. The recommended method for programming of the refractory period is that the refractory period should include the T wave and be slightly longer than the QT interval; however, dogs and cats with concurrent tachyarrhythmias may require programming with a slightly shorter refractory period to prevent noise reversion (an algorithm that causes the pacemaker to switch to asynchronous pacing when repetitive sensing at a high rate occurs).
- Although a pacemaker programmer is often necessary for trouble-shooting and thoroughly evaluating pacemaker function, a standard ECG recording may also be helpful. The ECG appearance of paced beats differs from that of endogenous beats. A paced beat includes a pacing stimulus artifact, a depolarization wave, and a repolarization wave. The pacing stimulus artifact is typically small with bipolar

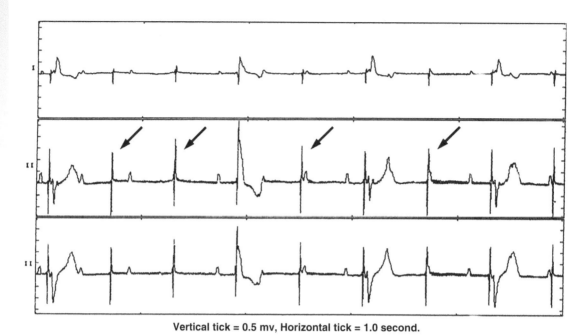

Vertical tick = 0.5 mv, Horizontal tick = 1.0 second.

Figure 22.11   A simultaneous lead I, II, and III electrocardiogram (ECG) recorded from a dog with complete atrioventricular block and a malfunctioning unipolar pacemaker. The ECG shows numerous pacing stimuli that do not depolarize the myocardium (intermittent failure to capture) (*arrows*).

pacing and relatively large with unipolar pacing (Figures 22.5 and 22.11). The QRS shape of a paced beat will depend on location of the ventricular pacing lead; transvenous pacing from the RV apex usually produces QRS complexes with a left bundle branch block configuration in the frontal plane leads (see Figure 22.5). If the pacing mode is VVI or VVIR, the paced beats are inhibited by sensed spontaneous beats, and the basic pacing cycle is reset.

- ECG abnormalities in patients with pacemakers may be broadly classified as failure to capture, failure of output, and abnormal sensing. Failure to capture is recognized as a pacing stimulus artifact without ventricular depolarization (see Figure 22.11). Causes of failure to capture include lead dislodgement, high thresholds with inadequately programmed output, partial lead fracture, insulation defect, impending battery depletion, poor or incompatible connection of the lead to the generator, and functional noncapture (pacing stimulus during the refractory period of a spontaneous beat).

- Failure to pace is recognized as failure of the generator to deliver an appropriately timed stimulus. This problem is often caused by oversensing, but it may be caused by true failure of the generator or circuit interruption (the electrical signal does not reach the heart). Reasons for true failure to output include circuit failure, complete or intermittent lead wire fracture, intermittent or permanent loose

screw set, incompatible lead, battery depletion, internal insulation fracture (bipolar lead), and lack of anodal contact (unipolar lead). When a pacemaker battery reaches the end state of depletion, either failure to capture because of reduced voltage output or failure to pace because of total battery depletion may occur.

- Sensing abnormalities, both under- and oversensing, may also be recognized on a surface ECG in many patients. Causes of sensing abnormalities include lead dislodgement or poor lead positioning, lead insulation failure, circuit failure, magnet application, malfunction of the generator (reed switch), EMI, and battery depletion.

FREQUENTLY ASK QUESTIONS

When and why should dual-chamber pacing be done?

Dual-chamber pacing provides AV synchrony, whereas single-chamber ventricular pacing does not. Pacing with AV synchrony reduces ventricular filling pressures and mitral regurgitation compared with VVI (or VVIR) pacing. Therefore dual-chamber pacing is preferable in patients with chronic valvular disease or myocardial disease. AV synchrony is also essential for high-level athletic activity, and therefore dual-chamber pacing should be considered in athletic dogs and working dogs. Placement of a VDD lead or two conventional transvenous leads is technically difficult, however, in animals weighing less than 10 kg.

What are the major advantages of atrial synchronous pacing (VDD pacing) compared with ventricular inhibited synchronous pacing (VVI pacing)?

Advantages of VDD pacing include chronotropic competence based on intrinsic sinus rate and restoration of AV synchrony. A disadvantage of this pacing mode is that it is appropriate only for treatment of patients with bradycardia caused by AV block. Therefore this method of pacing cannot be used in patients with atrial fibrillation, atrial standstill, or sinus node dysfunction. Furthermore, VDD pacing is limited to patients large enough to accommodate two leads or a special VDD lead.

What is an appropriate diagnostic approach for a patient with an implanted pacemaker that has recurrence of clinical signs suggestive of bradyarrhythmia?

A physical examination and standard ECG should be done. The physical examination will confirm bradycardia if the pacemaker dysfunction is continuous. Occasionally, event recording or Holter monitoring is needed to confirm bradycardia that is episodic as a result of intermittent pacemaker dysfunction. Physical examination may occasionally reveal a cause of pacemaker dysfunction, such as significant generator migration causing traction on a pacing lead. Standard ECG is used to identify the underlying rhythm, which, in turn, may confirm sustained pacemaker malfunction. In addition, standard ECG may help identify a specific cause of pacemaker malfunction. For example, regular pacing stimuli that occur at a rate below the lower programmed rate suggest battery depletion. Pacing stimuli with appropriate timing but without capture may indicate lead dislodgement, lead fracture, lead insulation defect, or inadequate capture threshold. Survey radiographs may confirm fractures or macrodislodgements of pacing leads. Use of a pacemaker programmer to evaluate output and sensing, to test lead impedance, and to determine capture thresholds is often necessary for definitive diagnosis of the cause of pacemaker dysfunction. Holter monitoring or event recording may be needed to confirm or refute intermittent tachyarrhythmias as the cause of the clinical signs if no evidence of pacemaker malfunction is found and ECG rhythm strips during tachycardia episodes are not available from the memory of the generator.

SUGGESTED READINGS

Bernstein AD, Daubert JC, Fletcher RD, et al: North American Society of Pacing and Electrophysiology/British Pacing and Electrophysiology Group: the revised NASPE/BPEG generic code for antibradycardia, adaptive-rate, and multisite pacing, Pacing Clin Electrophysiol 25:260, 2002.

Bonagura JD, Helphrey ML, Muir WW: Complications associated with permanent pacemaker implantation in the dog, J Am Vet Med Assoc 182:149, 1983.

Bulmer BJ, Oyama MA, Lamont LA, et al.: Implantation of a single-lead atrioventricular synchronous (VDD) pacemaker in a dog with naturally occurring 3rd-degree atrioventricular block, J Vet Intern Med 16:197, 2002.

Bulmer BJ, Oyama MA, Sisson DD: Acute hemodynamic consequences of physiologic VDD pacing in dogs with naturally occurring third degree atrioventricular block (abstract), J Vet Intern Med 16:341, 2002.

Estrada AH, Maisenbacher HW III, Prošek R, et al: Evaluation of pacing site in dogs with naturally occurring complete heart block, J Vet Cardiol 11:79, 2009.

Estrada AH, Pariaut R, Hemsley S, et al: Atrial-based pacing for sinus node dysfunction in dogs: initial results, J Vet Intern Med 26:558, 2012.

Genovese DW, Estrada AH, Maisenbacher HW, et al: Procedure times, complication rates, and survival times associated with single-chamber versus dual-chamber pacemaker implantation in dogs with clinical signs of bradyarrhythmia: 54 cases (2004-2009), J Am Vet Med Assoc 242:230, 2013.

Love CJ, Wilkoff BL, Byrd CH, et al: Recommendations for extraction of chronically implanted transvenous pacing and defibrillator leads: indications, facilities, training, PACE 23:544, 2000.

Oyama MA, Sisson DD, Lehmkuhl LB: Practices and outcome of artificial cardiac pacing in 154 dogs, J Vet Intern Med 15:229, 2001.

Petrie J-P: Permanent transvenous cardiac pacing, Clin Tech Small Anim Pract 20:164, 2005.

Phibbs B, Marriott HJ: Complications of permanent transvenous pacing, N Engl J Med 312:1428, 1985.

Sisson D, Thomas WP, Woodfield J, et al: Permanent transvenous pacemaker implantation in forty dogs, J Vet Intern Med 5:322, 1991.

23 Nutrition and Cardiovascular Disease

Lisa M. Freeman | John E. Rush

Research now supports the concept that optimal nutrition is an integral part of the overall medical treatment for cats and dogs with cardiac disease. Key nutritional concerns include maintenance of appetite and maintenance of optimal body condition, avoiding nutritional deficiencies and excesses (e.g., dietary sodium moderation), and gaining benefits of dietary supplementation. It also is becoming more apparent that the same diet is not optimal for every dog or every cat with cardiac disease, and that to optimize care for patients, it is important to individualize the nutritional plan, just as one individualizes the medication plan. General recommendations such as "feed a senior diet" or "give a renal diet" will typically result in suboptimal nutritional status and inferior outcomes.

GENERAL PRINCIPLES

NUTRIENTS OF CONCERN IN CARDIAC DISEASE

Dogs and cats with cardiac disease have a variety of pathophysiologic changes, such as activation of the renin-angiotensin-aldosterone system, sodium and water retention, and, depending on stage of disease and medication regimen, electrolyte alterations. As a result, nutritional alterations occur at various stages of cardiac disease. These nutrients are considered "nutrients of concern" in animals with cardiac disease.

COMMON NUTRITIONAL ALTERATIONS IN CARDIAC DISEASE

- Reduced calorie intake. Once congestive heart failure (CHF) arises, alterations in appetite are common. These can include a complete loss of appetite (anorexia), a reduction in food intake (hyporexia), or changes in food preferences (dysrexia). These all contribute to reduced food intake and resulting weight and muscle loss, which are common in CHF. These changes in appetite can be the result of increased production of inflammatory mediators (e.g., inflammatory cytokines,

oxidative stress), side effects of cardiac medications, or poor control of CHF signs. Although many animals with cardiac disease exhibit weight loss, particularly with more advanced disease, animals with cardiac disease also can be overweight or obese (with or without muscle loss). Interestingly, being overweight may actually be associated with a protective effect once CHF is present; this is known as the *obesity paradox.*

- Increased protein catabolism resulting in muscle loss. Muscle loss (cachexia) is common, particularly as the disease progresses. This muscle loss is unlike that seen in a healthy animal, which primarily loses fat. If an animal with CHF from any cause does not get sufficient calories and protein, the primary tissue lost is lean body mass. The loss of lean body mass in cardiac cachexia is a multifactorial process caused by anorexia, increased energy requirements, and increased production of inflammatory cytokines (e.g., tumor necrosis factor [TNF] and interleukin-1 [IL-1]). These cytokines cause anorexia, increase energy requirements, and increase the catabolism of lean body mass. In addition, TNF and IL-1 also cause cardiac myocyte hypertrophy and fibrosis and have negative inotropic effects. The term *cachexia* does not necessarily refer to an emaciated, end-stage patient. In fact, in the early stages, it can be very subtle and even may occur in obese animals. Loss of lean body mass usually is noted first in the epaxial, gluteal, scapular, or temporal muscles. Cardiac cachexia has deleterious effects on strength, immune function, and survival, so it is important to recognize this muscle loss at an early stage when there is a better opportunity to successfully manage it. Feeding a diet that is restricted in protein (e.g., renal diets) may contribute to unwanted muscle loss.

- Taurine deficiency. Taurine can play a role in the development of feline dilated cardiomyopathy (DCM) and in some cases of canine DCM. Taurine deficiency–induced DCM is now uncommon in cats but should be suspected if cats are eating diets that are vegetarian, home-prepared, or food made by a manufacturer with suspect quality control measures. Some dogs with DCM also can have taurine deficiency, and the index of suspicion should be higher in predisposed breeds (e.g., American Cocker Spaniels, St. Bernards, Newfoundlands, Golden Retrievers), particularly if they are eating lamb and rice, high-fiber, or very low-protein diets.

- Omega-3 fatty acid deficiency. In addition to serving as a source of calories and essential fatty acids, fat also can have significant benefits on inflammation, immune function, and hemodynamics. Most pet foods contain primarily omega-6 fatty acids (e.g., linoleic acid, arachidonic acids). The omega-3 fatty acids eicosapentaenoic acid (EPA) and docosahexaenoic acid (DHA) normally are found in very low concentrations in the cell membrane compared with the omega-6 fatty acids, but their level can be increased by consumption of a food or supplement enriched in omega-3 fatty acids. In one study, dogs with CHF had a relative deficiency of omega-3 fatty acids, which was corrected after supplementation of omega-3 fatty acids. However, omega-3 fatty acid status in cardiac disease may differ between breeds of dogs and between species. The benefit of having a higher concentration of omega-3 fatty acids in cell membranes is that breakdown products of the omega-3 fatty acids (eicosanoids) are less potent inflammatory mediators than eicosanoids derived from omega-6 fatty acids. This decreases the production of cytokines and other inflammatory mediators. Fish oil also reduces the production of TNF and IL-1 and improves muscle mass. In some animals fish oil supplementation also improves appetite. Another potential benefit is that omega-3 fatty acids have antiarrhythmic effects.
- Mineral excess or deficiency
  - Sodium. Increased retention of sodium and water is well recognized in animals with cardiac disease because of activation of the renin-angiotensin-aldosterone system and other neuroendocrine systems. In contrast, hyponatremia that develops in late-stage CHF due to excessive free water retention can be associated with adverse outcomes.
  - Potassium. Depending on the stage of disease and medications being administered, animals with cardiac disease can be hyperkalemic (with angiotensin-converting enzyme [ACE] inhibitors or aldosterone receptor antagonists), hypokalemic (with loop diuretics), or normokalemic. Hypokalemia can cause overall weakness and increase the risk for arrhythmia.

- Magnesium. High doses of diuretics can increase the risk for hypomagnesemia. Hypomagnesemia can increase the risk for arrhythmia. However, in animals with CHF and concurrent chronic kidney disease, hypermagnesemia may develop.
- Vitamin deficiency. Vitamin B deficiencies appear to be relatively common in humans with CHF and are likely caused by urinary losses secondary to diuretic use. Similar studies have not been published in dogs with CHF, but one study in cats with cardiomyopathies showed reduced serum concentrations of vitamins B_6 and B_{12}.

In addition to the above nutrients of concern, there are a number of other nutrients with potential pharmacologic effects (e.g., L-carnitine, coenzyme Q10, antioxidants, arginine) that are based on pathophysiologic changes in cardiac disease (e.g., altered myocardial energetics, increased oxidative stress, endothelial dysfunction). Some nutrients, such as omega-3 fatty acids and taurine, may act through pharmacologic and nutritional effects. For example, taurine, as an essential nutrient for cats, may have benefit by correcting a nutritional deficiency. However, taurine also has antioxidant and positive inotropic properties.

However, being a nutrient of concern does not mean that all cats with hypertrophic cardiomyopathy (HCM) or all dogs with chronic valvular disease (CVD) require modification of *all* of these nutrients or that they should be supplemented or restricted to the same levels. This would be similar to the concept of recommending furosemide for all dogs with CVD, no matter what the stage of disease, or prescribing an ACE inhibitor for every cat with HCM. Instead, one should consider the underlying disease (e.g., DCM, HCM, CVD, congenital heart disease) and the stage of disease (e.g., preclinical or mild, moderate, or severe heart failure), but also the following factors:

- Physical examination findings, especially body condition score [BCS], muscle condition score [MCS], and gain or loss in body weight.
- Laboratory results (e.g., hypoalbuminemia, azotemia, hypokalemia or hyperkalemia, hypomagnesemia).
- Concurrent diseases. Concurrent diseases are present in many animals with cardiac disease (61% of dogs and 56% of cats) and can have significant effects on the nutritional modifications that will be optimal for that patient.
- Animal preferences.
- Owner preferences

On the basis of all these factors, a nutritional plan can be individualized for each animal. For the development and execution of this plan, there are five key steps: (1) performing a nutritional assessment, (2) making individualized nutritional recommendations, (3) addressing all components of the diet, (4) communicating with the owner, and (5) reassessing nutritional needs at each recheck examination.

PERFORM A NUTRITIONAL ASSESSMENT ON EVERY PATIENT

A good nutritional assessment of the animal's current dietary intake and preferences should consider the following five questions:

1. Is the current diet contributing to the cardiac disease (or other medical conditions)? Examples include an animal with CHF eating a very high-sodium diet, a cat with DCM eating a vegetarian diet, or a dog with severe muscle loss eating a veterinary diet designed for animals with renal disease. Even if the diet is not directly affecting the cardiac disease, it could be contributing to suboptimal health (e.g., an unbalanced home-prepared diet, excessive calories contributing to obesity).
2. Is the current diet optimized for managing the cardiac disease?
3. Are all of the components of the animal's current diet known, including treats, supplements, and foods used to administer medications? The entire diet may be composed of pet food, but it more likely also includes home-prepared food, treats, table food, dietary supplements, rawhides or dental chews, and a variety of other sources of nutrients that must be addressed.
4. What are the animal's taste preferences? Recommending the preferred formulation (dry or canned) and flavor can be helpful for feeding the hospitalized animal, as well as for making long-term recommendations.
5. Are the owners' preferences understood, such as type of food, the importance of treats and table food, and the administration of medications?

Nutritional assessment consists of a screening evaluation and, if any "red flags" are identified, an extended evaluation should follow. The screening evaluation can quickly identify nutritional issues in the animal with cardiac disease that require further evaluation. The screening evaluation can be achieved by having the owner complete a short diet history form and by performing a physical examination.

- Diet history. Standardized diet history forms make gathering complete information more efficient and ensure that the required information is collected for every patient. A complete diet history includes the main pet food being provided (or the home-prepared diet recipe being used, if any), but also treats, table food, dietary supplements, and foods used for medication administration. Also, even if the dog or cat is discharged with an optimal diet plan, one should not assume that the owner is following these recommendations at subsequent visits; ask exactly what the owner is feeding at each visit. See Figure 23.1 for a cardiac-specific diet history form. Also see the World Small Animal Veterinary Association Nutrition Toolkit or the American College of Veterinary Nutrition websites for more general diet history forms.
- Body weight. Use the same scale at each visit to identify subtle changes in body weight, which may reflect altered nutritional status or fluid accumulation.
- BCS. Use a consistent method to assess BCS at each visit (either a 9- or a 5-point scale). The BCS evaluates body fat and can identify animals that are overweight or obese, as well as animals that are below ideal body weight.
- MCS. The MCS differs from the BCS in that the MCS evaluates muscle mass. Animals can be very obese (9/9) and have important muscle loss. Conversely, they can be thin (3/9) but have normal muscle mass. Evaluation of muscle mass includes visual examination and palpation over the temporal bones, scapulae, lumbar vertebrae, and pelvic bones. Muscle condition is graded as normal or as mild, moderate, or severe muscle loss (Figure 23.2). With an assessment of muscle condition at every visit, muscle loss can be identified at its early stages when intervention is more likely to be successful.
- Presence of other medical conditions that also require dietary modifications (e.g., gastrointestinal disease, feline lower urinary tract disease, chronic kidney disease).

If any of these issues are identified on the screening evaluation, an extended evaluation to gather necessary additional information is recommended, so that an optimal individualized nutritional plan can be developed.

MAKE INDIVIDUALIZED NUTRITIONAL RECOMMENDATIONS

The same diet will not be optimal for all animals with cardiac disease. For example, for a 9-year-old spayed female Cavalier King Charles Spaniel with CVD, well-controlled CHF, normal laboratory values, a BCS of 7/9, and no muscle loss, for which the owner prefers a combination of canned and dry food, the main nutrients of concern would be calories (reducing calories to achieve slow weight loss), protein (ensuring adequate protein intake), and

DIET HISTORY FORM FOR ANIMALS WITH HEART DISEASE

Please answer the following questions about your pet

Today's date: _____

Pet's name: _____ Owner's name : _____

1. How would you assess your pet's appetite? (mark the point on the line that best represents your pet's appetite)

    Poor   **Excellent**

    _____

2. Describe your pet's appetite over the last few weeks? (check all that apply)
    ☐Eats about the same amount as usual   ☐Eats less than usual   ☐Eats more than usual
    ☐Seems to prefer different foods than usual

3. Over the last few weeks, has your pet (check one)
    ☐Lost weight   ☐Gained weight ☐Stayed about the same weight ☐Don't know

4. Please list below the brands and product names (if applicable) and the amount of ALL foods, treats, snack, dental chews, rawhides, and any other food item that your pet currently eats.

Food	Form	Amount	How often?	Fed since
Examples:				
Purina Dog Chow	dry	1 ½ cups	2x/day	Jan, 2011
Science Diet Adult Gourmet Beef Entree	can	½ large can	1x/day	Jan, 2012
90% lean hamburger	microwaved	3 oz	1x/week	Jan, 2011
Milk Bone medium	dry	1	2x/day	Aug, 2010
Rawhide	dry	2x6" strip	3x/week	Dec, 2011

_____
_____
_____
_____
_____
_____
_____
_____

5. Do you give any dietary supplements to your pet (for example: vitamins, glucosamine, fatty acids, or any other supplements)?   ☐Yes ☐No   If yes, please list which ones and give brands and amounts:

		Brand	Dose
Taurine	☐Yes ☐No	_____	_____
Carnitine	☐Yes ☐No	_____	_____
Antioxidants	☐Yes ☐No	_____	_____
Multivitamin	☐Yes ☐No	_____	_____
Coenzyme Q10	☐Yes ☐No	_____	_____
Fish oil	☐Yes ☐No	_____	_____
Flaxseed, cod liver oil, or other fatty acids?	☐Yes ☐No	_____	_____
Other (please list)	☐Yes ☐No	_____	_____

6. How do you administer pills to your pet?
    ☐I do not give any medications
    ☐I give them without any food
    ☐I put them in my pet's dog/cat food
    ☐I put them in a Pill Pocket or similar product
    ☐I put them in other foods (such as cheese or lunch meat; please list foods):_____

Information below to be completed by the veterinarian:

Current body weight: _____kg Ideal body weight: _____kg

Current body condition score: _____/9

Muscle Condition Score: ☐normal muscle ☐mild muscle loss ☐moderate muscle loss ☐severe muscle loss

Figure 23.1 A sample diet history form designed to collect important nutritional information for dogs and cats with cardiac disease.

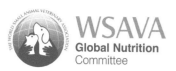

Muscle Condition Score

Muscle condition score is assessed by visualization and palpation of the spine, scapulae, skull, and wings of the ilia. Muscle loss is typically first noted in the epaxial muscles on each side of the spine; muscle loss at other sites can be more variable. Muscle condition score is graded as normal, mild loss, moderate loss, or severe loss. Note that animals can have significant muscle loss if they are overweight (body condition score > 5). Conversely, animals can have a low body condition score (< 4) but have minimal muscle loss. Therefore, assessing both body condition score and muscle condition score on every animal at every visit is important. Palpation is especially important when muscle loss is mild and in animals that are overweight. An example of each score is shown below.

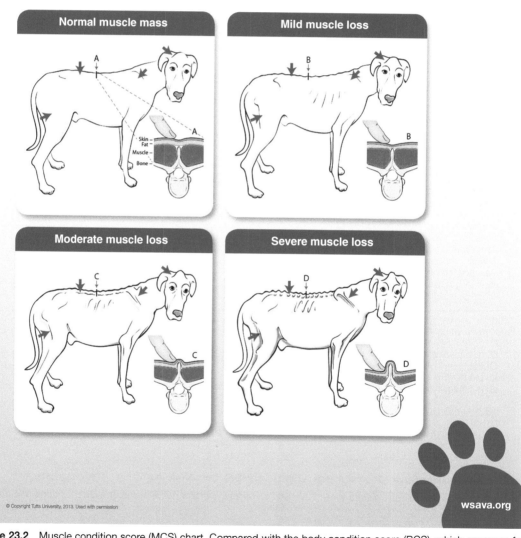

© Copyright Tufts University, 2013. Used with permission

wsava.org

Figure 23.2 Muscle condition score (MCS) chart. Compared with the body condition score (BCS), which assesses fat stores, the MCS assesses the animal's muscle, which can be affected by disease or aging. The MCS chart can be found in the Global Nutrition Committee Toolkit (World Small Animal Veterinary Association [http://www.wsava.org/nutrition-toolkit].) (Copyright Tufts University, 2013. Used with permission.)

mild sodium restriction (<100 mg/100 kcal). This would allow the clinician to make recommendations for several canned and dry options from which the owner could choose. However, if that same dog now had more severe CHF, with a BCS of 4/9, moderate muscle loss, picky appetite, hyperkalemia, and hypoalbuminemia, the nutrients of concern (and the levels to which nutrients should be modified) will be very different. In this situation, a high-calorie density and palatable diet, with increased protein (>6.5 g/100 kcal) and low to moderate potassium concentrations, would be ideal. Concurrent diseases also alter diet choice and are present in many animals with heart disease. The optimal diet for a cat with HCM alone is very different from that of a cat with HCM and chronic kidney disease or feline lower urinary tract disease. Finally, the animals' preferences and the owners' preferences (e.g., canned or dry, brand, type, and veterinary diet or over-the-counter) must be taken into consideration for good compliance and successful treatment.

On the basis of patient characteristics (and owner preferences), one or more diets can be selected. Animals with cardiac disease may be hyperkalemic, hypokalemic, or normokalemic, which influences the choice of diet. One general recommendation for heart disease is to avoid protein-restricted diets (e.g., renal diets or diets with protein <5.1 g/100 kcal for dogs or 6.5 g/100 kcal for cats), unless concurrent advanced kidney disease is present. Currently, two commercial veterinary cardiac diets for dogs are available in the United States. The specific characteristics of each diet differ, but both are moderately to severely sodium restricted (15 to 50 mg/100 kcal). They also vary widely in protein content (3.8 to 6.0 g/100 kcal, with an Association of American Feed Control Officials [AAFCO] minimum for dogs of 5.1 g/100 kcal). One cardiac diet also includes supplemental taurine, carnitine, arginine, antioxidants, and omega-3 fatty acids. There currently are no commercial veterinary diets designed for cats with cardiac disease in the United States. Nonetheless, there are a variety of diets, both veterinary diets marketed for other diseases and over-the-counter sodium-reduced diets, that may have the desired properties for individual patients with cardiac disease. We usually try to offer the owner several options so that they can determine which one the animal prefers. Having a number of choices is particularly beneficial for animals with CHF, a condition in which anorexia, hyporexia, and dysrexia are common.

Avoid common mistakes in nutritional recommendations:

- Be sure to make specific diet recommendations, not just "feed a low-sodium diet." It is difficult for owners to know which diets are low in sodium (because this is not required information on pet food label), and owners usually do not know what cutoff is specifically meant by low sodium.
- Avoid the general recommendation of "feed a senior diet." Although senior diets are assumed to be low in sodium, this is not always true. Some senior diets may be appropriate, but it is very important to look at the characteristics of the individual product. There is no legal definition for a senior diet, so the levels of calories, protein, sodium, and other nutrients can vary dramatically among products from different companies. In a recent study of 37 over-the-counter senior diets, the sodium content ranged from 33 to 412 mg/100 kcal (AAFCO sodium minimum for dogs is 17 mg/100 kcal, with a common over-the-counter adult dog food containing 105 mg/100 kcal sodium).

ADDRESS ALL COMPONENTS OF THE DIET

Including all sources of dietary sodium in the overall diet plan is important to achieve success with nutritional modifications.

- Treats. Over 90% of dogs and 30% of cats with heart disease receive treats. Most owners are not aware of what foods are high or low in sodium, and so they must be given very specific recommendations for appropriate treats and table food (and appropriate amounts). We typically provide a list of foods that are appropriate and foods to avoid as treats to assist the owner in wise selection. The HeartSmart website has an up-to-date listing of treats that are low in sodium.
- Foods used for medication administration. Most dog owners (57%) and many cat owners (34%) use food for medication administration, and the most commonly used foods are high in sodium (e.g., cheese, hot dogs, lunch meats). Therefore it is important to provide effective but appropriate foods for administering medications (Box 23.1).
- Dietary supplements. Ask at each visit if the owner is administering dietary supplements. If so, ensure that the supplements are safe, are not interacting with the diet or medications, and are being administered at an appropriate dose. Animals with cardiac disease (31% of dogs and 13% of cats) are more likely to be receiving dietary supplements than animals in the general pet population as "Internet surfing" for alternative treatments of cardiac disease is common. The clinician and pet owner should understand that dietary supplements can be marketed without proof of safety, efficacy, or

Box 23.1   Recommended Methods for Medication Administration

- Teach owners to administer pills without using foods (either by hand or using a device designed for this purpose, such as a pet piller or pet pill gun).
- A compounded liquid medication can be considered, although the pharmacokinetics of compounded medications may be significantly altered by compounding.
- Use low-sodium foods for medication administration.
  - Meat or fish (home cooked, without salt; not lunch meats)
  - Fresh fruit (e.g., banana, orange, melon, berries)
  - Low-sodium canned pet food
  - Peanut butter (labeled as "no salt added")
  - Pill administration treats also can be used but be sure to check the individual brand for sodium content and other nutrients of concern for an individual patient. This becomes particularly important the more these treats are used for daily medication administration.

quality control. Therefore careful consideration of the type, dose, and brand may be important to avoid toxicities or a complete lack of efficacy. Because there is little governmental regulation over dietary supplements, pet owners should consider selecting dietary supplements that have the Dietary Supplement Verification Program (DSVP) logo; this program tests supplements for ingredients, concentrations, dissolvability, and contaminants. Another resource is Consumerlab.com, which performs independent testing of health and nutrition products.

- Another important issue related to administration of dietary supplements is their use in place of standard cardiac medications. Animals with severe CHF may already be receiving many pills each day, and it may not be clear to owners that it is more important to give the cardiac medications than the dietary supplements. In situations in which pill administration is becoming overwhelming for an owner, the veterinarian can assist the owner in prioritizing dietary supplements (or encouraging them to discontinue all supplements).

COMMUNICATE WITH THE OWNER

- Be sure to understand "nonnegotiables" with the owners (e.g., they wish to continue giving treats, they want to feed a home-cooked diet, or they have to give medications in foods). Discuss the nutritional plan and answer questions (consider referring the owner to a board-certified

veterinary nutritionist for complicated cases or when owners have a large number of questions about nutrition).

- Warn owners of cyclical/variable appetite in animals with CHF. Animals with CHF often have periods of anorexia, hyporexia, and dysrexia. Altered appetite often heralds a change in CHF control or a need to change medications, but fluctuation in diet does happen even when CHF is well controlled. Owners often describe this as the animal preferring different foods than it used to or the animal eating one food well for a week and then not wanting it anymore (but they will eat a different food). It is helpful to warn the owner about appetite and to provide multiple appropriate diet options for the owner to feed (i.e., they can feed one diet for several days until the animal no longer has interest in that food and then switch to a different food. A cat will often be willing to eat the original food again, so owners can use a "rotation" of foods to keep the cat eating). It is important to advise the owner that if the animal is also acting lethargic, is tachypneic, will not eat *any* foods, or had been eating very well and then suddenly stops eating, this usually indicates the need for reassessment and adjustment of medications.

REASSESS THE PLAN

Monitoring the nutritional plan at each visit is important. This should include the following:

- Nutritional assessment
  - Clinical signs
  - Diet history
  - Body weight
  - BCS
  - MCS
  - Laboratory testing (e.g., electrolytes, blood urea nitrogen, creatinine, albumin)
  - Others, as indicated

NUTRITIONAL RECOMMENDATIONS BASED ON SEVERITY OF DISEASE

Nutritional recommendations will be considered with the severity of heart disease to emphasize the importance of considering different stages for nutrition (Table 23.1).

- Calories. Optimal calorie intake should be a goal for all stages of disease, as previously described.
- Protein. Ensuring adequate protein intake is important, as previously described. This should be a primary goal in animals with cardiac disease, particularly as CHF becomes more severe.

Table 23.1   Recommendations for Nutrients of Concern Based on Stage of Cardiac Disease*

Note that all of these nutrients may not be of concern for an individual animal (e.g., if an animal has normal serum potassium concentrations, modification of dietary potassium is not warranted). Conversely, if animals have concurrent disease (e.g., gastrointestinal disease, chronic kidney disease, cancer), additional nutrients will likely need to be modified. For some diet options, see the Tufts HeartSmart website or contact individual manufacturers for nutritional information. For complicated cases, consider consulting with a board-certified veterinary nutritionist (acvn.org or ecvcn.org).

Nutrient	No Heart Disease (but predisposed)	Preclinical	Mild or Compensated Heart Failure	Advanced Heart Failure
Calories	*Cats and dogs:* Calories sufficient to achieve and maintain BCS of 4-5 (on a 9-point scale). Try to prevent overweight/obesity and, if present, work to achieve successful weight loss.	*Cats and dogs:* Calories sufficient to achieve and maintain BCS of 5-6 (on a 9-point scale).	*Cats and dogs:* Calories sufficient to achieve and maintain BCS of 5-7 (on a 9-point scale).	*Cats and dogs:* Calories sufficient to achieve and maintain BCS of 5-7 (on a 9-point scale).
Protein	*Cats and dogs:* Minimum dietary protein of 5.1 g/100 kcal for dogs and 6.5 g/100 kcal for cats.	*Cats and dogs:* Minimum dietary protein of 5.1 g/100 kcal for dogs and 6.5 g/100 kcal for cats.	*Cats and dogs:* Minimum dietary protein of 6.1 g/100 kcal for dogs and 7.5 g/100 kcal for cats (unless concurrent kidney disease is present).	*Cats and dogs:* Minimum dietary protein of 6.1 g/100 kcal for dogs and 7.5 g/100 kcal for cats (unless concurrent kidney disease is present).
Fat Omega-3 fatty acids	*Cats and dogs:* No known benefits at this stage.	*Dogs:* Fish oil† (40 mg/kg EPA + 25 mg/kg DHA per day) if taste is acceptable to the animal or animal can be pilled.	*Dogs:* Fish oil† (40 mg/kg EPA + 25 mg/kg DHA per day) if taste is acceptable to the animal or animal can be pilled.	*Cats and dogs:* Fish oil† (40 mg/kg EPA + 25 mg/kg DHA per day) if taste is acceptable to the animal or animal can be pilled.
Minerals Sodium	*Cats and dogs:* <120 mg/100 kcal	*Cats and dogs:* <100 mg/100 kcal	*Cats and dogs:* <80 mg/100 kcal	*Cats and dogs:* <60 mg/100 kcal
Potassium	No known benefits of supplementation at this stage.	No known benefits of supplementation at this stage.	*Hypokalemia:* Check dietary K⁺ to ensure not a low K⁺ diet. Supplement if diet alone does not correct. *Hyperkalemia:* Lower dietary K⁺	*Hypokalemia:* Check dietary K⁺ to ensure not a low K⁺ diet. Supplement if diet alone does not correct. *Hyperkalemia:* Lower dietary K⁺
Magnesium	No known benefits of supplementation at this stage.	No known benefits of supplementation at this stage.	Ensure dietary intake if documented hypomagnesemia.	Ensure dietary intake if documented hypomagnesemia.
Vitamins B vitamins	*Cats and dogs:* No known benefits of supplementation at this stage.	*Cats and dogs:* No known benefits of supplementation at this stage.	*Cats and dogs:* Consider supplementation of B vitamin complex if on high-dose diuretics.	*Cats and dogs:* Supplement B vitamin complex if on high-dose diuretics or if anorexia or hyporexia is present.

Note: Home-prepared diets are strongly discouraged unless the recipe is formulated by a board-certified veterinary nutritionist (acvn.org, ecvcn.org, or www.esvcn.eu/college), the owner will follow the recipe exactly, and the animal/recipe will be reevaluated frequently.

†Consider quality control issues with all dietary supplements

BCS, Body condition score; *DHA,* docosahexaenoic acid; *EPA,* eicosapentaenoic acid.

- Amino acids
  - Taurine. Although most current cases of feline DCM appear to be independent of taurine status, taurine deficiency still should be suspected whenever the diagnosis of feline DCM is made. Plasma and whole blood taurine levels should be analyzed, and treatment with taurine (125 to 250 mg q12h PO) should begin concurrent with medical therapy. If the cat is eating an unconventional diet that is likely to be unbalanced or a food made by a small manufacturer, the owner also should be counseled to switch to a nutritionally balanced commercial cat food made by a well-known manufacturer.

As noted, for dogs with DCM, taurine concentrations should be tested in predisposed breeds (e.g., American Cocker Spaniels, St. Bernards, Newfoundlands, Golden Retrievers) or dogs eating lamb and rice, high-fiber, or very low-protein diets. The benefits of taurine supplementation are far less certain in canine DCM than in feline DCM associated with dietary deficiency. Although several small studies have shown that taurine supplementation can improve some clinical or echocardiographic parameters in taurine-deficient dogs, the response is generally not as dramatic as is seen in cats with taurine deficiency–induced DCM. Nonetheless, we recommend supplementing taurine until plasma and whole blood taurine concentrations for the patient are available. The optimal dose of taurine for correcting a deficiency has not been determined, but recommended dosages range from 250 to 1000 mg q12h.

- Fat. We currently recommend a daily dose of fish oil to provide 40 mg/kg of EPA and 25 mg/kg of DHA for dogs with anorexia or cachexia and also for most dogs with CHF if there are no contraindications (e.g., dietary fat intolerance, coagulopathies). Unless the diet is one of a few specially designed therapeutic diets, supplementation is necessary to achieve this omega-3 fatty acid dose. When fish oil supplements are used, it is important to know the exact amount of EPA and DHA in a specific fish oil brand because supplements vary widely. However, the most common formulation of fish oil is 1-g capsules that contain approximately 180 mg of EPA and 120 mg of DHA. At this concentration, fish oil can be administered at a dose of 1 capsule per 10 pounds of body weight per day to achieve the recommended EPA and DHA dosages. Fish oil supplements always should contain vitamin E as an antioxidant, but other nutrients should not be included to avoid toxicities. Cod liver oil and flaxseed oil should not be used to provide omega-3 fatty acids to dogs and cats. Understanding the potential benefits of fish oil supplementation for cats with cardiac disease and differences between dog breeds requires much additional research.

- Minerals
  - Sodium. Although sodium restriction is recommended for all stages of cardiac disease, the degree of restriction should vary with the stage of disease. We do not recommend severe sodium restriction in the early stages of disease (Table 23.1) because this can activate the renin-angiotensin-aldosterone system. Instead, we recommend mild restriction and using this time to begin to educate owners about nutrition and cardiac disease, particularly with respect to foods that are high in sodium. Most owners are unaware of the sodium content of pet and human foods and need very specific instructions regarding appropriate pet foods, acceptable low-salt treats, and methods for administering medications. Owners also should be counseled on specific foods to avoid, such as baby food, bread, canned vegetables (unless labeled "no salt added"), cheeses, condiments (e.g., ketchup, soy sauce), lunch meats and cold cuts (e.g., ham, corned beef, salami, sausages, bacon, hot dogs), most pet treats, rawhides and bully sticks, pickled foods, pizza, processed foods (e.g., potato mixes, rice mixes, macaroni and cheese), snack foods (e.g., potato chips, packaged popcorn, crackers), and soups (unless homemade without salt). As cardiac disease progresses, additional dietary sodium restriction is recommended.
  - Potassium. Commercial pet foods vary widely in their potassium content, and so, depending on the individual animal's serum potassium concentration, foods may exacerbate hypokalemia or hyperkalemia. Conversely, diets can be selected to help manage hypokalemia or hyperkalemia. Serum potassium should be monitored regularly in animals with CHF and addressed with diet, supplementation, or both.
  - Magnesium. Serum magnesium concentrations should be measured in animals with CHF, although serum magnesium concentrations are a poor indicator of total body stores. Nonetheless, serial evaluations in an individual patient may be useful, especially in patients with arrhythmias or in those receiving high doses of diuretics. Diets high in magnesium may be beneficial in a hypomagnesemic animal.
- Other nutrients
  - L-Carnitine. Carnitine is in high concentrations in the myocardium, and carnitine

deficiency syndromes can be associated with primary myocardial disease in humans. Carnitine deficiency was reported in a family of Boxers in 1991. Since that time, L-carnitine has been supplemented in some dogs with DCM, but no controlled prospective studies have been reported. Because of its important role in long-chain fatty acid metabolism and energy production, carnitine supplementation may have benefits for myocardial energy metabolism, even if a primary deficiency is not present. Diagnosis of L-carnitine deficiency is not clinically practical because plasma concentrations are often normal, even in the face of myocardial deficiency. Therefore L-carnitine supplementation is typically recommended empirically for owners of dogs with CHF who "wish to do everything." The optimal dose of L-carnitine is unknown, but 25 to 75 mg/kg q8-12h PO has been recommended.

- Coenzyme Q10. Coenzyme Q10 has been recommended as an adjunct treatment for DCM, although it is not clear whether any potential effects could be the result of correcting a deficiency (although this does not appear to be the case) or pharmacologic effects of coenzyme Q10. Other potential benefits of supplementation include improved myocardial metabolic efficiency and increased antioxidant protection. The current recommended (but empiric) dosage in dogs is 30 mg q12hr PO, although up to 90 mg q12h PO has been recommended for large dogs. Controlled prospective studies are needed to assess the efficacy of this supplement in dogs and cats.

- Antioxidants. Dogs with CHF have an imbalance between the levels of oxidants produced and the endogenous antioxidant protection available. The major antioxidants include enzymatic antioxidants (e.g., superoxide dismutase, catalase, glutathione peroxidase) and oxidant quenchers (e.g., vitamin C, vitamin E, and beta carotene). Supplemental antioxidants are now provided in many over-the-counter and veterinary diets, including at least one cardiac diet; however, the benefits of antioxidant supplementation in dogs and cats with CHF require much additional research.

FREQUENTLY ASKED QUESTIONS

What are some ways to improve appetite in a dog or cat with CHF and reduced food intake?

- Provide multiple diet options so owners can rotate foods if hyporexia or dysrexia occur.

- Change the temperature of the food. Cats often prefer the food to be warmed to body temperature before feeding, although individual dogs may prefer the food to be warmed, at room temperature, or cold.
- Feed several small frequent meals during the day rather than just one or two meals.
- Feed the animal from a different type of dish (e.g., a new food dish or a human dinner plate).
- Feed in a different location in the house.
- Add homemade chicken, beef, or fish broth to the food (even low-sodium store-bought broths are too high in sodium).
- Add a small amount (1 to 2 teaspoons) of cooked meat (hamburger, chicken, or fish) to the food. Be sure to instruct the owner not to use any prepared foods, such as rotisserie chicken, lunch meats, or canned meats or fish, because of their high sodium content. Cats typically prefer meat or fish as a palatability enhancer. Meat or fish also may enhance food intake in dogs, but some dogs prefer sweet flavors as a palatability enhancer (e.g., maple syrup, applesauce, fruit-flavored yogurt).
- Supplement fish oil, which is high in omega-3 fatty acids, reduces inflammatory cytokines and may have modest benefits for appetite (see later).

If I have just diagnosed CHF in a dog and am starting to medicate the dog, should I try to also change his diet before discharge to help improve compliance with nutritional recommendations?

Do not make major dietary changes while the animal is hospitalized or just getting started on new medications. Most animals with acute CHF will not eat but should begin eating when the CHF is better controlled. While hospitalized, avoid diets that are high in sodium, but do not make major dietary changes during hospitalization. At the time of discharge or at the time of initiating CHF medications, owners should be instructed to avoid high-sodium treats, people foods, and high-sodium pill administration techniques. Once the animal is home, feeling better, and stabilized on medications, a gradual change to a new and more optimal diet can be made. Forced dietary changes when the animal is sick can induce food aversions. Most animals started on diuretics need a recheck examination in 7 to 14 days to check kidney values, electrolytes, and response to treatment; this is an ideal time to reevaluate the nutritional status and to optimize the overall nutritional plan, especially if the animal is feeling better and eating well. It also is important to instruct the owner to notify the veterinarian if the patient does not eat adequate amounts of the new recommended foods so that other options can be devised.

Which patients should be taking fish oil supplements?

We currently recommend fish oil supplementation for dogs and cats with alterations in appetite or muscle loss. In addition, fish oil supplementation is also recommended for most dogs with CHF if there are no contraindications, such as dietary fat intolerance or coagulopathies, at a daily dose of 40 mg/kg of EPA and 25 mg/kg of DHA. Finally, animals with cardiac arrhythmias (e.g., ventricular arrhythmias or atrial fibrillation) may benefit from supplementation. This level of EPA and DHA can be achieved in a few specially formulated commercial diets or can be supplemented with carefully selected fish oil supplements.

SUGGESTED READINGS

American College of Veterinary Nutrition website. Retrieved from www.acvn.org.

Atkins C, Bonagura J, Ettinger S, et al: Guidelines for the diagnosis and treatment of canine chronic valvular heart disease, J Vet Intern Med 23:1142, 2009.

Finn E, Freeman LM, Rush JE, et al: The relationship between body weight, body condition, and survival in cats with heart failure, J Vet Intern Med 24:1369, 2010.

Freeman LM, Rush JE, Kehayias JJ, et al: Nutritional alterations and the effect of fish oil supplementation in dogs with heart failure, J Vet Intern Med 12:440, 1998.

Freeman LM, Rush JE, Cahalane AK, et al: Dietary patterns in dogs with cardiac disease, J Am Vet Med Assoc 223:1301, 2003.

Freeman LM, Rush JE, Farabaugh AE, et al: Assessment of health-related quality of life in dogs with cardiac disease, J Am Vet Med Assoc 226:2005, 1864.

Freeman LM, Rush JE, Milbury PE, et al: Antioxidant status and biomarkers of oxidative stress in dogs with congestive heart failure, J Vet Intern Med 19:537, 2005.

Freeman LM, Rush JE, Markwell PJ: Effects of dietary modification in dogs with early chronic valvular disease, J Vet Intern Med 20:1116, 2006.

Freeman LM: Beneficial effects of omega-3 fatty acids in cardiovascular disease, J Small Anim Pract 51:462, 2010.

Freeman LM: Cachexia and sarcopenia: Emerging syndromes of importance in dogs and cats, J Vet Intern Med 26:3, 2012.

Freeman LM, Rush JE, Oyama MA, et al.: Development and evaluation of a questionnaire for assessing health-related quality of life in cats with cardiac disease, J Am Vet Med Assoc 240:1188, 2012.

Freeman LM, Rush JE, Meurs KM, et al.: Body size and metabolic differences in Maine Coon cats with and without hypertrophic cardiomyopathy, J Feline Med Surg 5:74, 2013.

Hall DJ, Freeman LM, Rush JE, et al.: Comparison of serum fatty acid concentrations in cats with cardiomyopathy and healthy controls, J Feline Med Surg 16:631, 2013.

Hutchinson D, Freeman LM, Schreiner KE, et al.: Survey of opinions about nutritional requirements of senior dogs and analysis of nutrient profiles of commercially available diets for senior dogs, Intl J Vet Res Vet Med 9:68, 2011.

Mallery KF, Freeman LM, Harpster NK, et al.: Factors contributing to the euthanasia decision in dogs with congestive heart failure, J Am Vet Med Assoc 214:1201, 1999.

Rush JE, Freeman LM, Brown DJ, et al.: Clinical, echocardiographic, and neurohormonal effects of a low sodium diet in dogs with heart failure, J Vet Intern Med 14:513, 2000.

Slupe JL, Freeman LM, Rush JE: The relationship between body weight, body condition, and survival in dogs with heart failure, J Vet Intern Med 22:561, 2008.

Smith CE, Freeman LM, Rush JE, et al.: Omega-3 fatty acids in Boxer dogs with arrhythmogenic right ventricular cardiomyopathy, J Vet Intern Med 21:265, 2007.

Smith CE, Freeman LM, Meurs KM, et al.: Plasma fatty acid concentrations in Boxers and Doberman pinschers, Am J Vet Res 69:195, 2008.

Torin DS, Freeman LM, Rush JE: Dietary patterns of cats with cardiac disease, J Am Vet Med Assoc 230:862, 2007.

Tufts Cummings School of Veterinary Medicine. Heart Smart website. Retrieved from www.tufts.edu/vet/heartsmart.

World Small Animal Veterinary Association Global Nutrition Committee. Short diet history form. Retrieved from www.wsava.org/nutrition-toolkit.

World Small Animal Veterinary Association Global Nutrition Committee. Body condition score chart for cats. Retrieved from www.wsava.org/nutrition-toolkit.

World Small Animal Veterinary Association Global Nutrition Committee. Muscle condition score chart. Retrieved from www.wsava.org/nutrition-toolkit.

World Small Animal Veterinary Association Nutritional Assessment Guidelines Taskforce Freeman L, Becvarova I, Cave N, et al.: 2011. Nutritional Assessment Guidelines, J Small Anim Pract 52:385, 2011.

Yang VK, Freeman LM, Rush JE: Morphometric measurements and insulin-like growth factor in normal cats and cats with hypertrophic cardiomyopathy, Am J Vet Res 69:1061, 2008.

Canine and Feline Breed Predilections for Heart Disease

APPENDIX 1

Kathleen E. Cavanagh | Francis W. K. Smith, Jr.

Canine Breed	Disease
Affenpinscher	PDA (AU)
Afghan Hound	DCM
Airedale	PS
Akita	VSD
Basset Hound	PS
	VSD
Beagle	PS
	VSD
	Bundle branch block (AU)
	Tetralogy of Fallot (AU)
Bearded Collie	SAS (AU)
Bichon Frisé	PDA
	Degenerative valve disease
Bloodhound	SAS
Border Terrier	Aortic body tumors (AU)
	VSD (AU)
Boston Terrier	Degenerative valve disease
	DCM
	Chemodectoma (± pericardial effusion)
	PDA (AU)
Bouvier des Flandres	SAS
Boxer	SAS
	PS
	ASD
	DCM
	Arrhythmogenic right ventricular cardiomyopathy (Boxer cardiomyopathy)
	Chemodectoma (± pericardial effusion)
	Endocardial fibroelastosis (AU)
	HCM (Cambridge)
Boykin Spaniel	PS
	Degenerative valve disease
Brittany Spaniel	Persistent right aortic arch

ASD, Atrial septal defect; *AU,* author; *DCM,* Dilated cardiomyopathy; *HCM,* hypertrophic cardiomyopathy; *PDA,* patent ductus arteriosus; *PS,* pulmonic stenosis; *SAS,* subaortic stenosis; *VSD,* ventricular septal defect.

Canine Breed	Disease
British Bulldog	Arteriovenous fistula (AU)
	Mitral valve disease (AU)
	PS (AU)
Bullmastiff	PS
	DCM
Bull Terrier	Mitral valve dysplasia
	Mitral valve stenosis
	SAS
Cavalier King Charles Spaniel	Inherited ventricular arrhythmias
	Right atrial hemangiosarcoma (± pericardial effusion)
	PDA
	Degenerative (myxomatous mitral) valve disease
	Femoral artery occlusion (AU)
Chihuahua	PDA
	PS
	Degenerative valve disease
Chow Chow	PS
	VSD
Cocker Spaniel (American, English)	PDA (American, English)
	PS
	Degenerative valve disease
	DCM (American, English)
	Sick sinus syndrome (American, English)
Cocker Spaniel, American	Cardiomyopathy (AU)
	PDA (AU)
Collie (rough and smooth)	PDA
Dachshund	Degenerative valve disease
	Mitral valve prolapse
	Sick sinus syndrome
	PDA
Dalmatian	DCM
	Mitral valve dysplasia
Doberman Pinscher	ASD
	DCM
	Bundle of His degeneration
	Persistent right aortic arch (AU)
Dogue de Bordeaux	SAS

Continued

405

Canine Breed	Disease
English Bulldog (Bulldog)	PS
	Tetralogy of Fallot
	VSD
	SAS
	Chemodectoma (± pericardial effusion)
	Mitral valve dysplasia
	Persistent right aortic arch
English Sheepdog	DCM
English Springer Spaniel	PDA
	VSD
	Persistent atrial standstill
Estrela Mountain Dog	DCM (Cambridge)
Fox Terrier	Degenerative valve disease
	PS (wirehaired and smooth)
	Tetralogy of Fallot (wirehaired)
	Persistent right aortic arch (AU) (wirehaired and smooth)
French Bulldog	PS (Cambridge)
German Pinscher	Persistent right aortic arch
German Shepherd	SAS
	Mitral valve dysplasia
	Tricuspid valve dysplasia
	Persistent right aortic arch
	Inherited ventricular arrhythmia (tachycardia) (AU) (Cambridge Veterinary School Database) is Hereditary Ventricular Tachycardia
	Right atrial hemangiosarcoma (± pericardial effusion)
	Infective endocarditis
	DCM
	PDA
	Cardiomyopathy (AU)
German Shorthair Pointer	SAS
Golden Retriever	SAS
	Mitral valve dysplasia
	Tricuspid valve dysplasia
	Taurine deficient familial DCM
	Canine X-linked muscular dystrophy
	Pericardial effusion, idiopathic
	Right atrial hemangiosarcoma (± pericardial effusion)
Great Dane	Mitral valve dysplasia
	Tricuspid valve dysplasia
	SAS
	PS
	Persistent right aortic arch
	DCM
	Lone atrial fibrillation
Great Pyrenees	Tricuspid valve dysplasia
Greyhound	Persistent right aortic arch
Husky	VSD

Canine Breed	Disease
Irish Setter	Persistent right aortic arch
	DCM
	Right atrial hemangiosarcoma (± pericardial effusion)
	Tricuspid dysplasia (Cambridge)
Irish Wolfhound	DCM
	Lone atrial fibrillation
Italian Greyhound	Persistent right aortic arch (AU)
Keeshond (Keeshonden)	Conotruncal defects (CTD) includes conal septum, conal VSD, tetralogy of Fallot, and persistent truncus arteriosus
	PDA
	PS
	Mitral valve dysplasia
Kerry Blue Terrier	PDA
Labrador Retriever	Tricuspid valve dysplasia
	PDA
	PS
	DCM
	Pericardial effusion, idiopathic
	Right atrial hemangiosarcoma (± pericardial effusion)
	Supraventricular tachycardia (Cambridge)
Lakeland Terrier	VSD
Lhasa Apso	Degenerative valve disease
Maltese	PDA
	Mitral dysplasia (Cambridge)
Mastiff	Mitral valve dysplasia
	PS
	Tricuspid valve dysplasia (Cambridge)
Miniature Pinscher	Degenerative valve disease
Newfoundland	SAS
	Mitral valve dysplasia
	Mitral valve stenosis
	PDA
	PS
	DCM
	ASD
	VSD (AU)
New Zealand Huntaway Dog	DCM (Cambridge)
Norfolk Terrier	Mitral valve disease (AU)
	Syncope (AU)
Old English Sheepdog	Tricuspid valve dysplasia
	Persistent atrial standstill
	DCM
Pekingese	Degenerative valve disease
Pembroke Welsh Corgi	PDA (Cambridge)
Poodle	PDA (toy and miniature)
	Degenerative mitral valve disease (toy and miniature)
	VSD (toy and miniature) (AU)
	ASD (standard)
Pomeranian	PDA
	Degenerative valve disease
	Sick sinus syndrome

Canine Breed	Disease
Portuguese Water Dog	Juvenile DCM
Pug	Atrioventricular block (SYN: stenosis of the bundle of His as per Cambridge)
Rottweiler	SAS
	DCM
	HCM (Cambridge)
	Mitral dysplasia (Cambridge)
Saint Bernard	DCM
Saluki	PDA (Cambridge)
Samoyed	PS
	SAS
	ASD
Schnauzer, Miniature	PS
	PDA
	Degenerative valve disease
	Sick sinus syndrome
Schnauzer, Standard	PS (AU, Cambridge)
Scottish Deerhound	DCM
Scottish Terrier	PS
Shetland	PDA
Sheepdog	Degenerative valve disease
	Conotruncal heart malformation (AU)
Shih Tzu	VSD
	Degenerative valve disease
Springer Spaniel	DCM
Sussex Spaniel	Cardiomyopathy (AU)
Terriers (e.g., Fox Terrier, Mixed Terriers)	PS
	Degenerative valve disease
Weimaraner	Tricuspid valve dysplasia
	Peritoneopericardial diaphragmatic hernia
Welsh Corgi (Pembroke)	PDA (AU)
West Highland White Terrier	PS
	VSD
	Tetralogy of Fallot
	Degenerative valve disease
	Sick sinus syndrome (Cambridge)
Whippet	Degenerative valve disease
Yorkshire Terrier	PDA
	Degenerative valve disease

ASD, Atrial septal defect; *AU,* author; *DCM,* Dilated cardiomyopathy; *HCM,* hypertrophic cardiomyopathy; *PDA,* patent ductus arteriosus; *PS,* pulmonic stenosis; *SAS,* subaortic stenosis; *VSD,* ventricular septal defect.

RESOURCES

Alroy J, Rush JE, Freeman L, et al: Inherited infantile dilated cardiomyopathy in dogs: genetic, clinical, biochemical, and morphologic findings, Am J Med Genet 95:57–66, 2000.

Basso C, Fox PR, Meurs KM, et al: Arrhythmogenic right ventricular cardiomyopathy causing sudden cardiac death in boxer dogs: a new animal model of human disease, Circulation 109:1180–1185, 2004.

Bélanger MC, Ouellet M, Queney G, et al: Taurine-deficient dilated cardiomyopathy in a family of Golden Retrievers, J Am Anim Hosp Assoc 41:284–291, 2005.

Chetboul V, Charles V, et al: Retrospective study of 156 atrial septal defects in dogs and cats, J Vet Med A Physiol Pathol Clin Med 53:179–184, 2006.

Chetboul V, Trolle JM, et al: Congenital heart diseases in the Boxer dog: a retrospective study of 105 cases (1998-2005), J Vet Med A Physiol Pathol Clin Med 53:346–351, 2006.

Dambach DM, Lannon A, Sleeper MM, et al: Familial dilated cardiomyopathy of young Portuguese Water dogs, J Vet Intern Med 13:65, 1999.

Fox PR, Sisson D, Moïse NS, eds: Textbook of canine and feline cardiology, ed 2, Philadelphia, 1999, WB Saunders.

Gordon SG, Saunders AB, et al: Atrial septal defects in an extended family of standard poodles, In *Proceedings,* The Annual ACVIM Forum, p 730, 2006.

Gunby JM, Hardie RJ, Bjorling DE: Investigation of the potential heritability of persistent right aortic arch in Greyhounds, J Am Vet Med Assoc 224:1120–1122, 2004.

Hyun C, Lavulo L: Congenital heart diseases in small animals. I. Genetic pathways and potential candidate genes, Vet J 171:245–255, 2006. Comment in Vet J 171:195, 2006.

Hyun C, Park IC: Congenital heart diseases in small animals. II. Potential genetic aetiologies based on human genetic studies, Vet J 171:256, 2006. Comment in Vet J 171:195, 2006.

Kittleson MD, Kienle RD, eds: Small animal cardiovascular medicine, Philadelphia, 1998, Mosby.

MacDonald KA: Congenital heart diseases of puppies and kittens, Vet Clin North Am Small Anim Pract 36:503–531, 2006.

Meurs KM: Inherited heart disease in the dog, In *Proceedings,* 2003 Tufts Genetics Symposium, 2003.

Meurs KM: Update on Boxer arrhythmogenic right ventricular cardiomyopathy (ARVC), In *Proceedings,* The Annual ACVIM Forum, p 106, 2005.

Meurs KM, Fox PR, Nogard M, et al: A prospective genetic evaluation of familial dilated cardiomyopathy in the Doberman Pinscher, J Vet Intern Med 21:1016, 2007.

Meurs KM, Spier AW, Miller MW, et al: Familial ventricular arrhythmias in boxers, J Vet Intern Med 13:437–439, 1999.

Meurs KM, Spier AW, Wright NA, et al: Comparison of the effects of four antiarrhythmic treatments for familial ventricular arrhythmias in Boxers, J Am Vet Med Assoc 221:522, 2002.

Moïse NS: Update on inherited arrhythmias in German Shepherds, In *Proceedings,* The Annual ACVIM Forum, pp 67–68, 2005.

Olsen LH, Fredholm M, Pedersen HD: Epidemiology and inheritance of mitral valve prolapse in Dachshunds, J Vet Intern Med 13:448–456, 1999.

Phillip U, Menzel J, Distl O: A rare form of persistent right aorta arch in linkage disequilibrium with the DiGeorge critical region on CFA26 in German Pinschers, J Hered 102(Suppl 1):S68–S73, 2011.

Parker HG, Meurs KM, Ostrander EA: Finding cardiovascular disease genes in the dog, J Vet Cardiol 8:115–127, 2006.

Schober KE, Baade H: Doppler echocardiographic prediction of pulmonary hypertension in West Highland white terriers with chronic pulmonary disease, J Vet Intern Med 20:912, 2006.

Spier AW, Meurs KM, Muir WW, et al: Correlation of QT dispersion with indices used to evaluate the severity of familial ventricular arrhythmias in Boxers, Am J Vet Res 62:1481–1485, 2001.

Tidholm A: Retrospective study of congenital heart defects in 151 dogs, J Small Anim Pract 38:94–98, 2006.

Vollmar AC, Fox PR: Assessment of cardiovascular diseases in 527 Boxers, In Proceedings, The Annual ACVIM Forum, p 65, 2005.

Vollmar AC, Trötschel C: Cardiomyopathy in Irish Wolfhounds, In Proceedings, The Annual ACVIM Forum, p 66, 2005.

Werner P, Raducha MG, Prociuk U, et al: The Keeshond defect in cardiac conotruncal development is oligogenic, Human Genet 116:368–377, 2005.

GENETIC AND HEALTH DATABASES AND RESOURCES ACCESSED

Bell JS, Cavanagh KE, Tilley LP, Smith FWK: Veterinary medical guide to dog and cat breeds, Jackson, WY, 2012, Teton New Media.

Chetboul V, Petit A, Gouni V, et al: Prospective echocardiographic and tissue Doppler screening of a large Sphynx cat population: reference ranges, heart disease prevalence and genetic aspects, J Vet Cardiology 14:497–509, 2012.

National Institutes of Health Library: Retrieved from www.ncbi.nlm.nih.gov/pmc/.

Online mendelian inheritance in animals: Retrieved from http://omia.angis.org.au/home/.

Online mendelian inheritance in man: Retrieved from www.ncbi.nlm.nih.gov/omim.

Pub Med Literature Database: Retrieved from www.ncbi.nlm.nih.gov/pubmed/.

Sargan, DR: Cambridge Veterinary School Database: Retrieved from www.vet.cam.ac.uk/idid/ IDID: inherited diseases in dogs: web-based information for canine inherited disease genetics, Mamm Genome 15:503–506, 2004. (Cambridge).

University of Australia Faculty of Veterinary Medicine Database (LIDA): Retrieved from http://sydney.edu.au/vetscience/lida/ (AU).

UPEI Canine Inherited Disorders Database: Retrieved from www.upei.ca/cidd/intro.htm.

Feline	
Breed	**Disease**
Abyssinian	Subvalvular pulmonary stenosis
Birman	Systemic hypertension
British Shorthair	Hypertrophic cardiomyopathy Septal defect
Burmese	Septal defect Congenital heart defect
Chartreux	Septal defect Systemic hypertension
Devon Rex	Subvalvular pulmonary stenosis
Maine Coon	Hypertrophic cardiomyopathy Septal defect
Norwegian Forest	Hypertrophic cardiomyopathy
Persian	Systemic hypertension Septal defect
Ragdoll	Hypertrophic cardiomyopathy
Siamese	Systemic hypertension Septal defect Congenital heart defect Mitral valve stenosis PDA Subaortic stenosis Supravalvular aortic stenosis Tetralogy of Fallot Tricuspid stenosis
Siberian	Hypertrophic cardiomyopathy
Sphynx	HCM MVD

HCM, Hypertrophic cardiomyopathy; *MVD,* mitral valve disease; *PDA,* patent ductus arteriosus.

Cardiopulmonary Drug Formulary

APPENDIX 2

Francis W. K. Smith, Jr. | Larry P. Tilley | Mark A. Oyama | Meg M. Sleeper

DISCLOSURE

Advancing technology has provided clinicians with ever more powerful and effective drugs for treating diseases. As more drugs become available, it becomes progressively more difficult for practitioners to make rational choices between similar drugs. It is also difficult to be aware of the numerous side effects, contraindications, and drug interactions of the many cardiopulmonary drugs available. The following tables and charts have been designed and provided in the hope of facilitating rational drug selections for the treatment of cardiopulmonary disease.

An attempt has been made to make these tables as complete as possible, while focusing on the more common or serious side effects and drug interactions. For a more exhaustive review of individual drugs, the reader should refer to the package insert and chapters in this book. The reader should also follow the current veterinary literature because new dosing recommendations may become available as a result of clinical use and scientific research. This advice is especially appropriate for new or infrequently used drugs.

Medicine is a science that is constantly changing. Changes in treatment and drug therapy are required with new research and clinical experiences. The author, editor, and publisher of this book have made every effort to ensure that the drug dosage schedules are accurate. The drug dosages are based on the standards accepted at the time of publication. The product information sheet included in the package of each drug should be checked before the drug is administered to be certain that changes have not been made in the recommended dose of or in the contraindications for administration. Primary responsibility for decisions regarding treatment of patients remains with the attending clinician. All patients should be carefully monitored for desired efficacious and undesired toxic effects while instituting, titrating, and maintaining therapy.

Drugs are listed in alphabetical order by generic name. The order of presentation in no way reflects the preference for use. General recommendations for therapy may be found in the main body of this book.

KEY TO FORMULARY ABBREVIATIONS

ACE	angiotensin-converting enzyme
ACT	activated clotting time
ADP	adenosine diphosphate
APTT	activated partial thromboplastin time
BP	blood pressure
Cap	capsule
CHF	congestive heart failure
COPD	chronic obstructive pulmonary disease
CRI	continuous rate infusion
CPR	cardiopulmonary resuscitation
DCM	dilated cardiomyopathy
ECG	electrocardiogram
G	gram
GFR	glomerular filtration rate
GI	gastrointestinal
HCM	hypertrophic cardiomyopathy
IM	intramuscular
Inj	injectable
IO	intraosseous
IT	intratracheal
IV	intravenous
LRS	lactated Ringer solution
μg	micrograms
mg	milligram
mL	milliliter
PO	per os (oral)
PT	prothrombin time
q	every, as in q8h = every 8 hours
SC	subcutaneous
U	units

409

Cardiopulmonary Drugs—Formulations, Indications, and Dosages

DRUG TRADE NAME	FORMULATION	INDICATIONS	DOG DOSE (D) CAT DOSE (C)	COMMENTS
Acetylsalicylic acid Aspirin	Tab: 81, 325 mg	Prevention of thromboembolism	D: 5-10 mg/kg PO q24-48h C: 25 mg/kg PO q 3 days (81 mg/cat PO q48-72h)	Nonsteroidal antiinflammatory agent Platelet inhibitor Not effective in all animals May decrease efficacy of ACE inhibitors
Albuterol (Proventil, Ventolin, AccuNeb, Vospire, ProAir, generic)	Tab: 2, 4, 8 mg Syrup: 2mg/5mL Inhalation aerosol: 90 μg per actuation Nebulizing solution: 0.63, 1.25, and 2.5 mg/3 ml and 5 mg/ml	Bronchodilation in patients with reversible obstructive lung disease and asthma Collapsed trachea	D,C: 20-50 μg/kg PO q8h Emergency: 90 μg by metered dose inhalation every 30 min up to 4-6 hours	Beta-2 agonist bronchodilator Reduce dose by 50% first 4 days to prevent anxiety side-effect Decrease dose with renal disease Feline aerosol chamber (www.aerokat.com) can facilitate administration
Amiodarone (Cordarone, generic)	Tab: 200 mg Inj: 50 mg/mL	Indicated for severe refractory atrial and ventricular arrhythmias	D: Loading dose of 10 mg/kg PO q12h for 1 week; thereafter 5 mg/kg PO q12-24h C: None	Class III antiarrhythmic with some Class I, II, and IV effects Use as last resort for recurrent unstable ventricular tachycardia; takes weeks to achieve therapeutic levels Side effects include anorexia, liver, thyroid, and pulmonary dysfunction
Amlodipine besylate (Norvasc, generic)	Tab: 2.5, 5, 10 mg	Systemic hypertension, refractory heart failure	D: 2.5 mg/dog or 0.1 mg/kg PO q24h C: 0.18 mg/kg PO q24h (0.625-1.25 mg/cat q24h). Can increase to q12h in refractory cases	Dihydropyridine calcium channel blocker Arteral vasodilator; monitor for hypotension Ging val hyperplasia in small % of dogs Generally first choice for systemic hypertension in cats
Atenolol (Tenormin, generic)	Tab: 25, 50, 100 mg Oral suspension: 25 mg/ml Inj: 0.5 mg/ml	Atrial and ventricular arrhythmias, hypertrophic cardiomyopathy (outflow obstruction), systemic hypertension, aortic stenosis, cardiac manifestations of hyperthyroidism	D: 0.25-2.0 mg/kg PO q12-24h C: 6.25-12.5 mg PO q12-24h	Beta-1 selective beta blocker Less bronchoconstriction and vasoconstriction than nonselective beta blockers Taper dose when discontinuing therapy Avoid in CHF; can be cautiously used once congestion controlled
Atropine sulfate (generic)	Inj: 0.05, 0.1, 0.3, 0.4, 0.5, 0.8, 1.0 mg/mL	Sinus bradycardia, AV block, sick sinus syndrome, cardiac arrest	D: 0.01-0.04 mg/kg IV, IM, IO 0.02-0.04 mg/kg SC q6-8h (IT: double dose) C: Same	Anticholinergic May transiently worsen bradyarrhythmia Preoperatively, use with caution and only with bradycardia in cardiac cases

Drug	Formulations	Indications	Dosage	Notes
Benazepril (Fortekor, Lotensin, generic)	Tab: 5, 10, 20, 40 mg	Balanced vasodilation in CHF, systemic hypertension. Approved for feline renal disease in other countries	D: 0.25-0.5 mg/kg PO q24h; C: 0.25-0.5 mg/kg PO q24h (2.5 mg/cat/day)	Angiotensin-converting enzyme inhibitor. Monitor electrolytes and renal function. Excreted in bile and urine
Buprenorphine (Buprenex)	Inj: 0.324 mg/ml	Pain control following aortic thromboembolism	C: 0.005-0.1 mg/kg IV, IM	Opioid agonist
Butorphanol tartrate (Torbutrol, Stadol, generic)	Inj: 0.5, 1, 2 mg/m_ Tab: 1, 5, 10 mg (Torbutrol)	Nonproductive cough (COPD, tracheal collapse, left atrial compression of left mainstem bronchus)	D: 0.055-0.11 mg/kg SC q6-12h; 0.55 mg/kg PO q6-12h. C: None	Narcotic cough suppressant. More potent than dextromethorphan
Calcium gluconate	Inj: 100 mg/ml (10%), 230 mg/ml (23%)	Acute management of severe cardiac manifestations of hyperkalemia	D, C: 50-20 mg/kg slow IV (5-15 min)	Normalizes ionic gradients in myocytes without altering potassium levels. Monitor ECG while administering; discontinue if QT shortening, VPCs, or sudden slowing of the heart rate occur
Carnitine (Carnitor, generic)	Tab: 330 mg. Can be purchased in bulk as a powder	Canine dilated cardiomyopathy accompanied by carnitine deficiency	D: 50-100 mg/kg PO q8h; C: None	Amino acid. L isomer is active form. Not effective in all cases
Carvedilol (Coreg, generic)	Tab: 3.125, 6.25, 12.5, 25 mg. Cap (Extended Release): 10, 20, 40, 80 mg. Pharmacokinetics of extended release caps has not been evaluated in dogs	Myocardial failure	D: 0.2-0.4 mg/kg q12h (based on pharmacokinetic studies may be able to titrate to 1.5 mg/kg PO q12h if tolerated). Start slowly at 0.05-0.1 mg/kg PO q12h for 2 weeks; up-titrate the dose every 2-4 weeks. C: Not established	Alpha and nonselective beta blocker. Do not use with AV block. Monitor closely for worsening of heart failure. Absorption highly variable in dogs
Chlorothiazide (Diuril, generic)	Tab: 250, 500 mg. Oral suspension 50 mg/mL	Diseases associated with fluid retention (CHF, hepatic disease, nephrotic syndrome), end stage heart failure (ascites)	D: 20-40 mg/kg PO q12h; C: Same	Thiazide diuretic. Less potent than loop diuretics. Not effective with low GFR (renal failure). Can use with loop diuretics for increased diuresis, but reduce initial thiazide dose by 50%. May precipitate hepatic encephalopathy in patients with severe liver disease

Continued

Cardiopulmonary Drugs—Formulations, Indications, and Dosages—cont'd

DRUG TRADE NAME	FORMULATION	INDICATIONS	DOG DOSE (D) CAT DOSE (C)	COMMENTS
Clopidogrel (Plavix, generic)	Tab: 75, 300 mg	Prevention of aortic thromboembolism in cats that have already had a thromboembolic event or are at high risk for thromboembolism	D: 0.5-1 mg/kg PO q24h Loading dose of 2-4 mg/kg may be followed with 1 mg/kg q24h C: 18.75 mg PO q24h; loading dose of 37.5 mg immediately following embolism	Platelet inhibitor (ADP receptor blocker) More effective than aspirin in preventing recurrence of aortic thromboembolism Can be used in combination with aspirin or heparin; be aware of possibility of hemorrhage when using combinations Low risk of hemorrhage as sole agent May cause ptyalism because of distaste
Dalteparin (Fragmin)	Inj: 16 mg (2500 U)/0.2 mL; 32 mg (5000 U)/0.02 mL prefilled syringes; 64 mg (10,000 U)/mL multidose vials	Antithrombotic	D: 100-150 U/kg SC q8h C: 180 U/kg SC q6h	Low molecular weight heparin Dose extrapolated from humans and pharmacokinetic studies in animals; optimal dose in dogs and cats is unknown Less likely to cause bleeding complications than warfarin Expensive
Digoxin (Lanoxin, generic)	Tab: 0.0625, 0.125, 0.1875, 0.25 mg Elixir: 0.05 mg/mL	Supraventricular arrhythmias (especially atrial fibrillation), myocardial failure	D: *Maintenance dose:* 0.003-0.005 mg/kg PO q12h. Max. dose for Dobermans 0.25 mg q12h *Oral loading dose:* Twice the maintenance dose for the first 24-48 hours C: 0.01 mg/kg PO q48h (tab preferred) 0.007 mg/kg PO q48h (w/furosemide and aspirin); rarely used	Digitalis glycoside Toxicity potentiated by hypokalemia, hyponatremia, hypercalcemia, hypothyroidism, hypoxia Dose on lean body weight, reduce dose 10%-15% with elixirs Therapeutic range 0.5-1 ng/mL 8 hours after a dose Often used in combination with diltiazem or a beta blocker for rate control of atrial fibrillation
Diltiazem (Cardizem, Dilacor, generic)	Tab: 30, 60, 90, 120 mg Inj: 0.45, 0.83, 1.0 mg/mL Cardizem CD: 120, 180, 240, 300, 360 mg Dilacor XR: 120, 180, 240 mg	Supraventricular arrhythmias, hypertrophic cardiomyopathy, systemic hypertension	D: 0.5-2 mg/kg PO q8h (consider higher dose of 5mg/kg based on recent studies) 0.1-0.2 mg/kg IV bolus, then 2-6 µg/kg/min IV CRI Dilacor XR: 3-4 mg/kg PO q24h C: 1.0-2.5 mg/kg PO q8h 0.1-0.2 mg/kg IV bolus, then 2-6 µg/kg/min IV CRI Dilacor XR: 30-60 mg PO q24h	Calcium channel blocker Less myocardial depression than verapamil Dilacor XR capsules contain 60-mg tablets that are used for dosing cats Extended release formulations have unpredictable bioavailability and are often associated with anorexia, vomiting, weight loss, lethargy, and hepatopathy in cats Not as effective as beta blockers for treatment of left ventricular outflow tract obstruction

Drug	Indication	How supplied	Dosage	Comments
Dobutamine HCl (generic)	Short-term management of severe myocardial failure	Inj: 12.5 mg/mL	D: 2.5-20 μg/kg/min (titrate up to effect); administer in D5W C: 2-10 μg/kg/min (titrate up to effect); administer in D5W	Beta-adrenergic agonist Monitor ECG, BP, and pulse quality Preferable to dopamine in CHF but more expensive Inotropic effect is dose dependent Less arrhythmogenic than most other catecholamines Use with caution in cats; may cause seizures
Dopamine HCl (generic)	Shock, short-term management of severe myocardial failure Anuric or oliguric renal failure	Inj: 40, 80, or 160 mg/mL	D: 2-10 μg/kg/min (titrate up to effect); administer in D5W, saline, or LRS C: Same	Dopaminergic agonist Monitor ECG, blood pressure, and pulse quality; adjust dose based on response May cause tissue necrosis if extravasation occurs Can administer intraosseously
Doxycycline (Vibramycin and generic)	Adjunctive treatment for heartworm disease	Tab: 25, 75, 100, 150 mg Cap: 40, 50, 75, 100, 150 mg Oral suspension: 10 mg/mL Inj: 100, 200 mg vial	Heartworm treatment: 10 mg/kg PO q12h for 4 weeks before administering melarsomine	Tetracycline antibiotic effective against Wolbachia coinfection in heartworm disease Effect against Wolbachia enhanced by macrocyclic lactones Reduces disease associated with dead heartworms Disrupts heartworm transmission Enhances adulticide activity of macrocyclic lactones
Enalapril maleate (Enacard, Vasotec, generic)	Balanced vasodilation in CHF, systemic hypertension	Tab: 1, 2.5, 5, 10, 20 mg	D: 0.5 mg/kg PO q12-24h (titrate up to effect) C: 0.25-0.5 mg/kg PO q24-48h (titrate up to effect)	Angiotensin-converting enzyme inhibitor Monitor renal function and electrolytes Increased survival in heart failure patients Decrease dose with renal disease
Enoxaparin (Lovenox, generic)	Antithrombotic	Inj: 30mg/0.3 mL	D: 0.8 mg/kg SC q12h C: 1.25 mg/kg SC q12h	Low molecular weight heparin Dose extrapolated from humans and pharmacokinetic studies in animals; optimal dose in dogs and cats is unknown Less likely to cause bleeding complications than warfarin
Epinephrine (Adrenalin, generic)	Cardiac arrest	Inj: 1:1000 conc (1 mg/mL) 1:10000 conc (0.1 mg/mL)	D: 0.1-0.2 mg/kg IV, IO q3-5 min Double dose for IT administration C: Same	Beta-adrenergic agonist Previously recommended dose of 0.01-0.02 mg/kg may be a safer starting dose if a defibrillator is not available Vasopressin may be more effective

Continued

Cardiopulmonary Drugs—Formulations, Indications, and Dosages—cont'd

DRUG TRADE NAME	FORMULATION	INDICATIONS	DOG DOSE (D) CAT DOSE (C)	COMMENTS
Esmolol (Brevibloc, generic)	Inj: 10 mg/mL	Short-term management of supraventricular tachyarrhythmias, ventricular tachycardia, and systemic hypertension	D,C: 50-100 μg/kg IV bolus every 5 min (up to 500 μg/kg max) 25-200 μg/kg/min CRI	Ultra-short-acting beta-1 selective beta-adrenergic blocker
Fluticasone (Flovent)	Metered dose inhaler: 44, 110, 220 μg/actuation	Feline asthma, chronic bronchitis	D: <20 kg, 110 μg via metered dose (activation) q12h; >20 kg, 220 μg via metered dose q12 C: 110-220 μg via metered dose (activation) q12h (higher dose reserved for severe disease); or 220 μg via metered dose q24	Corticosteroid Feline aerosol chamber (www.aerokat.com) can facilitate administration
Furosemide (Lasix, generic)	Tab: 12.5, 20, 40, 50, 80 mg Inj: 10 and 50 mg/mL Oral solution: 10 mg/mL	Diseases associated with fluid retention (CHF, hepatic disease, nephrotic syndrome), systemic hypertension	D: 2-6 mg/kg PO, IM, IV q8-48h 2-8 mg/kg IV q1-2h for severe pulmonary edema CRI: 0.66 mg/kg IV bolus followed by 0.66 mg/kg/h IV C: 1-4 mg/kg PO, IM, IV q12-48h Titrate to lowest effective dose for maintenance	Loop diuretic Decreased oral absorption in decompensated CHF Monitor hydration and electrolytes; hypokalemia uncommon in dogs unless anorexic or high dose Bioavailability reduced with food Cats usually dislike taste of oral solution Can use in combination with other classes of diuretics in refractory CHF
Glycopyrrolate (Robinul, Cuvposa, Glycate, generic)	Inj: 0.2 mg/mL	Sinus bradycardia, AV block, sick sinus syndrome	D: 0.005-0.01 mg/kg IV, IM, 0.01-0.02 mg/kg SC C: Same	Anticholinergic Longer duration of action Preoperatively, use with caution and only with bradycardia in cardiac cases
Heparin (Calciparine, Liquaemin, generic)	Inj: 1000, 5000, 10,000 U/mL	Short-term prevention of thromboembolism	D: Loading dose: 100-500 U/kg SC q8h Chronic dose: 10-50 U/kg q6-8h C: Loading dose: 100-300 U/kg SC q8h Chronic dose: 10-50 U/kg q6-8h	Anticoagulant Antidote: Protamine sulfate Maintain APTT or ACT at 2-2.5 times the pretreatment values

Drug	Formulation	Indication	Dose	Comments
Hydralazine HCl (Apresoline, generic)	Tab: 10, 25, 50, 100 mg Inj: 20 mg/mL	Arterial dilation in CHF, systemic hypertension	D: 1-3 mg/kg PO q12h (titrate up to effect) C: 0.5-0.8 mg/kg PO q12h	Direct acting arterial vasodilator Causes sodium retention, requiring increased diuretic doses Reflex tachycardia can be controlled with digitalis Decreasing dose 50%-75% for 1-2 weeks and then titrating upward may reduce risk of vomiting Can use injectable formulation orally for more accurate dosing in small patients Use largely replaced by amlodipine because of superior efficacy and tolerability
Hydrochlorothiazide (Microzide, generic)	Tab: 12.5, 25, 50, 100 mg Cap: 12.5	Diseases associated with fluid retention (CHF, hepatic disease, nephrotic syndrome), systemic hypertension, end stage heart failure (ascites)	D: 2-4 mg/kg PO q12h C: Same	Thiazide diuretic Less potent than loop diuretics Not effective with low GFR (renal failure) Can use with loop diuretics for increased diuresis, but reduce initial thiazide dose by 50%
Hydrocodone bitartrate (Tussigon, generic)	Tab: 5 mg Syrup: 1 mg/mL	Nonproductive cough (COPD, tracheal collapse, left atrial compression of the mainstem bronchus)	D: 0.22 mg/kg PO q6-12h C: Do not use	Narcotic antagonist More potent than dextromethorphan
Hyoscyamine (Anaspaz, Cystospaz, Donnamar, Levsin, generic)	Tab: 0.125 mg	Rate control in sick sinus syndrome and AV block	D: 0.003-0.006 mg/kg PO q8h	Anticholinergic
Imidapril (Prilium [Europe, Canada])	Oral liquid: 5, 10 mg/ml	Balanced vasodilation in CHF, systemic hypertension	D: 0.25-0.5 mg/kg q24h C: 0.5 mg/kg PO q24h	Angiotensin–converting enzyme inhibitor Monitor renal function and electrolytes Decrease dose with renal disease
Isoproterenol (Isuprel, generic)	Inj: 1:5000 (0.2 mg/mL)	Short-term management of severe bradycardia unresponsive to atropine (sinus bradycardia, AV block, sick sinus syndrome)	D: 0.04-0.09 µg/kg/min IV (titrate up to effect) 10 µg/kg/min IM, SC q6h C: Same	Sympathomimetic agent Used as an emergency treatment until artificial pacing can be accomplished
Isosorbide dinitrate (Isordil Titradose, Isochron, generic)	Tab: 5, 10, 20, 30, 40 mg	End stage CHF	D: 0.2-1.0 mg/kg PO q12h C: Same	Nitrate venodilator Can combine with hydralazine for balanced vasodilation Schedule 12-hour drug-free period to try and avoid tolerance Efficacy uncertain

Continued

Cardiopulmonary Drugs—Formulations, Indications, and Dosages—cont'd

DRUG TRADE NAME	FORMULATION	INDICATIONS	DOG DOSE (D) CAT DOSE (C)	COMMENTS
Lidocaine (Xylocaine, generic)	Inj: 5, 10, 15, 20 mg/mL (without epinephrine)	Ventricular arrhythmias	D: 2 mg/kg slowly IV or IO (double the dose IT) in 2 mg/kg boluses followed by IV drip at 30-80 (occasionally up to 100) μg/kg/min CRI C: 0.25-0.75 mg/kg IV over 5 min	Class I antiarrhythmic Use with caution in cats as may cause seizures Drug of choice for initial control of ventricular tachycardia Effects increased by high potassium and decreased by low potassium
Lisinopril (Prinivil, Zestril, generic)	Tab: 2.5, 5, 10, 20, 30, 40 mg	Balanced vasodilation in CHF, systemic hypertension	D: 0.25-0.5 mg/kg PO q12-24h	Angiotensin-converting enzyme inhibitor Monitor renal function and electrolytes Decrease dose with renal disease
Magnesium (generic)	20% MgCl₂ solution for injection (contains 1.97 mEq of Mg++ per mL)	Refractory ventricular arrhythmias; torsade de pointes	D: 0.75-1 mEq/kg/24h IV infusion (50% of total dose can be given in 2-4 hours if necessary); for ventricular fibrillation: 0.15-0.30 mEq/kg IV over 5-10 min	Electrolyte Hypomagnesemia may potentiate ventricular tachycardia
Melarsomine (Immiticide)	Inj: 25 mg/mL	Heartworm disease	D: 2.5 mg/kg IM give a single injection of 2.5 mg/kg and then in one month give two additional doses 24 hours apart C: None	Heartworm adulticide Administer via deep IM injection Many heartworm experts recommend split dose (as for Class III patients) also for Class I and II Doxycycline may be administered for 4 weeks before melarsomine treatment to reduce pulmonary reaction
Methoxamine (Vasoxyl)	Inj: 20 mg/mL injection	Used primarily in critical care patients or during anesthesia to increase peripheral resistance and increase blood pressure	D, C: 200-250 μg/kg IM, or 40-80 μg/kg IV; repeat dose as needed	Sympathomimetic. Alpha-1 adrenergic agonist Short onset and duration of action Adverse effects related to excessive stimulation of alpha-1 receptor (prolonged peripheral vasoconstriction) Reflex bradycardia may occur
Metoprolol (Lopressor, generic)	Tab: 25, 50, 100 mg Inj: 1 mg/mL	Atrial and ventricular arrhythmias, hypertrophic cardiomyopathy, systemic hypertension, myocardial failure	D: 0.25-1.0 mg/kg PO q8h C: Same	Beta-1 selective beta blocker Less bronchoconstriction and interference with insulin therapy than with nonselective beta blockers Taper dose when stopping Dose should be slowly titrated over several weeks in dogs with myocardial failure

Drug	Formulation	Indication	Dose	Comments
Mexiletine (generic)	Cap: 150, 200, 250 mg	Ventricular arrhythmias	D: 4-8 mg/kg PO q8-12h C: None	Class I antiarrhythmic Reduce dose with liver disease Take with food to reduce GI side effects
Nitroglycerin (Nitro-BID, Nitroquick, Nitrostat, Nitrolingual, Nitro-Dur, Minitran, generic)	2% ointment (1 inch = 15 mg) Transdermal patch: 0.1, 0.2, 0.3, 0.4, 0.6, 0.8 mg/hour	Usually used for short-term management of acute CHF End-stage CHF	D: 0.25 inch/5 kg cutaneously q6-8h; Patch: 2.5-10 mg (small-giant dog) C: 1/8-1/4 inch cutaneously q6-8h	Nitrate venodilator Can combine with hydralazine for balanced vasodilation Apply to ears if warm to touch, otherwise use shaved area in inguinal or axillary region (use gloves when applying) Schedule 12-hour drug-free period to try and avoid tolerance Efficacy uncertain
Nitroprusside sodium (Nitropress, generic)	Inj: 50 mg/vial	Short-term balanced vasodilation in severe CHF	D: 1-10 µg/kg/min in D5W; start with 2 µg/kg/min and increase gradually until desired blood pressure is achieved C: Unknown	Nitrate vasodilator Protect solution from light Adjust drip rate to maintain mean arterial pressure of approximately 70 mm Hg Discontinue if metabolic acidosis develops Large dose or prolonged use may cause cyanide toxicity
Omega-3 fatty acids (ALA, EPA and DHA)	Cap: concentrations of EPA and DHA vary with product	Heart failure (to counter cachexia and reduce inflammatory mediators); arrhythmias	D: 40 mg/kg EPA and 25 mg/kg DHA PO q24h C: Same	Fatty acid Side effects rare
Phenoxybenzamine (Dibenzyline)	Cap: 10 mg	Systemic hypertension, especially secondary to a pheochromocytoma	D: 0.25-2.5 mg/kg PO q12h; start at 0.25 mg/kg and titrate upward to effect C: Same	Alpha-1 adrenergic blocker Direct acting vasodilator
Phenylephrine hydrochloride (generic)	Inj: 10 mg/ml	Acute hypotension	D: 1-3 µg/kg/min IV CRI; start low and titrate to effect or 0.01 mg/kg IV q15 minutes C: Same	Alpha-1 adrenergic agonist Vasopressor
Pimobendan (Vetmedin)	Chewable tab: 1.25, 5.0 mg Cap: 1.25, 2.5, 5.0 mg (Canada, Australia, and Europe)	Licensed for treating signs of mild, moderate, or severe CHF (Class II, III, & IV) from dilated cardiomyopathy or valvular insufficiency in dogs Occult DCM in Doberman Pinschers	D: 0.25-0.30 mg/kg PO q12h C: 1.25 mg/cat q12h PO (off-label use for DCM, HCM with heart failure, or restrictive/unclassified cardiomyopathy refractory to standard therapy)	Phosphodiesterase III inhibitor and a calcium sensitizer that acts as an inotropic vasodilator Do not use in aortic stenosis, HCM (dogs), HCM cats without heart failure, or when augmentation of cardiac output is inappropriate

Continued

Cardiopulmonary Drugs—Formulations, Indications, and Dosages—cont'd

DRUG TRADE NAME	FORMULATION	INDICATIONS	DOG DOSE (D) CAT DOSE (C)	COMMENTS
Prazosin HCl (Minipress, generic)	Cap: 1, 2, 5 mg	Balanced vasodilation in CHF, systemic hypertension	D: 1 mg/15 kg PO q8h Titrate to effect C: 0.25-0.5 mg/cat PO q24h	Alpha-1 adrenergic blocker Direct-acting vasodilator Tolerance develops
Procainamide (generic)	Cap: 250, 375, 500 mg Tab: 250, 375, 500 mg Tab: CR, SR: 250, 500, 750, 1000 mg Inj: 100, 500 mg/mL Some oral formulations may be unavailable	Ventricular and supraventricular arrhythmias, WPW	D: 10-30 mg/kg IM, PO q6h 2 mg/kg IV over 3-5 min up to total dose of 15 mg/kg 25-50 µg/kg/min CRI C: 2-5 mg/kg PO q6-8h	Class 1 antiarrhythmic agent Beware hypotension with IV administration Effects increased by high potassium and decreased by low potassium Monitor ECG; 25% prolongation of QRS is sign of toxicity May be difficult to obtain Use with caution in cats Reduce dose with severe renal and liver disease
Propantheline bromide (Pro-Banthine, generic)	Tab: 7.5, 15 mg	Rate control in sick sinus syndrome and AV block	D, C: 0.25-0.5 mg/kg PO q8-12h	Anticholinergic
Propranolol (Inderal, generic)	Tab: 10, 20, 40, 60, 80 mg Cap: 60, 80, 120, 160 mg Inj: 1 mg/mL Solution: 4 mg/mL	Atrial and ventricular arrhythmias, hypertrophic cardiomyopathy, systemic hypertension, thyrotoxicosis	D: 0.2-1.0 mg/kg PO q8h 0.02-0.06 mg/kg IV over 5-10 minutes C: <4.5 kg: 2.5-5 mg PO q8-12h >4.5 kg: 5 mg PO q8-12h 0.02-0.06 mg/kg IV over 5-10 minutes	Nonselective beta-blocker Start with low dose and titrate to effect Taper dose when discontinue therapy Reduce dose with liver disease Beware of possible bronchoconstriction
Quinidine gluconate (generic) Quinidine sulfate (generic)	Tab SR: 324 mg Inj: 80 mg/mL Tab SR: 300 mg	Ventricular and supraventricular arrhythmias, WPW, conversion of atrial fibrillation	D: 6-20 mg/kg PO, IM q6h 6-20 mg/kg PO q8h with sustained release products 5-10 mg/kg IV (very slowly) C: None Note: Dose calculated for quinidine base equivalent; see comment section	Rarely used; replaced by mexiletine and sotalol for managing ventricular arrhythmias Class 1 antiarrhythmic Reduce dose in CHF, hepatic disease, and hypoalbuminemia Quinidine base in each quinidine salt; quinidine gluconate: 324 mg tab = 200 mg quinidine; quinidine sulfate: 300 mg tab = 250 mg quinidine
Ramipril (Vasotop. Altace, generic)	Tab: 0.625, 1.25, 2.5, 5, 10 mg Cap: 0.625, 1.25, 2.5, 5, 10 mg	Balanced vasodilation in CHF; systemic hypertension	D: 0.125 mg/kg PO q12h C: 0.5 mg/kg PO q24h	Angiotensin-converting enzyme inhibitor Long duration of effect in cats No consistent effect on blood pressure in cats

Drug	Available Forms	Indications	Dosage	Comments
Sildenafil (Viagra, Revatio)	Tab: 25, 50, 130 mg Tab (Revatio): 20 mg	Pulmonary hypertension	D: 2 mg/kg PO q12h but dose interval may range from 8-24h C: 1 mg/kg PO q8h	Phosphodiesterase-5 inhibitor Arterial vasodilator that preferentially dilates the pulmonary vasculature Expensive Can cause hypotension
Sotalol (Betapace, generic)	Tab: 80, 120, 160 mg	Atrial and ventricular arrhythmias	D: 1-2 mg/kg PO q12h (medium-size dogs: start with 40 mg per dog, then increase to 80 mg, if needed) C: 2 mg/kg PO q12h	Antiarrhythmic agent with class II (beta blocking) and class III effects Monitor closely with CHF because of negative inotropic properties
Spironolactone (Aldactone, generic)	Tab: 25, 50, 100 mg	Diseases associated with fluid retention (CHF, hepatic disease, nephrotic syndrome), systemic hypertension, hypokalemia	D: 1-2 mg/kg PO q12h 2 mg/kg/day (cardiac antiremodeling) (European labeled dose: 2 mg/kg PO q24h) C: 1-2 mg/kg PO q12h	Aldosterone antagonist Potassium-sparing diuretic 2-3 days to achieve peak effect Weak diuretic so usually combined with a loop diuretic No effect on cardiac remodeling in Maine Coon cats with HCM Ulcerative facial dermatitis developed in $\frac{1}{3}$ of Maine Coon cats treated with 2 mg/kg q12h dose
Tadalafil (Cialis)	Tab: 2.5, 5, 10, 20 mg	Pulmonary hypertension	D: 1 mg/kg PO q24h	Phosphodiesterase-5 inhibitor Arterial vasodilator that preferentially dilates the pulmonary vasculature Expensive Can cause hypotension
Taurine (generic)	Tab: 250 mg Cap: 500	Dilated cardiomyopathy: cats and selective cases in dogs (esp. American Cocker Spaniel)	D: 500 mg PO q12h C: 250 mg PO q12h	Amino acid Clinical improvements noted in 4-10 days Echo improvement usually by 6 weeks Continue supplement for 12-16 weeks while correcting diet
Terbutaline (generic)	Tab: 2.5, 5 mg Inj: 1 mg/mL	Asthma, COPD, symptomatic bradycardia (AV block, sick sinus syndrome)	D: 1.25-5 mg/dog PO q8-12h C: 0.1 mg/kg PO q8h or 0.625-1.25 mg/cat q12h; 0.05 mg/kg SC, IM, IV	Beta-2 agonist bronchodilator Reduce dose by 50% first 4 days to prevent restless behavior Decrease dose with renal disease

Continued

Cardiopulmonary Drugs—Formulations, Indications, and Dosages—cont'd

DRUG TRADE NAME	FORMULATION	INDICATIONS	DOG DOSE (D) CAT DOSE (C)	COMMENTS
Theophylline (Extended Release generic)	Tab: 100, 200, 300, 450 mg Cap: 50, 75, 125, 200 mg (Availability of extended-release formulations may be variable)	Asthma, COPD, sick sinus syndrome	D: 9 mg/kg PO q8-12h Extended release: 10 mg/kg PO q12h C: 4 mg/kg PO q12h Extended release: 19 mg/kg PO q24h at night	Methylxanthine bronchodilator Reduce dose with CHF, liver disease, cimetidine, orbifloxacin, enrofloxacin Reduce dose by 50% first 4 days to prevent anxiety side-effect Therapeutic range: 10-20 µg/mL Dose on lean body weight
Torsemide (Demadex, generic)	Tab: 5, 10, 20 mg Cap: 100 mg Inj: 10 mg/ml	Refractory CHF with blunted response to furosemide	D: 0.1-0.3 mg/kg PO q12h C: 0.1-0.3 mg/kg PO q24h Titrate to effect	Loop diuretic Longer duration of action, decreased susceptibility to diuretic resistance, and adjunctive aldosterone antagonist properties compared with furosemide Monitor for electrolyte disturbances, azotemia, and dehydration
Triamterene (Dyrenium, generic)	Cap: 50, 100 mg	Diseases associated with fluid retention (CHF, hepatic disease, nephrotic syndrome), systemic hypertension, hypokalemia	D: 1-2 mg/kg PO q12h C: Same	Potassium-sparing diuretic Weak diuretic Usually combined with loop diuretic Does not block aldosterone
Vasopressin (generic)	Inj: 20 U/mL	Treatment of hypotension and cardiac arrest (CPR)	D: Vasopressor 0.01-0.04 U/kg/min CRI; CPR: 0.2-0.8 U/kg IV (can repeat at 3-5 minute intervals and alternate with epinephrine) C: Same	Noncatecholamine vasopressor peptide Potential advantages over epinephrine: Longer half-life Effective in acidosis No harmful beta-adrenergic effects
Verapamil (Calan, Isoptin, generic)	Tab: 40, 80, 120 mg Inj: 2.5 mg/mL	Supraventricular arrhythmias	D: 0.05 mg/kg slow IV (1-2 min) boluses given at 10-30 minute intervals (to effect) to a maximum cumulative dose of 0.2 mg/kg C: 0.05 mg/kg slow IV, may repeat twice as described for dog	Calcium channel blocker Diltiazem is a safer alternative in heart failure Potent vasodilator and negative inotrope
Warfarin (Coumadin, generic)	Tab: 1, 2, 2.5, 3, 4, 5, 6, 7.5, 10 mg	Prevention of thromboembolism (does not lyse existing thrombi)	D: 0.1-0.2 mg/kg PO q24h C: Same	Anticoagulant Initiate therapy with 4 days of heparin to prevent initial hypercoagulable state Control animal's lifestyle and environment to minimize risk of trauma Adjust dose to maintain PT at 1.5-2 times baseline value or INR of 2-3

CALCULATING A CONTINUOUS RATE INFUSION FOR LIDOCAINE

A CRI dosage of 25 to 75 µg/kg/min of lidocaine can be used in dogs with an intravenous loading dose of 1 to 2 mg/kg. In cats, various sources support a CRI dosage of 10 to 40 µg/kg/min of lidocaine with an intravenous loading dose of 0.25 to 0.75 mg/kg.

Lidocaine solution is made up by replacing 75 mL of fluid from a liter bag with 75 ml of 2% lidocaine (half the amount if 500-ml bag). Using the appropriate body weight and corresponding fluid rate in the table below will achieve a CRI dosage of 50 µg/kg/min.

BW (kg)	mL/hr
5	10
10	20
20	40
30	60
40	80
50	100
60	120
70	140

SOURCES OF DRUG INFORMATION IN ADDITION TO CHAPTERS IN THIS BOOK

Bonagura JD, Twedt DC: Current veterinary therapy XV, ed 15, St Louis, 2014, Elsevier Saunders.

Cote E, MacDonald KA, Meurs KM, Sleeper MM: Feline Cardiology, Ames, Iowa, 2011, Wiley-Blackwell.

Norsworthy G, Crystal M, Fooshee S, Tilley LP: The feline patient, ed 4, Ames, Iowa, 2010, Wiley-Blackwell.

Papich MG: Saunders handbook of veterinary drugs, ed 3, St Louis, 2011, Elsevier Saunders.

Plumb DC: Plumb's veterinary drug handbook, ed 7, Stockholm, Wisconsin, 2011, Pharma Vet Inc.

Tilley L.P., Smith F.W.K.: Essentials of electrocardiography. Interpretation and treatment, ed 4, Ames, Iowa 2015, Wiley-Blackwell. (In preparation).

Tilley LP, Smith FWK: The Five-Minute Veterinary Consult Canine and Feline, ed 5, Ames, Iowa, 2011, Wiley-Blackwell. Textbook, CD-ROM.

Echocardiographic Normal Values

Normal Canine Echocardiographic Values*

Parameter	Weight (kg)										
	3	5	7	10	15	20	25	30	35	40	50
LVID$_d$ (mm)	24.6	27.4	30.0	32.7	37.1	41.4	44.8	48.3	51.7	54.8	60.7
	(6.2)	(5.2)	(4.5)	(3.5)	(2.4)	(2.2)	(2.9)	(3.9)	(5.0)	(6.1)	(8.3)
LVID$_s$ (mm)	13.6	16.0	17.9	20.6	24.3	28.0	31.0	33.9	36.9	39.6	44.6
	(5.5)	(4.7)	(4.0)	(3.1)	(2.1)	(2.0)	(2.5)	(3.4)	(4.5)	(5.4)	(7.4)
LVPW$_d$ (mm)	5.0	5.4	5.7	6.2	6.8	7.4	7.9	8.4	8.9	9.3	10.2
	(2.1)	(1.7)	(1.5)	(1.2)	(0.8)	(0.7)	(1.0)	(1.3)	(1.7)	(2.0)	(2.8)
LVPW$_s$ (mm)	7.2	7.9	8.4	9.2	10.2	11.3	12.1	13.0	13.8	14.5	16.0
	(1.7)	(1.6)	(1.4)	(1.3)	(1.1)	(1.1)	(1.2)	(1.3)	(1.5)	(1.7)	(2.2)
IVS$_d$ (mm)	5.8	6.2	6.5	7.0	7.6	8.2	8.7	9.2	9.7	10.2	11.0
	(2.1)	(1.7)	(1.5)	(1.2)	(0.8)	(0.7)	(0.9)	(1.3)	(1.7)	(2.0)	(2.7)
IVS$_s$ (mm)	9.8	10.2	10.4	10.9	11.5	12.3	13.0	13.9	14.6	15.4	—
	(2.6)	(2.2)	(2.0)	(1.7)	(1.2)	(1.1)	(1.5)	(2.3)	(2.6)	(3.5)	
LA (mm)	12.7	14.0	15.0	16.3	18.3	20.2	21.8	23.3	24.8	26.2	28.8
	(5.3)	(4.5)	(3.8)	(3.0)	(2.0)	(1.9)	(2.4)	(3.3)	(4.3)	(5.2)	(7.1)
Ao (mm)	13.8	15.3	16.4	18.1	20.4	22.8	24.6	26.4	28.3	30.0	33.1
	(3.6)	(3.0)	(2.6)	(2.0)	(1.4)	(1.3)	(1.6)	(2.2)	(2.9)	(3.5)	(4.8)

From Ware WA: Diagnostic tests for the cardiovascular system. In Nelson RW, Couto CG, eds: Essentials of small animal internal medicine. St. Louis, 1992, Mosby. Data from Bonagura JD, O'Grady MR, Herring DS: Echocardiography: principles of interpretation, Vet Clin North Am Small Anim Pract 15:1177, 1985.

*Fractional shortening: 28% to 40%; mitral valve E point to septal separation: <5 to 6 mm. Mean values ± SD in parentheses

Ao, Aortic root (diastole); *IVS$_d$*, interventricular septum at end diastole; *IVS$_s$*, interventricular septum at end systole; *LA*, left atrium (systole); *LVID$_d$*, left ventricular internal dimension at end diastole; *LVID$_s$*, left ventricular internal dimension at end systole; *LVPW$_d$*, left ventricular posterior wall at end diastole; *LVPW$_s$*, left ventricular posterior wall at end systole.

Normal M-mode Average Values and Prediction Intervals for Dogs of Varying Weights*

Body weight (kg)	LVID$_d$	LVID$_s$	LVW$_d$	LVW$_s$	IVST$_d$	IVST$_s$	Ao	LA
3	2.1	1.3	0.5	0.8	0.5	0.8	1.1	1.1
	1.8-2.6	1.0-1.8	0.4-0.8	0.6-1.1	0.4-0.8	0.6-1.0	0.9-1.4	0.9-1.4
4	2.3	1.5	0.6	0.9	0.6	0.8	1.3	1.2
	1.9-2.8	1.1-1.9	0.4-0.8	0.7-1.2	0.4-0.8	0.6-1.1	1.0-1.5	1.0-1.6
6	2.6	1.7	0.6	1.0	0.6	0.9	1.4	1.4
	2.2-3.1	1.2-2-2	0.4-0.9	0.7-1.3	0.4-0.9	0.7-1.2	1.2-1.8	1.1-1.8
9	2.9	1.9	0.7	1.0	0.7	1.0	1.7	1.6
	2.4-3.4	1.4-2.5	0.5-1.0	0.8-1.4	0.5-1.0	0.7-1.3	1.3-2.0	1.3-2.1
11	3.1	2.0	0.7	1.1	0.7	1.0	1.8	1.7
	2.6-3.7	1.5-2.7	0.5-1.0	0.8-1.5	0.5-1.1	0.8-1.4	1.4-2.2	1.3-2.2
15	3.4	2.2	0.8	1.2	0.8	1.1	2.0	1.9
	2.8-4.1	1.7-3.0	0.5-1.1	0.9-1.6	0.6-1.1	0.8-1.5	1.6-2.4	1.6-2.5
20	3.7	2.4	0.8	1.2	0.8	1.2	2.2	2.1
	3.1-4.5	1.8-3.2	0.6-1.2	0.9-1.7	0.6-1.2	0.9-1.6	1.7-2.7	1.7-2.7
25	3.9	2.6	0.9	1.3	0.9	1.3	2.3	2.3
	3.3-4.8	2.0-3.5	0.6-1.3	1.0-1.8	0.6-1.3	0.9-1.7	1.9-2.9	1.8-2.9
30	4.2	2.8	0.9	1.4	0.9	1.3	2.5	2.5
	3.5-5.0	2.1-3.7	0.6-1.3	1.0-1.9	0.7-1.3	1.0-1.8	2.0-3.1	1.9-3.1
35	4.4	2.9	1.0	1.4	1.0	1.4	2.6	2.6
	3.6-5.3	2.2-3.9	0.7-1.4	1.1-1.9	0.7-1.4	1.0-1.9	2.1-3.2	2.0-3.3
40	4.5	3.0	1.0	1.5	1.0	1.4	2.7	2.7
	3.8-5.5	2.3-4.0	0.7-1.4	1.1-2.0	0.7-1.4	1.0-1.9	2.2-3.4	2.1-3.5
50	4.8	3.3	1.0	1.5	1.1	1.5	3.0	2.9
	4.0-5.8	2.4-4.3	0.7-1.5	1.1-2.1	0.7-1.5	1.1-2.0	2.4-3.6	2.3-3.7
60	5.1	3.5	1.1	1.6	1.1	1.5	3.2	3.1
	4.2-6.2	2.6-4.6	0.7-1.6	1.2-2.2	0.8-1.6	1.1-2.1	2.5-3.9	2.4-4.0
70	5.3	3.6	1.1	1.6	1.1	1.6	3.3	3.3
	4.4-6.5	2.7-4.8	0.8-1.6	1.2-2.2	0.8-1.6	1.2-2.2	2.7-4.1	2.6-4.2

From Cornell CC, Kittleson MD, Torre PD, et al: Allometric scaling of M-mode cardiac measurements in normal adult dogs, J Vet Intern Med 18:311-321, 2008.

*Mean and 95% prediction interval (cm).

Ao, Aortic root diameter; *IVST$_d$*, interventricular septal thickness in diastole; *IVST$_s$*, interventricular septal thickness in systole; *LA*, left atrial diameter; *LVID$_d$*, left ventricular end diastolic diameter; *LVID$_s$*, left ventricular end systolic diameter; *LVW$_d$*, left ventricular free wall thickness in diastole; *LVW$_s$*, left ventricular free wall thickness in systole.

Canine Normalized M-mode Values

Normalized M-mode Values*	Inner 90% Range
LV end-diastolic dimension (LVIDd/BW$^{0.294}$):	1.35-1.73
LV end-systolic dimension (LVIDs/BW$^{0.315}$):	0.79-1.14
Interventricular septum end-diastolic wall thickness (IVSd/BW$^{0.241}$):	0.33-0.52
Interventricular septum end-systolic wall thickness (IVSs/BW$^{0.240}$):	0.48-0.71
Left ventricular posterior wall end-diastolic thickness (LVPWd/BW$^{0.232}$):	0.33-0.53
Left ventricular posterior wall end-systolic thickness (LVPWs/BW$^{0.222}$):	0.53-0.78
Left atrial diameter (LAd/BW$^{0.345}$):	0.64-0.90
Aortic root diameter (Aod/BW$^{0.341}$):	0.68-0.89

From Cornell CC, Kittleson MD, Torre PD, et al: Allometric scaling of M-mode cardiac measurements in normal adult dogs, J Vet Intern Med 18:311-321, 2008.

*Values achieved by taking the specific echocardiographic measurement (cm) and dividing by the body weight (BW) in kg raised to the power shown in parenthesis. If the value falls within the 90% range, it is normal.

Example: A 10-kg dog is measured as having a 4.3-cm LVIDd on M-mode. To obtain the normalized value, follow this equation: 4.3 cm/10 kg^ 0.294 = 4.3/1.968 = 2.18. This value is greater than the 90% upper reference value for normalized LVIDd (1.73) and indicative of LV dilation.

Echocardiographic Ratio Indices

Reference	Breed	N	Weight (kg)	wIVSd	wLVIDd	wLVWd	wIVSs	wLVIDs	wLVWs	wAo	wLA	FS
Morrison[3]	Miniature Poodle	20	3.0 ± 2.0	0.44±0.05	1.74±0.28	0.44±0.05	0.70±0.09	0.87±0.19	0.70±0.09	0.87±0.12	1.05±0.23	0.47±0.06
				1.06 (0.11)	1.01 (0.16)	1.09 (0.11)	1.23 (0.13)	0.76 (0.21)	1.20 (0.13)	0.88 (0.13)	1.03 (0.22)	1.38 (0.13)
Yamato[7]	Miniature Poodle	30	4.5 ± 1.4	0.39±0.05	1.76±0.20	0.39±0.05	0.65±0.08	1.04±0.15	0.64±0.08	1.00±0.10	1.08±0.09	0.41±0.04
				0.96 (0.12)	1.02 (0.12)	0.99 (0.12)	1.14 (0.12)	0.91 (0.14)	1.11 (0.13)	1.01 (0.10)	1.06 (0.09)	1.21 (0.10)
Della Torre[4]*	Italian GH	20	5.4 ± 1.5	0.46±0.06	1.61±0.18	0.51±0.05	0.66±0.07	0.93±0.17	0.74±0.07			0.43±0.07
				1.12 (0.13)	0.93 (0.11)	1.29 (0.10)	1.16 (0.11)	0.81 (0.18)	1.28 (0.09)			1.26 (0.16)
Crippa[8]	Beagle	20	8.9 ± 1.5	0.41±0.07	1.60±0.22	0.50±0.12	0.58±0.10	0.95±0.22	0.69±0.12			0.40±0.10
				0.99 (0.18)	0.92 (0.14)	1.25 (0.25)	1.02 (0.17)	0.83 (0.23)	1.19 (0.18)			1.18 (0.24)
Cornell[9]*	CKCS	57	8.9 ± 1.4		1.78±0.16	0.42±0.05		1.19±0.14		0.98±0.09	0.97±0.10	0.33±0.05
					1.03 (0.09)	1.06 (0.12)		1.04 (0.12)		0.96 (0.10)	0.96 (0.10)	0.97 (0.14)
Cornell[9]*	Dachshund	33	9.5 ± 1.9	0.42±0.05	1.70±0.19	0.41±0.07	0.57±0.06	1.12±0.16	0.61±0.08	1.08±0.09	0.98±0.14	0.34±0.07
				1.03 (0.13)	0.98 (0.11)†	1.02 (0.16)	0.99 (0.11)†	0.98 (0.14)	1.04 (0.13)	1.09 (0.09)	0.96 (0.14)	0.99 (0.22)
Une[10]	Japanese Beagle	19	9.9 ± 2.6	0.38±0.05	1.82±0.23	0.37±0.04	0.55±0.08	1.21±0.18	0.52±0.07	0.89±0.08	0.91±0.09	0.33±0.03
				0.94 (0.14)	1.05 (0.13)	0.92 (0.11)	0.96 (0.14)	1.05 (0.15)	0.89 (0.13)	0.90 (0.09)	0.90 (0.10)	0.97 (0.09)
Baade[11]	Westie	24	10.3 ± 0.9	0.40±0.08	1.66±0.34	0.37±0.07	0.59±0.15	1.16±0.22	0.57±0.08			0.35±0.07
				0.97 (0.21)	0.96 (0.20)	0.93 (0.19)	1.04 (0.25)	1.00 (0.19)	0.98 (0.14)			1.03 (0.21)
Gooding[12]*	English Cocker	12	12.2 ± 2.4	0.45±0.08	1.85±0.14	0.44±0.08		1.22±0.14				0.34±0.05
				1.10 (0.19)	1.07 (0.07)	1.10 (0.19)		1.06 (0.12)				1.01 (0.14)
Della Torre[4]	Whippet	20	14.5 ± 2.1	0.44±0.05	1.86±0.12	0.46±0.05	0.64±0.06	1.25±0.14	0.67±0.10			0.33±0.05
				1.08 (0.12)	1.07 (0.06)	1.16 (0.10)	1.12 (0.10)	1.09 (0.11)	1.15 (0.15)†			0.96 (0.15)
Morrison[3]	Welsh Corgi	20	15.0 ± 2.9	0.41±0.04	1.63±0.16	0.41±0.05	0.61±0.05	0.97±0.15	0.61±0.07	0.92±0.10	1.07±0.16	0.44±0.06
				1.00 (0.10)	0.94 (0.10)	1.00 (0.12)	1.08 (0.09)	0.84 (0.16)	1.05 (0.11)	0.92 (0.10)	1.06 (0.15)	1.29 (0.15)
Mashiro[13]*	Generic	16	1.76 ± 3.1	0.31±0.04	1.81±0.12	0.30±0.03	0.50±0.05	1.25±0.10	0.54±0.06			0.31±0.04
				0.75 (0.12)	1.04 (0.07)	0.76 (0.11)	0.88 (0.09)	1.08 (0.08)	0.93 (0.11)			0.91 (0.13)
Sisson[2]	Pointer	16	19.2 ± 2.8	0.32±0.05	1.84±0.11	0.33±0.03	0.56±0.11	1.19±0.11	0.57±0.09			0.36±0.04
				0.79 (0.16)	1.06 (0.06)	0.83 (0.10)	0.98 (0.20)†	1.03 (0.09)	0.99 (0.15)			1.04 (0.11)
Cornell[9]*	Generic	47	20.8 ± 13.0	0.40±0.06	1.75±0.16	0.40±0.05	0.57±0.12	1.16±0.19	0.53±0.11	1.13±0.08	1.06±0.09	0.34±0.09
				0.99 (0.15)	1.01 (0.09)	1.00 (0.12)	1.01 (0.21)	1.01 (0.16)†	0.91 (0.20)	1.14 (0.07)	1.05 (0.09)	0.99 (0.27)†
Morrison[3]	Afghan	20	23.0 ± 5.1	0.57±0.12	1.86±0.22	0.40±0.05	0.52±0.07	1.24±0.20	0.51±0.09	1.15±0.17	1.15±0.20	0.33±0.06
				1.40 (0.21)	1.07 (0.12)	1.00 (0.12)	0.91 (0.14)	1.08 (0.16)	0.87 (0.17)	1.16 (0.14)	1.13 (0.18)	0.97 (0.19)
De Madron[14]*	Generic	27	24.4 ± 19.2	0.36±0.08	1.91±0.16	0.33±0.07	0.59±0.09	1.29±0.16	0.60±0.08	1.06±0.15	1.05±0.17	0.33±0.06
				0.88 (0.21)	1.10 (0.08)	0.82 (0.20)	1.04 (0.15)	1.12 (0.12)	1.04 (0.14)	1.07 (0.15)	1.03 (0.16)†	0.96 (0.18)
Brown[6]*	Generic	50	25.2 ± 17.4	0.44±0.06	1.59±0.15	0.41±0.06	0.56±0.11	1.04±0.16	0.64±0.09	1.00±0.12	1.01±0.11	0.34±0.07
				1.06 (0.12)	0.92 (0.10)†	1.02 (0.14)	0.99 (0.19)	0.91 (0.15)	1.11 (0.15)	1.01 (0.12)	0.99 (0.11)	1.01 (0.19)†
Page[15]	Greyhound	16	26.6 ± 3.5	0.45±0.07	1.86±0.12	0.51±0.07		1.37±0.15				0.25±0.06
				1.09 (0.16)	1.07 (0.06)	1.28 (0.14)		1.19 (0.11)				0.75 (0.25)
Della Torre[4]*	Greyhound	20	26.9 ± 3.3	0.50±0.04	1.79±0.13	0.54±0.04	0.66±0.04	1.35±0.10	0.72±0.05			0.25±0.04
				1.22 (0.09)	1.04 (0.07)	1.36 (0.07)	1.16 (0.07)	1.17 (0.07)	1.24 (0.07)†			0.72 (0.15)

Reference	Breed	n	Age									
Goncalves[16]*	Generic	70	27.7 ± 19.5	0.52±0.08	1.52±0.14	0.41±0.06	0.70±0.09	0.95±0.13	0.63±0.10	0.93±0.12	1.13±0.14	0.38±0.06
				1.28 (0.14)†	0.88 (0.09)	1.02 (0.15)	1.24 (0.13)	0.82 (0.13)	1.08 (0.15)	0.94 (0.12)†	1.12 (0.12)	1.11(0.16)†
Herrtage[17]	Boxer	30	28.0 ± 7.1	0.37±0.08	1.66±0.21	0.41±0.08	0.54±0.08		0.62±0.08	0.91±0.08	0.95±0.08	0.33±0.08
				0.91 (0.22)	0.96 (0.13)	1.04 (0.20)	0.95 (0.15)		1.07 (0.13)	0.92 (0.09)	0.94 (0.09)	0.97 (0.24)
Snyder[18]*	Greyhound	11	29.1 ± 3.7	0.55±0.07	1.92±0.12	0.48±0.06		1.37±0.11				0.29±0.04
				1.34 (0.12)	1.11 (0.06)	1.19 (0.13)		1.19 (0.08)				0.85 (0.14)
Schober[19]	Boxer	66	30.0 ± 4.0	0.39±0.06	1.76±0.19	0.39±0.06	0.54±0.08	1.20±0.15	0.56±0.09			0.32±0.06
				0.96 (0.15)	1.02 (0.11)	0.98 (0.15)	0.95 (0.15)	1.04 (0.12)	0.96 (0.16)			0.94 (0.19)
Cornell[9]*	Generic	23	30.1 ± 7.8		1.76±0.17	0.42±0.04		1.10±0.13		1.01±0.08	0.98±0.13	0.38±0.05
					1.02 (0.10)	1.05 (0.11)		0.95 (0.12)		1.02 (0.08)	0.97 (0.13)	1.11 (0.14)
Muzzi[20]	German Shepherd	60	30.2 ± 4.0	0.39±0.04	1.68±0.20	0.36±0.04	0.57±0.04	1.25±0.21	0.53±0.05	1.02±0.06	0.98±0.08	0.29±0.07
				0.95 (0.09)	0.97 (0.12)	0.89 (0.13)	0.99 (0.06)	1.09 (0.16)	0.90 (0.09)	1.02 (0.06)	0.97 (0.09)	0.84 (0.23)
Cornell[9]*	Boxer	75	31.0 ± 4.8	0.39±0.06	1.66±0.14	0.40±0.05	0.55±0.08	1.12±0.12	0.59±0.07	0.92±0.08	0.99±0.11	0.33±0.04
				0.95 (0.15)	0.96 (0.09)	0.99 (0.12)	0.97 (0.15)†	0.97 (0.11)	1.01 (0.12)	0.92 (0.09)	0.97 (0.12)	0.96 (0.11)
Morrison[3]	Golden Retriever	20	32.0 ± 4.8	0.40±0.05	1.78±0.15	0.40±0.04	0.55±0.07	1.07±0.18	0.59±0.14	0.95±0.14	1.07±0.17	0.39±0.07
				0.97 (0.13)	1.03 (0.08)	0.99 (0.11)	0.98 (0.13)	0.93 (0.17)	1.02 (0.16)	0.96 (0.15)	1.05 (0.16)	1.15 (0.19)
Kayar[21]	German Shepherd	50	34.6 ± 2.7	0.38±0.06	1.74±0.18	0.37±0.05	0.55±0.06	1.32±0.13	0.52±0.04	1.05±0.07	0.95±0.09	0.31±0.03
				0.92 (0.11)	1.00 (0.10)	0.92 (0.13)	0.96 (0.11)	1.15 (0.10)	0.90 (0.08)	1.06 (0.07)	0.94 (0.10)	0.92 (0.11)
Calvert[22]	Doberman Pinscher	21	36.0 ± 2.9	0.37±0.02	1.78±0.14	0.37±0.01	0.54±0.02	1.17±0.11	0.54±0.02	1.14±0.07	1.01±0.06	0.34±0.02
				0.89 (0.06)	1.03 (0.08)	0.91 (0.03)	0.96 (0.04)	1.02 (0.09)	0.93 (0.04)	1.15 (0.06)	1.00 (0.06)	1.00 (0.05)
Vollmar[23]	Deerhound	21	41.3 ± 4.9	0.33±0.10	1.86±0.18	0.36±0.07	0.53±0.15	1.24±0.19	0.56±0.08	1.08±0.13	1.03±0.14	0.34±0.06
				0.81 (0.31)	1.08 (0.10)	0.91 (0.18)	0.93 (0.28)	1.08 (0.15)	0.96 (0.14)	1.08 (0.13)	1.02 (0.14)	0.98 (0.17)
Bayon[24]	Spanish Mastiff	12	52.4 ± 3.3	0.33±0.05	1.60±0.16	0.33±0.04	0.53±0.06	0.97±0.12	0.51±0.05	0.93±0.09	0.96±0.11	0.39±0.02
				0.80 (0.15)	0.93 (0.10)	0.82 (0.13)	0.92 (0.11)	0.85 (0.13)	0.88 (0.10)	0.93 (0.10)	0.94 (0.11)	1.15 (0.04)
Koch[25]	Newfoundland	27	61.0 ± 5.6	0.37±0.06	1.60±0.13	0.32±0.04	0.48±0.07	1.13±0.12	0.48±0.04	0.93±0.06	0.96±0.07	0.30±0.04
				0.90 (0.17)	0.92 (0.08)	0.80 (0.13)	0.84 (0.15)	0.99 (0.11)	0.83 (0.08)	0.93 (0.06)	0.94 (0.08)	0.88 (0.13)
Koch[25]	Great Dane	15	62.0 ± 6.6	0.46±0.04	1.68±0.14	0.40±0.05	0.52±0.05	1.26±0.10	0.51±0.07	0.94±0.05	1.05±0.16	0.25±0.05
				1.12 (0.08)	0.97 (0.08)	0.99 (0.14)	0.92 (0.09)	1.09 (0.08)	0.88 (0.14)	0.94 (0.06)	1.03 (0.16)	0.73 (0.21)
Vollmar[26]*	Irish WH	144	63.5 ± 8.3	0.35±0.06	1.60±0.12	0.33±0.05	0.49±0.07	1.06±0.11	0.50±0.06	1.04±0.09	1.01±0.11	0.34±0.04
				0.86 (0.17)	0.93 (0.08)	0.84 (0.15)	0.86 (0.14)	0.92 (0.10)	0.86 (0.12)†	1.05 (0.08)†	0.99 (0.11)	1.00 (0.12)
Koch[25]	Irish WH	20	68.5 ± 8.0	0.37±0.05	1.54±0.11	0.31±0.03	0.46±0.05	1.11±0.10	0.43±0.05	0.92±0.02	0.95±0.11	0.28±0.04
				0.90 (0.12)	0.89 (0.07)	0.77 (0.11)	0.81 (0.11)	0.96 (0.09)	0.74 (0.11)	0.93 (0.02)	0.94 (0.11)	0.82 (0.13)
Global mean±SD				0.410± 0.062	1.731± 0.109	0.399± 0.059	0.569± 0.061	1.151± 0.131	0.581± 0.076	0.994± 0.083	1.014± 0.061	0.340± 0.051

Continued

Echocardiographic Ratio Indices—cont'd

From Hall DJ, Cornell BS Crawford S, Brown DJ: Meta-analysis of normal canine echocardiographic dimensional data using radio indices, J Vet Card 10: 11-23, 2008.

Results are presented as two rows for each group. The first row represents the mean group ERI ± SD. The second row represents the group ERI compared to the global mean with the group coefficient of variation in parentheses. The global mean ± SD is listed in the bottom row.

*Individualized data.

†Non-normal distribution.

CKCS, Cavalier King Charles Spaniel; FS, fractional shortening; GH, Greyhound; Irish WH, Irish Wolfhound; wAo = Aom/AO$_w$, index of aortic root dimension, M-mode; wLA = LA/AO$_w$, index of left atrial dimension, M-mode; wIVSd = IVSd/AO$_w$, index of interventricular septal, thickness, diastole, M-mode; wLVIDd = LVIDd/AO$_w$, index of left ventricular internal dimension, diastole, M-mode; wLVIDs = LVIDs/AO$_w$, index of left ventricular internal dimension, systole, M-mode; wIVSs = IVSs/AO$_w$, index of interventricular septal, thickness, systole, M-mode; wLVWs = LVWs/AO$_w$, index of left ventricular wall, thickness, diastole, M-mode.

[2]Sisson D, Schaeffer D: Changes in linear dimensions of the heart, relative to body weight, as measured by M-mode echocardiography in growing dogs, Am J Vet Res 52:1591-1596, 1991.

[3]Morrison SA, Moise NS, Scarlett J, et al: Effect of breed and body weight on echocardiographic values in four breeds of dogs of differing somatotype, J Vet Intern Med 6:220-224, 1992.

[4]Della Torre PK, Kirby AC, Church DB, et al: Echocardiographic measurements in greyhounds, whippets, and Italian greyhounds—dogs with a similar conformation but different size, Aust Vet J 78:49-55, 2000.

[6]Brown DJ, Rush JE, MacGregor J, et al: Rand M-mode echocardiographic ratio indices in normal dogs, cats, and horses: a novel quantitative method, J Vet Intern Med 17:653-662, 2003.

[7]Yamato RJ, Larsson MHMA, Mirandola RMS, et al: Echocardiographic parameters in unidimensional mode from clinically normal miniature poodle dogs, Ciencia Rural 36:142-148, 2006.

[8]Crippa L, Ferro E, Melloni E, et al: Echocardiographic parameters and indices in the normal beagle dog, Lab Anim 26:190-195, 1992.

[9]Cornell CC, Kittleson MD, Della Torre P, et al: Allometric scaling of M-mode variables in normal adult dogs, J Vet Intern Med 18:311-321, 2004.

[10]Une S, Terashita A, Nakaichi M, et al: Morphological and functional standard parameters of echocardiogram in beagles, J Jpn Vet Med Assoc 57:793-798, 2004.

[11]Baade H, Schober K, Oechtering G: Echocardiographic reference values in West Highland white terriers with special regard to right heart function, Tierarztl Prax 30:172-179, 2002.

[12]Gooding JP, Robinson WF, Mews GC: Echocardiographic assessment of left ventricular dimensions in clinically normal English cocker spaniels, Am J Vet Res 47:296-300, 1986.

[13]Mashiro I, Nelson RR, Cohn JN: Ventricular dimensions measured noninvasively by echocardiography in the awake dog, J Appl Physiol 41:953-959, 1976.

[14]de Madron E: M-mode echocardiography in the normal dog [L'echocardiographie en mode M chez le chien normal], Ecole Nationale Veterinare d'Alfort 76:1983.

[15]Page A, Edmunds G, Atwell RB: Echocardiographic values in the greyhound, Aust Vet J 70:361-364, 1993.

[16]Goncalves AC, Orton EC, Boon JA: Linear, logarithmic, and polynomial models of M-mode echocardiographic measurements in dogs, Am J Vet Res 63:994-999, 2002.

[17]Herritage ME: Echocardiographic measurements in the normal boxer (abstract). In: Proceedings of the Fourth European Society of Veterinary Internal Medicine Congress, 172: 1994.

[18]Snyder S, Sato T, Atkins OE: A comparison of echocardiographic indices of the nonracing healthy greyhound to reference values from other breeds, Vet Radiol Ultrasound 36:387-392, 1995.

[19]Schober K, Fuentes VL, Baade H: Echocardiographic reference values in boxer dogs, Tierarztl Prax 30:417-426, 2002.

[20]Muzzi RAL, Muzzi LAL, Baracat de Araujo M: Echocardiographic indices in normal German shepherd dogs, J Vet Sci 7:193-198, 2006.

[21]Kayar A, Gonul R, Or ME: M-mode echocardiographic parameters and indices in the normal German shepherd dog, Vet Radiol Ultrasound 47:482-486, 2006.

[22]Calvert CA, Brown J: Use of M-mode echocardiography in the diagnosis of congestive cardiomyopathy in Doberman pinschers, J Am Vet Med Assoc 189:293-297, 1986.

[23]Vollmar A: Echocardiographic examinations in Deerhounds, reference values for echocardiography, Kleintierpraxis 43:497-508, 1998.

[24]Bayon A, Fernandez del Palacio MJ, Montes AM: M-mode echocardiography study in growing Spanish mastiffs, J Small Anim Pract 35:473-479, 1994.

[25]Koch J, Pedersen HD, Jensen AL: M-mode echocardiographic diagnosis of dilated cardiomyopathy in giant breed dogs, J Vet Med 43:297-304, 1996.

[26]Vollmar AC: Echocardiographic measurements in the Irish wolfhund: reference values for the breed, J Am Anim Hosp Assoc 35:271-277, 1999.

Normal Feline Echocardiographic Values

Parameter	Range (Unsedated)* (N = 30)	Range (Sedated With Ketamine)† (N = 30)
$RVID_d$ (mm)	2.7-9.4	1.2-7.5
$LVID_d$ (mm)	12.0-19.8	10.7-17.3
$LVID_s$ (mm)	5.2-10.8	4.9-11.6
SF (%)	39.0-61.0	30-60
$LVPW_d$ (mm)	2.2-4.4	2.1-4.5
$LVPW_s$ (mm)	5.4-8.1	—
IVS_d (mm)	2.2-4.0	2.2-4.9
IVS_s (mm)	4.7-7.0	—
LA (mm)	9.3-15.1	7.2-13.3
Ao (mm)	7.2-11.9	7.1-11.5
LA/Ao	.95-1.65	.73-1.64
EPSS (mm)	.17-.21	—
PEP (s)	—	.024-.058
LVET (s)	.10-.18	.093-0.176
PEP/LVET	—	.228-.513
Vcf (circumf/s)	2.35-4.95	2.27-5.17

*Data from Jacobs G, Knight DH: M-Mode echocardiographic measurements in nonanesthetized healthy cats: effects of body weight, heart rate, and other variables, Am J Vet Res 46:1705, 1985.

†Data from Fox PR, Bond BR, Peterson ME: Echocardiographic reference values in healthy cats sedated with ketamine hydrochloride, Am J Vet Res 46:1479, 1985.

Ao, Aortic root (end diastole); *IVS_d*, interventricular septum at end diastole; *IVS_s*, interventricular septum at end systole; *LVET (s)*, left ventricular ejection time (seconds); *LVID_d*, left ventricular internal dimension at end diastole; *LVID_s*, left ventricular internal dimension at end systole; *LVPW_d*, left ventricular posterior wall at end diastole; *LVPW_s*, left ventricular posterior wall at end systole; *PEP (s)*, pre-ejection period (seconds); *RVID_d*, right ventricular internal dimension at end diastole; *SF*, shortening fraction; *Vcf (circumf/s)*, velocity of circumferential fiber shortening.

APPENDIX 4

Available Canine and Feline Genetic Tests for Breed-Specific Cardiac Diseases

Note that there are genotypic tests (gene test where the gene is identified, or the less definitive linkage tests where there is an identified gene close to the gene of interest) and phenotypic tests such as an echocardiogram that can be used to characterize inherited disorders. There are cardiac diseases that are present in multiple breeds with different mutations at their core, and congenital disorders with no proven genetic basis.

This appendix covers available gene and linkage testing. This list will change quickly as new tests come to market.

Breed	Condition	Tests/Laboratory
Canine		
Boxer	ARVC (arrhythmogenic right ventricular cardiomyopathy) Mutation: c.*3063del 8 bp CATACACA Chromosome: 17 Gene: STRN (striatin) OMIM 107970 OMIA: 000878-9615 Reference: 1 Myocardial protein calstabin2 is reduced in ARVC Boxers Reference: 2 Mode of inheritance: AD Reference: 3	NCSU Veterinary Cardiac Genetics Laboratory Bldg. 460 1060 William Moore Dr. Raleigh, NC 27607 USA www.cvm.ncsu.edu/vhc/csds/vcgl/index.html vcgl@lists.ncsu.edu (WSU lab moved here) www.ncstatevets.org/genetics/submitdna/ 919 513-8279 Laboklin Steubenstraße 4 PO Box 1810 Bad Kissingen D-97688 DEU www.laboklin.de info@laboklin.de +49 971 720 20
Doberman Pinscher	DCM (dilated cardiomyopathy) Mutation: c.1115+1_1115+16del Chromosome: 5 Gene: PDK4 OMIM 107970,115200 OMIA 000162-9615 References: 4, 5	NCSU Veterinary Cardiac Genetics Laboratory Bldg. 460 1060 William Moore Dr. Raleigh, NC 27607 USA www.cvm.ncsu.edu/vhc/csds/vcgl/index.html vcgl@lists.ncsu.edu (WSU lab moved here) www.ncstatevets.org/genetics/submitdna/ 919 513-8279 VetGen Suite #1 3728 Plaza Drive Ann Arbor, MI 48108 USA (Dobe panel includes DCM in association with Dr. Meurs) www.vetgen.com/canine-dob-panel-testing.html www.vetgen.com vetgen@vetgen.com 734 669-8440 or toll free 800 483-8436 (USA/Canada)

Breed	Condition	Tests/Laboratory
Doberman Pinscher—cont'd		Van Haeringen AgroBusiness Park 100 P.P Box 408 6700 AK Wageningen, Netherlands www.vhlgenetics.com info@vhlgenetics.com +31 0317 416 402
Newfoundland	SAS (Subaortic stenosis) (co-dominant with lethal homozygosity and penetrance of .33 in the heterozygote) Reference: 6	NCSU Veterinary Cardiac Genetics Laboratory Bldg. 460 1060 William Moore Dr. Raleigh, NC 27607 USA www.cvm.ncsu.edu/vhc/csds/vcgl/index.html vcgl@lists.ncsu.edu (WSU lab moved here) www.ncstatevets.org/genetics/submitdna/ 919 513-8279
Portuguese Water Dog	JDCM (Juvenile onset DCM) Gene: Linked marker Disease code: JDCM Chromosome: 8 OMIA: 000160-9615 Reference: 7	Van Haeringen AgroBusiness Park 100 P.P Box 408 6700 AK Wageningen, Netherlands www.vhlgenetics.com info@vhlgenetics.com +31 0317 416 402
		JDCM Testing Laboratory 3900 Delancey Street, Rm. 4022 Philadelphia, PA 19104 USA JDCMtest@vet.upenn.edu (affiliated with UPenn but not on website) 215 898-5703
Feline		
Maine Coon	HCM (hypertrophic cardiomyopathy) Myosin-binding protein C Inheritance: AD Mutation: c.31G>C (MYBPC3-A31P) @ 31st codon (ALA to PRO) Gene: MYBPC Disease Code: HCM-RD Chromosome: E2 OMIM: 192600 OMIA: 000515-9685 Reference: 8, 9, 10, 11, 12	Langford Veterinary Langford House, Langford Bristol, UK BS40 5DU www.langfordvets.co.uk/lab_pcrnews.htm genetic.test@langfordvets.co.uk 0117 928 9420
		UC Davis Veterinary Genetics Laboratory One Shields Avenue Davis, CA 95617 USA www.vgl.ucdavis.edu custserv@vgl.ucdavis.edu 530 752-2211
		NCSU Veterinary Cardiac Genetics Laboratory Bldg. 460 1060 William Moore Dr. Raleigh, NC 27607 USA www.cvm.ncsu.edu/vhc/csds/vcgl/index.html vcgl@lists.edu (WSU lab moved here) www.ncstatevets.org/genetics/submitdna/ 919 513-8279

Continued

Breed	Condition	Tests/Laboratory
Maine Coon— cont'd		Van Haeringen AgroBusiness Park 100 P.P Box 408 6700 AK Wageningen, Netherlands www.vhlgenetics.com info@vhlgenetics.com +31 0317 416 402 K725 (HCM1)
		Vetogene Via Celoria, 10 20133 Milano, IT (Università degli Studi di Milano, Faculty of Veterinary Medicine) or Viale Ortles 22/24 20139 Milano IT www.vetogene.com info@vetogene.com +39 327 4784676
		Antagene 6 allée du Levant CS60001 La Tour de Salvagny 69890 FR www.antagene.com contact@antagene.com +33 (0) 4 37 49 90 03
		Genomia s.r.o Janáĉkova 51 32300 Pizeň Czech Republic www.genomia.cz/en laborator@genomia.cz test for Meurs (A31P) and Koch (A74T) +420 373 749 999 +420 373 317 478
		Genindexe 6 rue de sports CS 30345 La Rochelle 17000 FR www.genindexe.com/uk/index.php contact@genindexe.com 05 46 30 69 66
		Progenus 2 rue des Praules Gembloux, Belgium 5030 www.progenus.be info@progenus.be +32-(0) 81-616901
Ragdoll	HCM (hyphertrophic cardiomyopathy) Myosin binding protein C Mutation: c.2460C > T (@ 820th codon (ARG to TYR)) Gene: MYBPC Disease code: HCM-RD OMIM: 192600 OMIA: 000515-9685 Inheritance: AD Chromosome: E2 References: 13	CatDNA.org C/O Animal Genetics Laboratory Texas A&M University Veterinary Integrated Biosciences, CVM 4458 TAMU College Station, TX 77843-4458 USA www.catdnatest.org gcothran@cvm.tamu.edu 979 845-0229
		UC Davis Veterinary Genetics Laboratory One Shields Avenue Davis CA 95617 USA www.vgl.ucdavis.edu custserv@vgl.ucdavis.edu 530 752-2211

Breed	Condition	Tests/Laboratory
Ragdoll—cont'd		NCSU Veterinary Cardiac Genetics Laboratory Bldg. 460 1060 William Moore Dr. Raleigh, NC 27607 USA www.cvm.ncsu.edu/vhc/csds/vcgl/index.html vcgl@lists.ncsu.edu 919 513-8279 (WSU lab moved here)
		Antagene 6 allée du Levant CS 60001 69890 La tour de Salvagny, FR www.antagene.com contact@antagene.com +33 (0) 4 37 49 90 03
		Genomia s.r.o Janáčkova 51 32300 Pizeň Czech Republic www.genomia.cz/en laborator@genomia.cz test for Meurs (A31P) and Koch (A74T) +420 373 749 999 +420 373 317 478
		Progenus 2, rue des Praules Gembloux, Belgium 5030 www.progenus.be info@progenus.be +32 (0) 81-616901
		Van Haeringen AgroBusiness Park 100 P.P Box 408 6700 AK Wageningen, Netherlands www.vhlgenetics.com info@vhlgenetics.com +31 0317 416 402 K725 (HCM1), K799 (HCM3)
		Vetogene Via Celoria, 10 20133 Milano, IT (Università degli Studi di Milano, Faculty of Veterinary Medicine) or Viale Ortles 22/24 20139 Milano, IT www.vetogene.com info@vetogene.com +39 327 4784676
		Langford Veterinary Langford House, Langford Bristol, UK BS40 5DU www.langfordvets.co.uk/lab_pcrnews.htm genetic.test@langfordvets.co.uk 0117 928 9420
Norwegian Forest, Birman, British Longhair, Devon Rex	HCM Test K764 (Test HCM2) Not offered internationally	Van Haeringen AgroBusiness Park 100 P.P Box 408 6700 AK Wageningen, Netherlands www.vhlgenetics.com info@vhlgenetics.com +31 0317 416 402

REFERENCES

1. Meurs KM, Mauceli E, Lahmers S, et al: Genome-wide association identifies a deletion in the 3' untranslated region of striatin in a canine model of arrhythmogenic right ventricular cardiomyopathy, Hum Genet 128:315–324, 2010.
2. Oyama MA, Reiken S, Lehnart SE, et al: Arrhythmogenic right ventricular cardiomyopathy in Boxer dogs is associated with calstabin2 deficiency, J Vet Cardiol 10:1–10, 2008.
3. Meurs KM, Spier AW, Miller MW, et al: Familial ventricular arrhythmias in boxers, J Vet Intern Med 13:437–439, 1999.
4. Mausberg T, Wess G, Simak J, et al: A locus on chromosome 5 is associated with dilated cardiomyopathy in Doberman Pinschers, PLoSOne, 6: e20042.
5. Meurs KM, Lahmers S, Keene BW, et al: A splice site mutation in a gene encoding for PDK4, a mitochondrial protein, is associated with development of dilated cardiomyopathy in the Doberman Pinscher, Hum Genet. 131:1319–1325, 2012.
6. Reist-Marti SB, Dolf G, Leeb T, et al: Genetic evidence of subaortic stenosis in the Newfoundland dog, Vet Rec 170:597, 2012.
7. Werner P, Raducha MG, Prociuk U, et al: A novel locus for dilated cardiomyopathy maps to canine chromosome 8, Genomics 91:517–521, 2008.
8. Mary J, Chetboul V, Sampedrano CC, et al: Prevalence of the MYBPC3-A31P mutation in a large European feline population and association with hypertrophic cardiomyopathy in the Maine Coon breed, J Vet Cardiol 12:155–161, 2010.
9. Meurs KM, Sanchez X, David RM, et al: A cardiac myosin binding protein C mutation in the Maine Coon cat with familial hypertrophic cardiomyopathy, Hum Mol Genet 14:3587–3593, 2005.
10. Carlos Sampedrano C, Chetboul V, Mary J, et al: Prospective echocardiographic and tissue Doppler imaging screening of a population of Maine Coon cats tested for the A31P mutation in the myosin-binding protein C gene: a specific analysis of the heterozygous status, J Vet Intern Med 23:91–99, 2009.
11. Kittleson MD, Meurs KM, Munro MJ, et al: Familial hypertrophic cardiomyopathy in Maine Coon cats: an animal model of human disease, Circulation 99: 3172–3180, 1999.
12. Meurs KM, Kuan M: Differential methylation of CpG sites in two isoforms of myosin binding protein C, an important hypertrophic cardiomyopathy gene, Environ Mol Mutagen 2:161–164, 2011.
13. Meurs KM, Norgard MM, Ederer MM, et al: A substitution mutation in the myosin binding protein C gene in ragdoll hypertrophic cardiomyopathy, Genomics 90:261–264, 2007.

Reported genetic cardiac disorders for which no test is available (as of the time of writing):

CANINE

CAVALIER KING CHARLES SPANIEL

MYXOMATOUS MITRAL VALVE DISEASE

Details: 2 loci identified, a1.58 Mb region of CFA13 and 1.68 Mb region of CFA14.

Reference: Madsen MB, Olsen LH, Häggström J, et al: Identification of 2 loci associated with the development of myxomatous mitral valve disease in Cavalier King Charles Spaniels, J Hered 102:S62, 2011.

GREAT DANE

DILATED CARDIOMYOPATHY

Details: X-linked recessive according to Meurs, et al, using pedigree analysis.

Reference: Muers KM, Miller MW, Wright NA: Clinical features of dilated cardiomyopathy in Great Danes and results of a pedigree analysis: 17 cases (1990-2000), J Am Vet Med Assoc 218:729, 2001.

IRISH WOLFHOUND

DILATED CARDIOMYOPATHY

Details: Polygenic inheritance is associated with DCM in this breed.

Reference: Phillip U, Vollmar A, Häggström J, et al: Multiple loci are associated with dilated cardiomyopathy in Irish Wolfhounds, PLosOne 7: e36691, 2012 www.iwclubofamerica.com states in one European dog study, 1/4 of dogs had DCM suggestive of AD inheritance see www.iwclubofamerica.org/Health/Brenneman.pdf

KEESHOND

CONOTRUNCAL DEFECT

Details: Three different chromosomes suggestive of being polygenic, using gene linkage testing.

Reference: Werner P, Raducha MG, Prociuk U, et al: The Keeshond defect in cardiac conotruncal development is oligogenic, Hum Genet 116:368, 2005.

LABRADOR RETRIEVER

TRICUSPID VALVE DYSPLASIA

Details: Proposed to be AD.

Reference: Famula TR, Siemens LM, Davidson AP, Packard M: Evaluation of the genetic basis of tricuspid valve dysplasia in Labrador Retrievers, Am J Vet Res 63:816, 2002.

Details: Later reported where the authors used gene linkage on chromosome #9 (CFA$_9$), but had to assume 70% penetrance to confirm hypothesis findings.

Reference: Andelfinger G, Wright KN, Lee HS, et al: Canine tricuspid valve malformation, a model of human Ebstein anomaly, maps to dog chromosome 9, J Med Genet 40:320, 2003.

FELINE

DEVON REX AND SPHYNX CAT BREEDS

HYPERTROPHIC CARDIOMYOPATHY

Details: pedigree studies suggest AD, incomplete penetrance.

References: Chetboul V, Petit A, Gouni V, et al: Prospective echocardiographic and tissue Doppler screening of a large Sphynx cat population: reference ranges, heart disease prevalence and genetic aspects, J Vet Cardiol 14:497, 2012.

Silverman SJ, Stern JA, Meurs KM: Hypertrophic cardiomyopathy in the Sphynx cat: a retrospective evaluation of clinical presentation and heritable etiology, J Fel Med Surg 14:246, 2012.

Index

Page numbers followed by *f* indicate figures; *t,* tables; *b,* boxes.